Need-to-Know N...

Nonalcoholic fatty liver disease (NAFLD) is the hepatic manifestation of the obesity and metabolic syndrome epidemics, which this up-to-date book deals with comprehensively. The contents outline disease mechanisms, diagnostic tests, management, varying manifestations and special populations. It covers the mechanistic pathways that contribute to NAFLD development, including the role of genetic variants and the gut microbiome. It elaborates on noninvasive diagnostic tests to screen for NAFLD, determine its severity, and monitor response to lifestyle intervention and pharmacologic treatment. This book helps clinicians to diagnose and treat this common and potentially deadly disease.

Key Features:

- Reviews current drugs in development and provides practical advice to clinicians on the diagnosis and management of fatty liver.

- Proves attractive to primary care providers who are on the front line of managing patients with NAFLD, to gastroenterologists and hepatologists who would benefit from updated data on how to risk-stratify patients and identify those who will be eligible for pharmacologic treatment, and other specialists such as cardiologists, endocrinologists and nephrologists who will find this book to be a useful reference on the extrahepatic manifestations of NAFLD.

- Focuses on extrahepatic manifestations and new insights on the mechanistic drivers of the disease.

Need-to-Know NAFLD

The Complete Guide to Nonalcoholic Fatty Liver Disease

Edited by

Naim Alkhouri and Stephen A. Harrison

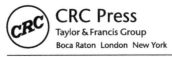

CRC Press
Taylor & Francis Group
Boca Raton London New York

CRC Press is an imprint of the
Taylor & Francis Group, an **informa** business

Designed cover image: Editors

First edition published 2024
by CRC Press
6000 Broken Sound Parkway NW, Suite 300, Boca Raton, FL 33487–2742

and by CRC Press
4 Park Square, Milton Park, Abingdon, Oxon, OX14 4RN

CRC Press is an imprint of Taylor & Francis Group, LLC

ISBN: 978-1-032-47949-1 (hbk)
ISBN: 978-1-032-47948-4 (pbk)
ISBN: 978-1-003-38669-8 (ebk)

DOI: 10.1201/9781003386698

Typeset in Palatino
by Apex CoVantage, LLC

*To my two daughters, Giada and Tala: you are the light that guides me in my
journey through life. I hope that you find me to be a cool dad one day.*

Naim Alkhouri

*This book is dedicated to my loving wife, Renee, and my two amazing children, Taylor and Anna-Lauren.
Your love and support have been amazing. I also want to thank the many patients with NAFLD/NASH who
have given me hope and inspiration to push forward and continue to advance the field.*

Stephen A. Harrison

Contents

Preface

Nonalcoholic fatty liver disease (NAFLD) is the hepatic manifestation of the obesity and metabolic syndrome epidemics. It is the most common form of chronic liver disease, affecting 25% of the global population. NAFLD has become a leading cause for cirrhosis, liver cancer, and the need for liver transplantation. It also contributes significantly to the development of cardiovascular disease, diabetes and chronic kidney disease. Our understanding of mechanistic pathways that contribute to NAFLD development and progression has expanded exponentially, including the role for genetic variants and the gut microbiome. Several advancements have been made over the past decade in noninvasive diagnostic tests to screen for NAFLD, determine its severity, and monitor response to lifestyle intervention and pharmacologic treatment.

Several agents are in phase 3 clinical trials with expected FDA approval by 2023 providing a rationale for a reference book that clinicians can use to diagnose and treat this common and potentially deadly disease.

We hope that this book will be attractive to primary care providers who are on the front line of managing patients with NAFLD. Gastroenterologists and hepatologists will find this book of interest in terms of providing the most updated data on how to risk-stratify patients and identify those who will be eligible for pharmacologic treatment. Other specialists such as cardiologists, endocrinologists and nephrologists will find this book to be a useful reference on the extrahepatic manifestations of NAFLD.

Naim Alkhouri and Stephen A. Harrison

Editors

Naim Alkhouri, MD, is the Chief Medical Officer (CMO), Chief of Transplant Hepatology, and Director of the Fatty Liver Program at Arizona Liver Health (ALH) in Phoenix, Arizona. Prior to joining ALH, Dr. Alkhouri served as the director of the Metabolic Health Center at the Texas Liver Institute and Associate Professor of Medicine and Pediatrics at the University of Texas (UT) Health in San Antonio, Texas. Dr. Alkhouri completed his Gastroenterology and Transplant Hepatology training at the renowned Cleveland Clinic in Cleveland, Ohio, where he was also appointed Assistant Professor of Medicine and Director of the Metabolic Liver Disease Clinic at the Cleveland Clinic Digestive Disease and Surgery Institute. Dr. Alkhouri is a key opinion leader in the field of NASH therapeutics and an advisor/consultant to many pharmaceutical and biomarker development companies. He is Principal Investigator on several multicenter global NASH trials and a member of the AASLD NASH Special Interest Group (NASH SIG).

Dr. Alkhouri has been published in more than 200 publications including the *New England Journal of Medicine, Lancet, JAMA, Gastroenterology, Hepatology,* and *Journal of Hepatology.* He presents his work at both national and international medical conferences. Among many research awards, Dr. Alkhouri received the American College of Gastroenterology Junior Faculty Development Award to study the analysis of breath volatile organic compounds to diagnose nonalcoholic fatty liver disease.

Stephen A. Harrison, MD, is the Founder and Chairman of Pinnacle Clinical Research and Cofounder and Chairman of Summit Clinical Research, LLC in San Antonio, Texas. He is board-certified in Internal Medicine and Gastroenterology. Dr. Harrison earned his medical degree from the University of Mississippi School of Medicine. He completed his internal medicine residency and gastroenterology fellowship at Brooke Army Medical Center before completing a 4-year advanced liver disease fellowship at Saint Louis University. Dr. Harrison served as a Professor of Medicine at the Uniformed Services University of the Health Sciences and is currently a Visiting Professor of Hepatology at Radcliffe Department of Medicine, University of Oxford.

Dr. Harrison served as a colonel in the United States Army. Retiring in 2016, he concluded 20 years of dedicated service to his country. During his army tenure, he served as the Director of Graduate Medical Education at Brooke Army Medical Center, Associate Dean for the San Antonio Uniformed Services Health Education Consortium and Gastroenterology Consultant to the Army Surgeon General. He is a past Associate Editor for *Hepatology* and *Alimentary Pharmacology & Therapeutics* journals. He is internationally known for studies in nonalcoholic fatty liver disease (NAFLD) with more than 300 peer-reviewed publications in top-tier journals including the *New England Journal of Medicine, Nature Medicine, Lancet, JAMA, Gastroenterology, Journal of Hepatology,* and *Hepatology.* He has an H-Index of 93.

Contributors

Nezam H. Afdhal
Division of Gastroenterology and Hepatology
Beth Israel Deaconess Medical Center and Harvard
  Medical School
Boston, Massachusetts, USA

Joseph C. Ahn
Division of Gastroenterology and Hepatology
Mayo Clinic
Rochester, Minnesota, USA

Angelo Armandi
Metabolic Liver Disease Research Program
I. Department of Medicine
University Medical Center of the Johannes
  Gutenberg–University
Mainz, Germany
Division of Gastroenterology and Hepatology
Department of Medical Sciences
University of Turin
Turin, Italy

Imad Asaad
Cleveland Clinic Foundation
Cleveland, Ohio, USA

Cristiana Bianco
Precision Medicine–Department of Transfusion Medicine
  and Hematology
Fondazione IRCCS Ca' Granda Ospedale Maggiore
  Policlinico
Milan, Italy

Rinjal Brahmbhatt
North Shore Gastroenterology & Endoscopy Centers
Westlake, Ohio, USA

Dania Brigham
Children's Hospital Colorado
University of Colorado Hospital
Aurora, Colorado, USA

Sven M. A. Francque
Department of Gastroenterology and Hepatology
Antwerp University Hospital
Antwerp, Belgium
Laboratory of Experimental Medicine and Paediatrics
  (LEMP)
Faculty of Medicine and Health Sciences
University of Antwerp
Antwerp, Belgium
InflaMed Centre of Excellence
University of Antwerp
Antwerp, Belgium
Translational Sciences in Inflammation and Immunology
University of Antwerp
Antwerp, Belgium
European Reference Network on Hepatological Diseases
  (ERN RARE-LIVER)

Daniel Garrido
Department of Medicine
Division of Gastroenterology and Hepatology

Thomas Jefferson University at Sidney Kimmel Medical
  College
Philadelphia, Pennsylvania, USA

Samer Gawrieh
Division of Gastroenterology and Hepatology
Department of Medicine
Indiana University School of Medicine
Indianapolis, Indiana, USA

Dina Halegoua-DeMarzio
Department of Medicine
Division of Gastroenterology and Hepatology
Thomas Jefferson University at Sidney Kimmel Medical
  College
Philadelphia, Pennsylvania, USA

Rukaiya Bashir Hamidu
Department of Medicine
Division of Gastroenterology and Hepatology
Thomas Jefferson University at Sidney Kimmel Medical
  College
Philadelphia, Pennsylvania, USA

Linda Henry
Betty and Guy Beatty Center for Integrated Research
Inova Health System
Falls Church, Virginia, USA
Inova Medicine, Inova Health System
Falls Church, Virginia, USA
Center for Outcomes Research in Liver Disease
Washington, DC, USA

Maryam Ibrahim
Department of Medicine
Massachusetts General Hospital
Boston, Massachusetts, USA
Harvard Medical School
Boston, Massachusetts, USA

Samar H. Ibrahim
Mayo Clinic
Rochester, Minnesota, USA

Scott Isaacs
Emory University School of Medicine
Atlanta, Georgia, USA

Manhal Izzy
Division of Gastroenterology
Hepatology and Nutrition
Vanderbilt University
Nashville, Tennessee, USA

Mohammad Qasim Khan
Division of Gastroenterology
University of Western Ontario
London, Ontario, Canada

Donghee Kim
Division of Gastroenterology and Hepatology
Stanford University School of Medicine
Stanford, California, USA

Rohit Kohli
Children's Hospital Los Angeles
Los Angeles, California, USA

Michelle J. Lai
Division of Gastroenterology and Hepatology
Beth Israel Deaconess Medical Center and Harvard
    Medical School
Boston, Massachusetts, USA

Victor de Lédinghen
Hepatology and Liver Transplantation Unit
CHU Bordeaux and INSERM U1312
Bordeaux University
Bordeaux, France

Julio Leey
Division of Endocrinology
Diabetes and Metabolism
University of Florida
Gainesville, Florida, USA

Michelle T. Long
Section of Gastroenterology
Department of Medicine
Boston University School of Medicine
Boston, Massachusetts, USA

Harmeet Malhi
Division of Gastroenterology and Hepatology
Mayo Clinic
Rochester, Minnesota, USA

Brent A. Neuschwander-Tetri
Department of Gastroenterology and Hepatology
Saint Louis University
St. Louis, Missouri, USA

Gopanandan Parthasarathy
Division of Gastroenterology and Hepatology
Mayo Clinic
Rochester, Minnesota, USA

Carlos J. Pirola
Systems Biology of Complex Diseases
Centro de Altos Estudios en Ciencias Humanas y de la
    Salud (CAECIHS)
Universidad Abierta Interamericana
Consejo Nacional de Investigaciones Científicas y Técnicas
    (CONICET)
Buenos Aires, Argentina
Clinical and Molecular Hepatology
Centro de Altos Estudios en Ciencias Humanas y de la
    Salud (CAECIHS)
Universidad Abierta Interamericana
Consejo Nacional de Investigaciones Científicas y Técnicas
    (CONICET)
Buenos Aires, Argentina

Jörn M. Schattenberg
Metabolic Liver Disease Research Program
I. Department of Medicine
University Medical Center of the Johannes
    Gutenberg–University
Mainz, Germany

Giada Sebastiani
Chronic Viral Illness Service
McGill University Health Centre
Montreal, Québec, Canada
Division of Gastroenterology and Hepatology
Royal Victoria Hospital
McGill University Health Centre
Montreal, Québec, Canada

Tracey G. Simon
Division of Gastroenterology and Hepatology
Massachusetts General Hospital
Boston, Massachusetts, USA
Clinical and Translational Epidemiology Unit (CTEU)
Massachusetts General Hospital
Boston, Massachusetts, USA

Silvia Sookoian
Systems Biology of Complex Diseases
Centro de Altos Estudios en Ciencias Humanas y de la
    Salud (CAECIHS)
Universidad Abierta Interamericana
Consejo Nacional de Investigaciones Científicas y Técnicas
    (CONICET)
Buenos Aires, Argentina
Clinical and Molecular Hepatology
Centro de Altos Estudios en Ciencias Humanas y de la
    Salud (CAECIHS)
Universidad Abierta Interamericana
Consejo Nacional de Investigaciones Científicas y Técnicas
    (CONICET)
Buenos Aires, Argentina

Shikha S. Sundaram
Children's Hospital Colorado
University of Colorado Hospital
Aurora, Colorado, USA

Mousab Tabbaa
North Shore Gastroenterology & Endoscopy Centers
Westlake, Ohio, USA

Vikas Taneja
Division of Gastroenterology and Hepatology
Beth Israel Deaconess Medical Center and Harvard
    Medical School
Boston, Massachusetts, USA

Norah Terrault
Keck Medicine at University of Southern California
Los Angeles, California, USA

Monica Tincopa
Transplant Hepatology
Department of Internal Medicine
Division of Digestive Diseases
University of California Los Angeles
Santa Monica, California, USA

Luca Valenti
Precision Medicine–Department of Transfusion Medicine
    and Hematology
Fondazione IRCCS Ca' Granda Ospedale Maggiore
    Policlinico
Milan, Italy

Department of Pathophysiology and Transplantation
Università Degli Studi di Milano
Milan, Italy

Kymberly D. Watt
Division of Gastroenterology and Hepatology
Mayo Clinic
Rochester, Minnesota, USA

Vincent Wai-Sun Wong
Department of Medicine and Therapeutics
The Chinese University of Hong Kong
Hong Kong

Xixi Xu
Department of Medicine
Boston University School of Medicine
Boston, Massachusetts, USA

Zobair M. Younossi
Betty and Guy Beatty Center for Integrated Research
Inova Medicine, Inova Health System
Falls Church, Virginia, USA
Center for Outcomes Research in Liver Disease
Washington, DC, USA
Center for Liver Disease
Department of Medicine
Inova Fairfax Medical Campus
Fairfax, Virginia, USA

Liyun Yuan
Keck Medicine at University of Southern California
Los Angeles, California, USA

MECHANISMS OF NAFLD DEVELOPMENT

1 Historical Perspectives and Clinical Presentation

Imad Asaad and Naim Alkhouri

CONTENTS

1.1 INTRODUCTION

Nonalcoholic fatty liver disease (NAFLD) is currently the most prominent cause of chronic liver disease worldwide. NAFLD is defined by the presence of hepatic steatosis by imaging or histology, affecting at least 5% of hepatocytes in individuals without secondary causes of hepatic fat accumulation such as significant alcohol consumption, viral hepatitis, steatogenic medications (e.g., tamoxifen, amiodarone, methotrexate), or lipodystrophy[1].

NAFLD can be categorized histologically into nonalcoholic fatty liver (NAFL), the potentially nonprogressive subtype of NAFLD, as well as nonalcoholic steatohepatitis (NASH), the potentially progressive subtype of NAFLD that can lead to advanced fibrosis and cirrhosis, as well as liver-related morbidity and mortality. NASH is defined histologically by the presence of hepatic steatosis with evidence for hepatocyte damage and liver inflammation[1,2].

Nonalcoholic fatty liver disease (NAFLD) is the most common cause of chronic liver disease worldwide, with a global prevalence of 25.24%[3]. In a cross-sectional study from 2011 to 2014, the overall prevalence of NAFLD among US adults was 21.9%, representing 51.6 million individuls[4]. And NASH-related cirrhosis is currently the second most common indication for liver transplants in the United States[5].

The prevalence of NAFLD in patients with components of metabolic syndrome is higher. For instance, NAFLD has been reported in over 76% of type 2 diabetics. Furthermore, over 90% of severely obese patients undergoing bariatric surgery have NAFLD[6].

A high burden of metabolic comorbidities is associated with NAFLD creating implications for clinical management of the disease. Given the common risk factors between NAFLD and cardiovascular disease (CVD), cardiac-related death is one of the leading causes of death for NAFLD patients. Patients with NAFLD have increased overall mortality compared to matched control populations without NAFLD, and patients with histological NASH have an increased liver-related mortality rate[7].

NAFLD is now considered the third most common cause of hepatocellular carcinoma (HCC) in the United States, likely related to the increasing prevalence of this condition. Extrahepatic cancer-related mortality is among the top three causes of death in subjects with NAFLD[1].

The significant prevalence and burden of the disease have led to major efforts during the last two decades in the development of diagnostics and treatments. However, NAFLD is a heterogeneous disease that has multiple metabolic and genetic factors contributing to its progression. It is largely asymptomatic in the early stages but can lead to significant clinical outcomes in the late stages. This variability in NAFLD natural history has led to substantial challenges in biomarkers discovery and drug development.

Learning the history of the disease will help provide better understanding about its pathophysiology and natural history, which are the cornerstones in the development of diagnostic testing and therapeutics.

The history of NAFLD has multiple major milestones. This chapter will provide an overview of the most important landmark discoveries and studies in the history of NAFLD that have formed our current understanding of this disease.

These are the major areas discussed in this chapter:

1. Historical perspectives of terminology and histopathology

2. Historical perspectives of pathophysiology, natural history and the association with metabolic syndrome

   a. Association between metabolic syndrome components

   b. Association of NAFLD and metabolic syndrome

   c. Apoptosis, lipid and bile acid metabolism

   d. Inflammatory response

   e. Genetics of NAFLD

3. Historical perspectives of diagnostic testing

4. Historical perspectives of therapeutics

1.2 HISTORICAL PERSPECTIVES OF TERMINOLOGY AND HISTOPATHOLOGY

In the 1800s, multiple pathologists reported fatty infiltration of the liver in individuals with diabetes and obesity similar to those with alcoholic liver disease[8–10]. In 1962, the link between fat accumulation in the liver and liver injury was first recognize by Thaler[11].

DOI: 10.1201/9781003386698-2

In 1980, Ludwig and colleagues at the Mayo Clinic introduced the term "nonalcoholic steatohepatitis" (NASH) based on histological features. They studied liver biopsies of 20 patients who had hepatitis of unknown cause and did not consume alcohol or consumed alcohol in quantities not considered harmful to the liver. Biopsy specimens had histological findings similar to alcoholic hepatitis characterized by the presence of fatty changes with evidence of lobular hepatitis, focal necrosis with mixed inflammatory infiltrates, Mallory bodies and evidence of fibrosis[12].

In 1983, Moran reported the presence of steatohepatitis in three obese children who presented with nonspecific abdominal pain and abnormal liver function tests[13].

Then the term "nonalcoholic fatty liver disease" (NAFLD) was first introduced by Schaffner and Thaler in 1986[14].

In 2020, multiple experts reached consensus that the terminology "nonalcoholic" overemphasizes "alcohol" and underemphasizes metabolic risk factors. So a name change from NAFLD to metabolic-associated fatty liver disease (MAFLD) has been proposed[15]. Subsequent studies afterward showed that MAFLD is associated with an increased risk of all-cause mortality and increased risk of cardiovascular disease[16,17]. However, this proposal was considered by other experts to be premature and suggested that a change will be justified when a more scientific and complete understanding of the disease pathogenesis, risk stratification, molecular phenotyping and related therapeutic approaches are elucidated[18].

1.3 HISTORICAL PERSPECTIVES OF PATHOPHYSIOLOGY, NATURAL HISTORY AND ASSOCIATION WITH METABOLIC SYNDROME

1.3.1 Association between Metabolic Syndrome Components

In 1765, J.B. Morgagni was the first to identify the association between components of metabolic syndrome. He clearly described the association between visceral obesity, hypertension, hyperuricemia, atherosclerosis and obstructive sleep apnea long before the modern recognition of this syndrome[19].

In the early twentieth century, obesity incidence was increasing and accompanied by a rising incidence of diabetes. Elliott Joslin was the first US doctor to specialize in diabetes. In 1924, Joslin noted: "Diabetes is 15 times as common among adults and 20 times as common among the fat"[20].

In 1939, Harold Himsworth identified the two different types of diabetes: The insulin-sensitive type, which is what we call now type 1, and the insulin-insensitive type, which is what we call now type 2. Himsworth described that insensitive diabetics tend to be elderly and obese and to have hypertension and arteriosclerosis[20].

Then multiple European scientists in 1900s described the very common coexistence of the various components of the syndrome, including hypertension obesity, hypertension and hyperlipidemia[21–23].

In 1988, Raevan introduced the term "Syndrome X" and further described the role of insulin resistance in the development and progression of T2D, HTN and CAD[24].

1.3.2 Association of NAFLD and Metabolic Syndrome

In 1932, Zelman described the presence of liver damage in obesity[25]. Then in 1970, Beringer and Thaler reported NAFLD association with obesity and diabetes in a study including 465 liver biopsies of diabetic patients[26].

In 1979, Itoh reported five cases of nonalcoholic diabetic women with obesity and hyperglycemia who had histological findings consistent with micronodular cirrhosis[27].

In 1980, study by Ludwig et al. that introduced the term NASH, most of the study's 20 patients were women with obesity and type 2 diabetes[12].

In 1990, Elizabeth Powell and colleagues identified obesity, hyperlipidemia and T2DM as risk factors for nonalcoholic steatohepatitis. In this study, 42 patients with nonalcoholic steatohepatitis were followed for a median of 4.5 years (range = 1.5–21.5 years). Except for two patients with lipodystrophy, all were obese; 35 of 42 were women, 26 of 32 were hyperlipidemic and 15 were hyperglycemic[28,29].

In 1994, Bruce Bacan analyzed a series of 33 patients with NASH. He noted in his study that NASH spectrum should be expanded as compared to Ludwig's initial description and should no longer be considered a disease predominantly seen in obese women with diabetes[30].

A study by Marchesini and colleagues in 1999 reported the association between nonalcoholic fatty liver disease and insulin resistance even in the absence of diabetes and obesity[31].

Another study by Aron Sanyal and colleagues indicated that peripheral insulin resistance, increased fatty acid beta-oxidation and hepatic oxidative stress are present in both fatty liver and NASH, but NASH alone is associated with mitochondrial structural defects[32].

In 2007, Kotronen evaluated liver fat content by proton magnetic resonance spectroscopy in 271 nondiabetic subjects and found that liver fat content is significantly (4-fold higher) increased in subjects with the metabolic syndrome as compared with those without the syndrome, independently of age, gender and body mass index[33].

In 2010, Vanni was one of the first to describe the bidirectional relationship linking NAFLD with metabolic syndrome and indicated that hyperinsulinemia is probably the consequence rather than cause of NAFLD[34]. Then Zhang in 2015 described further the bidirectional relationship; his study findings suggested a reciprocal causality between NAFLD and metabolic syndrome[35].

1.3.3 Apoptosis, Lipid and Bile Acid Metabolism

In 2003, Gregory Gore and colleagues concluded that hepatocyte apoptosis is significantly increased in patients with nonalcoholic steatohepatitis and that it correlates with disease severity[36]. This study demonstrated that saturated fatty acids could induce apoptosis and were increased in patients with NASH.

Another study in 2012 showed inappropriate increase in hepatic synthesis and dysregulation of cholesterol metabolism being associated with NAFLD especially elevated free cholesterol levels[37].

In 2011, Lima Cabello and colleagues described the potential role of liver X receptero (LXRα), a nuclear receptor that binds ligands such as cholesterol derivatives and polyunsaturated fatty acids, in the pathogenesis of NAFLD. This study showed increased hepatic expression levels of LXRα and related lipogenic and inflammatory mediators compared to farnesoid X receptor (FXR), another nuclear receptor that binds bile acids (Bas) as ligands with pleotrpic effects in the liver[38].

Insulin resistance, the principal risk factor for NAFLD, was found to be associated with a shift in the circulating BA profile toward a more trihydroxylic one, which has weaker FXR agonist effects compared to more hydrophobic bile acids[39].

These studies have provided the basis for the use of FXR agonists for the treatment of nonalcoholic steatohepatitis.

1.3.4 Inflammatory Response

In 1988, the 2-hit hypothesis was proposed by Day and colleagues, and it provided the basis for the current understanding of NAFLD pathophysiology, i.e., steatosis as the first hit and the inflammatory response leading to cell death as the second hit [40].

In the early 2000s, multiple studies investigated the role of mitochondrial abnormalities in NAFLD. In 2000, Robertson indicated that CYPs 2E1 and 4A, which are the microsomal oxidases involved with fatty acid oxidation, could generate the "second hit" of cellular injury by creating oxidative stress when antioxidant reserve is depleted[41]. In 2001 a study by Sanyal et al. showed that peripheral insulin resistance, increased fatty acid beta-oxidation and hepatic oxidative stress are present in both fatty liver and NASH, but NASH alone is associated with mitochondrial structural defects[32].

In 2005, Zobair M. Younossi published a study describing the molecular pathogenesis and the genomic/proteomic analysis of NAFLD. The study was done on liver biopsy specimens from 98 bariatric surgery patients who were classified as normal, steatosis alone, steatosis with nonspecific inflammation and NASH. The genomic/proteomic analysis of these specimens suggested differential expression of several genes and protein peaks in patients within the spectrum of NAFLD[42].

In 2004 and 2005, two studies reported lower plasma adiponectin concentration in NAFLD. Adiponectin is an adipokine with anti-inflammatory and anti-steatotic properties. In 2006, Giovanni Targher conducted a cross-sectional study investigating the role of adiponectin in NAFLD pathogenesis. The study enrolled 60 NAFLD patients and 60 age-, sex- and body mass index (BMI)-matched healthy controls. NAFLD patients had markedly lower plasma adiponectin concentrations than control subjects. Hypoadiponectinemia was also associated with the severity of the histologic features of NASH[43–45].

Development of NASH involves the innate immune system and is mediated by Kupffer cells and hepatic stellate cells (HSCs). Gyorgy Baffy was one of the first to describe the role of Kupffer cells in the progression of NAFLD. His paper in 2009 indicated that toll-like receptors, in particular TLR4, represent a major conduit for danger recognition linked to Kupffer cell activation. A toll-like receptor is a pattern recognition receptor that recognizes bacteria-derived cytosine phosphate guanine (CpG)-containing DNA and DNA from damaged cells to activate innate immunity[46].

A study done by Miura K. Kodama and colleagues in 2010 showed that in a mouse model of NASH, TLR9 signaling induces production of interleukin IL-1beta by Kupffer cells, leading to steatosis, inflammation and fibrosis[47].

Another study by Miura and colleagues concluded in 2012 that the CC-chemokine receptor (CCR)2 and Kupffer cells contribute to the progression of NASH by recruiting bone marrow-derived monocytes[48].

1.3.5 Genetics of NAFLD

The heritability of NAFLD is supported by a body of evidence derived from epidemiological studies and genetic studies.

Epidemiological studies demonstrate large interethnic variability in an individual's susceptibility to NAFLD and NASH. A retrospective study by Stephen Caldwell in 2002 showed that the prevalence of cirrhosis attributed to NAFLD differs between different ethnic groups[49]. Then another study by Jeffrey Browning in 2004 showed that the ethnic differences in the frequency of hepatic steatosis mirror those observed previously for NAFLD-related cirrhosis (Hispanics > Whites > Blacks)[50].

A meta-analysis by Zobair M. Younossi in 2016 showed that the global prevalence of NAFLD is 25.24% (95% CI: 22.10–28.65). The highest prevalence of NAFLD is reported from the Middle East (31.79% [95% CI, 13.48–58.23]) and South America (30.45% [95% CI, 22.74–39.440]), whereas the lowest prevalence rate is reported from Africa (13.48% [5.69–28.69])[3].

A study done by Schwimmer and colleagues in 2009 showed that fatty liver was significantly more common in siblings (59%) and parents (78%) of children with NAFLD. The association was independent of adiposity and led to estimates that between 38 and 100% of hepatic fat content and NAFLD variability are due to inherited factors[51].

A cross-sectional analysis by Rohit Loomba in 2015 including 60 pairs of twins showed that the presence of hepatic steatosis and the level of hepatic fibrosis, as measured using magnetic resonance imaging, are correlated between monozygotic twins but not between dizygotic twins[52].

Multiple genome-wide association studies (GWAS) were done during the last 20 years that have expanded the understanding of genetic background contributing to variation in NAFLD susceptibility, progression and outcomes.

The first genome-wide association study of GWAS in hepatology aimed at investigating the genetic basis of susceptibility to NAFLD dates back to 2008. A study by Stephano Romeo and colleagues showed an allele in the patatin-like phospholipase domain-containing protein 3 (PNPLA3 — rs738409[G], encoding I148M) strongly associated with increased hepatic fat levels and with hepatic inflammation. The allele was most common in Hispanics, the group most susceptible to NAFLD; hepatic fat content was more than 2-fold higher in PNPLA3 rs738409[G] homozygotes than in noncarriers. Resequencing revealed another allele of PNPLA3 (rs6006460[T], encoding S453I) that was associated with lower hepatic fat content in African Americans, the group at lowest risk of NAFLD[53].

Since 2008, other variants in different genes were found to be associated with the development of NAFLD (Table 1.1). All these genes encode proteins involved in the regulation of hepatic lipid metabolism. These include patatin-like phospholipase domain-containing protein 3 (PNPLA3), transmembrane 6 superfamily member 2 (TM6SF2), glucokinase regulator (GCKR) and membrane-bound O acyltransferase 7 (MBOAT7)[54].

Clinical implementation of genetics in NAFLD has a great potential. The rapidly growing knowledge of the genetic background will help accelerate the development of pharmacotherapies and identify targets that are likely to translate to clinical benefit. NAFLD genetics have also been incorporated into diagnostic and prognostic models and polygenic scores[54,55].

Table 1.1: Genetic Variants That Are Associated with the Development and Progression on NAFLD

Gene	Variant	Function	Phenotype
PNPLA3	rs738409 C>G	Lipid droplets remodeling	↑NAFLD, NASH, fibrosis, HCC
TM6SF2	rs58542926 C>T	VLDL secretion	↑NAFLD, NASH, fibrosis
GCKR	rs1260326 C>T	Regulation of de novo lipogenesis	↑NAFLD, NASH, fibrosis
MBOAT7	rs641738 C>T	Fatty acid remodeling	↑NAFLD, NASH, fibrosis, HCC

1.4 HISTORICAL PERSPECTIVES OF DIAGNOSTIC TESTING

Diagnosis of steatosis can be done accurately using noninvasive tests[56,57]. However, diagnosis of steatohepatitis still requires liver biopsy. Liver biopsy has also traditionally been considered the reference method for evaluation of hepatic fibrosis.

In 1999, the first grading and staging system for histologic diagnosis of NASH was developed by Brunt and colleagues. It included 10 histological variables of disease activity based on an observed progressive increase in steatosis, ballooning and lobular inflammation and a staging score for fibrosis[58].

In 2005, the Pathology Committee of the NASH Clinical Research Network designed and validated a histological feature scoring system that addresses the full spectrum of lesions of NAFLD and proposed the NAFLD activity score (NAS) to diagnose NASH especially for clinical trials (Table 1.2). The scoring system comprised 14 histological features, 4 of which were evaluated semiquantitatively: steatosis (0–3), lobular inflammation (0–2), hepatocellular ballooning (0–2) and fibrosis (0–4). NAS of > or = 5 correlated with a diagnosis of NASH, and biopsies with scores of less than 3 were diagnosed as "not NASH"[59].

In 2012, another scoring system for histological severity of NAFLD was developed, called the "SAF score," which stands for steatosis, activity and fibrosis. The SAF score used the same components as NAS, including steatosis (0–3), activity grade (A, 0–4) calculated by the unweighted addition of hepatocyte ballooning (0–2) and lobular inflammation (0–2), and the fibrosis stage (0–4). However, it is reported with subscripts for each component, i.e., S (0–3) A (0–4) F (0–4), whereas the NAS is reported as a single numeric value, the unweighted sum of steatosis + lobular inflammation + ballooning. Diagnosis of NASH was based on fatty liver inhibition of progression (FLIP) algorithm (Figure 1.1). The FLIP algorithm based on the SAF score has been shown to decrease interobserver variations among pathologists compared to NAS[60].

In 2012, Alkhouri and colleagues introduced a histological grading score for pediatric NAFLD to account for the fact that portal-based injury is a key feature of the disease in children. The score was based on steatosis, lobular inflammation, ballooning and portal inflammation. These histological feature were scored: steatosis (0–3), lobular inflammation (0–3), ballooning (0–2) and portal inflammation (0–2). This score was called the Pediatric NAFLD Histological Score (PNHS)[61].

Although liver biopsy is the most reliable approach for identifying the presence of steatohepatitis (SH) and fibrosis in patients with NAFLD, the biopsy specimen size has to be long enough and has to be interpreted by experts to provide reliable information[62]. It has also been shown that

Table 1.2: NAFLD Activity Score (NAS) and Its Components

NAFLD Activity Score (NAS)

Histologic Feature	Score
Steatosis	0 <5%
	1 5–33%
	2 34–66%
	3 >66%
Hepatocyte ballooning	0 None
	1 Few
	2 Many
Lobular inflammation	0 None
	1 1–2 foci per 20× field
	2 2–4 foci per 20× field
	3 >4 foci per 20× field
Fibrosis stage	0 No fibrosis
	1a Zone 3 mild perisinusoidal fibrosis
	1b Zone 3 moderate perisinusoidal fibrosis
	1c portal or periportal fibrosis
	2 Zone 3 and portal/periportal fibrosis
	3 Bridging fibrosis
	4 Cirrhosis

there is variability among hepatopathologists' readings for NASH histologic features and overall diagnosis[63]. Besides technical problems, liver biopsy remains a costly and an invasive procedure. These limitations led to the evolution of noninvasive testing for assessment of liver disease severity and fibrosis.

Noninvasive tests can be classified into (1) blood-based tests and (2) imaging methods assessing physical properties of the liver tissue, including stiffness attenuation and viscosity.

Numerous recent publications have reported on the accuracy of existing and novel NITs to assess liver diseases. These will be discussed in detail in another chapter.

1.5 HISTORICAL PERSPECTIVES OF THERAPEUTICS

As our understanding of NAFLD pathophysiology is advancing rapidly, the development of therapeutics that can affect a variety of new targets has been progressing.

The treatment of NAFLD can be divided into lifestyle modifications to induce weight loss and pharmacological treatments.

In a meta-analysis of eight randomized, controlled trials (RCTs), published in 2012, 5% weight loss led to improvement in steatosis, whereas 7% weight loss was associated with an improved NAS and resolution of NASH[64]. Another study published in 2015 of 293 patients

Steatosis ⟶	Ballooning ⟶	Lobular Inflammation	Diagnosis

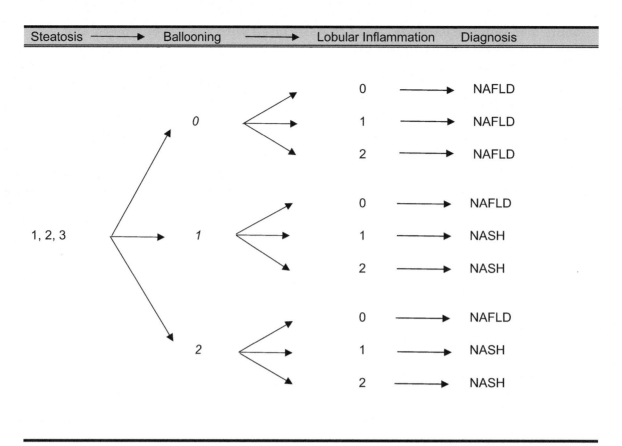

Figure 1.1 Fatty liver inhibition of progression (FLIP) algorithm based on the steatosis/activity/fibrosis (SAF) score

with histologically proven NASH showed that the highest rates of NAS reduction, NASH resolution and fibrosis regression occurred in patients with weight losses ≥10%[65]. However, only 50% of patients achieved 7% or more weight loss at 12 months and only 10% of patients lost ≥10%.

Given that patients with NAFLD without SH or any fibrosis have an excellent prognosis from a liver standpoint, pharmacological treatments aimed primarily at improving liver disease should generally be limited to those with biopsy-proven NASH and fibrosis[1].

The antioxidant vitamin E was one of the first drugs to be tested for NASH. A pilot study in 2000 showed that vitamin E administration normalized serum aminotransferases and alkaline phosphatase levels in children. Another pilot study in 2004 studied the combination of antioxidant (vitamin E) and an insulin sensitizer (pioglitazone) and showed that vitamin E alone produced a significant decrease in steatosis, whereas combination treatment produced improvement in NASH histology including decrease in steatosis cytological ballooning and pericellular fibrosis[66,67].

The PEVINS trial in 2010 included 247 individuals with NASH and without diabetes who were randomly assigned to receive pioglitazone (30 mg daily), vitamin E (800 IU daily) or placebo. Vitamin E was associated with a higher rate of improvement in NAS by 2 points or more than placebo, whereas the rate of improvement with pioglitazone was not significant. Individuals who received pioglitazone gained more weight than those

who received vitamin E or placebo. Otherwise, other the side effects were similar[68].

The widespread use of vitamin E was limited due to concerns about the association with hemorrhagic stroke risk in observational studies[69]. Another concern was the association with prostate cancer observed from continued follow-up of individuals in the SELECT trial, which showed that the absolute increase in risk of prostate cancer per 1000 person-years was 1.6 for vitamin E translating into a 17% incrased risk[70]. Weight gain, which is the most common side effect of pioglitazone, and the possible association of pioglitazone with bladder cancer and bone loss have limited the use of pioglitazone by providers[71,72].

Omega-3 fatty acids have been investigated to treat NAFLD. In a literature review in 2010 by Masterton and colleagues, animal studies demonstrated that omega-3 fatty acids reduced hepatic steatosis, improved insulin sensitivity and reduced markers of inflammation; however, clinical trials in human subjects were limited by small sample size and methodological flaws[73]. Two other studies failed to show convincing therapeutic benefit for omega-3 fatty acids[74,75].

The American Association for the Study of Liver Disease (AASLD) NAFLD guidelines recommend against using Omega-3 fatty acids as a specific treatment of NAFLD or NASH, but they may be considered to treat hypertriglyceridemia in patients with NAFLD[1].

Currently, several emerging therapies have progressed to phase II and beyond, and they will be discussed in detail in another chapter.

REFERENCES

1. Chalasani, N. *et al.* The diagnosis and management of nonalcoholic fatty liver disease: Practice guidance from the American association for the study of liver diseases. *Hepatology* **67**, 328–357 (2017). http://doi.org/10.1002/hep.29367/suppinfo.

2. Li, Z. *et al.* Prevalence of nonalcoholic fatty liver disease in mainland of China: A meta-analysis of published studies. *Journal of Gastroenterology and Hepatology* **29**, 42–51 (2014).

3. Younossi, Z. M. *et al.* Global epidemiology of nonalcoholic fatty liver disease-Meta-analytic assessment of prevalence, incidence, and outcomes. *Hepatology (Baltimore, Md.)* **64**, 73–84 (2016).

4. Wong, R. J., Liu, B. & Bhuket, T. Significant burden of nonalcoholic fatty liver disease with advanced fibrosis in the US: A cross-sectional analysis of 2011–2014 National Health and Nutrition Examination Survey. *Alimentary Pharmacology & Therapeutics* **46**, 974–980 (2017).

5. Wong, R. J. *et al.* Nonalcoholic steatohepatitis is the second leading etiology of liver disease among adults awaiting liver transplantation in the United States. *Gastroenterology* **148**, 547–555 (2015).

6. Portillo Sanchez, P. *et al.* High prevalence of nonalcoholic fatty liver disease in patients with type 2 diabetes mellitus and normal plasma aminotransferase levels. *The Journal of Clinical Endocrinology and Metabolism* **100** (2014).

7. Stepanova, M. *et al.* Predictors of all-cause mortality and liver-related mortality in patients with nonalcoholic fatty liver disease (NAFLD). *Digestive Diseases and Sciences* **58**, 3017–3023 (2013).

8. Connor, C. L. Fatty infiltration of the liver and the development of cirrhosis in diabetes and chronic alcoholism. *The American Journal of Pathology* **14**, 347–364 (1938).

9. Pepper, W. *A System of Practical Medicine by American Authors.* Lea Brothers & Co.: Philadelphia, PA, 1885; Volume II, p. 1050.

10. Pepper, W. Saccharine diabetes. *Medication Reconciliation* **25**, 9–12 (1884).

11. Thaler, H. The fatty liver and its pathogenetic relation to liver cirrhosis. *Virchows Archiv fur Pathologische Anatomie und Physiologie und fur Klinische Medizin* **335**, 180–210 (1962).

12. Ludwig, J., Viggiano, T. R., McGill, D. B. & Oh, B. J. Nonalcoholic steatohepatitis: Mayo Clinic experiences with a hitherto unnamed disease. *Mayo Clinic Proceedings* **55**, 434–438 (1980).

13. Moran, J. R., Ghishan, F. K., Halter, S. A. & Greene, H. L. Steatohepatitis in obese children: A cause of chronic liver dysfunction. *The American Journal of Gastroenterology* **78**, 374–377 (1983).

14. Schaffner, F. & Thaler, H. Nonalcoholic fatty liver disease. *Progress in Liver Diseases* **8**, 283–298 (1986).

15. Eslam, M., Sanyal, A. J., George, J. & International Consensus Panel. MAFLD: A consensus-driven proposed nomenclature for metabolic associated fatty liver disease. *Gastroenterology* **158**, 1999–2014.e1 (2020).

16. Lee, H., Lee, Y.-H., Kim, S. U. & Kim, H. C. Metabolic dysfunction-associated fatty liver disease and incident cardiovascular disease risk: A nationwide cohort study. *Clinical Gastroenterology and Hepatology: The Official Clinical Practice Journal of the American Gastroenterological Association* **19**, 2138–2147.e10 (2021).

17. Kim, D. *et al.* Metabolic dysfunction-associated fatty liver disease is associated with increased all-cause mortality in the United States. *Journal of Hepatology* **75**, 1284–1291 (2021).

18. Younossi, Z. M. *et al.* From NAFLD to MAFLD: Implications of a premature change in terminology. *Hepatology (Baltimore, Md.)* **73**, 1194–1198 (2021).

19. Enzi, G., Busetto, L., Inelmen, E. M., Coin, A. & Sergi, G. Historical perspective: Visceral obesity and related comorbidity in Joannes Baptista Morgagni's "De sedibus et causis morborum per anatomen indagata". *International Journal of Obesity and Related Metabolic Disorders : Journal of the International Association for the Study of Obesity* **27**, 534–535 (2003).

20. Haslam, D. *Diabesity-a historical perspective: Part II Article points.*

21. Avogaro, P., Crepaldi, G., Enzi, G. & Tiengo, A. Associazione di iperlipemia, diabete mellito e obesita' di mediogrado. *Acta Diabetologica Latina* **4**, 572–590 (1967).

22. Feldman, R., Sender, A. J. & Siegelaub, A. B. Difference in diabetic and nondiabetic fat distribution patterns by skinfold measurements. *Diabetes* **18**, 478–486 (1969).

23. Kissebah, A. H. *et al.* Relation of body fat distribution to metabolic complications of obesity. *The Journal of Clinical Endocrinology and Metabolism* **54**, 254–260 (1982).

24. Reaven, G. M. Banting lecture 1988. Role of insulin resistance in human disease. *Diabetes* **37**, 1595–1607 (1988).

25. Zelman, S. The liver in obesity. *A.M.A. Archives of Internal Medicine* **90**, 141–156 (1952).

26. Beringer, A. & Thaler, H. Relationships between diabetes mellitus and fatty liver. *Deutsche medizinische Wochenschrift (1946)* **95**, 836–838 (1970).

27. Itoh, S., Tsukada, Y., Motomura, Y. & Ichinoe, A. Five patients with nonalcoholic diabetic cirrhosis. *Acta hepato-gastroenterologica* **26**, 90–97 (1979).

28. Powell, E. E. *et al.* The natural history of nonalcoholic steatohepatitis: A follow-up study of forty-two patients for up to 21 years. *Hepatology (Baltimore, Md.)* **11**, 74–80 (1990).

29. Powell, E. E., Searle, J. & Mortimer, R. Steatohepatitis associated with limb lipodystrophy. *Gastroenterology* **97**, 1022–1024 (1989).

30. Bacon, B. R., Farahvash, M. J., Janney, C. G. & Neuschwander-Tetri, B. A. Nonalcoholic steatohepatitis: An expanded clinical entity. *Gastroenterology* **107**, 1103–1109 (1994).

31. Marchesini, G. *et al.* Association of nonalcoholic fatty liver disease with insulin resistance. *The American Journal of Medicine* **107**, 450–455 (1999).

32. Sanyal, A. J. *et al.* Nonalcoholic steatohepatitis: Association of insulin resistance and mitochondrial abnormalities. *Gastroenterology* **120**, 1183–1192 (2001).

33. Kotronen, A., Westerbacka, J., Bergholm, R., Pietiläinen, K. H. & Yki-Järvinen, H. Liver fat in the metabolic syndrome. *The Journal of Clinical Endocrinology and Metabolism* **92**, 3490–3497 (2007).

34. Vanni, E. *et al.* From the metabolic syndrome to NAFLD or vice versa? *Digestive and Liver Disease: Official Journal of the Italian Society of Gastroenterology and the Italian Association for the Study of the Liver* **42**, 320–330 (2010).

35. Zhang, Y. *et al.* Identification of reciprocal causality between non-alcoholic fatty liver disease and metabolic syndrome by a simplified Bayesian network in a Chinese population. *BMJ Open* **5**, e008204 (2015).

36. Feldstein, A. E. *et al.* Hepatocyte apoptosis and Fas expression are prominent features of human nonalcoholic steatohepatitis. *Gastroenterology* **125**, 437–443 (2003).

37. Min, H. K. *et al.* Increased hepatic synthesis and dysregulation of cholesterol metabolism is associated with the severity of nonalcoholic fatty liver disease. *Cell Metabolism* **15**, 665–674 (2012).

38. Lima-Cabello, E. *et al.* Enhanced expression of proinflammatory mediators and liver X-receptor-regulated lipogenic genes in non-alcoholic fatty liver disease and hepatitis C. *Clinical Science (London, England: 1979)* **120**, 239–250 (2011).

39. Haeusler, R. A., Astiarraga, B., Camastra, S., Accili, D. & Ferrannini, E. Human insulin resistance is associated with increased plasma levels of 12α-hydroxylated bile acids. *Diabetes* **62**, 4184–4191 (2013).

40. Day, C. P. & James, O. F. Steatohepatitis: A tale of two "hits"? *Gastroenterology* **114**, 842–845 (1998).

41. Robertson, G., Leclercq, I. & Farrell, G. C. Nonalcoholic steatosis and steatohepatitis. II. Cytochrome P-450 enzymes and oxidative stress. *American Journal of Physiology. Gastrointestinal and Liver Physiology* **281**, G1135–G1139 (2001).

42. Younossi, Z. M. *et al.* A genomic and proteomic study of the spectrum of nonalcoholic fatty liver disease. *Hepatology (Baltimore, Md.)* **42**, 665–674 (2005).

43. Hui, J. M. *et al.* Beyond insulin resistance in NASH: TNF-alpha or adiponectin? *Hepatology (Baltimore, Md.)* **40**, 46–54 (2004).

44. Pagano, C. *et al.* Plasma adiponectin is decreased in nonalcoholic fatty liver disease. *European Journal of Endocrinology* **152**, 113–118 (2005).

45. Targher, G. *et al.* Associations between plasma adiponectin concentrations and liver histology in patients with nonalcoholic fatty liver disease. *Clinical Endocrinology* **64**, 679–683 (2006).

46. Baffy, G. Kupffer cells in non-alcoholic fatty liver disease: The emerging view. *Journal of Hepatology* **51**, 212–223 (2009).

47. Miura, K. *et al.* Toll-like receptor 9 promotes steatohepatitis by induction of interleukin-1beta in mice. *Gastroenterology* **139**, 323–334.e7 (2010).

48. Miura, K., Yang, L., van Rooijen, N., Ohnishi, H. & Seki, E. Hepatic recruitment of macrophages promotes nonalcoholic steatohepatitis through CCR2. *American Journal of Physiology. Gastrointestinal and Liver Physiology* **302**, G1310–G1321 (2012).

49. Caldwell, S. H., Harris, D. M., Patrie, J. T. & Hespenheide, E. E. Is NASH underdiagnosed among African Americans? *The American Journal of Gastroenterology* **97**, 1496–1500 (2002).

50. Browning, J. D. *et al.* Prevalence of hepatic steatosis in an urban population in the United States: Impact of ethnicity. *Hepatology (Baltimore, Md.)* **40**, 1387–1395 (2004).

51. Schwimmer, J. B. *et al.* Heritability of nonalcoholic fatty liver disease. *Gastroenterology* **136**, 1585–1592 (2009).

52. Loomba, R. *et al.* Heritability of hepatic fibrosis and steatosis based on a prospective twin study. *Gastroenterology* **149**, 1784–1793 (2015).

53. Romeo, S. *et al.* Genetic variation in PNPLA3 confers susceptibility to nonalcoholic fatty liver disease. *Nature Genetics* **40**, 1461–1465 (2008).

54. Eslam, M., Valenti, L. & Romeo, S. Genetics and epigenetics of NAFLD and NASH: Clinical impact. *Journal of Hepatology* **68**, 268–279 (2018).

55. Eslam, M. *et al.* FibroGENE: A gene-based model for staging liver fibrosis. *Journal of Hepatology* **64**, 390–398 (2016).

56. Idilman, I. S. *et al.* Hepatic steatosis: Quantification by proton density fat fraction with MR imaging versus liver biopsy. *Radiology* **267**, 767–775 (2013).

57. Siddiqui, M. S. *et al.* Vibration-controlled transient elastography to assess fibrosis and steatosis in patients with nonalcoholic fatty liver disease. *Clinical Gastroenterology and Hepatology* **17**, 156–163.e2 (2019).

58. Brunt, E. M., Janney, C. G., di Bisceglie, A. M., Neuschwander-Tetri, B. A. & Bacon, B. R. Nonalcoholic steatohepatitis: A proposal for grading and staging the histological lesions. *The American Journal of Gastroenterology* **94**, 2467–2474 (1999).

59. Kleiner, D. E. *et al.* Design and validation of a histological scoring system for nonalcoholic fatty liver disease. *Hepatology (Baltimore, Md.)* **41**, 1313–1321 (2005).

60. Bedossa, P. & FLIP Pathology Consortium. Utility and appropriateness of the fatty liver inhibition of progression (FLIP) algorithm and steatosis, activity, and fibrosis (SAF) score in the evaluation of biopsies of nonalcoholic fatty liver disease. *Hepatology (Baltimore, Md.)* **60**, 565–575 (2014).

61. Alkhouri, N. *et al.* Development and validation of a new histological score for pediatric non-alcoholic fatty liver disease. *Journal of Hepatology* **57**, 1312–1318 (2012).

62. Bedossa, P., Dargère, D. & Paradis, V. Sampling variability of liver fibrosis in chronic hepatitis C. *Hepatology (Baltimore, Md.)* **38**, 1449–1457 (2003).

63. Davison, B. A. *et al.* Suboptimal reliability of liver biopsy evaluation has implications for randomized clinical trials. *Journal of Hepatology* **73**, 1322–1332 (2020).

64. Musso, G., Cassader, M., Rosina, F. & Gambino, R. Impact of current treatments on liver disease, glucose metabolism and cardiovascular risk in non-alcoholic fatty liver disease (NAFLD): A systematic review and meta-analysis of randomised trials. *Diabetologia* **55**, 885–904 (2012).

65. Vilar-Gomez, E. *et al.* Weight loss through lifestyle modification significantly reduces features of nonalcoholic steatohepatitis. *Gastroenterology* **149**, 367–378.e5; quiz e14–15 (2015).

66. Sanyal, A. J. *et al.* A pilot study of vitamin E versus vitamin E and pioglitazone for the treatment of nonalcoholic steatohepatitis. *Clinical Gastroenterology and Hepatology: The Official Clinical Practice Journal of the American Gastroenterological Association* **2**, 1107–1115 (2004).

67. Lavine, J. E. Vitamin E treatment of nonalcoholic steatohepatitis in children: A pilot study. *The Journal of Pediatrics* **136**, 734–738 (2000).

68. Sanyal, A. J. *et al.* Pioglitazone, vitamin E, or placebo for nonalcoholic steatohepatitis. *The New England Journal of Medicine* **362**, 1675–1685 (2010).

69. Keli, S. O., Hertog, M. G., Feskens, E. J. & Kromhout, D. Dietary flavonoids, antioxidant vitamins, and incidence of stroke: The Zutphen study. *Archives of Internal Medicine* **156**, 637–642 (1996).

70. Klein, E. A. *et al.* Vitamin E and the risk of prostate cancer: The Selenium and Vitamin E Cancer Prevention Trial (SELECT). *JAMA* **306**, 1549–1556 (2011).

71. Tang, H. *et al.* Pioglitazone and bladder cancer risk: A systematic review and meta-analysis. *Cancer Medicine* **7**, 1070–1080 (2018).

72. Yau, H., Rivera, K., Lomonaco, R. & Cusi, K. The future of thiazolidinedione therapy in the management of type 2 diabetes mellitus. *Current Diabetes Reports* **13**, 329–341 (2013).

73. Masterton, G. S., Plevris, J. N. & Hayes, P. C. Review article: Omega-3 fatty acids—a promising novel therapy for non-alcoholic fatty liver disease. *Alimentary Pharmacology & Therapeutics* **31**, 679–692 (2010).

74. Sanyal, A. J. *et al.* No significant effects of ethyl-eicosapentanoic acid on histologic features of nonalcoholic steatohepatitis in a phase 2 trial. *Gastroenterology* **147**, 377–384.e1 (2014).

75. Scorletti, E. *et al.* Effects of purified eicosapentaenoic and docosahexaenoic acids in nonalcoholic fatty liver disease: Results from the Welcome* study. *Hepatology (Baltimore, Md.)* **60**, 1211–1221 (2014).

2 Epidemiology and Natural History of Nonalcoholic Fatty Liver Disease and Nonalcoholic Steatohepatitis

Linda Henry and Zobair M. Younossi

CONTENTS

2.1 GENERAL PREVALENCE OF NAFLD AND NASH

Nonalcoholic fatty liver disease (NAFLD) is described as a spectrum of fatty liver disease that is associated with components of metabolic syndrome including obesity, insulin resistance, type 2 diabetes mellitus (T2DM), hypertension, and dyslipidemia. [1,2] NAFLD is diagnosed when the presence of hepatic steatosis affects at least 5% of liver hepatocytes in the absence of other causes of liver disease and excess alcohol consumption. [3] The histologic spectrum includes simple hepatic steatosis without other histologic changes (NAFL) as well as nonalcoholic steatohepatitis (NASH), which includes hepatic steatosis in addition to ongoing liver cell injury that can potentially lead to fibrosis, cirrhosis and hepatocellular carcinoma (HCC). [1–3]

Presence of insulin resistance, type 2 diabetes mellitus (T2DM) and visceral obesity not only increases the risk of hepatic steatosis but also is associated with the severity of liver disease, including development of NASH and increasing the stage of hepatic fibrosis. In this context, the relationship of T2DM and NAFLD is bidirectional. For example, one recent meta-analysis determined that NAFLD is associated with an almost 2.2-fold increased risk of incident diabetes and that this risk rises as NAFLD becomes severe. [4] In addition, diseases that are associated with T2DM are also more common in patients with NAFLD. In this context, several other studies recently reported that NAFLD is associated with a 1.5 times increased risk for the development of chronic kidney disease (CKD) ≥ stage 3 and an almost 1.5- to 2.0-fold increased risk for the development of extrahepatic cancers (GI cancers, breast cancer and gynecological cancers). [5,6]

Given this association and the dramatic increase in the prevalence of obesity and T2DM over the past several decades as well as improvements in care of viral hepatitis, NAFLD is now poised to become the most common chronic liver disease in many regions of the world. [7,8] Currently, it is estimated that 25–30% of the global general adult population has NAFLD. [9] Additionally, it is estimated that the prevalence of NASH in the general population is approximately 5–6%. [1,10,11]

It is important to note that these rates are significantly higher among some patient populations. In fact, among those undergoing weight reduction surgeries, the prevalence of NAFLD can be over 80%, while among those with type 2 diabetes mellitus, the prevalence of NAFLD is over 55% with over a third (37.3%) of diabetics estimated to

have NASH and 17% estimated to have advanced fibrosis. [12,13] As better and more accurate noninvasive tests for NASH become available, our understanding of the true prevalence and incidence of this disease state will be forthcoming.

In addition to negative impact on clinical outcomes, NAFLD has been shown to have a negative impact of patient reported outcomes (PROs), including health-related quality of life, the ability to be physically active, the ability to be present at work, increased fatigue and depression. [14–22] Furthermore, the economic burden of NAFLD has been reported to be quite substantial especially among those with NASH and fibrosis. [23–29]

However, there are geographic variations in the prevalence of NAFLD (Figure 2.1).[30] The overall prevalence of NAFLD in Asia is estimated to be 29.6%. [31] The prevalence in China is reported to be approximately 29.2%, whereas Japan also now reports a prevalence of between 25 and 35%, an over 2-fold increase from the 1990s. [32] The overall NASH prevalence is estimated to be between 1.9 and 2.7% among the general population, but this rate may be very underreported given the difficulties in the diagnosis of NASH, i.e., liver biopsy. [33] The rates of NASH are much higher in those with NAFLD. For example, one study from China reported that the prevalence of NASH in patients with biopsy-proven NAFLD was 58.9%, while others reported NASH prevalence rates as high as 97.4 and 93.8% in Singaporean and Japanese NAFLD cohorts, respectively. [34]

In addition to the East Asian countries, the prevalence of NAFLD and NASH has also been reported from South Asia. [10,35–40] India has a reported prevalence rate that ranges from 8.7 to 32.6%, depending on whether patients were from rural or urban areas, respectively. [37] In urban Sri Lanka, the prevalence of NAFLD was reported to be 32.6%. [38]

The overall prevalence in the Middle East has been reported to range from 20 to 30%. [41,42] The prevalence of NAFLD in Kuwait, Saudi Arabia, South of Iran and North of Iran was reported as 33.3, 16.6, 21.5 and 43.8%, respectively. [41,42] Israel reports a NAFLD prevalence of 30%. [43] A recent study completed in Nigeria found that the overall prevalence of NAFLD was 8.7%, while for Sudan the reported rate was 20%. [44,45] These results are in line with what has been reported in a prior study in which the NAFLD prevalence for Africa was estimated at 13–14%. [9]

DOI: 10.1201/9781003386698-3

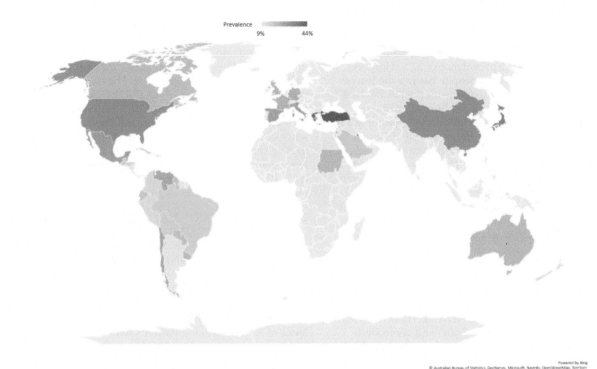

Figure 2.1 Geographic variations in the prevalence of NAFLD

In Europe, the prevalence of NAFLD is around 24%. [9] There is a wide range of prevalence rates reported from different European countries. Greece reports NAFLD prevalence of 41%, while Spain reported a prevalence of NAFLD of 33% in men and 20% in women. [46,47] In Australia, the prevalence of NAFLD has been reported to be 20–30% and is the most common liver disease in Australia. [48] In New Zealand, the prevalence of NAFLD was reported to be 28% in 2015. [49] Cuba reports a prevalence of approximately 17%. [50] Current estimates suggest the prevalence of NASH is approximately 5–6% among the general population. [9,40]

Although most of the data regarding the epidemiology of NAFLD in North America come from studies carried out in the United States (US), the estimated NAFLD prevalence rate is 24.13%. [9,10] The prevalence of NAFLD in the United States ranges between 18.8 and 40%. [11,30,50–53] On the other hand, based on limited ultrasound data, the prevalence of NAFLD in Mexico ranges between 14.4 and 62.9%. [54–56] Similarly, the prevalence of NAFLD (diagnosed by imaging) in Canada is estimated to be around 24.7%. [13,57] Recent data from Central and South America are lacking, but one study suggested that, based on the rates of obesity, the prevalence of NAFLD was estimated as 26% in Mexico; between 15 and 20% in Central America; 28% in Belize and Barbados; 24% in Venezuela and Chile; 20% in Uruguay; 18% in Guyana, Paraguay and Ecuador; and ≤16% in the other countries. [58]

As noted, the true prevalence of NASH by geographical region is not known from population-based studies; however, to fill the gap, investigators have undertaken the use of modeling to determine the NASH prevalence. One such study conducted in 2016 demonstrated that the prevalence of NASH within the general population (to include children) ranged from 2.4% for China to 5.3% for the US, while among those with NAFLD, the prevalence

of NASH ranged from 13.4% for China to 20.3% for the US, but rates were forecasted to be 7.6% in the general US population, followed by 6.3% for Italy and 3.4% for China. [59] In 2017, using the same modeling techniques for Saudi Arabia and the United Arab Emirates (UAE), the NASH prevalence was estimated to be 4.2 and 4.1%. [60] Similar studies have been done for Hong Kong, Singapore, South Korea, Taiwan, Australia, Canada and Switzerland, with all studies noting that if the rates of obesity and type 2 diabetes mellitus continue to increase, the prevalence of NAFLD and NASH will increase as well, and in some cases the incidence of NASH will outpace that of NAFLD. [61–64] The investigators also reported that by 2030, NASH in the general population is expected to be greater than 6% an increase between 87 and 96%. [65]

2.2 PREVALENCE OF NAFLD ACCORDING TO AGE, GENDER AND ETHNICITY

The consensus is that the prevalence of NAFLD increases with age. The peak prevalence of NAFLD for males is between ages 50 and 60 years (29.3%) [64], while for females the peak time is noted for those over the age of 65 (25.4%). [66,67] Based on NHANES III data, the prevalence rates for males by age have been cited as 16.1% in those aged 30–40 years old and 22.3% in those aged 41–50 years old, and 27.6% in those over 60 years old. [68] For women, the prevalence of NAFLD was 12.5% in those aged 30–40 years old and 16.1% in those aged 41–50 years old and 21.6% for those 51–60 years. [68] Assessment of disease burden according to gender, researchers found that women 50 years and older were 17% more likely to develop NASH and 56% more likely to develop advanced fibrosis compared to males of similar ages. [69]

Ethnicity can also impact the prevalence and severity of NAFLD. In the United States, one study found the overall NAFLD prevalence was 32.6% and was highest among

Mexican Americans at 48.4% and lowest in non-Hispanic Blacks (18.0%) and Asians (18.1%), while non-Hispanic whites had a prevalence of 33% and Hispanics outside of Mexican Americans had a prevalence of 32%. However, a disturbing finding was that, despite having the lowest prevalence of NAFLD, non-Hispanic Blacks (28.5%) had the highest prevalence of advanced fibrosis, while non-Hispanic Asians had the lowest (2.7%).[70] Another study that explored the NAFLD prevalence among different subgroups of minorities (Japanese Americans, Whites, Latinos, African Americans and Native Hawaiians) in the United States found that NAFLD accounted for over 50% of the cases of chronic liver disease (CLD) and that 63.6% of the Japanese Americans with CLD had NAFLD, followed by 57.8% of Native Hawaiians, 45.6% of Latinos, 40.7% of whites and 39.2% of African Americans. [71] NALFD was also the most common cause of cirrhosis, accounting for over 32% of cases. When stratified by race/ethnicity, NAFLD accounted for 32.3% of cirrhosis cases in Japanese Americans, 31.5% in Native Hawaiians, and 31.9% in Latinos.

Interestingly, in a study using NHANES data in which NAFLD was diagnosed by FibroScan® and controlled attenuation parameter, Mexican Americans had the highest prevalence of moderate to severe steatosis, while African Americans had the lowest, but when the investigators looked by gender, it was male Mexican Americans that had a higher likelihood of having moderate to severe steatosis. [72] In a meta-analysis, similar results were found where Hispanics had the higher prevalence of both NAFLD and NASH, but the proportion of patients with significant fibrosis did not significantly differ among racial or ethnic groups. [73] The role of ethnicity was also explored outside the United States. In a recent meta-analysis from China, the NAFLD prevalence of 29.2% by ethnicity found the Hui had the highest NAFLD prevalence of 53.8%, followed by the Uygur at 46.6%, then Taiwan at 39.9% and northwest China at 39.9%. [33] (See Figure 2.2.)

Finally, among the younger age groups, a recent meta-analysis of 14 studies of the prevalence of NAFLD among children and adolescents reported an overall prevalence of 7.4% regardless of the diagnostic method used and 8.8% when ultrasound was used. The investigators also reported the prevalence of NAFLD by global areas and found a NAFLD prevalence of 8.5% for North America, 7.0% for Asia and 1.7% for Europe. Like adults, the prevalence of NAFLD was higher among those with obesity at 52.5%. Their trend analysis indicated that NAFLD prevalence is increasing at 0.26% per year, and it forecasts that by 2040, the NAFLD prevalence among the youth will be almost 31%. [74]

2.3 PREVALENCE OF NAFLD IN SUBPOPULATIONS (DIABETES MELLITUS, OBESE, METABOLIC SYNDROME, LEAN) (FIGURE 2.3)

Although the prevalence of NAFLD and NASH is quite high in the general population, it is even higher in specific cohorts, such as those with T2DM and the severely obese. In a systematic review of studies, the overall global prevalence of NAFLD among patients with T2DM was 61.1%. [13] The prevalence of NASH among those with diabetes and NAFLD was found to be as high 64.0%. Furthermore, the prevalence of advanced fibrosis (fibrosis, ≥ F3) was also found to be high at 10.4%. [13] In a study from China, the prevalence of NAFLD among those with T2DM was 51.8% as compared to 30.8% in nondiabetics. [75] NAFLD has also been reported for those with type 1 diabetes. A meta-analysis of studies conducted for those with type 1 diabetes found an overall pooled NAFLD prevalence of 19.3% in which the prevalence was 22.0% in adults only and 7.9% in children/adolescents. [76]

In a study conducted among morbidly obese patients undergoing weight reduction surgery, the prevalence of NAFLD was found to be 95%. [77] Furthermore, a study from China noted that the prevalence of NAFLD among

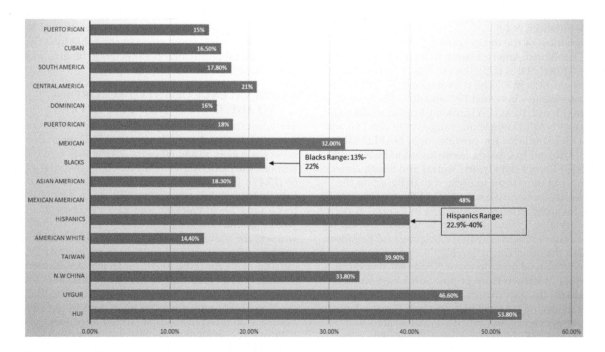

Figure 2.2 NAFLD prevalence by ethnicity

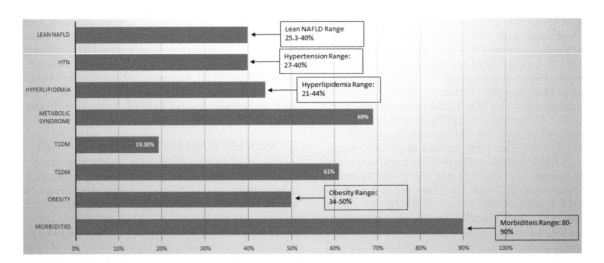

Figure 2.3 NAFLD prevalence by subgroups

those with obesity was 66.2% compared to only 11.7% in those of normal weight and that the higher prevalence of NAFLD was found in the areas with a higher gross domestic product. [75]

NAFLD has also been reported in those considered nonobese or "lean" with a reported prevalence of 11.2% in the general population and a reported prevalence among those with NAFLD of 25.3% with a range of 19.2% among the lean and 41% among the nonobese (lean and overweight). The prevalence also varied by geographical area from 25% or lower in some countries (e.g., Malaysia and Pakistan) to higher than 50% in others (e.g., Austria, Mexico and Sweden). [78] This group appears to carry a higher burden of comorbidities as well as a higher risk of mortality than those without NAFLD. [79–82] Although the lean group has less severe histologic findings, including hepatocyte ballooning, lobular inflammation, NAFLD activity score and fibrosis stage, they may be at higher risk for severe liver disease and possibly mortality suggesting that lean NAFLD is a distinct entity with metabolic, biochemical and inflammatory abnormalities compared to healthy subjects. [79] In fact, a recent meta-analysis reported that, among those with lean (nonobese) NAFLD, 39% had NASH, 29% had fibrosis stage ≥2, and 3.2% had cirrhosis, along with a reported incidence for all-cause mortality at 12.1 per 1000 person-years, liver-related mortality at 4.1 per 1000 person-years, cardiovascular-related mortality at 4.0 per 1000 person-years, new-onset diabetes at 12.6 per 1000 person-years, and new-onset hypertension at 56.0 per 1000 person-years. [80]

2.4 PREVALENCE OF FIBROSIS IN NAFLD

Since the fibrosis stage is the most important predictor for adverse outcomes in those with NAFLD, recognizing the prevalence rate among those with NAFLD is imperative so that timely treatment and referrals can be initiated. [83] In a study using data from NHANES (2005–2016), the prevalence of NAFLD-related advanced fibrosis doubled over a decade with a steady increase in the prevalence noted for Hispanics and non-Hispanic Whites but not for non-Hispanic Blacks. [84] Similar studies conducted in Asia reported rates of advanced fibrosis among those with NAFLD ranging between 4 up to 25%. [33,85] In a study of over 1000 residents in Cuba, cirrhosis was diagnosed

in 3.5% of the patients at the time of their NAFLD diagnosis. [86] A meta-analysis from South Korea found that, although NAFLD and NASH were quite prevalent, the prevalence of advanced fibrosis was low (18%) but that over time the progression of disease may occur, increasing the disease burden. [87]

The prevalence of advanced fibrosis among those with NASH and NASH HCC has also been studied and reported to range from 21 to 50% for patients with NASH and from 44 to 80% of patients with NASH-HCC. [88,89] The major independent predictors of having advanced fibrosis found in global studies were increasing age (OR:1.11) and diabetes (OR:2.28). [90] Other investigators have also suggested that it was the presence of a higher percentage of body fat and waist circumference that were significantly associated with worsening of fibrosis as measured with the NAFLD fibrosis score. [90]

In a study of the global burden of cirrhosis, investigators found that over a 30-year period, the number of prevalent cases for compensated cirrhosis due to NASH doubled while the number for decompensated cirrhosis due to NASH tripled. Another study assessing the burden of NAFLD/NASH-related burden using the same Global Burden of Disease database revealed that between 2007 and 2017, cirrhosis DALY (disability-adjusted life years) due to NAFLD/NASH increased by 23.4%, while liver cancer DALY due to NAFLD/NASH increased by 37.5%. [8,91]

2.5 INCIDENCE OF NAFLD, NASH AND RELATED FIBROSIS

Studies on the incidence of NAFLD are sparse partly due to the length of time it takes for the disease to be identified and progress. In one relatively long-term study, it was noted that, during 348,193.5 person-years of follow-up, 10,340 of the participants developed NAFLD, providing an incidence rate of 29.7 per 1000 person-years. In this same study, the investigators found that those who were overweight were at 2 times the risk for developing NAFLD, while those considered obese were at almost four times the odds. [93] The presence of metabolic risk factors further increased the risk of developing NAFLD by at least 2 times even among those with normal weight. [93]

In a recently reported meta-analysis, the researchers recorded several incident rates for the progression of fibrosis, NASH, HCC and mortality. They found that almost 41% of those with NASH experienced fibrosis progression with an annual rate of progression of 0.09%. HCC incidence among NAFLD patients was noted at 0.44 per 1000 person-years with a range of 0.29–0.66 per 1000 person-years. Liver-specific mortality among those with NAFLD was reported as 0.77 per 1000 person-years with a range of 0.33–1.77 compared to 11.77 per 1000 person-years with a range of 7.10–19.53 per 1000 person-years for those with NASH. On the other hand, overall mortality among those with NAFLD was found to be 15.44 per 1000 person-years with a range of 11.72–20.34 per 1000 person-years, and for NASH it was 25.56 per 1000 person-years with a range of 6.29–103.80 per 1000 person-years. [9]

The incidence of NAFLD in the nonobese population (without NAFLD at baseline) was 24.6 (95% CI 13·4–39·2) per 1000 person-years. These rates, though lower, are still worrisome given this is a population not heavily associated with the development of NAFLD but does help raise awareness about the potential prevalence of NAFLD across the general population and not just those considered to be obese. [31]

2.6 NATURAL HISTORY OF NAFLD AND NASH (FIGURE 2.4)

NAFLD is a complex disease with significant variability between different patients in regard to disease development, progression, and regression. Our current understanding of the disease suggests that a minority of patients with NAFLD progress to liver fibrosis or cirrhosis. Nevertheless, 10–20% of patients with NASH can progress and some of these patients can be rapid progressors. [94] Adding to the complexity of this disease is that the progression of NAFLD and NASH is not linear. In this context, some patients will progress for a period of time followed by stability or regression. In fact, it is important to note that the majority of progressors are those with insulin resistance and T2DM. [95,96,97] In one prospective study, 23% of patients with simple steatosis at baseline developed NASH in the follow-up. [98] Recently the 20%

rule was suggested in that 20% of those with NASH and F3/F4 will progress over 2.5 years. [99] Furthermore, a recent systematic review reported that 64% of those with NAFL progressed to NASH after a mean follow-up of 3.7 years (SD 2.1). [100] Although patients with NAFLD seem to have a relatively nonprogressive course, some may develop fibrosis albeit at a significantly slower pace than patients with NASH. [95,101,102]

2.7 RISK FACTORS FOR NAFLD AND NASH

As previously noted, NAFLD is closely associated with metabolic disorders of obesity, insulin resistance, T2DM, hypertension, mixed hyperlipidemia, and hypercholesterolemia in addition to older age and male sex. Recent studies have reported that between 28 and 66% of patients with NAFLD have metabolic syndrome. [103–107] The presence of metabolic syndrome can increase the rate of liver fibrosis progression, leading to cirrhosis, HCC, and/or death. In fact, the more components of metabolic syndrome there are, the higher the risk of mortality will be. [104,105] In fact, a review of patients with NAFLD on the waiting list for liver transplant confirmed the high prevalence of metabolic comorbidities especially for obesity, T2DM and hypertension. [108] Similar rates have been reported from other parts of the world to include Middle East, Africa, China, Cuba and Spain. [109–111]

NAFLD in children is also associated with metabolic comorbidities, which include type 2 diabetes, sleep disorders, osteoporosis, vitamin D deficiency, hypertension and dyslipidemia. [112] However, there is evidence for familial clustering of NAFLD. In fact, as many as 27% of cases of NAFLD may be related to familial clustering, suggesting a genetic predisposition for NAFLD and NASH development and progression. [112] More research studying NAFLD in children and families is warranted.

As noted previously, ethnicity also appears to play a considerable role in the development of NAFLD, which may be partially attributed to differences in genetic background. In North America, the highest prevalence

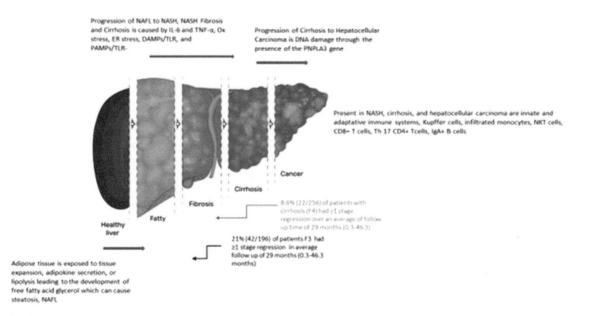

Figure 2.4 Natural history of NAFLD

of NAFLD has been observed in Hispanics, followed by non-Hispanic white individuals, while African Americans appear to have a very low prevalence rate but a much higher mortality rate if present. [113–115] Among Hispanic patients, the genetic marker from the serpin family E member 1 (PAI-1, a marker of fibrosis) is only associated with NAFLD in Hispanic patients, whereas serum levels of adiponectin are associated with NAFLD in African Americans. [113–119] Other studies have shown that fructose malabsorption (ingestion of high amounts of fructose are associated with NAFLD) is greater in African Americans than in Hispanics. [120] The increased levels of adiponectin among African Americans may be attributed to the gene patatin-like phospholipase domain-containing protein-3 (PNPLA3). [116] This gene encodes adiponutrin, a triacylglycerol lipase important in fatty acid hydrolysis in adipocytes. A polymorphism of I148M PNPLA3 has been associated with a higher probability of developing NAFLD. [116–119] African Americans tend to have a lower genotype distribution of PNPLA3, which may partly explain why the prevalence of NAFLD is higher in Hispanics and lower in African Americans in the United States. [115]

Given the rapid increase in the prevalence of NAFLD in China, studies are also investigating the genetic link. As such, recent studies from Asia have shown a number of gene polymorphisms associated with NAFLD. [32] In particular, the *PNPLA3* with the rs738409 gene has been consistently shown to increase the risk of severe steatosis, NASH and liver fibrosis in adults and appears to be more common among East Asians than Caucasians. This may be the reason behind the high NAFLD prevalence in East Asia despite a lower metabolic burden. Other genetic variants significantly associated with NAFLD include those in *NCAN*, *GCKR* and *LYPLAL1*, as well as the polymorphisms C-482T and T-455C in APOC, which has also been associated with insulin resistance. [32,116–119]

Gut dysbiosis has also been implicated in the development of NAFLD. Although studies continue to further our understanding of all the mechanisms involved with the effect of gut microbiota on the organs outside the intestinal system, it is now known that these effects are achieved by various bacterial metabolites, which include bile acids, short-chain fatty acids, amino acids, choline, and ethanol. These metabolites appear to cause a chronic inflammatory state and a dysregulation of lipids and branched chain amino acids. Changes in the gut flora also correspond to the state of NAFLD and NASH. [121–123] A study of children found that, among the children that had NAFLD, the alpha-diversity of gut microbiota was lower compared with their healthy controls and those with NASH had the lowest alpha-diversity. [124] Studies in this area are ongoing especially with respect to what intervention may be appropriate for a healthy gut microbiome.

2.8 NAFLD MORTALITY

The progressive potential for NAFLD can confer increase mortality. Although liver-related mortality is higher among patients with NASH, the most common cause of death among patients with NAFLD is cardiovascular mortality. In this context, the overall mortality rate for NAFLD is estimated to be 15.44 per 1000 person-years, while it was 25.56 per 1000 person-years for those with NASH. Liver-specific mortality among patients with NAFLD has been reported to be at a rate of 0.77 per 1000 person-years, while the rate is approximately 15 times higher among those

with NASH (11.77 per 1000 person-years). [9] Recent studies have shown that for patients with NAFLD and stage F0, the HR for overall mortality was 1.9 but increased to HR of 104.9 for those with F4 (cirrhosis) fibrosis and that those with F3–F4 fibrosis incurred a 3-fold higher overall mortality than those without liver disease. [102]

A study conducted in 2017 found there were 184,905 deaths from liver complications due to NAFLD, which translated into an age standard rate (ASR) of NAFLD liver deaths of 2.32 per 100,000 persons. From 1990 to 2017, investigators using global data reported that the age-standardized DALY rate (ASDR) for cirrhosis-NAFLD also increased at an annual percentage change (APC) of 0.3% while the ASR for compensated and decompensated cirrhosis due to NASH increased more than for any other cause of cirrhosis (by 33.2% for compensated cirrhosis and 54.8% for decompensated cirrhosis) for the study period of 1990–2017. [92]

HCC is an important complication of CLD and NAFLD and is now the third-leading cause of cancer death worldwide due to its very poor prognosis. [125] As a result, incidence and mortality rates are roughly equivalent. In 2018, the estimated global incidence rate of liver cancer per 100,000 person-years was 9.3, while the corresponding mortality rate was 8.5. [126] In patients with NAFLD, the annual incidence of HCC has been reported to be 1.8 cases per 1000 person-years with an overall mortality rate of 5.3 deaths per 1000 person-years. [80] Others have reported NAFLD increasing annually by 1.42% from 2012 to 2017, with the age-standardized death rate (ASDR) for NAFLD and liver cancer also increasing over the same period. [127] Similar reports have come from Asia, the Middle East and North Africa region where investigators studied the liver complications of cirrhosis and liver cancer. They reported that Asia accounted for 48.3% of the global incidence of NAFLD liver complications and for 46.2% of deaths attributable to NAFLD liver complications, while the MENA regions accounted for 8.9% of the global incidence of NAFLD and liver complications and 8.6% deaths attributable to NAFLD and liver complications. [128] HCC related to NAFLD and NASH in Japan is the most common malignancy and cause of death among patients with NAFLD/NASH with higher mortality observed among those with advanced disease (up to 40% in almost 3 years). [129] Prevention of NAFLD may be even more relevant as recent studies have found that HCC can develop in those with NAFLD without having developed fibrosis. [130]

As noted previously, cardiovascular mortality is the most common cause of death among NAFLD. In this context, the presence of T2DM, very low-density lipids, hepatic overproduction of glucose, inflammatory factors, C-reactive protein, coagulation factors and insulin resistance, which are commonly found among patients with NAFLD, can contribute to the increased risk of death from cardiovascular diseases. [131–133] It has been estimated that 5–10% of patients with NAFLD die from cardiovascular disease and have a 2-fold increase in risk for cardiovascular disease. Interestingly, recent data suggest that the stage of fibrosis may be associated with CVD even in the presence of cardiometabolic risk factors. [134] These data suggest that the underlying pathophysiology that hastens the development of fibrosis in NAFLD may also promote the development of CVD. [135–138] In fact, this may help explain recent findings that NAFLD was not directly related to CVD mortality but rather was associated with both the prevalence and incidence of coronary heart disease, atherosclerosis and hypertension, suggesting that the presence of NAFLD can indirectly increase the risk for CVD mortality through its affect on CVD related risk factors. [135] Findings from this study were further enhanced in a more recent meta-analysis where investigators found that those with NAFLD were at 1.5 times higher long-term risk for fatal or nonfatal CVD events, especially in those with advanced liver disease and higher fibrosis stages. [139]

In addition to CVD and liver-specific death, cancer-related deaths are also increased among NAFLD. [140–142] In a recent meta-analysis, researchers determined that NAFLD was significantly intertwined with extrahepatic cancers. From their analysis, these investigators determined that the odds of developing colorectal cancer (CRC) in patients with NAFLD were almost doubled, while the odds for developing intrahepatic cholangiocarcinoma and extrahepatic cholangiocarcinoma in patients with NAFLD were increased 2.5 times compared to those without NAFLD. Furthermore, the odds of developing breast cancer gastric cancer, pancreatic cancer, prostate cancer and esophageal cancer were also found to be significantly increased. [141] These data suggest an association between NAFLD and extrahepatic malignancy and related mortality.

Most recently, attention has been given to the association of sarcopenia, NAFLD and mortality. Sarcopenia is defined as the loss of muscle mass and strength, which has generally been associated with the elderly, although it is highly prevalent in persons with end-stage liver disease. The exact pathophysiologic mechanisms in which NAFLD and sarcopenia interact are still to be investigated; however, the current understanding is that the presence of insulin resistance, low vitamin D levels, inflammatory myokines and physical inactivity, all present in NAFLD, contribute to increased proteolysis, myosteatosis, increased oxidative stress and decreased uptake of glucose in the muscle, which contributes to the development of sarcopenia. On the other hand, these factors are also present in those with sarcopenia, suggesting a shared pathway for the development of each. Although most studies to date have been carried out among persons from Asia, several studies showed that those with sarcopenia had a 2.3- to 3.3-fold increased risk of NAFLD and a 2-fold increased risk of fibrosis, independent of obesity or IR. [143–145] In this light, the presence of sarcopenia in those with NAFLD has also been linked with an almost 2 times higher risk for all-cause mortality, a 3 times higher risk for cardiac-related mortality and 2 times higher risk for cancer-related mortality. [146]

2.9 CONCLUSIONS

Due to the increasing global prevalence of obesity and T2DM, the prevalence of NAFLD and its associated adverse disease outcomes is increasing. The only proven treatments are weight loss and increased physical activity, which are hard to achieve and sustain, especially if the social determinants of health are not part of the comprehensive management plan. This increasing disease burden and limited treatment options are further compounded by lack of awareness among patients, health care providers and policy makers. It is only through a comprehensive multiprong approach that the challenge of NAFLD can be met at both the local and the global levels to change the trajectory of this important liver disease.

REFERENCES

1. Ludwig J, Viggiano TR, McGill DB, Oh BJ. Nonalcoholic steatohepatitis: Mayo Clinic experiences with a hitherto unnamed disease. *Mayo Clin Proc.* 1980;55:434–438.

2. Schaffner F, Thaler, H. Nonalcoholic fatty liver disease. *Prog. Liver Dis.* 1986;8:283–298.

3. Chalasani N, Younossi Z, Lavine JE, Charlton M, Cusi K, Rinella M, Harrison SA, Brunt EM, Sanyal AJ. The diagnosis and management of nonalcoholic fatty liver disease: practice guidance from the American Association for the Study of Liver Diseases. *Hepatology.* 2018;67(1):328–357. http://doi.org/10.1002/hep.29367. Epub 2017 Sep 29. PMID: 28714183.

4. Mantovani A, Petracca G, Beatrice G, Tilg H, Byrne CD, Targher G. Non-alcoholic fatty liver disease and risk of incident diabetes mellitus: an updated meta-analysis of 501 022 adult individuals. *Gut.* 2021;70(5):962–969. http://doi.org/10.1136/gutjnl-2020-322572. Epub 2020 Sep 16. PMID: 32938692.

5. Mantovani A, Petracca G, Beatrice G, Csermely A, Lonardo A, Schattenberg JM, Tilg H, Byrne CD, Targher G. Non-alcoholic fatty liver disease and risk of incident chronic kidney disease: an updated meta-analysis. *Gut.* 2022;71(1):156–162. http://doi.org/10.1136/gutjnl-2020-323082. Epub 2020 Dec 10. PMID: 33303564.

6. Mantovani A, Petracca G, Beatrice G, Csermely A, Tilg H, Byrne CD, Targher G. Non-alcoholic fatty liver disease and increased risk of incident extrahepatic cancers: a meta-analysis of observational cohort studies. *Gut.* 2021;71(4):778–788. http://doi.org/10.1136/gutjnl-2021-324191. Epub ahead of print. PMID: 33685968.

7. Paik JM, Golabi P, Younossi Y, Mishra A, Younossi ZM. Changes in the global burden of chronic liver diseases from 2012 to 2017: the growing impact of NAFLD. *Hepatology.* 2020;72(5):1605–1616. http://doi.org/10.1002/hep.31173. Epub 2020 Oct 27. PMID: 32043613.

8. Younossi ZM, Stepanova M, Younossi Y, Golabi P, Mishra A, Rafiq N, Henry L. Epidemiology of chronic liver diseases in the USA in the past three decades. *Gut.* 2020;69(3):564–568. http://doi.org/10.1136/gutjnl-2019-318813. Epub 2019 Jul 31. PMID: 31366455.

9. Younossi ZM, Koenig AB, Abdelatif D, Fazel Y, Henry L, Wymer M. Global epidemiology of nonalcoholic fatty liver disease-Meta-analytic assessment of prevalence, incidence, and outcomes. *Hepatology.* 2016;64(1):73–84. http://doi.org/10.1002/hep.28431. Epub 2016 Feb 22. PMID: 26707365.

10. Sayiner M, Koenig A, Henry L, Younossi ZM. Epidemiology of nonalcoholic fatty liver disease and nonalcoholic steatohepatitis in the United States and the rest of the world. *Clin Liver Dis.* 2016;20(2):205–214. http://doi.org/10.1016/j.cld.2015.10.001. Epub 2015 Dec 14. PMID: 27063264.

11. Fazel Y, Koenig AB, Sayiner M, Goodman ZD, Younossi ZM. Epidemiology and natural history of non-alcoholic fatty liver disease. *Metabolism.* 2016;65(8):1017–1025. http://doi.org/10.1016/j.metabol.2016.01.012. Epub 2016 Jan 29. PMID: 26997539.

12. Soresi M, Cabibi D, Giglio RV, Martorana S, Guercio G, Porcasi R, Terranova A, Lazzaro LA, Emma MR, Augello G, Cervello M, Pantuso G, Montalto

G, Giannitrapani L. The prevalence of NAFLD and fibrosis in bariatric surgery patients and the reliability of noninvasive diagnostic methods. *Biomed Res Int*. 2020;2020:5023157. http://doi.org/10.1155/2020/5023157. PMID: 32420347; PMCID: PMC7201516.

13. Younossi ZM, Golabi P, de Avila L, Paik JM, Srishord M, Fukui N, Qiu Y, Burns L, Afendy A, Nader F. The global epidemiology of NAFLD and NASH in patients with type 2 diabetes: a systematic review and meta-analysis. *J Hepatol*. 2019;71(4):793–801. http://doi.org/10.1016/j.jhep.2019.06.021. Epub 2019 Jul 4. PMID: 31279902.

14. Dan AA, Kallman JB, Wheeler A, Younoszai Z, Collantes R, Bondini S, Gerber L, Younossi ZM. Health-related quality of life in patients with non-alcoholic fatty liver disease. *Aliment Pharmacol Ther*. 2007;26(6):815–820. http://doi.org/10.1111/j.1365-2036.2007.03426.x. PMID: 17767465.

15. Younossi ZM, Stepanova M, Lawitz EJ, Reddy KR, Wai-Sun Wong V, Mangia A, Muir AJ, Jacobson I, Djedjos CS, Gaggar A, Myers RP, Younossi I, Nader F, Racila A. Patients with nonalcoholic steatohepatitis experience severe impairment of health-related quality of life. *Am J Gastroenterol*. 2019;114(10):1636–1641. http://doi.org/10.14309/ajg.0000000000000375. PMID: 31464743.

16. Younossi ZM, Stepanova M, Younossi I, Racila A. Validation of chronic liver disease questionnaire for nonalcoholic steatohepatitis in patients with biopsy-proven nonalcoholic steatohepatitis. *Clin Gastroenterol Hepatol*. 2019;17(10):2093–2100.e3. http://doi.org/10.1016/j.cgh.2019.01.001. Epub 2019 Jan 11. PMID: 30639779.

17. Younossi ZM, Stepanova M, Noureddin M, Kowdley KV, Strasser SI, Kohli A, Ruane P, Shiffman ML, Sheikh A, Gunn N, Caldwell SH, Huss RS, Myers RP, Wai-Sun Wong V, Alkhouri N, Goodman Z, Loomba R. Improvements of fibrosis and disease activity are associated with improvement of patient-reported outcomes in patients with advanced fibrosis due to nonalcoholic steatohepatitis. *Hepatol Commun*. 2021;5(7):1201–1211. http://doi.org/10.1002/hep4.1710. PMID: 34278169; PMCID: PMC8279457.

18. Younossi ZM, Stepanova M, Nader F, Loomba R, Anstee QM, Ratziu V, et al. REGENERATE study investigators. obeticholic acid impact on quality of life in patients with nonalcoholic steatohepatitis: regenerate 18-month interim analysis. *Clin Gastroenterol Hepatol*. 2021;S1542–3565(21)00751–5. http://doi.org/10.1016/j.cgh.2021.07.020. Epub ahead of print. PMID: 34274514.

19. Weinstein AA, Kallman Price J, Stepanova M, Poms LW, Fang Y, Moon J, Nader F, Younossi ZM. Depression in patients with nonalcoholic fatty liver disease and chronic viral hepatitis B and C. *Psychosomatics*. 2011;52(2):127–132. http://doi.org/10.1016/j.psym.2010.12.019. PMID: 21397104.

20. Gerber LH, Weinstein AA, Mehta R, Younossi ZM. Importance of fatigue and its measurement in chronic liver disease. *World J Gastroenterol*. 2019;25(28):3669–3683. http://doi.org/10.3748/wjg.v25.i28.3669. PMID: 31391765; PMCID: PMC6676553.

21. Newton JL, Jones DE, Henderson E, Kane L, Wilton K, Burt AD, Day CP. Fatigue in non-alcoholic fatty liver disease (NAFLD) is significant and associates with inactivity and excessive daytime sleepiness but not with liver disease severity or insulin resistance. *Gut*. 2008;57(6):807–813. http://doi.org/10.1136/gut.2007.139303. Epub 2008 Feb 12. PMID: 18270241.

22. Geier A, Rinella ME, Balp MM, McKenna SJ, Brass CA, Przybysz R, et al. Real-world burden of non-alcoholic steatohepatitis. *Clin Gastroenterol Hepatol*. 2021;19(5):1020–1029.e7. http://doi.org/10.1016/j.cgh.2020.06.064. Epub 2020 Jul 4. PMID: 32634622.

23. Younossi ZM, Blissett D, Blissett R, Henry L, Stepanova M, Younossi Y, Racila A, Hunt S, Beckerman R. The economic and clinical burden of nonalcoholic fatty liver disease in the United States and Europe. *Hepatology*. 2016;64(5):1577–1586. http://doi.org/10.1002/hep.28785. Epub 2016 Sep 26. PMID: 27543837.

24. Younossi ZM, Tampi R, Priyadarshini M, Nader F, Younossi IM, Racila A. Burden of illness and economic model for patients with nonalcoholic steatohepatitis in the United States. *Hepatology*. 2019;69(2):564–572. http://doi.org/10.1002/hep.30254. Epub 2019 Jan 8. PMID: 30180285.

25. Tampi RP, Wong VW, Wong GL, Shu SS, Chan HL, Fung J, Stepanova M, Younossi ZM. Modelling the economic and clinical burden of non-alcoholic steatohepatitis in East Asia: data from Hong Kong. *Hepatol Res*. 2020;50(9):1024–1031. http://doi.org/10.1111/hepr.13535. Epub 2020 Jul 20. PMID: 32537840.

26. Younossi ZM, Tampi RP, Racila A, Qiu Y, Burns L, Younossi I, Nader F. Economic and clinical burden of nonalcoholic steatohepatitis in patients with type 2 diabetes in the U.S. *Diabetes Care*. 2020;43(2):283–289. http://doi.org/10.2337/dc19-1113. Epub 2019 Oct 28. PMID: 31658974.

27. Younossi ZM, Blissett D, Blissett R, Henry L, Stepanova M, Younossi Y, Racila A, Hunt S, Beckerman R. The economic and clinical burden of nonalcoholic fatty liver disease in the United States and Europe. *Hepatology*. 2016;64(5):1577–1586. http://doi.org/10.1002/hep.28785. Epub 2016 Sep 26. PMID: 27543837.

28. Phisalprapa P, Prasitwarachot R, Kositamongkol C, Hengswat P, Srivanichakorn W, Washirasaksiri C, et al. Economic burden of non-alcoholic steatohepatitis with significant fibrosis in Thailand. *BMC Gastroenterol*. 2021;21(1):135. http://doi.org/10.1186/s12876-021-01720-w. PMID: 33765931; PMCID: PMC7992785.

29. Schattenberg JM, Lazarus JV, Newsome PN, Serfaty L, Aghemo A, Augustin S, et al. Disease burden and economic impact of diagnosed non-alcoholic steatohepatitis in five European countries in 2018: a cost-of-illness analysis. *Liver Int*. 2021;41(6):1227–1242. http://doi.org/10.1111/liv.14825. Epub 2021 Mar 18. PMID: 33590598; PMCID: PMC8252761.

30. Younossi ZM, Stepanova M, Younossi Y, Golabi P, Mishra A, Rafiq N, Henry L. Epidemiology of chronic liver diseases in the USA in the past three decades. *Gut*. 2020;69(3):564–568. http://doi.org/10.1136/gutjnl-2019-318813. Epub 2019 Jul 31. PMID: 31366455.

31. Li J, Zou B, Yeo YH, Feng Y, Xie X, Lee DH, et al. Prevalence, incidence, and outcome of non-alcoholic fatty liver disease in Asia, 1999–2019: a systematic review and meta-analysis. *Lancet Gastroenterol Hepatol*. 2019;4(5):389–398. http://doi.org/10.1016/S2468-1253(19)30039-1. Epub 2019 Mar 20. PMID: 30902670.

32. Ito T, Ishigami M, Zou B, Tanaka T, Takahashi H, Kurosaki M, et al. The epidemiology of NAFLD and lean NAFLD in Japan: a meta-analysis with individual

and forecasting analysis, 1995–2040. *Hepatol Int.* 2021;15(2):366–379. http://doi.org/10.1007/s12072-021-10143-4. Epub 2021 Feb 12. PMID: 33580453.

33. Zhou F, Zhou J, Wang W, Zhang XJ, Ji YX, Zhang P, She ZG, Zhu L, Cai J, Li H. Unexpected rapid increase in the burden of NAFLD in China from 2008 to 2018: a systematic review and meta-analysis. *Hepatology.* 2019;70(4):1119–1133. http://doi.org/10.1002/hep.30702. PMID: 31070259.

34. Chan WK, Treeprasertsuk S, Imajo K, Nakajima A, Seki Y, Kasama K, Kakizaki S, Fan JG, Song MJ, Yoon SK, Dan YY, Lesmana L, Ho KY, Goh KL, Wong VW. Clinical features and treatment of nonalcoholic fatty liver disease across the Asia Pacific region- the GO ASIA initiative. *Aliment Pharmacol Ther.* 2018;47(6):816–825. http://doi.org/10.1111/apt.14506. Epub 2018 Jan 14. PMID: 29333610.

35. Younossi Z, Tacke F, Arrese M, Chander Sharma B, Mostafa I, Bugianesi E, Wai-Sun Wong V, Yilmaz Y, George J, Fan J, Vos MB. Global perspectives on non-alcoholic fatty liver disease and nonalcoholic steato-hepatitis. *Hepatology.* 2019;69(6):2672–2682. http://doi.org/10.1002/hep.30251. PMID: 30179269.

36. Browning JD, Szczepaniak LS, Dobbins R, Nuremberg P, Horton JD, Cohen JC, Grundy SM, Hobbs HH. Prevalence of hepatic steatosis in an urban population in the United States: impact of ethnicity. *Hepatology.* 2004;40(6):1387–1395. http://doi.org/10.1002/hep.20466. PMID: 15565570.

37. Das K, Das K, Mukherjee PS, Ghosh A, Ghosh S, Mridha AR, Dhibar T, Bhattacharya B, Bhattacharya D, Manna B, Dhali GK, Santra A, Chowdhury A. Nonobese population in a developing country has a high prevalence of nonalcoholic fatty liver and significant liver disease. *Hepatology.* 2010;51(5):1593–1602. http://doi.org/10.1002/hep.23567. PMID: 20222092.

38. Dassanayake AS, Kasturiratne A, Rajindrajith S, Kalubowila U, Chakrawarthi S, De Silva AP, Makaya M, Mizoue T, Kato N, Wickremasinghe AR, de Silva HJ. Prevalence and risk factors for non-alcoholic fatty liver disease among adults in an urban Sri Lankan population. *J Gastroenterol Hepatol.* 2009;24(7):1284–1288. http://doi.org/10.1111/j.1440-1746.2009.05831.x. Epub 2009 May 19. PMID: 19476560.

39. Association TGSoAAL. *The economic cost and health burden of liver diseases in Australia.* Sydney: Deloitte Access Economics. 2012.

40. Younossi Z, Anstee QM, Marietti M, Hardy T, Henry L, Eslam M, George J, Bugianesi E. Global burden of NAFLD and NASH: trends, predictions, risk factors and prevention. *Nat Rev Gastroenterol Hepatol.* 2018;15(1):11–20. http://doi.org/10.1038/nrgastro.2017.109. Epub 2017 Sep 20. PMID: 28930295.

41. Ramezani-Binabaj M, Motalebi M, Karimi-Sari H, Rezaee-Zavareh MS, Alavian SM. Are women with polycystic ovarian syndrome at a high risk of non-alcoholic Fatty liver disease; a meta-analysis. *Hepat Mon.* 2014;14(11):e23235. http://doi.org/10.5812/hepatmon.23235. PMID: 25598791; PMCID: PMC4286712.

42. Sohrabpour A, Rezvan H, Amini-Kafiabad S, Dayhim M, Merat S, Pourshams A. Prevalence of nonalcoholic steatohepatitis in Iran: a population based study. *Middle East J Dig Dis.* 2010;2(1):14–19. PMID: 25197507; PMCID: PMC4154901.

43. Zelber-Sagi S, Lotan R, Shlomai A, Webb M, Harrari G, Buch A, Nitzan Kaluski D, Halpern Z, Oren R. Predictors for incidence and remission of NAFLD in the general population during a seven-year prospective follow-up. *J Hepatol.* 2012;56(5):1145–1151. http://doi.org/10.1016/j.jhep.2011.12.011. Epub 2012 Jan 13. PMID: 22245895.

44. Almobarak AO, Barakat S, Khalifa MH, Elhoweris MH, Elhassan TM, Ahmed MH. Non alcoholic fatty liver disease (NAFLD) in a Sudanese population: what is the prevalence and risk factors? *Arab J Gastroenterol.* 2014;15(1):12–15. http://doi.org/10.1016/j.ajg.2014.01.008. Epub 2014 Feb 12. PMID: 24630507.

45. Almobarak AO, Barakat S, Suliman EA, Elmadhoun WM, Mohamed NA, Abobaker IO, Noor SK. et al. Prevalence of and predictive factors for nonalcoholic fatty liver disease in Sudanese individuals with type 2 diabetes: is metabolic syndrome the culprit? *Arab J Gastroenterol.* 2015;16(2):54–58. http://doi.org/10.1016/j.ajg.2015.06.001.

46. Zois CD, Baltayiannis GH, Bekiari A, et al. Steatosis and steatohepatitis in postmortem material from Northwestern Greece. *World J Gastroenterol: WJG.* 2010;16(31):3944–3949. http://doi.org/10.3748/wjg.v16.i31.3944.

47. Caballería L, Pera G, Auladell MA, Torán P, Muñoz L, Miranda D, et al. Prevalence and factors associated with the presence of nonalcoholic fatty liver disease in an adult population in Spain. *Eur J Gastroenterol Hepatol.* 2010;22(1):24–32.

48. Adams LA, Roberts SK, Strasser SI, Mahady SE, Powell E, Estes C, Razavi H, George J. Nonalcoholic fatty liver disease burden: Australia, 2019–2030. *J Gastroenterol Hepatol.* 2020;35:1628—1635. https://doi.org/10.1111/jgh.15009.

49. Coppell KJ, Miller JC, Gray AR, Schultz M, Mann JI, Parnell WR. Obesity and the extent of liver damage among adult New Zealanders: findings from a national survey. *Obes Sci Pract.* 2015;1(2):67–77. http://doi.org/10.1002/osp4.13

50. Barreto-Suárez E, Díaz-Elías JO, Corrales-Alonso S, Morales-Martínez L, Morales-Martínez I, Cedeño-Ramírez E, et al. Non-alcoholic fatty liver disease in Cuba. *MEDICC Rev.* 2021;23(1):64–71.

51. Bellentani S. The epidemiology of non-alcoholic fatty liver disease. *Liver Int.* 2017;37(Suppl 1):81–84.

52. Arshad T, Golabi P, Paik J, Mishra A, Younossi ZM. Prevalence of nonalcoholic fatty liver disease in the female population. *Hepatol Commun.* 2019;3:74–83.

53. Golabi P, Paik J, Reddy R, Bugianesi E, Trimble G, Younossi ZM. Prevalence and long-term outcomes of non-alcoholic fatty liver disease among elderly individuals from the United States. *BMC Gastroenterol.* 2019;19:56.

54. Bernal-Reyes R, Castro-Narro G, Malé-Velázquez R, Carmona-Sánchez R, González-Huezo MS, García-Juárez I, et al. The Mexican consensus on nonalcoholic fatty liver disease. *Rev Gastroenterol Mex (Engl Ed).* 2019;84:69–99.

55. Lizardi-Cervera J, Laparra DIB, Chávez-Tapia NC, Ramos DM, Esquivel MU. Prevalencia de hígado graso no alcohólico y síndrome metabólico en población asintomática. *Acta médica Grupo Ángeles.* 2006;4.

56. Martínez SGM, Flores A, Torre AG. Estudio epidemiológico de la enfermedad por hígado graso en población mexicana. *Revista de Gastroenterología de México.* 2017:17–21.

57. Wells MM, Li Z, Addeman B, McKenzie CA, Mujoomdar A, Beaton M, et al. Computed tomography measurement of hepatic steatosis: prevalence of hepatic steatosis in a canadian population. *Can J Gastroenterol Hepatol*. 2016;2016:4930987.

58. López-Velázquez JA, Silva-Vidal KV, Ponciano-Rodríguez G, Chávez-Tapia NC, Arrese M, Uribe M, Méndez-Sánchez N. The prevalence of nonalcoholic fatty liver disease in the Americas. *Ann Hepatol*. 2014;13(2):166–178. PMID: 24552858.

59. Estes C, Anstee QM, Arias-Loste MT, Bantel H, Bellentani S, Caballeria J, et al. Modeling NAFLD disease burden in China, France, Germany, Italy, Japan, Spain, United Kingdom, and United States for the period 2016–2030. *J Hepatol*. 2018:S0168–8278(18)32121–4. http://doi.org/10.1016/j.jhep.2018.05.036 [Epub ahead of print].

60. Alswat K, Aljumah AA, Sanai FM, Abaalkhail F, Alghamdi M, Al Hamoudi WK, et al. Nonalcoholic fatty liver disease burden—Saudi Arabia and United Arab Emirates, 2017–2030. *Saudi J Gastroenterol*. 2018;24(4):211–219. http://doi.org/10.4103/sjg.SJG_122_18

61. Estes C, Chan HLY, Chien RN, Chuang WL, Fung J, Goh GB, Hu TH, Huang JF, Jang BK, Jun DW, Kao JH, Lee JW, Lin HC, Razavi-Shearer K, Seto WK, Wong GL, Wong VW, Razavi H. Modelling NAFLD disease burden in four Asian regions-2019–2030. *Aliment Pharmacol Ther*. 2020;51(8):801–811. http://doi.org/10.1111/apt.15673. Epub 2020 Mar 4. PMID: 32133676; PMCID: PMC7154715.

62. Adams LA, Roberts SK, Strasser SI, Mahady SE, Powell E, Estes C, Razavi H, George J. Nonalcoholic fatty liver disease burden: Australia, 2019–2030. *J Gastroenterol Hepatol*. 2020;35(9):1628–1635. http://doi.org/10.1111/jgh.15009. Epub 2020 Feb 26. PMID: 32048317; PMCID: PMC7540570.

63. Swain MG, Ramji A, Patel K, Sebastiani G, Shaheen AA, Tam E, Marotta P, Elkhashab M, Bajaj HS, Estes C, Razavi H. Burden of nonalcoholic fatty liver disease in Canada, 2019–2030: a modelling study. *CMAJ Open*. 2020;8(2):E429–E436.

64. Goossens N, Bellentani S, Cerny A, Dufour JF, Jornayvaz FR, Mertens J, Moriggia A, Muellhaupt B, Negro F, Razavi H, Semela D, Estes C. Nonalcoholic fatty liver disease burden—Switzerland 2018–2030. *Swiss Med Wkly*. 2019;149:w20152.

65. Estes C, Razavi H, Loomba R, Younossi Z, Sanyal AJ. Modeling the epidemic of nonalcoholic fatty liver disease demonstrates an exponential increase in burden of disease. *Hepatology*. 2018;67(1):123–133.

66. Perumpail BJ, Khan MA, Yoo ER, Cholankeril G, Kim D, Ahmed A. Clinical epidemiology and disease burden of nonalcoholic fatty liver disease. *World J Gastroenterol*. 2017;23(47):8263–8276. http://doi.org/10.3748/wjg.v23.i47.8263. PMID: 29307986; PMCID: PMC5743497.

67. Frith J, Day CP, Henderson E, Burt AD, Newton JL. Non-alcoholic fatty liver disease in older people. *Gerontology*. 2009;55:607–613.

68. Lazo M, Hernaez R, Eberhardt MS, Bonekamp S, Kamel I, Guallar E, Koteish A, Brancati FL, Clark JM. Prevalence of nonalcoholic fatty liver disease in the United States: the Third National Health and Nutrition Examination Survey, 1988–1994. *Am J Epidemiol*. 2013;178(1):38–45. http://doi.org/10.1093/aje/kws448. Epub 2013 May 23. PMID: 23703888; PMCID: PMC3698993.

69. Balakrishnan M, Patel P, Dunn-Valadez S, Dao C, Khan V, Ali H, et al. Women have a lower risk of nonalcoholic fatty liver disease but a higher risk of progression vs men: a systematic review and meta-analysis. *Clin Gastroenterol Hepatol*. 2021;19(1):61–71.e15.

70. Le MH, Yeo YH, Cheung R, Wong VW, Nguyen MH. Ethnic influence on nonalcoholic fatty liver disease prevalence and lack of disease awareness in the United States, 2011–2016. *J Intern Med*. 2020;287(6):711–722. http://doi.org/10.1111/joim.13035. Epub 2020 Mar 4. PMID: 32128904.

71. Setiawan VW, Stram DO, Porcel J, Lu SC, Le Marchand L, Noureddin M. Prevalence of chronic liver disease and cirrhosis by underlying cause in understudied ethnic groups: the multiethnic cohort. *Hepatology*. 2016;64(6):1969–1977.

72. Shaheen M, Schrode KM, Pan D, Kermah D, Puri V, Zarrinpar A, Elisha D, Najjar SM, Friedman TC. Sex-specific differences in the association between race/ethnicity and NAFLD among US population. *Front Med (Lausanne)*. 2021;8:795421. http://doi.org/10.3389/fmed.2021.795421. PMID: 34926533; PMCID: PMC8674562.

73. Rich NE, Oji S, Mufti AR, Browning JD, Parikh ND, Odewole M, et al. Racial and ethnic disparities in nonalcoholic fatty liver disease prevalence, severity, and outcomes in the United States: a systematic review and meta-analysis. *Clin Gastroenterol Hepatol*. 2018;16(2):198–210.e2.

74. Li J, Ha A, Rui F, Zou B, Yang H, Xue Q, et al. Meta-analysis: global prevalence, trend and forecasting of non-alcoholic fatty liver disease in children and adolescents, 2000–2021. *Aliment Pharmacol Ther*. 2022. http://doi.org/10.1111/apt.17096. Epub ahead of print. PMID: 35736008.

75. Wu Y, Zheng Q, Zou B, Yeo YH, Li X, Li J, Xie X, Feng Y, Stave CD, Zhu Q, Cheung R, Nguyen MH. The epidemiology of NAFLD in Mainland China with analysis by adjusted gross regional domestic product: a meta-analysis. *Hepatol Int*. 2020;14(2):259–269. http://doi.org/10.1007/s12072-020-10023-3. Epub 2020 Mar 4. PMID: 32130675.

76. de Vries M, Westerink J, Kaasjager KHAH, de Valk HW. Prevalence of Nonalcoholic Fatty Liver Disease (NAFLD) in patients with type 1 diabetes mellitus: a systematic review and meta-analysis. *J Clin Endocrinol Metab*. 2020;105(12):3842–3853. http://doi.org/10.1210/clinem/dgaa575. PMID: 32827432; PMCID: PMC7526735.

77. Soresi M, Cabibi D, Giglio RV, Martorana S, Guercio G, Porcasi R, Terranova A, Lazzaro LA, Emma MR, Augello G, Cervello M, Pantuso G, Montalto G, Giannitrapani L. The prevalence of NAFLD and fibrosis in bariatric surgery patients and the reliability of noninvasive diagnostic methods. *Biomed Res Int*. 2020;2020:5023157.

78. Young S, Tariq R, Provenza J, Satapathy SK, Faisal K, Choudhry A, Friedman SL, Singal AK. Prevalence and profile of nonalcoholic fatty liver disease in lean adults: systematic review and meta-analysis. *Hepatol Commun*. 2020;4(7):953–972. http://doi.org/10.1002/hep4.1519. PMID: 32626829; PMCID: PMC7327210.

79. Sookoian S, Pirola CJ. Systematic review with meta-analysis: risk factors for non-alcoholic fatty liver disease suggest a shared altered metabolic and cardiovascular profile between lean and obese patients. *Aliment Pharmacol Ther.* 2017;46(2):85–95. http://doi.org/10.1111/apt.14112. Epub 2017 May 2. PMID: 28464369.

80. Ye Q, Zou B, Yeo YH, Li J, Huang DQ, Wu Y, et al. Global prevalence, incidence, and outcomes of non-obese or lean non-alcoholic fatty liver disease: a systematic review and meta-analysis. *Lancet Gastroenterol Hepatol.* 2020;5(8):739–752. http://doi.org/10.1016/S2468-1253(20)30077-7. Epub 2020 May 12. PMID: 32413340.

81. Feng RN, Du SS, Wang C, Li YC, Liu LY, Guo FC, Sun CH. Lean-non-alcoholic fatty liver disease increases risk for metabolic disorders in a normal weight Chinese population. *World J Gastroenterol.* 2014;20(47):17932–17940. http://doi.org/10.3748/wjg.v20.i47.17932. PMID: 25548491; PMCID: PMC4273143.

82. Lu FB, Zheng KI, Rios RS, Targher G, Byrne CD, Zheng MH. Global epidemiology of lean non-alcoholic fatty liver disease: a systematic review and meta-analysis. *J Gastroenterol Hepatol.* 2020;35(12):2041–2050. http://doi.org/10.1111/jgh.15156. Epub 2020 Jul 7. PMID: 32573017.

83. Hagström H, Nasr P, Ekstedt M, Hammar U, Stål P, Hultcrantz R, Kechagias S. Fibrosis stage but not NASH predicts mortality and time to development of severe liver disease in biopsy-proven NAFLD. *J Hepatol.* 2017;67(6):1265–1273. http://doi.org/10.1016/j.jhep.2017.07.027. Epub 2017 Aug 10. PMID: 28803953.

84. Kim D, Kim W, Adejumo AC, Cholankeril G, Tighe SP, Wong RJ, Gonzalez SA, Harrison SA, Younossi ZM, Ahmed A. Race/ethnicity-based temporal changes in prevalence of NAFLD-related advanced fibrosis in the United States, 2005–2016. *Hepatol Int.* 2019;13(2):205–213. http://doi.org/10.1007/s12072-018-09926-z. Epub 2019 Jan 29. PMID: 30694445.

85. Golabi P, Paik J, Hwang JP, Wang S, Lee HM, Younossi ZM. Prevalence and outcomes of non-alcoholic fatty liver disease (NAFLD) among Asian American adults in the United States. *Liver Int.* 2019;39(4):748–757. http://doi.org/10.1111/liv.14038. Epub 2019 Feb 13. PMID: 30597715.

86. Castellanos-Fernández MI, Crespo-Ramírez E, Del Valle-Díaz S, Barreto-Suárez E, Díaz-Elías JO, Corrales-Alonso S, et al. Non-alcoholic fatty liver disease in Cuba. *MEDICC Rev.* 2021;23(1):64–71.

87. Tutunchi H, Naeini F, Ebrahimi-Mameghani M, Najafipour F, Mobasseri M, Ostadrahimi A. Metabolically healthy and unhealthy obesity and the progression of liver fibrosis: a cross-sectional study. *Clin Res Hepatol Gastroenterol.* 2021;45(6):101754. http://doi.org/10.1016/j.clinre.2021.101754. Epub 2021 Jul 22. PMID: 34303827.

88. Park J, Lee EY, Li J, Jun MJ, Yoon E, Ahn SB,. NASH/Liver fibrosis prevalence and incidence of nonliver comorbidities among people with NAFLD and incidence of NAFLD by metabolic comorbidities: lessons from South Korea. *Dig Dis.* 2021;39(6):634–645.

89. GBD 2017 Cirrhosis collaborators. The global, regional, and national burden of cirrhosis by cause in 195 countries and territories, 1990–2017: a systematic analysis for the Global Burden of Disease Study 2017. *Lancet Gastroenterol Hepatol.* 2020;5(3):245–266. https://www.thelancet.com/journals/langas/article/PIIS2468-1253(19)30349-8/fulltext

90. McPherson S, Hardy T, Henderson E, Burt AD, Day CP, Anstee QM. Evidence of NAFLD progression from steatosis to fibrosing-steatohepatitis using paired biopsies: implications for prognosis and clinical management. *J Hepatol.* 2015;62:1148–1155.

91. Golabi P, Paik JM, Arshad T, Younossi Y, Mishra A, Younossi ZM. Mortality of NAFLD according to the body composition and presence of metabolic abnormalities. *Hepatol Commun.* 2020;4(8):1136–1148. http://doi.org/10.1002/hep4.1534. PMID: 32766474; PMCID: PMC7395070.

92. Paik JM, Golabi P, Younossi Y, Srishord M, Mishra A, Younossi ZM. The growing burden of disability related to nonalcoholic fatty liver disease: data from the global burden of disease 2007–2017. *Hepatol Commun.* 2020;4(12):1769–1780.

93. Chang Y, Jung HS, Cho J, Zhang Y, Yun KE, Lazo M, et al. Metabolically healthy obesity and the development of nonalcoholic fatty liver disease. *Am J Gastroenterol.* 2016;111(8):1133–1140.

94. Singh S, Allen AM, Wang Z, Prokop LJ, Murad MH, Loomba R. Fibrosis progression in nonalcoholic fatty liver vs nonalcoholic steatohepatitis: a systematic review and meta-analysis of paired-biopsy studies. *Clin Gastroenterol Hepatol.* 2015;13(4):643–654.e1–9;

95. Sanyal AJ, Harrison SA, Ratziu V, Abdelmalek MF, Diehl AM, et al. The natural history of advanced fibrosis due to nonalcoholic steatohepatitis: data from the simtuzumab trials. *Hepatology.* 2019;70(6):1913–1927. http://doi.org/10.1002/hep.30664. Epub 2019 May 28. PMID: 30993748.

96. Machado MV, Diehl AM. Pathogenesis of nonalcoholic steatohepatitis. *Gastroenterology.* 2016;150:1769–1777. https://doi.org/10.1053/j.gastro.2016.02.066.

97. Angulo P, Machado MV, Diehl AM. Fibrosis in non-alcoholic fatty liver disease: mechanisms and clinical implications. *Semin Liver Dis.* 2015;35:132–145. https://doi.org/10.1055/s-0035-1550065.

98. Dongiovanni P, Stender S, Pietrelli A, Mancina RM, Cespiati A, Petta S, Pelusi S, Pingitore P, Badiali S, Maggioni M, et al. Causal relationship of hepatic fat with liver damage and insulin resistance in nonalcoholic fatty liver. *J Intern Med.* 2018;283:356–370. http://doi.org/10.1111/joim.12719.

99. Loomba R, Adams LA. The 20% rule of NASH progression: the natural history of advanced fibrosis and cirrhosis caused by NASH. *Hepatology.* 2019;70(6):1885–1888. http://doi.org/10.1002/hep.30946. PMID: 31520407; PMCID: PMC7504908.

100. Singh S, Allen AM, Wang Z, Prokop LJ, Murad MH, Loomba R. Fibrosis progression in nonalcoholic fatty liver vs nonalcoholic steatohepatitis: a systematic review and meta-analysis of paired-biopsy studies. *Clin Gastroenterol Hepatol.* 2015;13(4):643–654.e1–9.

101. Kleiner DE, Brunt EM, Wilson LA, Behling C, Guy C, Contos M, et al. Nonalcoholic steatohepatitis clinical research network. Association of histologic disease activity with progression of nonalcoholic fatty liver disease. *JAMA Netw Open.* 2019;2(10): e1912565.

102. Hagström H, Nasr P, Ekstedt M, Hammar U, Stål P, Hultcrantz R, Kechagias S. Fibrosis stage but not NASH predicts mortality and time to development of severe liver disease in biopsy-proven NAFLD. *J Hepatol*. 2017;67(6):1265–1273.

103. Vusirikala A, Thomas T, Bhala N, Tahrani AA, Thomas GN, Nirantharakumar K. Impact of obesity and metabolic health status in the development of non-alcoholic fatty liver disease (NAFLD): a United Kingdom population-based cohort study using the health improvement network (THIN). *BMC Endocr Disord*. 2020;20(1):96.

104. Golabi P, Otgonsuren M, de Avila L, Sayiner M, Rafiq N, Younossi ZM. Components of metabolic syndrome increase the risk of mortality in nonalcoholic fatty liver disease (NAFLD). *Medicine (Baltimore)*. 2018;97(13):e0214.

105. Stepanova M, Rafiq N, Younossi ZM. Components of metabolic syndrome are independent predictors of mortality in patients with chronic liver disease: a population-based study. *Gut*. 2010;59(10):1410–1415.

106. Rodriguez-Hernandez H, Cervantes-Huerta M, Luis Gonzalez J, Dolores Marquez-Ramirez M, Rodriguez-Moran M, Guerrero-Romero F. Nonalcoholic fatty liver disease in asymptomatic obese women. The work was originated in the Biomedical Research Unit of the Mexican Social Security Institute at Durango, Mex. *J Hepatol*. 2010;9:144–149.

107. Jinjuvadia R, Antaki F, Lohia P, Liangpunsakul S. The association between nonalcoholic fatty liver disease and metabolic abnormalities in the United States population. *J Clin Gastroenterol*. 2017;51:160–166.

108. Burra P, Becchetti C, Germani G. NAFLD and liver transplantation: disease burden, current management and future challenges. *JHEP Rep*. 2020;2(6):100192.

109. Ahmed MH, Noor SK, Bushara SO, Husain NE, Elmadhoun WM, Ginawi IA, et al. Non-alcoholic fatty liver disease in Africa and Middle East: an attempt to predict the present and future implications on the healthcare system. *Gastroenterology Res*. 2017;10(5):271–279.

110. Kalia HS, Gaglio PJ. The prevalence and pathobiology of nonalcoholic fatty liver disease in patients of different races or ethnicities. *Clin Liver Dis*. 2016;20(2):215–224.

111. Messiah SE, Vidot DC, Baeker B, Jordan A, Kristopher L, Khorgami Z, De La Cruz-Muñoz N. Ethnic and gender differences in the prevalence of nonalcoholic steatohepatitis among bariatric surgery patients. *Bariatr Surg Pract Patient Care*. 2016;11(4). https://doi.org/10.1089/bari.2016.0018

112. Selvakumar PKC, Kabbany MN, Nobili V, Alkhouri N. Nonalcoholic fatty liver disease in children: hepatic and extrahepatic complications. *Pediatr Clin North Am*. 2017;64(3):659–675.

113. Kotronen A, Johansson LE, Johansson LM, et al. A common variant in PNPLA3, which encodes adiponutrin, is associated with liver fat content in humans. *Diabetologia*. 2009;52:1056–1060.

114. Chinchilla-López P, Ramírez-Pérez O, Cruz-Ramón V, Canizales-Quinteros S, Domínguez-López A, Ponciano-Rodríguez G, et al. More evidence for the genetic susceptibility of Mexican population to nonalcoholic fatty liver disease through PNPLA3. *Ann Hepatol*. 2018;17:250–255.

115. Martínez LA, Larrieta E, Kershenobich D, Torre A. The expression of PNPLA3 polymorphism could be the key for severe liver disease in NAFLD in hispanic population. *Ann Hepatol*. 2017;16:909–915.

116. Sookoian S, Pirola CJ. Meta-analysis of the influence of I148M variant of patatin-like phospholipase domain containing 3 gene (PNPLA3) on the susceptibility and histological severity of nonalcoholic fatty liver disease. *Hepatology*. 2011;53:1883–1894.

117. Barbara M, Scott A, Alkhouri N. New insights into genetic predisposition and novel therapeutic targets for nonalcoholic fatty liver disease [Internet]. *Hepatobiliary Surg Nutr*. 2018;7:372–381. http://doi.org/10.21037/hbsn.2018.08.05

118. Sliz E, Sebert S, Würtz P, Kangas AJ, Soininen P, Lehtimäki T, et al. NAFLD risk alleles in PNPLA3, TM6SF2, GCKR and LYPLAL1 show divergent metabolic effects. *Hum Mol Genet* [Internet]. 2018;27:2214–2223. http://doi.org/10.1093/hmg/ddy124

119. Anstee QM, Day CP. The genetics of NAFLD [Internet]. *Nat Rev Gastroenterol Hepatol*. 2013;10:645–655.

120. Walker RW, Lê KA, Davis J, Alderete TL, Cherry R, Lebel S, Goran MI. High rates of fructose malabsorption are associated with reduced liver fat in obese African Americans. *J Am Coll Nutr*. 2012;31(5):369–374.

121. Mouzaki M, Loomba R. Insights into the evolving role of the gut microbiome in nonalcoholic fatty liver disease: rationale and prospects for therapeutic intervention. *Therap Adv Gastroenterol*. 2019;12:1756284819858470. http://doi.org/10.1177/1756284819858470. PMID: 31258623; PMCID: PMC6591661.

122. Leung C, Rivera L, Furness JB, Angus PW. The role of the gut microbiota in NAFLD. *Nat Rev Gastroenterol Hepatol*. 2016;13(7):412–425. http://doi.org/10.1038/nrgastro.2016.85. Epub 2016 Jun 8. PMID: 27273168.

123. Aron-Wisnewsky J, Vigliotti C, Witjes J, Le P, Holleboom AG, Verheij J, Nieuwdorp M, Clément K. Gut microbiota and human NAFLD: disentangling microbial signatures from metabolic disorders. *Nat Rev Gastroenterol Hepatol*. 2020;17(5):279–297. http://doi.org/10.1038/s41575-020-0269-9. Epub 2020 Mar 9. PMID: 32152478.

124. Schwimmer JB, Johnson JS, Angeles JE, Behling C, Belt PH, Borecki I, et al. Microbiome signatures associated with steatohepatitis and moderate to severe fibrosis in children with nonalcoholic fatty liver disease. *Gastroenterology*. 2019;157:1109–1122.

125. World Health Organization (WHO). *World cancer mortality*. Obtained from the world wide web at: www.who.int/news-room/fact-sheets/detail/cancer. Last accessed on 4/7/22.

126. Bray F, Ferlay J, Soerjomataram I, Siegel RL, Torre LA, Jemal A. Global cancer statistics 2018: GLOBOCAN estimates of incidence and mortality worldwide for 36 cancers in 185 countries. *CA Cancer J Clin*. 2018;68:394–424.

127. Paik JM, Golabi P, Biswas R, Alqahtani S, Venkatesan C, Younossi ZM. Nonalcoholic fatty liver disease and alcoholic liver disease are major drivers of liver mortality in the United States. *Hepatol Commun*. 2020;4(6):890–903.

128. Golabi P, Paik JM, AlQahtani S, Younossi Y, Tuncer G, Younossi ZM. Burden of non-alcoholic fatty liver

disease in Asia, the Middle East and North Africa: data from Global Burden of disease 2009–2019. *J Hepatol*. 2021;75(4):795–809. http://doi.org/10.1016/j.jhep.2021.05.022. Epub 2021 May 31. PMID: 34081959.

129. Eguchi Y, Wong G, Lee IH, Akhtar O, Lopes R, Sumida Y. Hepatocellular carcinoma and other complications of non-alcoholic fatty liver disease and non-alcoholic steatohepatitis in Japan: a structured review of published works. *Hepatol Res*. 2021;51(1):19–30. http://doi.org/10.1111/hepr.13583. Epub 2020 Dec 9. PMID: 33091191.

130. White DL, Kanwal F, El-Serag HB. Association between nonalcoholic fatty liver disease and risk for hepatocellular cancer, based on systematic review. *Clin Gastroenterol Hepatol*. 2012;10:1342–1359.e2.

131. Targher G. Non-alcoholic fatty liver disease, the metabolic syndrome and the risk of cardiovascular disease: the plot thickens. *Diabet Med*. 2007;24:1–6.

132. Bhatia LS, Curzen NP, Calder PC, Byrne CD. Non-alcoholic fatty liver disease: a new and important cardiovascular risk factor? *Eur Heart J*. 2012;33(10):1190–1200. http://doi.org/10.1093/eurheartj/ehr453. Epub 2012 Mar 8. PMID: 22408036.

133. Marchesini G, Bugianesi E, Forlani G, Cerrelli F, Lenzi M, Manini R, et al. Nonalcoholic fatty liver, steatohepatitis, and the metabolic syndrome. *Hepatology*.2003;37:917–923.

134. Taylor R, Taylor R, Bayliss S et al. Association between fibrosis stage and outcomes of patients with non-alcoholic fatty liver disease: a systematic review and meta-analysis. *Gastroenteorlogy*. 2020;20:30137.

135. Wu S, Wu F, Ding Y, et al. Association of non-alcoholic fatty liver disease with major adverse cardiovascular events: a systematic review and meta-analysis. *Sci Rep*. 2016;6:1–14.

136. Zhou Y, Zhou X, Wu S, et al. Synergistic increase in cardiovascular risk in diabetes mellitus with non-alcoholic fatty liver disease: a meta-analysis. *Eur J Gastroenterol Hepatol*. 2018;30:631–636.

137. Stefan N, Häring H, Cusi K. Non-alcoholic fatty liver disease: causes, diagnosis, cardiometabolic consequences, and treatment strategies. *Lancet Diabetes Endocrinol*. 2019;7:313–324.

138. Paik JM, Henry L, De Avila L, Younossi E, Racila A, Younossi ZM. Mortality related to nonalcoholic fatty liver disease is increasing in the United States. *Hepatol Commun*. 2019;3(11):1459–1471. http://doi.org/10.1002/hep4.1419. PMID: 31701070; PMCID: PMC6824058.

139. Mantovani A, Csermely A, Petracca G, Beatrice G, Corey KE, Simon TG, Byrne CD, Targher G. Non-alcoholic fatty liver disease and risk of fatal and non-fatal cardiovascular events: an updated systematic review and meta-analysis. *Lancet Gastroenterol Hepatol*. 2021;6(11):903–913.

140. Wu K, Zhai MZ, Weltzien EK, Cespedes Feliciano EM, Meyerhardt JA, Giovannucci E, Caan BJ. Non-alcoholic fatty liver disease and colorectal cancer survival. *Cancer Causes Control*. 2019;30(2):165–168. http://doi.org/10.1007/s10552-018-1095-z. Epub 2018 Nov 15. PMID: 30443695; PMCID: PMC6613648.

141. Liu SS, Ma XF, Zhao J, Du SX, Zhang J, Dong MZ, Xin YN. Association between nonalcoholic fatty liver disease and extrahepatic cancers: a systematic review and meta-analysis. *Lipids Health Dis*. 2020;19(1):118. http://doi.org/10.1186/s12944-020-01288-6. PMID: 32475354; PMCID: PMC7262754.

142. Simon TG, Roelstraete B, Sharma R, Khalili H, Hagström H, Ludvigsson JF. Cancer risk in patients with biopsy-confirmed nonalcoholic fatty liver disease: a population-based cohort study. *Hepatology*. 2021;74(5):2410–2423. http://doi.org/10.1002/hep.31845. Epub 2021 Aug 25. PMID: 33811766.

143. Lee YH, Kim SU, Song K, Park JY, Kim do Y, Ahn SH, et al. Sarcopenia is associated with significant liver fibrosis independently ofobesity and insulin resistance in nonalcoholic fatty liver disease: nationwide surveys (KNHANES 2008–2011). *Hepatology*. 2016;63:776–786.

144. Lee YH, Jung KS, Kim SU, Yoon HJ, Yun YJ, Lee BW, et al. Sarcopaenia is associated with NAFLD independently of obesity and insulin resistance: nationwide surveys (KNHANES 2008–2011). *J Hepatol*. 2015;63:486–493.

145. Li AA, Kim D, Ahmed A. Association of sarcopenia and NAFLD: an overview. *Clin Liver Dis (Hoboken)*. 2020;16(2):73–76. http://doi.org/10.1002/cld.900. PMID: 32922754; PMCID: PMC7474147.

146. Golabi P, Gerber L, Paik JM, Deshpande R, de Avila L, Younossi ZM. Contribution of sarcopenia and physical inactivity to mortality in people with non-alcoholic fatty liver disease. *JHEP Rep*. 2020;2(6):100171. http://doi.org/10.1016/j.jhepr.2020.100171. PMID: 32964202; PMCID: PMC7490851.

3 Genetics of NAFLD

Luca Valenti and Cristiana Bianco

CONTENTS

Key Points

- NAFLD is a complex trait, and the susceptibility to develop the disease depends on the interaction between inherited and environmental factors.

- Variants in gene-regulating hepatic handling of lipid metabolism play a key role in the pathogenesis of hepatic fat accumulation and NAFLD.

- Genetic factors modulating hepatic fat drive the progression toward cirrhosis and hepatocellular carcinoma.

3.1 INTRODUCTION

Nonalcoholic fatty liver disease (NAFLD) is now the most frequent liver disease, affecting about a quarter of the population globally, and it has become a leading cause of liver-related morbidity and mortality. The term includes a large spectrum of clinical entities, from simple steatosis to progressive steatohepatitis, cirrhosis and hepatocellular carcinoma (HCC). It is a complex trait, whose risk of onset and progression varies among individuals. Inherited factors, metabolic status (type 2 diabetes [T2D] and obesity, overall) and lifestyle contribute to disease susceptibility and the heterogeneity of clinical presentation.

In the last 15 years, genome-wide association studies (GWAS), whole-exome sequencing (WES) and whole-genome sequencing (WGS) have allowed us to identify an initial set of genetic variants and deranged biological pathways implicated in the genetic susceptibility to NAFLD, improving the comprehension of disease pathophysiology.

3.2 HERITABILITY OF NAFLD

Genetic predisposition (or susceptibility) can be defined as an increased likelihood of developing a disease based on a person's genetic architecture. Common diseases are complex traits that depend on the interaction between genetic predisposition and environmental factors. According to the commonest view, several common genetic variants with a small individual impact on the phenotype contribute to the development of common traits, but more recent data suggest that rarer variants with a large effect size can contribute as well.

Several research approaches support the notion that hepatic fat accumulation and NAFLD variability are strongly influenced by inherited factors.[1] First, twin studies showed that more than a half of the variability of hepatic fat content and circulating liver enzymes (such as alanine aminotransferase [ALT] levels) depends on heritability.[2,3] From these studies, it also emerged that liver fat and hepatic fibrosis are shared traits, suggesting that hepatic fat accumulation has a causal role in progressive liver disease. More recent general population studies employing magnetic resonance imaging to quantify liver fat and elastometry to estimate liver fibrosis led to the same conclusion.[2–4] Second, family studies showed that the risk of NAFLD and progressive liver disease is higher in relatives of patients affected by cirrhotic NAFLD as compared to the general population, independently of metabolic comorbidities.[5] Lastly, multiethnic cohort studies demonstrated a marked interethnic variability in NAFLD susceptibility, which is higher in Hispanics, followed by East Asians, intermediate in Europeans and lower in African Americans independently of confounding factors.[6]

3.3 GENETIC ARCHITECTURE OF NAFLD

3.3.1 Main Common Genetic Variants Associated with NAFLD

The mapping of the genetic architecture of common diseases started with the development and application of approaches based on GWAS, complemented by candidate gene association studies. Indeed, starting from large and well-characterized cohorts, GWAS permit the identification of the main common genetic variants associated with a trait (e.g., hepatic fat accumulation) or a condition (e.g., NAFLD). The idea is that susceptibility to complex diseases is accounted for by common genetic variants (with a minor allele frequency [MAF] ≥5%), each of which explains a small part of the risk in the general population. Studies conducted in recent years have allowed us to identify a handful of common genetic determinants of hepatic fat accumulation that contribute to explaining the interindividual and interethnic variability of this condition (Figure 3.1). Notably, most of the main genetic variants implicated in NAFLD pathogenesis affect proteins implicated in lipid metabolism, determining quantitative or qualitative changes of lipids within hepatic deposits (Table 3.1).

The largest fraction of genetic predisposition to NAFLD and progressive liver disease is accounted for the rs738409 C>G single-nucleotide polymorphism (SNP), encoding for an aminoacidic substitution of methionine for isoleucine at position 148 (I148M protein variant) of patatin-like phospholipase domain containing3 (*PNPLA3*). The I148M

DOI: 10.1201/9781003386698-4

Table 3.1: List of Common and Rare Variants Associated with NAFLD

Gene	Function	Variant	Impact on Protein	Effect of the Variant	Phenotype
PNPLA3	Lipid droplets remodeling	rs738409 C>G	p.I148M	Loss plus gain of function	↑NAFLD, NASH, fibrosis, HCC
TM6SF2	VLDL secretion	rs58542926 C>T	p.E167K	Loss of function	↑NAFLD, NASH, fibrosis, HCC
MBOAT7	Lipid droplets remodeling, phospholipid metabolism	rs641738 C>T	Linked to 3'-UTR	Reduced expression	↑NAFLD, NASH, fibrosis, HCC
GCKR	Regulation of de novo lipogenesis	rs1260326 T>C	p.P446L	Loss of function	↑NAFLD, NASH, fibrosis
HSD17B13	Hepatic retinol metabolism ?	rs72613567 T > TA	Alternate splicing	Loss of function	↓NASH, fibrosis, HCC
PPP1R3B	Glycogen synthesis	rs4841132 G > A		Gain of function	↓NAFLD, NASH, fibrosis, HCC
IFNL4	Innate immunity	rs368234815 TT > dG	Alternative protein translation site	Alternative protein	↓NASH, fibrosis
MERTK	Innate immunity, HSCs activation	rs4374383 G > A	Noncoding variant	Reduced expression	↓Fibrosis
PCSK7	Lipoprotein remodeling	rs236918 G > C	Noncoding variant	Gain of function	↑NAFLD, NASH, fibrosis
UCP2	Mitochondrial lipid metabolism, oxidative phosphorylation	rs695366 G > A	Promoter variant	Gain of function	↓NASH
SOD2	Mitochondrial antioxidant	rs4880 C > T	p.A16V	Loss of function	↑Fibrosis
MARC1	Oxidative stress?		p.M187K p.A165T	Loss of function	↓NAFLD, fibrosis
APOE	Lipoprotein remodeling	rs429358 T > C	p.C112R		↓NAFLD
GPAM	Lipid synthesis	rs2792751 C > T	p.V43I		↑NAFLD
LEPR	Leptin signaling	rs12077210 C > T	Intronic variant		↑NAFLD, NASH
PYGO1	Adiposity and glucose metabolism, unclear	rs11858624 G > T	p.P299H		↓NAFLD
HFE	Iron metabolism	rs1800562 G > A	p.C282Y	Loss of function	↑Fibrosis
CP	Iron metabolism			Loss of function	↑Fibrosis
SERPINA1	Immunomodulation, ER stress		p.E342K	Loss of function	↑Fibrosis
APOB	VLDL secretion	Several	Protein change	Loss of function	↑NAFLD, NASH, fibrosis, HCC
LIPA	Lipid catabolism	Several	Protein change	Loss of function	↑NAFLD
TERT	Cellular senescence	Several		Loss of function	↑Fibrosis. HCC
ATG7	Autophagy	rs143545741 C>T rs36117895 T>C	p.P426L p.V471A	Loss of function	↑NASH

variant predisposes to the whole spectrum of NAFLD, including development of steatohepatitis (NASH), progression to severe fibrosis-cirrhosis and HCC onset independently of fibrosis.[7–9] Interestingly, the presence of the *PNPLA3* variant is responsible for the 15–27% of the population attributable fraction of severe NAFLD, namely cirrhosis and HCC.[10] PNPLA3 is a protein expressed on the surface of lipid droplets (LDs) with hydrolytic activity on glycerolipids, but it also has an acyltransferase activity, resulting in the remodeling of phospholipids and triglycerides (TGs) within LDs. The I148M variant induces a loss of function in protein's enzymatic activity by reducing the substrate access to the enzyme's active site; in addition, the mutated protein acquires the ability of evading ubiquitylation and avoiding proteasomal degradation. Thus the nonfunctional protein accumulates on LDs and inhibits the metabolization of TGs, promoting their storage and LDs enlargement.[11,12] *PNPLA3* is also

highly expressed in hepatic stellate cells (HSCs), where it is responsible for the hydrolysis of retinyl esters. Here, the loss of function induced by the I148M variant determines the retention of retinol and HSCs, as a response to chronic inflammation, are activated to myofibroblast-like cells and secrete collagen, leading to liver fibrosis.[11] The phenotypic expression of this variant is mainly promoted by obesity and insulin resistance. Indeed, *PNPLA3* expression is induced by insulin through the activation of the transcription factor sterol regulatory element binding protein 1c (SREBP1c) and carbohydrate response element binding protein (ChREBP).[12,13]

The rs58542926 C>T in the transmembrane 6 superfamily member 2 (*TM6SF2*) is a missense mutation encoding for the E167K variant that has been associated with NAFLD, NASH and hepatic fibrosis.[14,15] TM6SF2 protein localizes in the endoplasmic reticulum and ER-Golgi intermediate compartment, where it is involved in the secretion and/or

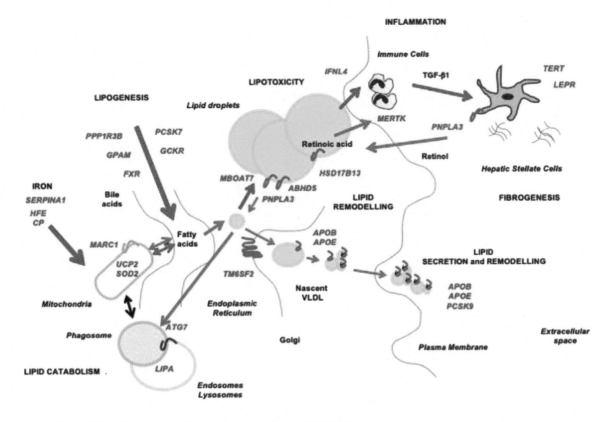

Figure 3.1 Genetic loci involved in the pathophysiology of NAFLD

ABHD5: Abhydrolase domain containing 5; APOB: Apolipoprotein B; APOE: Apolipoprotein E; ATG7: Autophagy-related-7; CP: Ceruloplasmin; FXR: Farnesoid X receptor; GCKR: Glucokinase regulator; GPAM: Glycerol-3-phosphate aminotransferase; HFE: Hemochromatosis gene; HSD17B13: 17-beta hydroxysteroid dehydrogenase 13; IFNL4: Interferon lambda 4; LEPR: Leptin receptor; LIPA: Lysosomal acid lipase; MARC1: Mitochondrial amidoxime reducing component 1; MBOAT7: Membrane bound O-acyl transferase 7; MERTK: Mer T kinase; PCSK7: Proprotein convertase subtilisin/kexin 7; PCSK9: Proprotein convertase subtilisin/kexin 9; PNPLA3: Patatin-like phospholipase domain-containing 3; PPP1R3B: Protein phosphatase 1 regulatory subunit 3B; SERPINA1: Serpin family A member 1; SOD2: mitochondrial Superoxide dismutase; TERT: human Telomerase reverse transcriptase; TGF-b1: Transforming growth factor beta 1; TM6SF2: Transmembrane 6 superfamily member 2; UCP2: Uncoupling protein 2; VLDL: very-low-density lipoproteins.

Genetic variants are classified according to the biological mechanism by which the encoded proteins contribute to the development of liver disease. Green arrows indicate beneficial pathways, while red arrows indicate pathological process/lipid fluxes.

lipidation of very-low-density lipoprotein (VLDL). Indeed, some of the liver lipids deriving from de novo lipogenesis or absorption of remnant lipoprotein particles and fatty acids from the circulation are secreted back in the bloodstream in the form of VLDL. The variant induces a loss of function of the protein and thus impairs VLDL secretion, determines TGs accumulation and increases susceptibility to liver damage.[16,17] Interestingly, the variant has a paradoxical effect in liver and heart; indeed, reducing circulating lipids confers a more favorable plasmatic lipid profile that provides protection against cardiovascular diseases.[16]

A number of studies have confirmed the impact of the variant rs641738 C>T in the membrane-bound O-acyltransferase domain containing 7 (*MBOAT7*) gene on the full spectrum of NAFLD, including NASH and progression to advanced fibrosis,[18] and on the risk of NAFLD-HCC development in patients without severe fibrosis[19]; recently, a new rare likely pathogenic variant has been identified in patients with NAFLD-HCC.[20] *MBOAT7* encodes

lysophosphatidyl-inositol acyltransferase 1 (LPIAT1), an endoplasmic reticulum membrane protein involved in the remodeling of phospholipid acyl-chain in the so-called Land's cycle[21]; the enzyme mediates the incorporation of arachidonic acid (AA) and other polyunsaturated fatty acids (PUFAs) into lysophosphatidyl-inositol (LPI) and other lysophospholipids. The rs641738 C>T variant induces a downregulation of *MBOAT7* transcription and translation, resulting in a reduction of AA containing phospholipids and accumulation of LPI, which is converted in TGs that accumulate in LDs.[22] In addition, it promotes the synthesis of phosphatidyl inositol and its degradation into diacylglycerol, fueling a vicious cycle of TGs generation and driving hepatic steatosis. On the other hand, some evidence suggest that downregulation of *MBOAT7* itself can trigger hepatic fibrosis inducing proinflammatory and profibrotic cytokines via LPI accumulation.[23,24]

Glucokinase regulator (GCKR) is a protein that acts as an inhibitor of glucokinase (GCK) in response to glucose levels; in fact, GCK is involved in the modulation of the influx of glucose in hepatocytes in response to insulin and activates glucose storage pathways including de novo lipogenesis and glycogen synthesis.[25] The common missense SNP rs1260326 C>T, encoding the P446L variant of *GCKR*, lacks the ability to inhibit glucokinase in response to fructose-6-phosphate, and therefore the hepatic uptake of glucose is constitutively activated.[26] The consequence is a decrease in fasting glycemia and insulin resistance, but at the same time glycolysis, de novo lipogenesis and hepatic steatosis are promoted.[25,27]

More recently, loss of function variants in the hydroxysteroid 17-beta dehydrogenase 13 (*HSD17B13*), such as rs143404524 and rs72613567, have been identified as protective factors against liver damage[28,29]; in particular, the rs72613567:TA encodes for a prematurely truncating and unstable protein with reduced enzymatic activity. The HSD17B family consists of catalytic enzymes acting toward 7β-hydroxy and -keto steroid substrates; most HSD17B family members are involved in the activation/inactivation of sex hormones. HSD17B13 is mainly expressed in the liver and localized on the surface of LDs in hepatocytes, where it exerts a retinoic dehydrogenase activity promoting the conversion of retinol to retinoic acid.[29] Although the molecular mechanisms have not been well-uncovered yet, it is known that the effect of these variants is not accounted for by protection against hepatic fat accumulation but involves direct modulation of inflammation and fibrogenesis.

3.3.2 Other Inherited Risk Variants for NAFLD

The genetics of NALFD is an ever changing field, and the list of genetic variants is increasing day by day.

The rs4841132 G>A variant in the protein phosphatase 1 regulatory subunit 3B (*PPP1R3B*) has been identifies as a protective factor against hepatic fat accumulation modulating hepatic lipid metabolism.[30]

Polymorphisms in genes that regulate innate immunity, fibrogenesis and oxidative stress may modify the effect of fat accumulating in hepatocytes. For example, variants in the interferon lambda 3/4 (*IFNL4*) locus encoding for the alternative interferon lambda-3 and lambda-4 proteins modulate the activation of innate immunity and necroinflammation.[31] The rs4374383 G>A in Mer tyrosine kinase (*MERTK*) reduces MERTK expression in hepatic myeloid cells and therefore the activation of HSCs, protecting from hepatic inflammation and fibrogenesis.[32] Conversely, the rs236918 G>C in proprotein convertase subtilisin/kexin type 7 (*PCSK7*) seems to be linked to lipid and iron metabolism and the promotion of fibrogenesis.[33] Variants in uncoupling protein 2 (*UCP2*) and mitochondrial manganese-dependent superoxidase dismutase 2 (*SOD2*), respectively the rs695366 G>A and the rs4880 C>T, influence fatty acid oxidation and oxidative stress in mitochondria,[34,35] whereas the p.M187K variant in mitochondrial amidoxime reducing component 1 (*MARC1*) has a protective role against disease progression and cirrhosis.[36]

More recent studies highlighted variants in apolipoprotein E (*APOE*) and glycerol-3-phosphate aminotransferase (*GPAM*), which regulate hepatic lipid metabolism, in the leptin receptor (*LEPR*), involved in the modulation of appetite and fibrogenesis and in pygopus homolog-1 (*PYGO1*), as risk factors for NAFLD and cirrhosis progression.[37,38]

In this list, other genes known to cause other inherited diseases should be added. Indeed, genetic variants known to influence iron metabolism (*HFE* C282Y, responsible for hereditary hemochromatosis) have been associated with more severe liver damage in patients with NAFLD, probably due to the predisposition to iron accumulation in hepatocytes.[39] Similarly, variations in the ceruloplasmin gene (*CP*) have been associated with increased hepatic iron stores and more advanced fibrosis in patients with NAFLD.[40] In addition, the PiZ variant in *SERPINA1* (responsible for alpha-1-antitrypsin deficiency) seems to impair lipid secretion and play a role in fat-associated liver damage.[41]

3.3.3 Role of Rare Genetic Variants

Genetic variants are defined as "rare" when present in the general population with a minor allele frequency (MAF) of less than 1%. There is initial evidence that rare missense or nonsense genetic variants with a strong impact on protein structure and function predispose with a large effect size to hepatic fat accumulation and liver damage.[20] These variants in key genes regulating hepatic lipid metabolism are responsible for disease clustering in families. As example, rare mutations on apolipoprotein B (*APOB*), responsible for familial hypobetalipoproteinemia, predispose to steatosis and severe progressive liver diseases because of the lipid compartmentalization in hepatocytes due to the inability to secrete VLDL.[42] Moreover, *APOB* mutations predispose to NAFLD-HCC.[20] APOB is also involved in chylomicrons secretion and may cause damage to the intestinal barrier due to lipid accumulation on enterocytes and malabsorption of liposoluble vitamins. It should be remembered that severe genetic disorders may manifest with NAFLD even in children, as in the case of mutations of *LIPA*; these are responsible for lysosomal acid lipase deficiency and cause the accumulation of triglycerides and cholesteryl esters in hepatocytes.[43]

Another key mechanism involved in the progression of liver disease is cell senescence related to telomerase shortening. Indeed, loss-of-function variants in telomerase reverse transcriptase (*TERT*) have been associated with progressive liver disease and HCC development.[44,45]

Finally, there is evidence that rare loss-of-function variants in autophagy-related-7 (*ATG7*) and the low-frequency hypomorphic V471A variant predispose to progressive NAFLD by impairing the autophagic flux, leading to the accumulation of fat and of the sequestome protein p62 in damaged hepatocytes, thereby triggering ballooning and hepatic inflammation.[46]

3.4 GENETIC AND ENVIRONMENTAL FACTORS: TWO SIDES OF THE SAME COIN

The phenotypic expression of complex traits, as NAFLD is, depends on the interaction between genetic background and environmental determinants. The magnitude of the effect of a given variant may be modulated by the number of alleles of another genetic variant (gene–gene interaction) or by an environmental factor (gene–environment interaction). At the general population level, being carriers of common genetic risk variants is not sufficient to develop NAFLD or progressive liver disease. The main environmental trigger of NAFLD is represented by adiposity, which is related to insulin resistance and hyperinsulinemia.[47,48] Indeed, the impact of genetic variants, as for example *PNPLA3* I148M, on hepatic fat and predisposition to cirrhosis increases with body mass index (BMI), being higher in obese and very obese individuals.[13] Similarly,

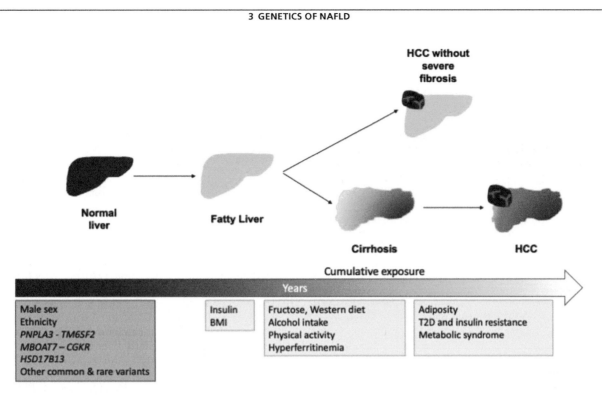

Figure 3.2 Inherited and acquire.d factors involved in the development and progression of NAFLD

BMI: Body mass index; GCKR: Glucokinase regulator; HCC: Hepatocellular carcinoma; MBOAT7: Membrane-bound O-acyl transferase 7; PNPLA3: Patatin-like phospholipase domain-containing 3; TM6SF2: Transmembrane 6 superfamily member 2; T2D: type 2 diabetes.

an interaction between BMI and *TM6SF2* E167K, *GCKR* P446L, and rare *ATG7* variants as well, but not with other BMI-associated phenotypes such as TGs levels, has been observed in a population cohort study.[13] The development of the disease in obese individuals is related to the concomitant insulin resistance and hyperinsulinemia, that for example amplify the *PNPLA3*-associated genetic risk of NAFLD.[49] Similarly, the susceptibility to NAFLD linked to *PNPLA3* is exacerbated by the consumption of industrial fructose in soft drinks, but the effect of genetic predisposition is positively modulated by a Mediterranean dietary pattern and physical activity.[50,51] In addition, high insulin levels induce downregulation of *MBOAT7*, and in the case of insulin resistance, this process promotes hepatic lipogenesis and steatosis, particularly in carriers of genetic risk variants.[22]

PNPLA3 offers the clearest example of the effect of gene–gene interaction in NAFLD pathogenesis.

An overview of the interaction between genetic and acquired factors involved in the development and progression of NAFLD is shown in Figure 3.2.

3.5 CLINICAL APPLICATIONS: PRECISION MEDICINE

The main focus of precision medicine is the individualized management of the disease from disease screening to follow-up strategy and treatment. Genetic predisposition has been often called upon for the development of a personalized health care approach.

Mendelian randomization studies that exploited as instruments the genetic risk variants for NAFLD just presented have provided data supporting the notion that hepatic fat accumulation is not an innocent bystander but a key driver of progressive liver disease, fibrosis and HCC.

Importantly, NAFLD-HCC develops in almost a half of noncirrhotic patients.[52] Identifying patients who may benefit from cost-effective surveillance program therefore remains a major challenge, and noninvasive tools able to discriminate individuals at risk of liver disease progression are urgently needed. A precision medicine approach using the knowledge emerging from human genomics partly meets this need. Although the genotyping of a risk variant is a relatively simple and cheap investigation, no single SNP permits an adequate risk stratification in complex traits, and the use of single variants (e.g., the variant with the higher impact in the natural history of the disease, *PNPLA3*[10]) for this purpose is not sufficiently accurate.[53] However, larger panels of genetic determinants included in polygenic risk scores (PRSs) could be a sensible approach.

PRSs capture the individual's genetic predisposition to develop a trait or an associated outcome and are calculated by summing the number of trait-associated alleles carried by an individual, which can be weighted by their effect size on the trait.[54] Contrary to imaging, circulating biomarkers or other favoring comorbidities that represent a punctual assessment of disease predisposition, PRSs capture the potential to develop the outcome during the whole lifetime in the presence of triggering factors and may be used for screening purposes, especially in younger individuals and for conditions amenable to treatment.

In the case of NAFLD, evidence supporting the possible utility of PRS is emerging. However, the diagnostic accuracy and the prognostic performance of these tools should be established in larger and prospective cohorts.

Weighted PRS combining genetic loci, previously associated with liver damage, oxidative stress and fibrogenesis, and common steatogenic risk variants, predict NAFLD and the full spectrum of liver damage in children and adults.[55] This is particularly relevant when HCC risk has to be evaluated. Slightly less than one NAFLD patient in two develops HCC in a noncirrhotic liver, and surveillance is not recommended in the absence of liver cirrhosis, resulting in a delayed diagnosis and the worsening of prognosis due to limited treatment options. Thus PRSs based on genetic variants associated with NAFLD-HCC onset may be useful tools to improve the stratification of the risk. Some weighted and unweighted scores suitable for this purpose have already been proposed,[56,57] and including common and rare variants identified by NGS in a model of acquired clinical factors may improve the ability to discriminate the disease and correctly reclassify a considerable number of patients.[20]

There is still a lack of drug therapies approved for NAFLD. Recent genetic discoveries may assist in identifying molecular pathways that predispose to the disease and in targeting variant proteins that play a role in the development of progressive NAFLD in subsets of patients with distinct disease genetics and pathophysiology. Besides, this approach has been successfully used in some forms of cancer. Although now there is consistent evidence about the robust correlation between common genetic variants and NAFLD, knowledge about the implicated metabolic, epigenetic and biological mechanisms is still uneven.[58]

3.6 CONCLUSION

Human genetics offers a privileged point of view on NAFLD. Identification of common and rare genetic risk variants has strengthened the understanding of the mechanisms at the base of the heterogeneous presentation of the disease. Furthermore, it has spurred the study of several pathogenic pathways implicated in hepatic fat accumulation, inflammation, fibrogenesis and carcinogenesis. This knowledge may eventually impact on clinical practice, through enabling a medicine approach based on improved individual risk stratification and the development of targeted therapies.

REFERENCES

1. Eslam M, Valenti L, Romeo S. Genetics and epigenetics of NAFLD and NASH: Clinical impact. *J Hepatol.* 2018;68(2):268–279. http://doi.org/10.1016/j.jhep.2017.09.003

2. Loomba R, Rao F, Zhang L, et al. Genetic covariance between γ-glutamyl transpeptidase and fatty liver risk factors: Role of β2-adrenergic receptor genetic variation in twins. *Gastroenterology.* 2010;139(3):836–845.e1. http://doi.org/10.1053/j.gastro.2010.06.009

3. Makkonen J, Pietiläinen KH, Rissanen A, Kaprio J, Yki-Järvinen H. Genetic factors contribute to variation in serum alanine aminotransferase activity independent of obesity and alcohol: A study in monozygotic and dizygotic twins. *J Hepatol.* 2009;50(5):1035–1042. http://doi.org/10.1016/j.jhep.2008.12.025

4. Loomba R, Schork N, Chen CH, et al. Heritability of hepatic fibrosis and steatosis based on a prospective twin study. *Gastroenterology.* 2015;149(7):1784–1793. http://doi.org/10.1053/j.gastro.2015.08.011

5. Long MT, Gurary EB, Massaro JM, et al. Parental non-alcoholic fatty liver disease increases risk of non-alcoholic fatty liver disease in offspring. *Liver Int.* 2019;39(4):740–747. http://doi.org/10.1111/liv.13956

6. Guerrero R, Vega GL, Grundy SM, Browning JD. Ethnic differences in hepatic steatosis: An insulin resistance paradox? *Hepatology.* 2009;49(3):791–801. http://doi.org/10.1002/hep.22726

7. Romeo S, Kozlitina J, Xing C, et al. Genetic variation in PNPLA3 confers susceptibility to nonalcoholic fatty liver disease. *Nat Genet.* 2008;40(12):1461–1465. http://doi.org/10.1038/ng.257

8. Valenti L, Al-Serri A, Daly AK, et al. Homozygosity for the patatin-like phospholipase-3/adiponutrin i148m polymorphism influences liver fibrosis in patients with nonalcoholic fatty liver disease. *Hepatology.* 2010;51(4):1209–1217. http://doi.org/10.1002/hep.23622

9. Liu YL, Patman GL, Leathart JBS, et al. Carriage of the PNPLA3 rs738409 C >g polymorphism confers an increased risk of non-alcoholic fatty liver disease associated hepatocellular carcinoma. *J Hepatol.* 2014;61(1):75–81. http://doi.org/10.1016/j.jhep.2014.02.030

10. Jamialahmadi O, Bianco C, Pelusi S, Romeo S, Valenti L. Reply to: Polygenic risk score: A promising predictor for hepatocellular carcinoma in the population with non-alcoholic fatty liver disease. *J Hepatol.* 2021;74(6):1494-1496. http://doi.org/10.1016/j.jhep.2021.02.030

11. Trépo E, Romeo S, Zucman-Rossi J, Nahon P. PNPLA3 gene in liver diseases. *J Hepatol.* 2016;65(2):399–412. http://doi.org/10.1016/j.jhep.2016.03.011

12. Cherubini A, Casirati E, Tomasi M, Valenti L. PNPLA3 as a therapeutic target for fatty liver disease: The evidence to date. *Expert Opin Ther Targets.* 2021;25(12):1033–1043. http://doi.org/10.1080/14728222.2021.2018418

13. Stender S, Kozlitina J, Nordestgaard BG, Tybjærg-Hansen A, Hobbs HH, Cohen JC. Adiposity amplifies the genetic risk of fatty liver disease conferred by multiple loci. *Nat Genet.* 2017;49(6):842–847. http://doi.org/10.1038/ng.3855

14. Kozlitina J, Smagris E, Stender S, et al. Exome-wide association study identifies a TM6SF2 variant that confers susceptibility to nonalcoholic fatty liver disease. *Nat Genet.* 2014;46(4):352–356. http://doi.org/10.1038/ng.2901

15. Dongiovanni P, Petta S, Maglio C, et al. Transmembrane 6 superfamily member 2 gene variant disentangles nonalcoholic steatohepatitis from cardiovascular disease. *Hepatology.* 2015;61(2):506–514. http://doi.org/10.1002/hep.27490

16. Luo F, Oldoni F, Das A. TM6SF2: A novel genetic player in nonalcoholic fatty liver and cardiovascular disease. *Hepatol Commun.* 2022;6(3):448–460. http://doi.org/10.1002/hep4.1822

17. Prill S, Caddeo A, Baselli G, et al. The TM6SF2 E167K genetic variant induces lipid biosynthesis and reduces apolipoprotein B secretion in human hepatic 3D spheroids. *Sci Rep.* 2019;9(1):1–12. http://doi.org/10.1038/s41598-019-47737-w

18. Teo K, Abeysekera KWM, Adams L, et al. rs641738C>T near MBOAT7 is associated with liver fat, ALT and fibrosis in NAFLD: A meta-analysis. *J Hepatol.* 2021;74(1):20–30. http://doi.org/10.1016/j.jhep.2020.08.027

19. Donati B, Dongiovanni P, Romeo S, et al. MBOAT7 rs641738 variant and hepatocellular carcinoma in non-cirrhotic individuals. *Sci Rep.* 2017;7(1):4492. http://doi.org/10.1038/s41598-017-04991-0

20. Pelusi S, Baselli G, Pietrelli A, et al. Rare pathogenic variants predispose to hepatocellular carcinoma in nonalcoholic fatty liver disease. *Sci Rep*. 2019;9(1):1–10. http://doi.org/10.1038/s41598-019-39998-2

21. Matsuda S, Inoue T, Lee HC, et al. Member of the membrane-bound O-acyltransferase (MBOAT) family encodes a lysophospholipid acyltransferase with broad substrate specificity. *Genes to Cells*. 2008;13(8):879–888. http://doi.org/10.1111/j.1365-2443.2008.01212.x

22. Bianco C, Casirati E, Malvestiti F, Valenti L. Genetic predisposition similarities between NASH and ASH: Identification of new therapeutic targets. *JHEP Reports*. 2021;3(3):100284. http://doi.org/10.1016/j.jhep.2021.100284

23. Meroni M, Dongiovanni P, Longo M, et al. Mboat7 down-regulation by hyper-insulinemia induces fat accumulation in hepatocytes: Mboat7 reduction and hepatic steatosis. *EBioMedicine*. 2020;52:102658. http://doi.org/10.1016/j.ebiom.2020.102658

24. Thangapandi VR, Knittelfelder O, Brosch M, et al. Loss of hepatic Mboat7 leads to liver fibrosis. *Gut*. 2020;70(5):940–950. http://doi.org/10.1136/gutjnl-2020-320853

25. Martin K, Hatab A, Athwal VS, Jokl E, Piper Hanley K. Genetic contribution to non-alcoholic fatty liver disease and prognostic implications. *Curr Diab Rep*. 2021;21(3):8. http://doi.org/10.1007/s11892-021-01377-5

26. Beer NL, Tribble ND, McCulloch LJ, et al. The P446L variant in GCKR associated with fasting plasma glucose and triglyceride levels exerts its effect through increased glucokinase activity in liver. *Hum Mol Genet*. 2009;18(21):4081–4088. http://doi.org/10.1093/hmg/ddp357

27. Speliotes EK, Yerges-Armstrong LM, Wu J, et al. Genome-wide association analysis identifies variants associated with nonalcoholic fatty liver disease that have distinct effects on metabolic traits. McCarthy MI, ed. *PLoS Genet*. 2011;7(3):e1001324. http://doi.org/10.1371/journal.pgen.1001324

28. Abul-Husn NS, Cheng X, Li AH, et al. A protein-truncating HSD17B13 variant and protection from chronic liver disease. *N Engl J Med*. 2018;378(12):1096–1106. http://doi.org/10.1056/NEJMoa1712191

29. Ma Y, Belyaeva OV, Brown PM, et al. 17-Beta hydroxysteroid dehydrogenase 13 is a hepatic retinol dehydrogenase associated with histological features of nonalcoholic fatty liver disease. *Hepatology*. 2019;69(4):1504–1519. http://doi.org/10.1002/hep.30350

30. Dongiovanni P, Meroni M, Mancina RM, et al. Protein phosphatase 1 regulatory subunit 3B gene variation protects against hepatic fat accumulation and fibrosis in individuals at high risk of nonalcoholic fatty liver disease. *Hepatol Commun*. 2018;2(6):666–675. http://doi.org/10.1002/hep4.1192

31. Petta S, Valenti L, Tuttolomondo A, et al. Interferon lambda 4 rs368234815 TT>δG variant is associated with liver damage in patients with nonalcoholic fatty liver disease. *Hepatology*. 2017;66(6):1885–1893. http://doi.org/10.1002/hep.29395

32. Petta S, Valenti L, Marra F, et al. MERTK rs4374383 polymorphism affects the severity of fibrosis in non-alcoholic fatty liver disease. *J Hepatol*. 2016;64(3):682–690. http://doi.org/10.1016/j.jhep.2015.10.016

33. Dongiovanni P, Meroni M, Baselli G, et al. PCSK7 gene variation bridges atherogenic dyslipidemia with hepatic inflammation in NAFLD patients. *J Lipid Res*. 2019;60(6):1144–1153. http://doi.org/10.1194/jlr.P090449

34. Fares R, Petta S, Lombardi R, et al. The UCP2–866 G>A promoter region polymorphism is associated with non-alcoholic steatohepatitis. *Liver Int*. 2015;35(5):1574–1580. http://doi.org/10.1111/liv.12707

35. Al-Serri A, Anstee QM, Valenti L, et al. The SOD2 C47T polymorphism influences NAFLD fibrosis severity: Evidence from case-control and intra-familial allele association studies. *J Hepatol*. 2012;56(2):448–454. http://doi.org/10.1016/j.jhep.2011.05.029

36. Luukkonen PK, Juuti A, Sammalkorpi H, et al. MARC1 variant rs2642438 increases hepatic phosphatidylcholines and decreases severity of non-alcoholic fatty liver disease in humans. *J Hepatol*. 2020;73(3):725–726. http://doi.org/10.1016/j.jhep.2020.04.021

37. Jamialahmadi O, Mancina RM, Ciociola E, et al. Exome-wide association study on alanine aminotransferase identifies sequence variants in the GPAM and APOE associated with fatty liver disease. *Gastroenterology*. 2021;160(5):1634–1646.e7.

38. Anstee QM, Darlay R, Cockell S, et al. Genome-wide association study of non-alcoholic fatty liver and steatohepatitis in a histologically characterised cohort☆. *J Hepatol*. 2020;73(3):505–515. http://doi.org/10.1016/j.jhep.2020.04.003

39. Valenti L, Canavesi E, Galmozzi E, et al. Beta-globin mutations are associated with parenchymal siderosis and fibrosis in patients with non-alcoholic fatty liver disease. *J Hepatol*. 2010;53(5):927–933. http://doi.org/10.1016/j.jhep.2010.05.023

40. Corradini E, Buzzetti E, Dongiovanni P, et al. Ceruloplasmin gene variants are associated with hyperferritinemia and increased liver iron in patients with NAFLD. *J Hepatol*. 2021;75(3):506–513. http://doi.org/10.1016/j.jhep.2021.03.014

41. Hamesch K, Mandorfer M, Pereira VM, et al. Liver fibrosis and metabolic alterations in adults with alpha-1-antitrypsin deficiency caused by the Pi*ZZ mutation. *Gastroenterology*. 2019;157(3):705–719.e18. http://doi.org/10.1053/j.gastro.2019.05.013

42. Di Filippo M, Moulin P, Roy P, et al. Homozygous MTTP and APOB mutations may lead to hepatic steatosis and fibrosis despite metabolic differences in congenital hypocholesterolemia. *J Hepatol*. 2014;61(4):891–902. http://doi.org/10.1016/j.jhep.2014.05.023

43. Carter A, Brackley SM, Gao J, Mann JP. The global prevalence and genetic spectrum of lysosomal acid lipase deficiency: A rare condition that mimics NAFLD. *J Hepatol*. 2019;70(1):142–150. http://doi.org/10.1016/j.jhep.2018.09.028

44. Hartmann D, Srivastava U, Thaler M, et al. Telomerase gene mutations are associated with cirrhosis formation. *Hepatology*. 2011;53(5):1608–1617. http://doi.org/10.1002/hep.24217

45. Donati B, Pietrelli A, Pingitore P, et al. Telomerase reverse transcriptase germline mutations and hepatocellular carcinoma in patients with nonalcoholic fatty liver disease. *Cancer Med*. 2017;6(8):1930–1940. http://doi.org/10.1002/cam4.1078

46. Baselli G, Jamialahmadi O, Pelusi S, et al. Rare ATG7 genetic variants predispose patients to severe fatty liver disease. *J Hepatol*. 2022; 77(3):596-606.

47. Valenti L, Bugianesi E, Pajvani U, Targher G. Nonalcoholic fatty liver disease: Cause or consequence of type 2 diabetes? *Liver Int*. 2016;36(11):1563–1579. http://doi.org/10.1111/liv.13185

48. Dongiovanni P, Stender S, Pietrelli A, et al. Causal relationship of hepatic fat with liver damage and insulin resistance in nonalcoholic fatty liver. *J Intern Med*. 2018;283(4):356–370. http://doi.org/10.1111/joim.12719

49. Barata L, Feitosa MF, Bielak LF, et al. Insulin resistance exacerbates genetic predisposition to nonalcoholic fatty liver disease in individuals without diabetes. *Hepatol Commun*. 2019;3(7):hep4.1353. http://doi.org/10.1002/hep4.1353

50. Nobili V, Liccardo D, Bedogni G, et al. Influence of dietary pattern, physical activity, and I148M PNPLA3 on steatosis severity in at-risk adolescents. *Genes Nutr*. 2014;9(3). http://doi.org/10.1007/s12263-014-0392-8

51. Ma J, Hennein R, Liu C, et al. Improved diet quality associates with reduction in liver fat, particularly in individuals with high genetic risk scores for nonalcoholic fatty liver disease. *Gastroenterology*. 2018;155(1):107–117. http://doi.org/10.1053/j.gastro.2018.03.038

52. Piscaglia F, Svegliati-Baroni G, Barchetti A, et al. Clinical patterns of hepatocellular carcinoma in nonalcoholic fatty liver disease: A multicenter prospective study. *Hepatology*. 2016;63(3):827–838. http://doi.org/10.1002/hep.28368

53. EASL–EASD–EASO Clinical Practice Guidelines for the management of non-alcoholic fatty liver disease. *J Hepatol*. 2016;64(6):1388–1402. http://doi.org/10.1016/j.jhep.2015.11.004

54. Wand H, Lambert SA, Tamburro C, et al. Improving reporting standards for polygenic scores in risk prediction studies. *Nature*. 2021;591(7849):211–219. http://doi.org/10.1038/s41586-021-03243-6

55. Bianco C, Tavaglione F, Romeo S, Valenti L. Genetic risk scores and personalization of care in fatty liver disease. *Curr Opin Pharmacol*. 2021;61:6–11. http://doi.org/10.1016/j.coph.2021.08.014

56. Gellert-Kristensen H, Richardson TG, Davey Smith G, Nordestgaard BG, Tybjærg-Hansen A, Stender S. Combined effect of PNPLA3, TM6SF2, and HSD17B13 variants on risk of cirrhosis and hepatocellular carcinoma in the general population. *Hepatology*. 2020;72(3):845–856. http://doi.org/10.1002/hep.31238

57. Bianco C, Jamialahmadi O, Pelusi S, et al. Non-invasive stratification of hepatocellular carcinoma risk in non-alcoholic fatty liver using polygenic risk scores. *J Hepatol*. 2021;74(4):775–782. http://doi.org/10.1016/j.jhep.2020.11.024

58. Sookoian S, Pirola CJ. Precision medicine in non-alcoholic fatty liver disease: New therapeutic insights from genetics and systems biology. *Clin Mol Hepatol*. 2020;26(4):461–475. http://doi.org/10.3350/cmh.2020.0136

4 Mechanisms of Hepatocyte Injury and Inflammation in NAFLD

Gopanandan Parthasarathy and Harmeet Malhi

CONTENTS

Key Points

- Bioactive and signaling lipids, such as saturated fatty acids, cholesterol and sphingolipids are hepatotoxic by activating organelle stress responses and proapoptotic signaling.

- Hepatocyte injury and death activate a cascade of inflammatory and reparative responses such as inflammasome activation, release of soluble mediators such as cytokines and secretion of extracellular vesicles.

- Genetic variants that influence lipid droplet dynamics and lipid metabolism modulate human NASH—for example, variants in PNPLA3, TM6SF or MBOAT7 exacerbate, while HSD17B13 modulates liver injury.

- The liver is rich in immune cells, and a complex network of immune-mediated liver injury is described in NASH. Innate immune cells such as macrophages are particularly important and mediate crosstalk with hepatocytes, other immune cells and stellate cells, thus amplifying inflammation, fibrosis and carcinogenesis.

- NASH occurs in the context of disordered organismal metabolism and inflammation, in that the liver communicates with the gut and adipose tissue in the form of metabolites, PAMPs, DAMPs, extracellular vesicles and immune cells, which create feed-forward loops of metabolic dysregulation and chronic inflammation.

4.1 INTRODUCTION

The existing definitions of nonalcoholic fatty liver (NAFL) and nonalcoholic steatohepatitis (NASH) rely on hepatocellular injury and inflammation as defining features. The focus of this chapter is the mechanisms that lead to injury and inflammation. Steatosis (discussed in other chapters) is largely dependent on increased delivery of free fatty acids (FFA) to the liver due to enhanced adipose tissue lipolysis in insulin resistance (IR), diet-derived FFA and de novo lipogenesis, which is in part driven by dietary sugars[1].

Mechanistic insights in NASH have been obtained from cellular and animal model systems (Figure 4.1) with correlative studies in human liver samples. These studies have demonstrated the key role of ectopically accumulated lipids in activating cell death pathways and organelle stress, whether mitochondrial, endoplasmic reticulum (ER) or lysosomal stress. It is also clear from accumulated data and unsurprising given the complex immune composition of the liver, that hepatocyte–immune cell crosstalk plays an important role in the sterile inflammatory response associated with NASH. The immune response in the liver is further modified by interorgan crosstalk, such as gut–liver and adipose tissue–liver crosstalk. In this chapter, we provide a synopsis of these injury and inflammation pathways.

4.2 LIPOTOXICITY

The concept of lipotoxicity was introduced in the context of the obesity-associated type 2 diabetes mellitus and rapidly expanded to the liver with the recognition that several lipid classes, including saturated FFA, lysophosphatidyl cholines (LPCs), cholesterol and sphingolipids (ceramides and sphingosine 1-phosphate, S1P) were deleterious in NASH by inducing organelle stress and activating cell death pathways[2]. The saturated FFA, palmitate (Figure 4.2) and stearate, are directly toxic to hepatocytes via activation of proapoptotic signaling[3]. Monounsaturated fatty acids (MUFA) such as oleate and palmitoleate are not directly toxic and may mitigate the toxicity of saturated FFA by increasing their partitioning into neutral triglycerides[3]. In fact, knockout (-/-) of stearoyl-CA desaturase-1 (SCD1) decreased hepatocyte steatosis but increased SFA-induced apoptosis, injury and inflammation[4]. Palmitate can drive the generation of LPC by phospholipase A2 and ceramides via de novo synthesis, thus it can be toxic directly or via lipid intermediaries[5,6]. LPC and ceramides can be generated by additional pathways, lecithin cholesterol acyltransferase and sphingolipid salvage pathway, respectively, which may also contribute to lipotoxicity. This interconnectedness of lipids may also explain why many of the same mechanistic pathways are activated by bioactive lipids. Crystals of free cholesterol, a distinct lipid class, are detected in patients with fibrosing NASH, and cholesterol content of mouse diets correlates with the fibrogenic potential of specific diets, suggesting a role for cholesterol toxicity in progressive NASH[7].

DOI: 10.1201/9781003386698-5

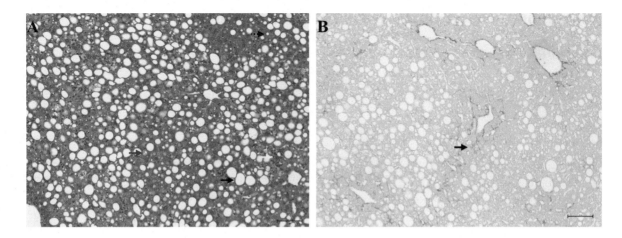

Figure 4.1 Mouse models recapitulate NASH histology

Representative images from liver sections from a mouse model of diet-induced NASH stained with hematoxylin and eosin (panel A) and picro-sirius red (panel B). (A) The arrows denote the features of NASH: macrovesicular steatosis (solid black arrow), microvesicular steatosis (dashed black arrow), ballooned hepatocyte (blue arrow), lobular inflammation (yellow arrow). (B) Pericellular fibrosis (solid black arrow).

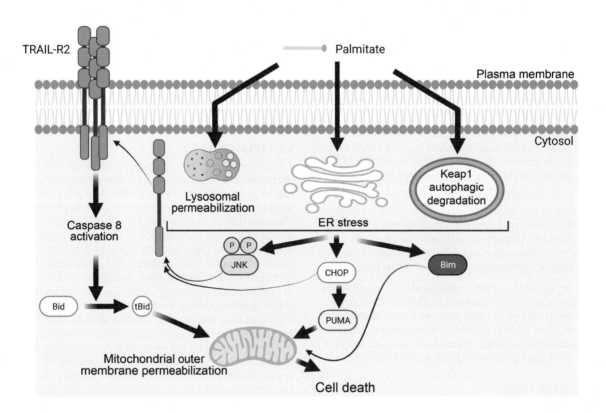

Figure 4.2 Palmitate activates the intrinsic and extrinsic apoptosis pathways in hepatocytes (This figure was created with BioRender.com.)

Excess palmitate activates organelle stress in many forms including lysosomal permeabilization, endoplasmic reticulum (ER) stress, and autophagic degradation of Kelch-like ECH-associated protein 1 (Keap1). These processes lead to the activation of c-jun N-terminal kinase (JNK), induction of C/EBP homologous protein (CHOP) and upregulation of proapoptotic proteins PUMA and Bim (intrinsic pathway), leading to mitochondrial outer membrane permeabilization (MOMP). JNK and CHOP also lead to the transcriptional upregulation of TRAIL-R2. Ligand independent oligomerization of TRAIL-R2 activates caspase 8 leading to the cleavage of Bid to tBid (extrinsic pathway) and MOMP.

SFAs and LPC activate proapoptotic signaling in hepatocytes via the mixed lineage kinase 3, c-Jun N-terminal kinase (JNK), and ER stress-induced induction of the proapoptotic transcription factor, C/EBP homologous protein (CHOP)[2,3,8]. These stress kinase and ER stress-induced pathways converge on mitochondria, and, indeed, SFAs shift the balance of proapoptotic and antiapoptotic Bcl-2 family proteins toward cell death, by increasing the expression of PUMA and Bim and inhibiting Mcl-1. Epigenetic mechanisms also regulate sensitivity to apoptosis as demonstrated by the microRNA, miR-296–5p, which inhibits the expression of PUMA and is inversely related to PUMA mRNA levels in NASH liver biopsies. Activation of autophagic degradation of Kelch-like ECH-associated protein 1 (Keap1) also contributes to an increase in the levels of PUMA and Bim with sensitization to apoptosis. Bim is also upregulated by phosphatase-driven dephosphorylation and activation of the transcription factor, FOXO3a in palmitate-treated hepatocytes. SFAs also induced the expression of death receptors and sensitize hepatocytes to death receptor-induced apoptosis. Palmitate induces the upregulation of the death receptor, TRAIL-R2, and leads to clustering and ligand-independent activation of TRAIL-R2 by changing the organization of its plasma membrane domains. Increased membrane rigidity in SFA-treated hepatocytes is also implicated in organelle stress, such as lipotoxic activation of the unfolded protein response sensors, IRE1α and PERK. Recent studies have demonstrated that hepatocytes release proinflammatory extracellular vesicles with distinct signaling cargoes as a response to lipotoxic endoplasmic reticulum stress[9].

Changes in membrane fluidity are also impacted by cholesterol[2,7]. In hepatocytes, increased accumulation of cholesterol in intracellular membranes leads to increased membrane rigidity and organelle stress. Impaired activity of sarcoplasmic-endoplasmic reticulum calcium ATPase by increases in ER membrane cholesterol content lead to ER stress and activation of the unfolded protein response. A reduction in mitochondrial 2-oxoglutarate carrier function due to increases in mitochondrial membrane cholesterol result in mitochondrial glutathione depletion. In macrophages, the accumulation of free cholesterol may activate the inflammasome (discussed later in the chapter). Ceramides are mechanistically linked to the development of IR. In addition, sphingosine 1-phosphate (S1P) is proinflammatory in the liver by recruiting monocyte-derived macrophages into the liver. Inhibitors of S1P receptors, such as FTY720, demonstrate a reduction in liver injury and inflammation in preclinical models[10].

Thus, many bioactive lipid species are directly or indirectly deleterious to the liver by activating cellular stress responses, activating inflammatory pathways or leading to cell death[3]. Mouse models that are deficient in pathways activated by lipotoxic signaling demonstrate attenuated NASH, such as mice deficient in the death receptor, TRAIL-R2, hepatocyte caspase 8 deficient or Bid silenced mice[11]. Markers of apoptosis such as apoptotic hepatocytes, cleaved caspases and death receptors are elevated in NASH human liver samples. Readouts of lipotoxic pathways may also serve as disease biomarkers in NASH. In this regard, hepatocyte-derived extracellular vesicles, the S1P content of extracellular vesicles and the caspase cleaved fragment of cytokeratin 18 (CK18 M30) have demonstrated utility in tracking NASH activity[12]. Lastly, several therapeutic agents that target various aspects of lipid homeostasis are in development. These include inhibitors of acetyl coenzyme A carboxylase mediated de novo lipogenesis, diacylglycerol transferase which catalyzes triglyceride synthesis, agonists of PPARs which modulate lipid utilization and flux, and FXR agonists which regulate lipid metabolism[13].

4.3 INFLAMMASOME ACTIVATION

Inflammasomes are cytosolic multiprotein complexes assembled downstream of pathogen-associated molecular patterns (PAMPs) and damage-associated molecular patterns (DAMP) binding to their respective pattern recognition receptors (PRRs). The canonical inflammasomes are multiprotein complexes containing PRRs such as NOD-like receptor (NLR) family members (NLRP1, NLRP3 and NLRC4), procaspase 1 and the adaptor apoptosis-associated speck-like protein containing a caspase recruitment domain (ASC). Downstream of PAMPs binding to toll-like receptors (TLRs), in a process called priming, the activation of the transcription factor nuclear factor κB (NF-κB) leads to production of cytokine precursors prointerleukin (IL)-1β and pro-IL-18. Proteolytic cleavage of procaspase 1 in the inflammasome generates caspase-1, which in turn is necessary for the proteolytic cleavage of these precursors into interleukin (IL)-1β and IL-18. Caspase 1 activation also leads to an inflammatory cell death, termed "pyroptosis," via cleavage-mediated activation of the membrane pore-forming protein gasdermin D (GSDMD). Association of the inflammasome component NLRP3 with the metabolic syndrome is well established in various cell types in the liver and adipose tissue[14]. In liver biopsies from patients with NAFLD, elevated mRNA levels of NLRP3 components and GSDMD expression were correlated with NASH severity[15,16]. Experimental evidence in mouse models of NASH described lipotoxicity-induced upregulation of NLRP3 inflammasome components at the transcriptional but not protein level. Conversely, in mice lacking NLRP3, ASC and caspase 1–inflammasome components, diet-induced NASH was attenuated[17]. NLRP3 and NLRP6 inflammasome deficiency in mice led to altered gut microbiota composition and greater influx of TLR4 and TLR9 agonists into the portal circulation, thus worsening NASH[18]. In NASH mice, both hepatic and macrophage AIM2 expression was increased, mediated by increased TLR9 ligands[19].

Ligands implicated in inflammasome activation include palmitate via TLR2, extracellular ATP via its cell membrane receptor–purinergic 2X7 receptor (P2X7R), cholesterol crystals, bile acids via their surface receptor TGR5 or their nuclear receptor FXR, ER stress, mitochondrial oxidative stress and mitochondrial DNA[19-22]. Conceivably, several approaches to target inflammasomes as therapeutic intervention in NASH have been attempted. Sulforaphane, a small molecule inhibitor of NLRP3 inflammasome activation attenuated diet-induced murine NASH[23]. Similarly, a P2RX7 inhibitor attenuated liver inflammation and fibrosis in a nonhuman primate model of NASH[22]. Thus inflammasome activation represents a crucial pathway in the pathogenesis of NASH and provides a link between cell death and inflammation. Further exploration of therapeutic targeting of the inflammasome in a cell type-specific manner is warranted.

4.4 GENETIC MODIFIERS OF LIPOTOXICITY

NASH pathogenesis involves a complex interplay of genetic and environmental factors. In the context of hepatocyte injury and liver inflammation, the functional mechanistic contribution for how the genetic variants may increase risk for liver injury or inflammation is known for a few of the many genetic risk factors. The patatin-like phospholipase domain-containing 3 (*PNPLA3*) gene encodes a protein associated with lipid droplets and has lipase activity. PNPLA3 I148M variant increases steatosis, fibrosis and HCC risk[24]. Lipotoxicity may be increased due to the I148M variant as it can inhibit the activity of adipose tissue triglyceride lipase. The TM6SF E167K variant impairs VLDL lipidation with accumulation of triglyceride and potentially other toxic lipids in the liver[25]. Glucokinase regulator (*GCKR*) P446L variant is a loss of function variant in which the ability to inhibit glucokinase is lost with an increase in de novo lipogenesis leading to increased hepatic steatosis. A genetic variant near membrane bound O-acyltransferase domain containing 7 (*MBOAT7*) is also associated with hepatic steatosis and fibrosis[26]. On the other hand, hydroxysteroid 17-beta dehydrogenase 13 (*HSD17B13*) loss-of-function variants (rs143404524 and rs72613567) are associated with a reduction in liver injury, suggesting that silencing or inhibiting HSD17B13 may be a potential therapeutic strategy for NASH[27]. While many of the reported variants are lipid droplet-associated proteins or impact lipid flux in the liver, it is not known whether these variants directly impact known toxic lipid mediators or shift lipid accumulation or flux to less harmful lipids. The variants could also, at a cellular level, shift the compartmental distribution of lipids, another potential area for future studies.

4.5 CROSSTALK WITH IMMUNE CELLS

The liver contains many innate and adaptive immune cells that uniquely interface with the cellular compartments of the liver due to the microanatomical architecture of hepatic sinusoids. Two-thirds of hepatic blood supply is from the portal circulation; the immune-cell rich hepatic microenvironment serves as a crucial immunologic firewall against gut-derived signals, including pathogens, PAMPs and DAMPs in both health and disease.

Long-liver resident cells include Kupffer cells (KCs), CD8+ tissue resident memory T (T$_{RM}$) cells and type 1 innate lymphoid cells (ILC1s), but other cell types circulate through the liver and serve a patrolling role, including natural killer (NK) cells, γδ T cells, CD4+ and CD8+ αβ T cells, monocytes, B cells, invariant NKT (iNKT) cells, mucosal-associated invariant T (MAIT) cells and dendritic cells (DCs). Intrahepatic blood flow in the portal to central direction constructs a gradient of nutrients, oxygen, gut derivatives, and, in response to these, a zonation of immune cells. Mechanistically, because of hepatocyte lipotoxicity and apoptosis, release of soluble mediators such as the DAMP, high-mobility group box 1 (HMGB1), FFA, PAMPs, and extracellular vesicles leads to recruitment and inflammatory activation of circulating immune cells (Figure 4.3). Subsequently, immune cells directly promote inflammation by secreting inflammatory cytokines including tumor necrosis factor-alpha and IL-1β but also promote a feed-forward loop of inciting hepatocyte injury, death, and further activation of other immune cells. Lastly, immune-mediated activation of hepatic stellate cells (HSCs) promotes fibrogenesis in NASH[28]. Alternatively, injury resolution models demonstrate that immune cells are also key for the termination of inflammation, regression of fibrosis and hepatocyte regeneration. Given the multicellular and context-specific roles of immune cells in NASH, we do not yet have an integrated understanding of the intrahepatic crosstalk, including spatiotemporal aspects and mechanistic insights; however, rapid advances

in single-cell multiomics and spatial analytics are expected to revolutionize our understanding of this crosstalk.

4.5.1 Macrophages

Macrophages are the most abundant immune cell type in the liver and can be classified into resident embryonic yolk sac-derived KCs and recruited bone marrow-derived macrophages (BMDMs), both of which are capable of self-renewal[29]. They have been extensively studied as a driver of NASH pathogenesis in human disease as well as animal models. In NASH, a lipotoxic environment impairs the survival and self-renewal of KCs[30], and this niche is repopulated by BMDMs, which do not fully recapitulate homeostatic KC functions and are considered more proinflammatory. The resulting intrahepatic macrophage population is heterogeneous, and many subsets have been characterized, including premonocyte-derived KCs, monocyte-derived KCs and hepatic lipid-associated macrophages (LAMs)[31]. LAMs are characterized by *Trem2* and *Cd9* expression, enriched in fibrotic zones, and possess differential lipid handling capabilities. A similar NASH-associated macrophage (NAM) subset has also been described, reminiscent of LAMs in adipose tissue[31], as well as scar-associated macrophages (SAM) in fibrotic human livers[31]. Microanatomical niche-derived signals that epigenetically educate macrophage identity and function have been described, for example reprogramming of liver X receptor (LXR) functions is implicated in promoting the *Trem2*+ macrophage phenotype[31]. Other examples implicated in macrophage activation include the transmembrane protein 173 (TMEM173 or STING) pathway[32], toll-like receptor 4 (TLR4)[33] and extracellular vesicles that mediate monocyte adhesion and recruitment[34]. Macrophages play a role in various stages of NASH by directly amplifying (1) steatosis by secretion of IL-1β, (2) inflammation by chemokines and cytokines, including tumor necrosis factor alpha (TNF-α) and IL-1β, (3) monocyte recruitment by chemokines such as CCL2[35], and (4) fibrosis by activating hepatic stellate cells[31].

4.5.2 Dendritic Cells

Dendritic cells are recognized for their role in inducing the innate immune system by presenting antigens to and inflammatory reprogramming of T cells, but they can also directly participate in the inflammatory response, downstream of pattern recognition receptors. Although dendritic cells represent a relatively rare population in the liver, constituting less than 5% of immune cells, all 3 subsets, plasmacytoid (pDCs) and conventional (cDC1 and 2), have been associated with NASH but with differential effects on NASH pathogenesis. Human transcriptomic study suggested that cDC2 correlated with NASH severity while cDC1 were protective in NASH[36], and, indeed, mice genetically deficient in cDC1 had worse diet-induced NASH[37]. In a recent study, XCR1+ cDC1s were increased in number in the blood and liver from patients with NASH, due to enhanced proliferation in the bone marrow. Mechanistically, analysis of DC–T cell pairs in liver-draining lymph nodes demonstrated cDCs potentiate CD8 T cell activation in NASH[38].

4.5.3 T Cells

During homeostasis, conventional T cells, including CD4+ and, more commonly, CD8+ αβ T cells, perform immune surveillance, along with a subset of liver-resident/memory CD8+ T cells. Influenced by innate immune cells and the

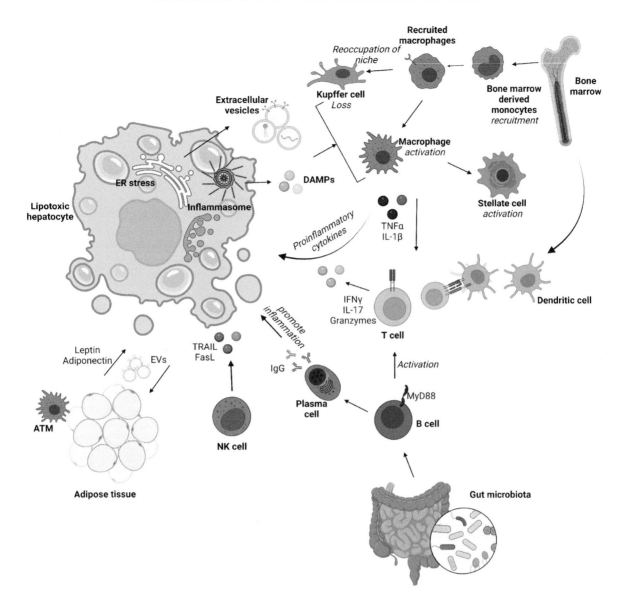

Figure 4.3 Liver-immune cell crosstalk mediates NASH (This figure was created with BioRender.com.)

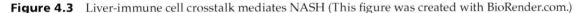

Signals released from lipotoxic hepatocytes in the form of extracellular vesicles (EVs) or damage-associated molecular patterns (DAMPs) recruit various bone marrow-derived immune cells. For example, loss of resident Kupffer cells is followed by reoccupation of the liver macrophage niche by bone marrow-derived monocytes. These cells release proinflammatory cytokines, such as TNFα, IL-1, mediate further hepatocellular injury directly and by crosstalk with other immune cells such as T cells, and activate stellate cells leading to fibrosis. Further, adipose tissue-derived adipokines or gut microbiota-derived products, respectively, lead to activation of intrahepatic proinflammatory macrophage and B cells.

local niche, CD4+ T cell subpopulations include T_H1, T_H2 and T_H17 cells and are characterized by the expression of interferon-γ (IFNγ), IL-4 and/or IL-13, and IL-17, respectively. Considered the prototypical T_H1 cytokine, IFNγ can also be produced by other cell types including NK cells, and IFN-γ-deficient mice were protected from NASH[39]. In human NAFLD, the CXC chemokine receptor 3 (CXCR3), implicated in the chemotaxis of T cells, was significantly upregulated in liver biopsies, and CXCR3 knockout mice were protected from NASH[40]. Cytokines released by T_H2 cells have also been studied in NASH; for example, serum levels of IL-13, implicated in HSC activation, are elevated in NASH patients. Intrahepatic T_H17 cells were more abundant and activated in human NASH and normalized after bariatric surgery. Mechanistically, murine models of NASH demonstrate increased glycolytic skewing in T_H17 cells and IL-17-induced hepatic lipotoxicity and myeloid infiltration[41]. Finally, in a humanized mouse model of NASH, circulating and intrahepatic CD4+ T cells were correlated with inflammation and fibrosis[42].

In addition to producing inflammatory cytokines, CD8+ T cells are directly cytotoxic via effector molecules such as granzymes and perforins. In human NASH, CD8+ accumulate in the liver and promote carcinogenesis by secreting TNF superfamily cytokines; CD8+ T cell depletion blunted murine NASH[43]. Recently, in both human and murine NASH, a tissue-resident CXCR6+ subset that simultaneously expressed effector (granzyme) and exhaustion (PD1) markers was described[44]. Intriguingly, these T cells were "autoaggressive" in that, their activation was antigen independent but susceptible to metabolic stimuli. Consequently, PD1 blockade caused exaggerated CD8+ T cell activation and worsened NASH. The liver also contains innate-like T cell populations, including γδ T cells, natural killer T (NKT) cells, which are abundant in mice, and mucosal-associated invariant T (MAIT) T cells in humans. Microbiota sustain proinflammatory intrahepatic γδ T cells[45] and invariant NKT (iNKT) cells in a CD1d-restricted lipid antigen manner. Notably, iNKT cells are variably abundant in mouse and human liver, representing up to 50% and <1% of all intrahepatic T cells[46]. Along with CD8+ T cells, NKT cells have been implicated in worsening steatosis[43] and fibrosis by secreting osteopontin and hedgehog ligands[47,48]. MAIT cells, which can represent 15–45% of intrahepatic T cells, directly recognize bacteria- derived vitamin B metabolites through MHC-related 1 (MR1) and are considered proinflammatory in obesity and NAFLD[49].

4.5.4 NK Cells

NK cells, along with innate lymphoid cell (ILC) subsets 1–3, are members of the innate immune system, that incite liver inflammation via direct cytotoxicity as well as cytokine secretion. Of these, NK cells are the most abundant, can constitute up to 50% of intrahepatic lymphocytes and possess adaptive immune features such as antigen-specific memory. In mouse models of NASH, they have been implicated to have a proinflammatory role by producing (TNF)-related apoptosis-inducing ligand (TRAIL) and Fas ligand[50], as well as an immunoregulatory role by IFN-γ mediated attenuation of liver fibrosis [51]. Recently, in 3 different dietary models of murine NASH, NK cells activated JAK-STAT1/3 and nuclear factor-κB signaling in hepatocytes, thus promoting NASH; conversely, genetically NK cell deficient mice were protected from NASH[52]. In human NAFLD, they are considered proinflammatory, but their specific roles in different stages of disease remain unclear.

4.5.5 B Cells

B lymphocytes are primarily divided into two subsets: B1 cells produce germline-encoded immunoglobulins (Ig) in the absence of antigenic stimulation, and B2 cells produce antigen-specific antibodies with the help of CD4+ T_H cells and can differentiate into long-lived antibody-producing plasma cells. Even in health, gut-associated lymphoid tissues are a source of B cells that respond to gut-derived antigens and populate the liver as plasma cells that produce IgA. In human NASH, these cells are more abundant in the liver and express programmed death ligand 1 (PD-L1) and interleukin-10 that lead to suppression of cytotoxic CD8+ T lymphocytes, thus dismantling a defense mechanism against carcinogenesis[53]. Indeed, serum IgA levels were correlated with disease severity and fibrosis stage among 285 patients with NAFLD[54]. Although a NASH-specific antigenic stimulus has not been identified, oxidative stress-derived epitopes have been implicated in B2 cell activation. In a murine model of NASH, intrahepatic B-cells were directly activated via the innate adaptor myeloid differentiation primary response protein 88 (MyD88) in response to microbiota-derived signals and either B-cell deficiency or B cell-specific deletion of MyD88 ameliorated NASH[55]. Alternatively, a subset of regulatory B1 cells that secrete interleukin (IL)-10 are anti-inflammatory in NASH but are lost in obesity.

Thus in the chronic sterile inflammatory state of NASH, the intrahepatic immunologic network is maladaptively remodeled into a dynamic interconnected network. Identifying the key nodes of regulation in this network will be crucial to better understanding immune mediated liver injury in NASH and will help in designing better therapeutic interventions.

4.6 INTERORGAN CROSSTALK

Obesity is a systemic disorder, and associated changes in other organs modify liver injury and inflammation. Liver crosstalk with the gut, the adipose tissue (AT) and the bone marrow modulates key pathogenic processes in NASH. Having discussed immune cells in previous sections, we focus here on gut–liver and AT–liver crosstalk in the context of liver injury and inflammation.

4.6.1 Gut–Liver Crosstalk

The role of the microbiome in NAFLD development is discussed in detail in Chapter 7. Here we highlight key mechanistic facets of intestinal barrier function, microbiome, bile acids, nuclear receptors and gut–liver immune crosstalk. Notably, there is significant interrelatedness in these disease-modifying pathways; perturbations in any one of them leads to secondary changes in the other.

The importance of intestinal barrier function in NASH pathogenesis has been demonstrated in several experimental models. Mice deficient in the gene F11r, which encodes the junctional adhesion molecule A (JAM-A), have increased intestinal and colonic permeability and develop exaggerated diet-induced steatohepatitis associated with dysbiosis and increased cecal bile acid concentration[56]. Observations in a preclinical model of galacatoside 2-alpha-L-fucosyltransferase 2 (Fut2) knockout mice (Fut2-/-) further highlight the importance of the intestinal barrier function in NASH. The Western diet-fed Fut2-/- mice are protected from diet-induced obesity and NASH while demonstrating an increase in calorie intake[57]. An increase in the bacterial enzyme 7-α-hydroxysteroid dehydrogenase was increased in Fut2-/- mice with a corresponding increase in secondary bile acids and a reduction in the bile acid pool. Interestingly, microbiota changes that occur in Fut2-/- mice are sufficient to transfer the protection to wildtype mice, and dietary supplementation of α1–2-fucosylated glycans negates the resistance of obesity and NASH conferred by Fut2 deficiency. Though Fut2 deficiency can itself lead to liver injury, and Fut2 nonsecretors are at increased risk of intestinal disease, these models illustrate the mechanistic crosstalk that occurs between the gut and the liver.

Primary bile acids, synthesized by hepatocytes and secreted as taurine or glycine conjugates, are deconjugated and converted to secondary bile acids by microbial enzymes[58]. This process increases the diversity of the bile acid pool and generates more hydrophobic bile acids. In the ileum, secondary bile acids function as agonists of the farnesoid X receptor (FXR). Upon bile acid binding, FXR induces the expression of Fgf15 in mice (FGF19 in humans), which reaches the liver via portal blood to activate fibroblast growth factor receptor 4 (FGFR4)/β-klotho and inhibit bile acid synthesis via inhibiting the expression of cholesterol 7α-hydroxylase (Cyp7a1). Intestinal FXR signaling plays an important role in NAFLD pathogenesis as demonstrated in a study where intestine-specific disruption of FXR led to a reduction in high-fat diet-induced hepatic steatosis mediated by a reduction in intestinal synthesis of ceramides[59]. Hepatocytes also express FXR at a high level, where bile acid-induced FXR activation leads to the upregulation of small heterodimer partner (SHP), which inhibits the expression of Cyp7a1. In addition to regulating bile acid homeostasis, FXR activation in the liver inhibits SREBP-1c expression suppressing de novo lipogenesis, increases fatty acid oxidation, decreases VLDL production and increases lipoprotein clearance[60]. Experimental models demonstrate that FXR agonists decrease lipotoxicity in hepatocytes concomitant with an increase in triglyceride storage[61]. The pleiotropic effects of hepatic FXR agonism thus mitigate lipotoxicity. Additionally, FXR has anti-inflammatory and antifibrotic effects in the liver[62]. FXR agonists, such as obeticholic acid, alter bile acid composition and gut microbiota and may prevent dysbiosis-driven disruption of the gut vascular barrier[63,64].

Kupffer cells in the liver clear intestinal commensal bacteria that escape mesenteric lymph nodes, and the zonal distribution of immune cells in the liver is driven by commensal microbiota[65]. Given this close relationship between intestinal bacteria and the liver immune response, dysbiosis has been mechanistically linked to the deleterious activation of the immune system in NASH. Correlative changes in gut microbiota, CD4[+] and CD8[+] lymphocyte depletion in the duodenum, widened duodenal tight junctions and disruption of duodenal microvilli have been reported in patients with NAFLD[66]. Gut-derived lymphocytes from mice with NAFLD, when adoptively transferred into recipient mice, migrated to the liver and induced liver injury[67]. Dysbiotic microbiota transplantation from human NAFLD donors into mice increased the intrahepatic activation of B cells[55]. Perturbations in bacterial sensing and immune activation in the liver may activate retrograde liver to gut crosstalk as demonstrated in mice lacking the nucleotide-binding oligomerization domain-containing (NOD)2 in hepatocytes[68]. These mice develop worse hepatic steatosis and fibrosis associated with the development of dysbiosis, though high-fat diet feeding can result in dysbiosis by itself. Thus, the immune response in the liver and the intestine depends on intestinal microbiota.

4.6.2 Adipose-Liver Crosstalk

Adipose tissue (AT) handling of lipids, inflammation and adipokine release have been implicated in modulating homeostasis in concert with the liver[69]. In mammals, two subtypes of adipose tissue—brown (BAT) and the more common white (WAT) exist. BAT contains more mitochondria and functions to dissipate stored energy in the form of heat, is present in the interscapular region of rodents but is thought to be restricted to infants in humans, though adipocytes with brown and white characteristics ("beige") have also been described in adults[70]. AT depots in mice and humans do not overlap perfectly—for example, omental fat is a major depot in humans but minimal in mice, and epididymal fat is commonly accessed in mice but is absent in men. Both visceral AT (VAT) and subcutaneous AT (SAT) inflammation has been correlated with IR and severity of NAFLD[69]. Genomic studies identified that impaired AT expansion is associated with IR and dyslipidemia and that the primary defects in AT triglyceride storage result in hepatic steatosis and lipotoxicity[71]. Downstream of inflammation, release of adipokines, such as leptin, adiponectin, neuregulin 4, retinol-binding protein 4 and resistin, as well as cytokines such as TNFα and IL-6, are implicated in interorgan crosstalk. In mouse models of obesity, levels of IL-1β are upregulated in AT, and the genetic deficiency of IL-1α and IL-1β ameliorated the high-fat diet-induced NASH[72]. In obese mice, proinflammatory tissue macrophages accumulated in AT (ATM) and expressed more neutrophil chemotaxis proteins such as CXCL14 and CXCL16, thus increasing circulating and hepatic neutrophil accumulation. Transplanting VAT from obese mice to mice on a chow diet worsened, causing hepatic macrophage accumulation and NASH. This correlation between macrophage accumulation in AT and the liver was also confirmed in paired human biopsies. This crosstalk appears to be bidirectional, as hepatic inflammation can lead to AT inflammation as demonstrated by hepatocyte derived dipeptidyl peptidase 4 leading to AT inflammation and IR [73].

Human samples from NASH patients had increased infiltrating macrophages in VAT, and higher levels of inflammatory cytokines produced by macrophages correlated with NASH severity[69]. Alanine aminotransferase elevation was correlated with SAT as well as VAT area. In a study with 40 nondiabetic patients with biopsy-proven NAFLD, activation of hepatic macrophages was correlated with elevated plasma FFA levels from AT lipolysis[74]. Indeed, in the PIVENS (pioglitazone vs. vitamin E vs. placebo for the treatment of nondiabetic patients with nonalcoholic dteatohepatitis [NASH]) trial, AT-IR was correlated with liver fibrosis, and the improvement in hepatocyte ballooning in patients treated with pioglitazone, a peroxisome proliferator-activated receptor-gamma agonist, was correlated with change in AT-IR[75].

Thus, the liver integrates signals from both the gut and AT in regulating the metabolic and inflammatory drivers of metabolic syndrome. These relationships are bidirectional and highlight the fact that NASH is characterized by the systemic dysregulation of metabolism and inflammation. Indeed, there are conserved mechanisms of injury across tissues, and thus identifying causal primacy and employing combinatorial approaches are crucial to developing successful therapeutic strategies in metabolic syndrome.

4.7 CONCLUSIONS

NASH is a multifactorial, multicellular and multiorgan disorder characterized by a disordered metabolic milieu and chronic inflammation. Hepatic lipotoxicity is the cornerstone of NASH pathogenesis, and crosstalk with the gut, adipose tissue and cells of the immune system, along with genetic predisposition, influences NASH progression. Given that several overlapping and redundant mechanisms can be in play, NASH must also be understood as a heterogeneous disorder with different pathways becoming more relevant in different stages of disease as well as in different patients. An integrated molecular understanding of this landscape is still evolving, which is crucial for developing disease modifying and mechanistically combinatorial therapies.

REFERENCES

1. Donnelly KL, Smith CI, Schwarzenberg SJ, Jessurun J, Boldt MD, Parks EJ. Sources of fatty acids stored in liver and secreted via lipoproteins in patients with nonalcoholic fatty liver disease. *J Clin Invest.* 2005;115(5):1343–1351.
2. Musso G, Cassader M, Paschetta E, Gambino R. Bioactive lipid species and metabolic pathways in progression and resolution of nonalcoholic steatohepatitis. *Gastroenterology.* 2018;155(2):282–302.e288.

3. Hirsova P, Ibrabim SH, Gores GJ, Malhi H. Lipotoxic lethal and sublethal stress signaling in hepatocytes: relevance to NASH pathogenesis. *J Lipid Res.* 2016;57(10):1758–1770.

4. Li ZZ, Berk M, McIntyre TM, Feldstein AE. Hepatic lipid partitioning and liver damage in nonalcoholic fatty liver disease: role of stearoyl-CoA desaturase. *J Biol Chem.* 2009;284(9):5637–5644.

5. Kakisaka K, Cazanave SC, Fingas CD, et al. Mechanisms of lysophosphatidylcholine-induced hepatocyte lipoapoptosis. *Am J Physiol Gastrointest Liver Physiol.* 2012;302(1):G77–G84.

6. Dasgupta D, Nakao Y, Mauer AS, et al. IRE1A stimulates hepatocyte-derived extracellular vesicles that promote inflammation in mice with steatohepatitis. *Gastroenterology.* 2020;159(4):1487–1503.e1417.

7. Ioannou GN, Landis CS, Jin G-Y, et al. Cholesterol crystals in hepatocyte lipid droplets are strongly associated with human nonalcoholic steatohepatitis. *Hepatol Commun.* 2019;3(6):776–791.

8. Malhi H, Gores GJ. Molecular mechanisms of lipotoxicity in nonalcoholic fatty liver disease. *Semin Liver Dis.* 2008;28(4):360–369.

9. Dasgupta D, Nakao Y, Mauer AS, et al. IRE1A stimulates hepatocyte-derived extracellular vesicles that promote inflammation in mice with steatohepatitis. *Gastroenterology.* 2020;159(4):1487–1503 e1417.

10. Mauer AS, Hirsova P, Maiers JL, Shah VH, Malhi H. Inhibition of sphingosine 1-phosphate signaling ameliorates murine nonalcoholic steatohepatitis. *Am J Physiol Gastrointest Liver Physiol.* 2017;312(3):G300–g313.

11. Idrissova L, Malhi H, Werneburg NW, et al. TRAIL receptor deletion in mice suppresses the inflammation of nutrient excess. *J Hepatol.* 2015;62(5):1156–1163.

12. Nakao Y, Amrollahi P, Parthasarathy G, et al. Circulating extracellular vesicles are a biomarker for NAFLD resolution and response to weight loss surgery. *Nanomedicine.* 2021;36:102430.

13. Vuppalanchi R, Noureddin M, Alkhouri N, Sanyal AJ. Therapeutic pipeline in nonalcoholic steatohepatitis. *Nat Rev Gastroenterol Hepatol.* 2021;18(6):373–392.

14. Vandanmagsar B, Youm YH, Ravussin A, et al. The NLRP3 inflammasome instigates obesity-induced inflammation and insulin resistance. *Nat Med.* 2011;17(2):179–188.

15. Mitsuyoshi H, Yasui K, Hara T, et al. Hepatic nucleotide binding oligomerization domain-like receptors pyrin domain-containing 3 inflammasomes are associated with the histologic severity of non-alcoholic fatty liver disease. *Hepatol Res.* 2017;47(13):1459–1468.

16. Xu B, Jiang M, Chu Y, et al. Gasdermin D plays a key role as a pyroptosis executor of non-alcoholic steatohepatitis in humans and mice. *J Hepatol.* 2018;68(4):773–782.

17. Dixon LJ, Flask CA, Papouchado BG, Feldstein AE, Nagy LE. Caspase-1 as a central regulator of high fat diet-induced non-alcoholic steatohepatitis. *PLoS ONE.* 2013;8(2):e56100.

18. Henao-Mejia J, Elinav E, Jin C, et al. Inflammasome-mediated dysbiosis regulates progression of NAFLD and obesity. *Nature.* 2012;482(7384):179–185.

19. Ganz M, Csak T, Szabo G. High fat diet feeding results in gender specific steatohepatitis and inflammasome activation. *World J Gastroenterol.* 2014;20(26):8525–8534.

20. Han CY, Rho HS, Kim A, et al. FXR inhibits endoplasmic reticulum stress-induced NLRP3 inflammasome in hepatocytes and ameliorates liver injury. *Cell Rep.* 2018;24(11):2985–2999.

21. Pan J, Ou Z, Cai C, et al. Fatty acid activates NLRP3 inflammasomes in mouse Kupffer cells through mitochondrial DNA release. *Cell Immunol.* 2018;332:111–120.

22. Baeza-Raja B, Goodyear A, Liu X, et al. Pharmacological inhibition of P2RX7 ameliorates liver injury by reducing inflammation and fibrosis. *PLoS ONE.* 2020;15(6):e0234038.

23. Yang G, Lee HE, Lee JY. A pharmacological inhibitor of NLRP3 inflammasome prevents non-alcoholic fatty liver disease in a mouse model induced by high fat diet. *Sci Rep.* 2016;6:24399.

24. Romeo S, Kozlitina J, Xing C, et al. Genetic variation in PNPLA3 confers susceptibility to nonalcoholic fatty liver disease. *Nat Genet.* 2008;40(12):1461–1465.

25. Kozlitina J, Smagris E, Stender S, et al. Exome-wide association study identifies a TM6SF2 variant that confers susceptibility to nonalcoholic fatty liver disease. *Nature Genetics.* 2014;46(4):352–356.

26. Mancina RM, Dongiovanni P, Petta S, et al. The MBOAT7-TMC4 variant rs641738 increases risk of non-alcoholic fatty liver disease in individuals of European descent. *Gastroenterology.* 2016;150(5):1219–1230.e1216.

27. Ma Y, Belyaeva OV, Brown PM, et al. 17-beta hydroxysteroid dehydrogenase 13 is a hepatic retinol dehydrogenase associated with histological features of nonalcoholic fatty liver disease. *Hepatology.* 2019;69(4):1504–1519.

28. Schwabe RF, Tabas I, Pajvani UB. Mechanisms of fibrosis development in nonalcoholic steatohepatitis. *Gastroenterology.* 2020;158(7):1913–1928.

29. Krenkel O, Tacke F. Liver macrophages in tissue homeostasis and disease. *Nat Rev Immunol.* 2017;17(5):306–321.

30. Tran S, Baba I, Poupel L, et al. Impaired Kupffer cell self-renewal alters the liver response to lipid overload during non-alcoholic steatohepatitis. *Immunity.* 2020;53(3):627–640 e625.

31. Parthasarathy G, Malhi H. Macrophage heterogeneity in NASH: More than just nomenclature. *Hepatology.* 2021;74(1):515–518.

32. Luo X, Li H, Ma L, et al. Expression of STING is increased in liver tissues from patients with NAFLD and promotes macrophage-mediated hepatic inflammation and fibrosis in mice. *Gastroenterology.* 2018;155(6):1971–1984 e1974.

33. Yang L, Miura K, Zhang B, et al. TRIF differentially regulates hepatic steatosis and inflammation/fibrosis in mice. *Cell Mol Gastroenterol Hepatol.* 2017;3(3):469–483.

34. Malhi H. Emerging role of extracellular vesicles in liver diseases. *Am J Physiol Gastrointest Liver Physiol.* 2019;317(5):G739–g749.

35. Baeck C, Wehr A, Karlmark KR, et al. Pharmacological inhibition of the chemokine CCL2 (MCP-1) diminishes liver macrophage infiltration and steatohepatitis in chronic hepatic injury. *Gut.* 2012;61(3):416–426.

36. Haas JT, Vonghia L, Mogilenko DA, et al. Transcriptional network analysis implicates altered hepatic immune function in NASH development and resolution. *Nat Metab.* 2019;1(6):604–614.

37. Heier EC, Meier A, Julich-Haertel H, et al. Murine CD103(+) dendritic cells protect against steatosis progression towards steatohepatitis. *J Hepatol*. 2017;66(6):1241–1250.

38. Deczkowska A, David E, Ramadori P, et al. XCR1(+) type 1 conventional dendritic cells drive liver pathology in non-alcoholic steatohepatitis. *Nat Med*. 2021;27(6):1043–1054.

39. Luo XY, Takahara T, Kawai K, et al. IFN-gamma deficiency attenuates hepatic inflammation and fibrosis in a steatohepatitis model induced by a methionine- and choline-deficient high-fat diet. *Am J Physiol Gastrointest Liver Physiol*. 2013;305(12):G891–899.

40. Zhang X, Han J, Man K, et al. CXC chemokine receptor 3 promotes steatohepatitis in mice through mediating inflammatory cytokines, macrophages and autophagy. *J Hepatol*. 2016;64(1):160–170.

41. Moreno-Fernandez ME, Giles DA, Oates JR, et al. PKM2-dependent metabolic skewing of hepatic Th17 cells regulates pathogenesis of non-alcoholic fatty liver disease. *Cell Metab*. 2021;33(6):1187–1204 e1189.

42. Her Z, Tan JHL, Lim YS, et al. CD4(+) T cells mediate the development of liver fibrosis in high fat diet-induced NAFLD in humanized mice. *Front Immunol*. 2020;11:580968.

43. Wolf MJ, Adili A, Piotrowitz K, et al. Metabolic activation of intrahepatic CD8+ T cells and NKT cells causes nonalcoholic steatohepatitis and liver cancer via cross-talk with hepatocytes. *Cancer Cell*. 2014;26(4):549–564.

44. Dudek M, Pfister D, Donakonda S, et al. Auto-aggressive CXCR6(+) CD8 T cells cause liver immune pathology in NASH. *Nature*. 2021;592(7854):444–449.

45. Li F, Hao X, Chen Y, et al. The microbiota maintain homeostasis of liver-resident gammadeltaT-17 cells in a lipid antigen/CD1d-dependent manner. *Nat Commun*. 2017;7:13839.

46. Hammond KJ, Pellicci DG, Poulton LD, et al. CD1d-restricted NKT cells: an interstrain comparison. *J Immunol*. 2001;167(3):1164–1173.

47. Syn WK, Agboola KM, Swiderska M, et al. NKT-associated hedgehog and osteopontin drive fibrogenesis in non-alcoholic fatty liver disease. *Gut*. 2012;61(9):1323–1329.

48. Syn WK, Oo YH, Pereira TA, et al. Accumulation of natural killer T cells in progressive nonalcoholic fatty liver disease. *Hepatology*. 2010;51(6):1998–2007.

49. Hegde P, Weiss E, Paradis V, et al. Mucosal-associated invariant T cells are a profibrogenic immune cell population in the liver. *Nat Commun*. 2018;9(1):2146.

50. Gomez-Santos L, Luka Z, Wagner C, et al. Inhibition of natural killer cells protects the liver against acute injury in the absence of glycine N-methyltransferase. *Hepatology*. 2012;56(2):747–759.

51. Tosello-Trampont AC, Krueger P, Narayanan S, Landes SG, Leitinger N, Hahn YS. NKp46(+) natural killer cells attenuate metabolism-induced hepatic fibrosis by regulating macrophage activation in mice. *Hepatology*. 2016;63(3):799–812.

52. Wang F, Zhang X, Liu W, et al. Activated natural killer cell promotes nonalcoholic steatohepatitis through mediating JAK/STAT pathway. *Cell Mol Gastroenterol Hepatol*. 2022;13(1):257–274.

53. Shalapour S, Lin XJ, Bastian IN, et al. Inflammation-induced IgA+ cells dismantle anti-liver cancer immunity. *Nature*. 2017;551(7680):340–345.

54. McPherson S, Henderson E, Burt AD, Day CP, Anstee QM. Serum immunoglobulin levels predict fibrosis in patients with non-alcoholic fatty liver disease. *J Hepatol*. 2014;60(5):1055–1062.

55. Barrow F, Khan S, Fredrickson G, et al. Microbiota-driven activation of intrahepatic B cells aggravates NASH through innate and adaptive signaling. *Hepatology*. 2021;74(2):704–722.

56. Rahman K, Desai C, Iyer SS, et al. Loss of junctional adhesion molecule A promotes severe steatohepatitis in mice on a diet high in saturated fat, fructose, and cholesterol. *Gastroenterology*. 2016;151(4):733–746. e712.

57. Zhou R, Llorente C, Cao J, et al. Intestinal α1–2-Fucosylation contributes to obesity and steatohepatitis in mice. *Cell Mol Gastroenterol Hepatol*. 2021;12(1):293–320.

58. Wahlström A, Sayin Sama I, Marschall H-U, Bäckhed F. Intestinal crosstalk between bile acids and microbiota and its impact on host metabolism. *Cell Metab*. 2016;24(1):41–50.

59. Jiang C, Xie C, Li F, et al. Intestinal farnesoid X receptor signaling promotes nonalcoholic fatty liver disease. *J Clin Invest*. 2015;125(1):386–402.

60. Jiao Y, Lu Y, Li X-y. Farnesoid X receptor: a master regulator of hepatic triglyceride and glucose homeostasis. *Acta Pharmacol Sin*. 2015;36(1):44–50.

61. Wu K, Zhao T, Hogstrand C, et al. FXR-mediated inhibition of autophagy contributes to FA-induced TG accumulation and accordingly reduces FA-induced lipotoxicity. *Cell Commun Signal*. 2020;18(1):47.

62. Armstrong LE, Guo GL. Role of FXR in liver inflammation during nonalcoholic steatohepatitis. *Curr Pharmacol Rep*. 2017;3(2):92–100.

63. Zhang DY, Zhu L, Liu HN, et al. The protective effect and mechanism of the FXR agonist obeticholic acid via targeting gut microbiota in non-alcoholic fatty liver disease. *Drug Des Devel Ther*. 2019;13:2249–2270.

64. Mouries J, Brescia P, Silvestri A, et al. Microbiota-driven gut vascular barrier disruption is a prerequisite for non-alcoholic steatohepatitis development. *J Hepatol*. 2019;71(6):1216–1228.

65. Gola A, Dorrington MG, Speranza E, et al. Commensal-driven immune zonation of the liver promotes host defence. *Nature*. 2021;589(7840):131–136.

66. Jiang W, Wu N, Wang X, et al. Dysbiosis gut microbiota associated with inflammation and impaired mucosal immune function in intestine of humans with non-alcoholic fatty liver disease. *Sci Rep*. 2015;5(1):8096.

67. Hu Y, Zhang H, Li J, et al. Gut-derived lymphocyte recruitment to liver and induce liver injury in non-alcoholic fatty liver disease mouse model. *J Gastroenterol Hepatol*. 2016;31(3):676–684.

68. Cavallari JF, Pokrajac NT, Zlitni S, Foley KP, Henriksbo BD, Schertzer JD. NOD2 in hepatocytes engages a liver-gut axis to protect against steatosis, fibrosis, and gut dysbiosis during fatty liver disease in mice. *Am J Physiol-Endocrinol Metab*. 2020;319(2):E305–E314.

69. du Plessis J, van Pelt J, Korf H, et al. Association of adipose tissue inflammation with histologic severity of nonalcoholic fatty liver disease. *Gastroenterology.* 2015;149(3):635–648 e614.

70. Wang W, Seale P. Control of brown and beige fat development. *Nat Rev Mol Cell Biol.* 2016;17(11):691–702.

71. Aryal B, Singh AK, Zhang X, et al. Absence of ANGPTL4 in adipose tissue improves glucose tolerance and attenuates atherogenesis. *JCI Insight.* 2018;3(6).

72. Kamari Y, Shaish A, Vax E, et al. Lack of interleukin-1alpha or interleukin-1beta inhibits transformation of steatosis to steatohepatitis and liver fibrosis in hypercholesterolemic mice. *J Hepatol.* 2011;55(5):1086–1094.

73. Ghorpade DS, Ozcan L, Zheng Z, et al. Hepatocyte-secreted DPP4 in obesity promotes adipose inflammation and insulin resistance. *Nature.* 2018;555(7698):673–677.

74. Rosso C, Kazankov K, Younes R, et al. Crosstalk between adipose tissue insulin resistance and liver macrophages in non-alcoholic fatty liver disease. *J Hepatol.* 2019;71(5):1012–1021.

75. Bell LN, Wang J, Muralidharan S, et al. Relationship between adipose tissue insulin resistance and liver histology in nonalcoholic steatohepatitis: a pioglitazone versus vitamin E versus placebo for the treatment of nondiabetic patients with nonalcoholic steatohepatitis trial follow-up study. *Hepatology.* 2012;56(4):1311–1318.

5 Role of the Microbiome

Carlos J. Pirola and Silvia Sookoian

CONTENTS

Key Points

- The pathogenesis of NAFLD, including its severe clinical forms, involves complex and multiscale processes across all levels of biological organization (from DNA to RNA, proteins, metabolites and the microbiome).

- Current evidence suggests that the human gastrointestinal microbiome exerts a key role in the biology of NAFLD.

- Multiple hits derived from microbial signals that interact with one another modulate liver metabolism and the immune and inflammatory response. These events trigger fibrogenesis signaling and eventually hepatocarcinogenesis.

- Gut dysbiosis might also drive the development of NAFLD by endogenous alcohol production.

- Manipulation of gut microbiota by phages offers an innovative solution for the treatment of liver diseases.

- The latest evidence from human studies showed that the liver tissue of NAFLD patients contains a diverse repertoire of bacterial DNA (up to 2.5×10^4 read counts). The liver metataxonomic signature may explain differences in the NAFLD pathogenic mechanisms and physiological functions of the host in the context of obesity degree.

- Genetic variation may influence the liver microbial DNA composition.

- These observations may represent potentially actionable mechanisms of disease.

5.1 WHY THE STUDY OF THE HUMAN MICROBIOME IS RELEVANT TO UNDERSTANDING THE BIOLOGY OF NAFLD?

This chapter seeks to summarize and illustrate the underlying biological and molecular processes that link the microbiome with the development of nonalcoholic fatty liver (NAFLD) and its progression toward severe histopathological and clinical forms, including nonalcoholic steatohepatitis (NASH) and NASH-fibrosis.

The pathogenesis of NAFLD and NASH involves complex and multiscale processes across all levels of biological organization—from DNA to RNA, to proteins and metabolites. This entailed complexity implicates stepwise perturbations of physiological processes that generally converge into liver metabolic distress. In addition, the underlying mechanisms associated with the disease pathogenesis entangle interconnections among all levels of biological organization that ultimately determine liver and systemic metabolic dysfunction.

The metagenome study—referred initially to the shotgun characterization of total microbial DNA, now being applied to studies of marker genes such as the 16s ribosomal RNA (16S rRNA) gene that captures bacterial diversity—uncovered a "hidden" but a relevant actor in the pathogenesis of NAFLD. The use of high-throughput sequencing, also known as next-generation sequencing technologies, has opened a door for understanding the interrelationship between the human microbiota and body function/dysfunction in health and disease, respectively.

Here, we highlight the role of the microbiota in the biology of NAFLD. We specifically focus the content of this chapter on recent advances from human studies that involve a robust phenotypic characterization of NAFLD and the profiling of diverse microbiotas, from gut to circulating and tissue microbiotas. In addition, we integrate information on the role of microbiota in NAFLD with other levels of biological complexity, for instance, the interplay between host genetics and the microbiome.

5.2 ROLE OF THE GUT MICROBIOTA IN THE BIOLOGY OF NAFLD

The collective genomes of our microbial symbionts (microbiomes) are known as the metagenomes, as initially described in *The human microbiome project*[1]. Nevertheless, this definition is constantly being reviewed as much as the field is evolving. There are arguments on what exactly comprises the microbiota and on whether, besides bacteria, other microorganisms like fungi, algae, phages, viruses, plasmids and mobile genetic elements and small protists should or should not be considered as members of the microbiome [2]. We will use the traditional definition of the microbiota, which is the assemblage of living microorganisms present in a defined environment[3].

DOI: 10.1201/9781003386698-6

Based on this definition, it is reckoned that the human microbiota consists of 10–100 trillion symbiotic microbial cells[1]. Likewise, estimates based on different approaches, for instance, multiplying measured concentrations of bacteria by the volume of each human organ, suggest that the number of bacteria residing in the body organs is of several orders of magnitude greater than the cells of the host[4]. For example, it is estimated that the concentration of bacteria residing in the human colon (large intestine)— over 1000 known species—is in the order of magnitude of 10^{14}, in the ileum (lower small intestine) 10^{11}, in the duodenum and jejunum (upper small intestine) 10^7, in the stomach 10^7, in dental plaque 10^{12}, and in skin 10^{11} order of magnitude[4].

The classical approach for characterizing the human gut microbiota is by profiling the bacteria composition in stool samples. With the explosion of knowledge in the field of metagenomics, novel concepts about the pathogenesis of NAFLD have emerged, including the putative role of the gut microbiota in modulating liver fat accumulation, inflammation and fibrogenesis[5–12] and liver cancer[13].

Targeted studies based on the analysis of the hypervariable region of the 16s rRNA gene, which is a part of the small subunit of the bacterial ribosome, showed diverse bacterial taxa associated with NAFLD and NASH. However, *Proteobacteria*, *Enterobacteriaceae* and *Escherichia* are the most enriched taxa in stool samples derived from NAFLD patients found in many studies[6,9,12,14,15].

A comprehensive description of the composition of the gut microbiota across diverse human studies with different designs, including adult and children's populations, has been recently reviewed elsewhere[16,17]. Together, it appears that the gut–liver axis plays a fundamental role in the initiation and progression of NAFLD, which seems largely explained by the anatomical relationship between the liver and the gut through the venous portal system. The liver acts as a key filtration system of the whole body by receiving blood from the hepatic artery and the portal vein. Therefore, microbes become entrapped in the complex liver anatomy, and, more importantly, the liver gets bacterially derived products that are potent stimuli for initiating the inflammatory response (Figure 5.1).

The evidence suggests that the human gastrointestinal microbiome exerts a complex role in NAFLD biology by multiple interacting hits, including microbial signals. These stimuli modulate the liver and whole-body metabolism at critical levels such as energy balance, fat storage/synthesis and glucose sensitivity, and activation of the immune response by *PAMPs* (pathogen-associated molecular patterns) and the inflammatory response by the release of proinflammatory signals (Figure 5.1). These processes are coupled to the gut microbiome dysbiosis, intestinal permeability and translocation of *MAMPs* (microbe-associated molecular patterns) and *DAMPs* (danger-associated molecular patterns) through the portal system (Figure 5.1). This cascade of events activates, in turn, the inflammasome and then perpetuates the vicious circle of inflammation and fibrogenesis.

The evidence also suggests that not only the presence of intact bacteria is needed to activate the immune system. On the contrary, the immune system also senses bacterial DNA, cell wall components of gram-positive and gram-negative bacteria, such as peptidoglycan, endotoxin or lipoteichoic acid[18]. The most commonly known component of bacterial cells that not only activate the immune system

but also may even evoke an immune response to the level of a 'septic shock' is the lipopolysaccharide (LPS)—a component of gram-negative bacteria.

Most importantly, it has been known for quite some time that bacterial DNA, which lacks methylation, is sensed by antigen-presenting cells of the immune system[18]. Therefore, bacterial DNA has been regarded as an efficient endotoxin that triggers the release of proinflammatory cytokines and activates macrophages and dendritic cells[18]. Interestingly, the concept of immunostimulatory DNA was borne in a long series of studies on BCG-mediated tumor resistance[19].

Earlier studies in mice demonstrated that endotoxins produced by gram-negative bacteria stimulate hepatic fibrogenesis[20]. Furthermore, Boursier et al. identified the abundance of *Bacteroides* as associated with NASH and *Ruminococcus* with significant fibrosis[5]. More recently, Loomba et al. showed that, compared to mild/moderate NAFLD, proteobacteria (*Escherichia coli at the species level)* abundance was higher in NAFLD patients with advanced fibrosis[9]. In addition, the investigators demonstrated that nine metabolites (associated with amino acids and carbon metabolism) and enzymes associated with butyrate, D-lactate, propionate and succinate were enriched in advanced fibrosis[9].

Re et al. showed that the phylum Actinobacteria as well as 13 genera including *Gemmiger* and *Parabacteroides* were increased in early stages of hepatocellular carcinoma (HCC)[21]. Further studies that investigated the association between gut dysbiosis, NAFLD and HCC suggested that alterations of the gut microbiota induced by obesity could promote the development of HCC[22]. More specifically, Yoshimoto et al. showed that deoxycholic acid (DCA), a gut bacterial metabolite known to cause DNA damage, may explain the development of obesity-associated HCC development in mice[22].

It is also postulated that the gut microbiota may modulate the immune response in HCC. Behary and coworkers used metagenomic and metabolomic studies to characterize the gut microbiota in patients with NAFLD-related cirrhosis, with or without HCC, and to evaluate its effect on the peripheral immune response[13]. Remarkably, the investigators found that gut dysbiosis is involved in the compositional and functional effects of the microbial profile associated with HCC development[13].

5.3 BEYOND THE GUT "BACTERIOME": The Role of Commensal Populations of Microorganisms in Shaping the NASH Phenotype

Besides bacteria, the human body hosts commensal populations of fungi, viruses, archaea, and protists. Thus, in addition to the term "bacteriome," the scientific literature also includes other terms, such as the "archaeome," "mycobiome," and "virome"[2].

The study of these diverse ecosystems in the pathogenesis of NAFLD is still in its infancy. However, recent evidence based on human samples of patients with NAFLD and with alcohol use disorder demonstrated that nonobese NAFLD patients with more advanced disease have a different fecal mycobiome composition than nonobese NAFLD patients with mild disease[23]. Specifically, Demir and coworkers found that the abundance of *Mucor* sp./*Saccharomyces cerevisiae* (*S. cerevisiae*) was particularly unbalanced in patients with NASH and F2-F4 fibrosis[23].

As expected, diet is a crucial factor, affecting the composition and variability of the gut mycobiome. For example, the abundance of *Candida* in the gut positively correlates with high-carbohydrate diets. Still, it inversely correlates with consumption of total saturated fatty acids, while recent intake of short-chain fatty acids reduced the abundance of *Aspergillus*[24]. *However, the interrelationship between the NAFLD mycobiome and environmental factors such as diet remains unexplored.*

As well, the healthy human gut hosts approximately 10^{15} bacteriophages that play an important role in maintaining the gut microbiome structure and function and thereby contributes significantly to human health[25].

The intestinal phageome consists of both prophages in bacterial cells and free virions or virus-like particles[26].

A recent longitudinal study of stool bacteriophages from healthy donors and subjects with metabolic syndrome before and after fecal microbiota transplantation treatment identified bacteriophage groups—for example Caudovirale—that could explain clinical differences between healthy and disease groups[27].

Of note, *Caudovirales* presents a mosaic genome, meaning that its presence can be detected either free or as prophages in the core of some bacteria[26].

A proof-of-concept study that explored the abundance of RNA and DNA virus-like particles from fecal samples of patients with NAFLD with fibrosis and cirrhosis and primary biliary cholangitis as control subjects showed that fecal viral diversity may affect disease severity[28]. For example, some viral species were less present (*Lactococcus* phages) or significantly more present (*Streptococcus* phages TP-J34) in stool samples of patients with more severe disease[28]. Several *Lactococcus* and *Leuconostoc* phages were significantly decreased in patients with NAFLD and higher degrees of liver fibrosis, whereas *Lactobacillus* phage phiAT3 was significantly increased[28].

There are several clinical trials involving phage-based therapy against bacterial infections in gastrointestinal diseases[26] suggesting that manipulation of gut microbiota by phages is a novel option not only to target diverse gastrointestinal diseases but also for the treatment of liver diseases. For example, an experimental study showed that the use of a phage cocktail involving three or four phages that target cytolytic *E. faecalis* abolished ethanol-induced liver disease in humanized mice[29].

While the study of the NAFLD "gut phageome" and the "gut mycobiome" might uncover some clues regarding disease progression, it is unclear how reproducible these findings are across different geographic regions and what factors drive the mentioned unbalanced viral and/or fungus diversity.

5.4 NONINTESTINAL MICROBIOTAS AND NAFLD: BACTERIAL BIOGEOGRAPHY DOES MATTER

Several studies in the field of liver diseases have demonstrated the importance of the nonintestinal microbiotas in the development and/or prognosis of different liver disease states, from metabolic, inflammatory and autoimmune diseases to liver cancer[17]. These nonintestinal microbiotas include, for instance, explorations of the microbial DNA composition of samples from the peripheral blood, bile and bile duct tissue, saliva and, more recently, the liver tissue, as recently reviewed[17]. It is important to highlight that the study of the nonintestinal microbiotas does not necessarily mean proof of the "culturability" and/or the

viability of the discovered microorganisms. However, it is undoubtedly very plausible to speculate that bacteria-related products such as bacterial DNA play a significant role in the biology of cardiometabolic diseases, including NAFLD.

For example, the circulating blood microbiome has been the focus of intense research in the field of cardiovascular diseases and type 2 diabetes[30,31]. *Proteobacteria* abundance was measured in blood collected at baseline from 3936 participants, including 73 incident cases of acute cardiovascular events and 30 myocardial infarctions, and it was linked to the incidence of atherothrombotic disease[30]. Likewise, blood microbiota dysbiosis was directly correlated with the onset of cardiovascular complications[30].

Lelouvier et al. investigated the relationship between the blood microbiota and liver fibrosis in patients with severe obesity and observed that changes in several taxa correlated with the fibrosis status, including the genera *Sphingomonas*, *Bosea* and *Variovorax*[32].

Puri and coworkers investigated the circulating microbiome signature in patients with alcoholic hepatitis and found that the relative abundance of the phylum *Bacteroidetes* was significantly decreased in alcohol-consuming patients[33]. In addition, the circulating microbiome of subjects consuming alcohol was significantly enriched with the gram-negative bacilli phylum *Fusobacteria* and its subclasses *Fusobacteriales* and *Leptotrichiaceae*[33].

Several subsequent studies explored the role of the circulating microbiota in cirrhosis and HCC[31,34,35].

Based on the profiling of salivary microbiota, Bajaj and coworkers[36] reported that salivary dysbiosis was greater in patients with cirrhosis who developed 90-day hospitalizations because of hepatic encephalopathy.

5.5 LIVER TISSUE MICROBIOTA IN NAFLD AND ITS ROLE IN THE DISEASE SEVERITY

More recently, we explored the liver tissue bacterial DNA composition in patients with NAFLD and different phenotypic and histological characteristics, and we found for the first time that the liver tissue of NAFLD patients contains a diverse repertoire of bacterial DNA (up to 2.5×10^4 read counts)[37]. More importantly, we observed that the liver metataxonomic signature may explain differences in the NAFLD pathogenic mechanisms as well as physiological functions of the host[37].

Based on previous knowledge of human bacterial biogeography[38], we speculated that, while some bacterial DNAs might be derived from the human intestinal tract, for example, *Bifidobacterium*, *Peptostreptococcus*, *Stenotrophomonas*, *Xanthomonadaceae*, *Lachnoclostridium* and *Ruminococcaceae*, some other taxa might be derived from the oral microbiome, for example, *Actinobacteria* and *Prevotella*, and some species of *Deltaproteobacteria*. In addition, we found some critical features that may help understand the role of the liver tissue microbiome in the disease progression. For example, we found that depletion of DNA from *Lachnospiraceae* family members was particularly associated with severe histological features[37]. Several members of the *Lachnospiraceae* family are butyrate producers, and microbial butyrate-producing communities are often reported as associated with healthy microbiota. More research should be done on this aspect, however, as higher levels of butyrate consumption and pathways related to butanoate synthesis may be associated with NAFLD[39].

Furthermore, we found that overabundance of DNA derived from gram-negative *Proteobacteria*, particularly *Gammaproteobacteria*, was a distinguishing feature of NASH and NASH-related severe histological outcomes[37]. For example, DNA derived from *Stenotrophomonas* showed a 3.1-fold increase in the liver of morbidly obese patients with NASH. Likewise, DNA derived from *Xanthomonadaceae* family members was consistently increased in all samples of NASH patients regardless of their body mass index status[37]. We also found that DNA from *Alpha-* and *Gammaproteobacteria* were consistently associated with increased lobular and portal inflammation scores[37].

5.6 MICROBIOTA, BIOACTIVE SECONDARY METABOLITES AND NAFLD

Numerous studies have proven the existence of derived metabolites from the human microbiota that are relevant to body physiology. These metabolites are not only bioactive molecules that can interfere with different biological processes, for example, energy metabolism and gut homeostasis, but also may trigger pathophysiological changes in many diseases.

Postler and Ghosh have summarized the metabolites derived from the human microbiota into three categories: (1) metabolites that are produced by bacteria directly from dietary components, (2) metabolites that are produced by the host and biochemically modified by gut bacteria, and (33) metabolites that are synthesized de novo by gut microbes[40].

Short-chain fatty acids (primarily acetate, propionate, butyrate) are among those metabolites produced by bacteria from dietary components. It was shown that the gut microbiota associated with type 2 diabetes produce lower levels of short-chain fatty acids (SCFAs) that can differentially regulate prostaglandins production and may play an important role in the mucoprotective effect of bacterial fermentation products[41]. Hence, it appears that the absence of SCFA production may cause an increase in the permeability of the intestinal mucosa increases that would allow gut bacteria to enter the bloodstream (Figure 5.1).

Secondary bile acids, which are among metabolites that are produced by the host and biochemically modified by gut bacteria, are relevant as immune modulators with key roles in inflammatory pathways[40,42].

For instance, some intestinal species in the genus of *Clostridium*, including *C. scindens*, *C. hiranonis*, *C. hylemonae* (Clostridium cluster XVIa), and *C. sordelli* (Clostridium cluster XI), may produce secondary bile acids[42].

Finally, Postler and Ghosh highlight polysaccharide A (PSA) as metabolites that are synthesized de novo by gut microbes[40].

Our group explored the predicted functionality of the liver microbial DNA composition and found that patients with NAFLD and metabolic syndrome presented overrepresentation of metabolic pathways linked to fatty acid metabolism, beta alanine and porfirin metabolism, and microbial metabolism in a diverse environment[37]. In liver specimens derived from morbidly obese patients with NAFLD, we found overenrichment of pathways associated

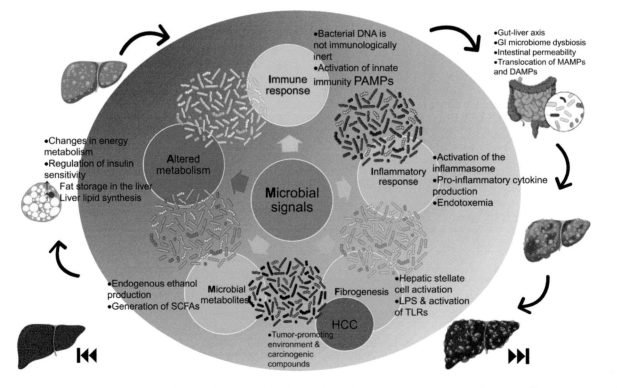

Figure 5.1 NAFLD and the microbiome: from microbial signals to disease progression, road map in the interaction of the gut microbiome and NAFLD pathogenesis

SCFAs: Short-chain fatty acids; PAMPs: Pathogen-associated molecular patterns; MAMPs: Microbial-associated molecular patterns; DAMPs: Danger-associated molecular patterns; LP: Lipopolysaccharide; TLR: Toll-like receptors; HCC: Hepatocellular carcinoma.

with biosynthesis of amino acids, pentose and glucoronate interconversions, pyrimidine metabolism, and amino sugar and nucleotide sugar metabolism[37].

Perhaps an overlooked pathway that may have a significant impact in the development and progression of NAFLD is the "KEGG KO Microbial metabolism in diverse environments," which involves several subpathways, including carbohydrate metabolism, energy metabolism, methane metabolism, sulfur metabolism, nitrogen metabolism and amino acid metabolism, among many others. An enzyme in this pathway has been shown to participate in several biological events linked to the NAFLD pathogenesis[43,44]: the alcohol dehydrogenase (ADH) (1.1.1.1). The ADH is an oxidoreductase enzyme that oxidizes alcohol to acetaldehyde while subsequently reducing an NAD^+ cofactor to NADH; this pathway probably evolved as a detoxification mechanism for environmental alcohols. In addition, ADH is involved in ethanol production, which will be discussed in detail in the next section of this chapter.

5.7 NAFLD, ENDOGENOUS ETHANOL PRODUCTION AND THE INTESTINAL MICROBIOTA

Pioneering studies in murine models showed that intestinally derived ethanol may contribute to the pathogenesis of NASH[45]. The hypothesis behind this observation was based on the concept that intestinal bacteria can produce ethanol. Cope et al. postulated that an indirect way of measuring endogenous ethanol, derived from gut bacterial metabolism, is by measuring the breath ethanol concentration[45]. By doing so, Nair et al. from the same group of researchers demonstrated that while the concentration of breath ethanol was unrelated to the severity of NAFLD, obese patients were more likely to have higher breath ethanol concentrations[46].

A subsequent study using 16S rRNA gene pyrosequencing that involved the analysis of the composition of gut bacterial communities in healthy subjects and NASH-obese children showed no differences in blood-ethanol concentrations between these two groups[12]. However, the investigators noted that NASH patients exhibited elevated blood ethanol levels[12].

Recent evidence from China has suggested that high-alcohol-producing Klebsiella pneumoniae was associated with up to 60% of individuals with NAFLD[47]. Yuan et al. transferred clinical isolates of Klebsiella pneumoniae by oral gavage into mice and found that this intervention induced NAFLD in rodents[47]. Likewise, the investigators observed that selective elimination of the Klebsiella pneumoniae strain before fecal microbiota transplant into mice prevented NAFLD in the recipient animals[47]. Further experimental investigations that extended the exploration of the mechanisms by which Klebsiella pneumoniae potentially produced alcohol-related NAFLD included the analysis of the proteome and metabolome[48]. The researchers showed 10 proteins and 6 major metabolites involved in the 2,3-butanediol fermentation pathway as increased during Klebsiella pneumoniae intestinal overgrowth[48]. The authors found that high amounts of endogenous alcohol were responsible for liver fat accumulation in mice and that carbohydrates from diet are catabolized to produce alcohol and 2,3-butanediol via the 2,3-butanediol fermentation pathway in mice colonized by Klebsiella pneumoniae[48].

Elshaghabee and coworkers evaluated the ethanol production of some gastrointestinal bacteria and a yeast strain under different conditions and concluded that ethanol is one of the dominating metabolites of heterolactic intestinal microbes[49].

The investigators observed that significant amounts of ethanol were produced in vitro from glucose and fructose by the Lactobacillus fermentum 92294 and the Weisella confusa NRRL-B-14171, which were associated with experimentally developed NAFLD[49]. Collectively, Elshaghabee et al. provided valuable evidence on the hypothesis that ethanol is one of the dominant metabolites of heterolactic intestinal microbes.

Of note, in addition to the stellar role of members of the ADH family of proteins in the biology of NAFLD and NASH[43,44], ADH is involved in bacteria-derived ethanol production. Specifically, ADH catalyzes both an acetaldehyde dehydrogenase reaction, which converts acetyl-coA to acetaldehyde, and an alcohol dehydrogenase inverse reaction, which converts the acetaldehyde to ethanol. For example, Figure 5.2a shows the pathway of heterolactic fermentation, and Figure 5.2b illustrates the "pyruvate fermentation to ethanol I" pathway that is one of the many related pathways that prove bacteria-derived ethanol production. There are other closely related pathways, for example, pyruvate fermentation to ethanol II, pyruvate fermentation to ethanol III and pyruvate fermentation to isobutanol. A full description of these pathways can be found in the MetaCyc web page (https://metacyc.org/), a curated database of experimentally elucidated metabolic pathways from all domains of life.

Hence, the participation of the ADH enzymes not only in ethanol degradation that begins with conversion of ethanol to acetaldehyde but also in "alcoholgenic" (formation of ethanol and butan-1-ol but not acetone) pathways—particularly in bacteria—suggests that ethanol formation from acetyl-CoA that is converted to ethanol via acetaldehyde is a highly plausible mechanism to explain how gut dysbiosis may drive the pathogenesis of NAFLD.

Some of the gut bacteria taxa that were associated with NAFLD and NASH in human studies are capable of producing ethanol, including gram-positive members of the class Actinobacteria (genus Bifidobacterium, an obligate aerobe) and the class Bacilli (genus Bacillus and Blautia, a facultative anaerobe and obligate anaerobe, respectively), and gram-negative members of the class Gammaproteobacteria (genus Acinetobacter, an aerobe bacteria) and the class Verrucomicrobiae (genus Akkermansia, an obligate anaerobe).

5.8 LIPOPOLYSACCHARIDE (LPS), NASH AND MODULATION OF IMMUNE RESPONSE

Lipopolysaccharide (LPS) is a major component of the outer membrane of gram-negative bacteria consisting of three domains: a hydrophobic anchor called lipid A, a non-repeating core oligosaccharide (OS) and a repetitive glycan polymer called O-antigen or O-polysaccharide (O-PS). The enzymes for the biosynthesis of lipid A are well-conserved among gram-negative bacterial species. O-antigen is the most variable part used for serotyping of pathogenic Escherichia coli, where about 170 types are known. All three domains are involved in toxicity, pathogenicity, antimicrobial resistance and other activities.

LPS derived from the gut though a process known as bacterial translocation has been directly linked to the pathogenesis of NAFLD[50] and alcoholic liver disease[51] by inducing chronic liver inflammation.

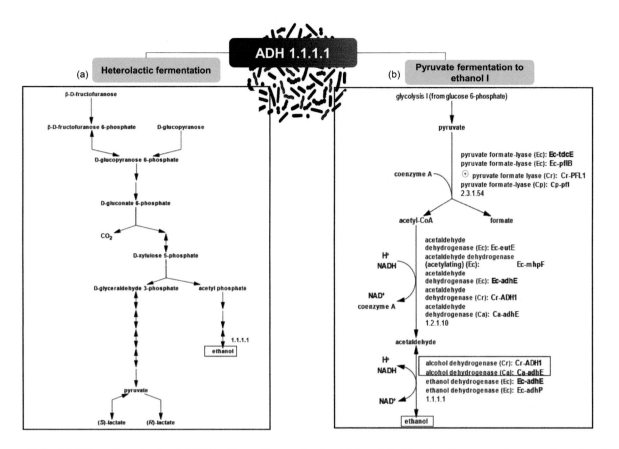

Figure 5.2 Multifunctional role of ADH in the pathway of microbial metabolism in diverse environments and endogenous ethanol formation by gut bacteria: key subpathways in which the enzyme EC 1.1.1.1 (alcohol dehydrogenase) is involved

(a) Enzymatic reaction of heterolactic fermentation (MetaCyc). The lactic acid bacteria (LAB) are a group of gram-positive bacteria that produce lactate as the major end product of the fermentation of carbohydrates. Some taxa known to possess this pathway are *Fructilactobacillus sanfranciscensis, Lacticaseibacillus casei, Lentilactobacillus buchneri, Leuconostoc lactis, Leuconostoc mesenteroides, Leuconostoc mesenteroides cremoris, Leuconostoc mesenteroides dextranicum, Levilactobacillus brevis, Limosilactobacillus fermentum, Limosilactobacillus reuteri, Oenococcus oeni, Weissella confusa, Weissella paramesenteroides*. When glucose is used as the carbon source, there is production of equimolar quantities of lactate, ethanol and carbon dioxide, with occasional traces of acetate. (b) Enzymatic involvement of ADH in the BioCyc ID: PWY-5480: pyruvic acid fermentation to ethanol I. During aerobic respiration in most organisms, most of the pyruvate that is formed by glycolysis is directed into the TCA cycle I (prokaryotic) after its conversion to acetyl-CoA by a large protein complex, the pyruvate decarboxylation to acetyl CoA I. Under anaerobic conditions, pyruvate is still formed by glycolysis, but since oxidative phosphorylation is not available, pyruvate is fermented to several end products by different fermentation routes. In *Escherichia coli* K–12, minutes after a shift to anaerobic conditions, the enzyme-activated pyruvate-formate lyase is expressed and is active. This enzyme converts pyruvate into acetyl-CoA by a different mechanism from the pyruvate dehydrogenase complex. It uses a two-step mechanism, first cleaving the C-C bond in the pyruvate molecule, generating formate and an acetylated-enzyme intermediate, and then reacts with coenzyme A, resulting in the formation of acetyl CoA. Acetyl-CoA can be used in several routes, leading to different end products (see mixed acid fermentation). One branch, mediated by the enzyme fused acetaldehyde-CoA dehydrogenase and iron-dependent alcohol dehydrogenase, leads to the formation of ethanol. Some taxa known to possess this pathway are *Chlamydomonas reinhardtii, Clostridium acetobutylicum ATCC 824, Clostridium pasteurianum, Escherichia coli K-12 substr. MG1655, Neocallimastix sp. LM-2, Streptococcus* (https://biocyc.org/).

Henao-Mejia J. and coworkers demonstrated that an altered microbiome triggering colonic inflammation and bacterial translocation causes simple hepatic steatosis to turn into NASH in mice[52].

Guo et al. showed for the first time that the LPS increases intestinal tight junction permeability and intestinal inflammation by TLR4-dependent activation of the FAK/MyD88/IL-1R-associated kinase 4 signaling pathway[53]. The cross talk between gut-derived LPS and the toll-like receptor signaling pathway is illustrated in Figure 5.3.

Finally, by examining by immunohistochemistry liver tissue specimens of patients with NAFLD across the entire spectrum of the disease severity, we demonstrated that LPS immunoreactivity in samples of NASH patients is predominantly localized in the portal tracts[37]. Notably, we found that the higher the level of LPS there is in the portal tracks, the higher the score of liver fibrosis will be[37].

5.9 NAFLD, HOST GENETICS AND THE MICROBIOME

While interpersonal variation in the microbiome can be considerable, each individual's microbiome appears to be remarkably stable, suggesting that the genetic profile of the host is a factor that maintains the composition of microbial communities throughout the body. On the one hand, the pioneering work of Goodrich et al. suggested that the heritability of microbiomes is lower than many other traits and is not evenly distributed among taxa (for example, with higher heritability among Firmicutes than Bacteroidetes)[54]. On the other hand, comparisons in previous studies between monozygotic and dizygotic twins have identified a set of microbial taxa with higher-than-expected heritability coefficients[55].

In the GWAS catalog (www.ebi.ac.uk), there are 1479 associations derived from 699 studies that explored the relationship between host genetics and the gut microbiome (Figure 5.4).

The large majority of associated loci are located in chromosome 2 (Figure 5.4), and variants are related to a diverse gene–protein functionality, from a set of conserved minichromosome maintenance proteins (MCM), which are essential for the initiation of eukaryotic genome replication, the ATP binding cassette subfamily A member 13 involved in ATP hydrolysis activity *and* cholesterol transfer activity, to a long intergenic nonprotein coding RNA 1887 of unknown function (Figure 5.4).

While there is a clear and biologically plausible interplay between microbiome and host genetics, the evidence in this regard is still weak. In the particular case of NAFLD and NASH, the evidence is very scarce.

Monga et al. investigated the potential relationship between gut microbiota composition and the rs738409 variant in *PNPLA3*—the major contributor of the disease severity[56–58]. By exploring samples from NAFLD-obese children, the authors found in the multivariate model that rs738409 genotypes, the taxa Gemmiger, and BMI z-score were predictors of hepatic fat content[59]. In addition, Monga et al. reported an additive effect between *Oscillospira* and *PNPLA3* rs738409 variant in conveying susceptibility to NAFLD, in which both factors independently affect hepatic fat content[59].

More recently, our group explored the hypothesis that the liver microbiota is shaped by host genetics. Thus we conducted candidate gene association analyses using as a proxy of NAFLD histological severity common variants in loci that impose either risk or protection against the disease (*PNPLA3*-*rs738409*[56–58], *TM6SF2*-*rs58542926*[60–63], *MBOAT7*-*rs641738*[64] and *HSD17B13*-*rs72613567*[65–67]. In addition, as a proxy of major dietary modifiers, we used a variant in a locus that has been reproducibly linked to high-carbohydrate intake and macronutrient preferences (*FGF21*-rs838133)[68].

We identified at least 18 bacterial taxa associated with variants in the selected loci. Members of the

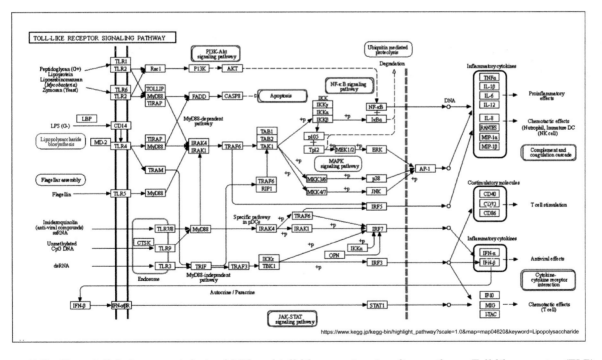

Figure 5.3 Cross talk between gut-derived LPS and toll-like receptor signaling pathway Toll-like receptor (TLR) signaling pathway. Specific families of pattern recognition receptors are responsible for detecting microbial pathogens and generating innate immune responses. Toll-like receptors are membrane-bound receptors identified as homologs of toll in *Drosophila*. Mammalian TLRs are expressed on innate immune cells, such as macrophages and dendritic cells, and they respond to the membrane components of gram-positive or gram-negative bacteria. Pathogen recognition by TLRs provokes rapid activation of innate immunity by inducing the production of proinflammatory cytokines and upregulation of costimulatory molecules. TLR signaling pathways are separated into two groups: an MyD88-dependent pathway that leads to the production of proinflammatory cytokines with the quick activation of NF-kB[68] and MAPK, and an MyD88-independent pathway associated with the induction of IFN-beta and IFN-inducible genes, and maturation of dendritic cells with slow activation of NF-kB[68] and MAPK.

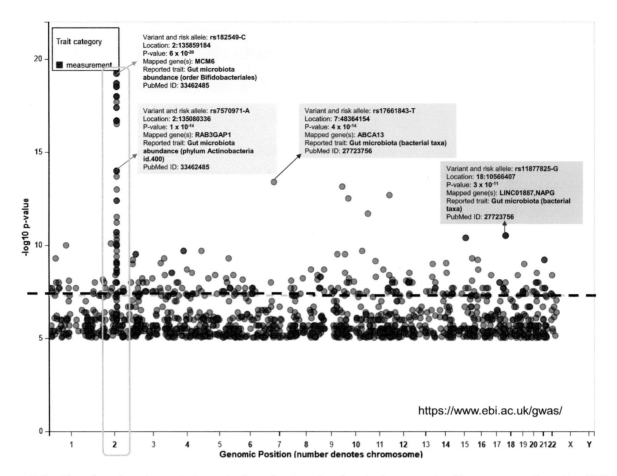

Figure 5.4 Plot of cataloged associations of selected traits related to the human microbiome across all studies (GWAS catalog [www.ebi.ac.uk/gwas/])

Quantification of some aspect of the individual's microbiome of the gut, involving 687 reported traits, 1479 associations, and 699 studies. Some examples of the most significantly associated variants, the rs id, the *p*-value for the association, the PubMed ID, and the trait whenever available. The most striking associations are located in chromosome 2.

Gammaproteobacteria class were significantly enriched in carriers of the rs738409 and rs58542926 risk-alleles, including *Enterobacter* (fold change [FC] = 6.2) and *Pseudoalteromonas* (FC = 2) genera, respectively. *Lawsonella* (1.6-FC), *Prevotella_9* (FC = 1.5), and *Staphylococcus* (FC = 1.3) genera were enriched in rs838133-minor allele carriers, which is linked to sugar consumption and carbohydrate intake. *Tyzzerella* abundance (FC = 2.64) exhibited the strongest association (*p* = 0.0019) with high polygenic risk scores (PRS) values (>4 risk alleles)[69].

Of note, the percentage of genus-level taxa variation explained by our NAFLD/NASH PRS was ~7.4%, which was independent of key covariate parameters that may affect this effect, including age, gender, steatosis score and obesity degree[69].To the best of our knowledge, our study is the first in exploring the interrelationship between the liver metataxonomic profile in patients with NAFLD across the entire spectrum of the disease severity and variants modifying either risk or protection against the disease and variants involved in carbohydrate intake and macronutrient preferences. Together, we have provided evidence that the liver microbiota depends in part on the host genetic background[69]. These observations may represent potentially actionable mechanisms of disease.

5.10 CONCLUSION/SUMMARY POINTS

Microbiome-derived bioactive molecules are key regulators of virtually every aspect of body physiology. In the context of NAFLD, microbially derived metabolites exert a myriad of modifications in the liver tissue that are relevant to the NAFLD biology, including activation of pathways associated with liver fat accumulation, inflammation and hepatic stellate cell activation. Gut dysbiosis might also drive the development of NAFLD by endogenous alcohol production. The discovery of the liver microbiome in samples of patents with NAFLD across the entire spectrum of the disease severity suggested key findings to explain the disease biology and probably a portion of the "missing heritability"[37]. Across major host phenotypic differences—from moderate to severe obesity—the study of the liver metataxonomic profile identified distinctive liver microbial DNA patterns associated with key histological features such as disease severity, liver inflammation and fibrosis. The strongest severe disease-associated imbalance in bacterial DNA was highly linked to obesity. Whereas overabundance of Proteobacteria (alpha or gamma) was predominantly seen in liver specimens of nonmorbidly obese patients, overrepresentation of Peptostreptococcus-,

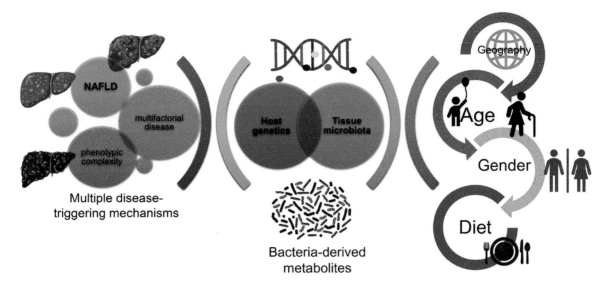

Figure 5.5 Conclusion/summary points

NAFLD is a multifactorial disease that denotes phenotypic complexity. The figure highlights the role of the interrelationship between the host-genome and the liver tissue microbiota, a novel mechanism that may explain the disease biology. There are relevant actors in this relationship, including ethnic diversity and geographic location, the age and gender of the affected patients, and the crucial role of the environmental factors, such as diet.

Verrucomicrobia-, Actinobacteria-, and Proteobacteria-derived DNA was more frequently observed in livers of morbidly obese patients. Notably, decreased amounts of bacterial DNA from the Lachnospiraceae family were associated with more severe histological features. This study suggests that therapeutic options, including probiotic selection, should be precisely defined according to specific clinical scenarios, including features of the host phenome.

Finally, it becomes clear that understanding the putative synergistic effect(s) between the microbiome and their by-products and the genetic background of the host may serve to predict and design novel personalized treatments[17].

The goal of future investigations in this field should be identifying novel pathways and interactions with microbial components that could provide effective therapies for NASH. Nevertheless, there are gaps in our *understanding* of how and by which mechanisms these putative interactions between the body microbiotas and the host-genetics impact on disease biology[17].

It is obvious that the microbiome research domain is driven by methodological advances. Thus future investigations will accelerate our ability to completely understand the role of the microbiome in the biology of NAFLD. Although progress has been made, unanswered questions remain. Nevertheless, this area of research has a bright future.

5.11 ACKNOWLEDGMENT

This study was partially supported by grants PICT 2018–889, PICT 2019–0528, PICT 2016–0135, PICT2018–00620 (Agencia Nacional de Promoción Científica y Tecnológica, FONCyT), CONICET Proyectos Unidades Ejecutoras 2017, PUE 0055.
Conflicts of interest: None

REFERENCES

1. Turnbaugh PJ, Ley RE, Hamady M, Fraser-Liggett CM, Knight R, Gordon JI. The human microbiome project. *Nature* 2007;449(7164):804–810.
2. Berg G, Rybakova D, Fischer D et al. Microbiome definition re-visited: old concepts and new challenges. *Microbiome* 2020;8(1):103.
3. Marchesi JR, Ravel J. The vocabulary of microbiome research: a proposal. *Microbiome* 2015;3:31.
4. Sender R, Fuchs S, Milo R. Revised estimates for the number of human and bacteria cells in the body. *PLoS Biol* 2016;14(8):e1002533.
5. Boursier J, Mueller O, Barret M et al. The severity of nonalcoholic fatty liver disease is associated with gut dysbiosis and shift in the metabolic function of the gut microbiota. *Hepatology* 2016;63(3):764–775.
6. Caussy C, Tripathi A, Humphrey G et al. A gut microbiome signature for cirrhosis due to nonalcoholic fatty liver disease. *Nat Commun* 2019;10(1):1406.
7. Da Silva HE, Teterina A, Comelli EM et al. Nonalcoholic fatty liver disease is associated with dysbiosis independent of body mass index and insulin resistance. *Sci Rep* 2018;8(1):1466.
8. Duarte SMB, Stefano JT, Miele L et al. Gut microbiome composition in lean patients with NASH is associated with liver damage independent of caloric intake: a prospective pilot study. *Nutr Metab Cardiovasc Dis* 2018;28(4):369–384.
9. Loomba R, Seguritan V, Li W et al. Gut microbiome-based metagenomic signature for non-invasive detection of advanced fibrosis in human nonalcoholic fatty liver disease. *Cell Metab* 2017;25(5):1054–1062.
10. Schwimmer JB, Johnson JS, Angeles JE et al. Microbiome signatures associated with steatohepatitis and moderate to severe fibrosis in children with nonalcoholic fatty liver disease. *Gastroenterology* 2019.

11. Wong VW, Tse CH, Lam TT et al. Molecular characterization of the fecal microbiota in patients with nonalcoholic steatohepatitis-a longitudinal study. *PLoS ONE* 2013;8(4):e62885.

12. Zhu L, Baker SS, Gill C et al. Characterization of gut microbiomes in nonalcoholic steatohepatitis (NASH) patients: a connection between endogenous alcohol and NASH. *Hepatology* 2013;57(2):601–609.

13. Behary J, Amorim N, Jiang XT et al. Gut microbiota impact on the peripheral immune response in non-alcoholic fatty liver disease related hepatocellular carcinoma. *Nat Commun* 2021;12(1):187.

14. Michail S, Lin M, Frey MR et al. Altered gut microbial energy and metabolism in children with non-alcoholic fatty liver disease. *FEMS Microbiol Ecol* 2015;91(2):1–9.

15. Ponziani FR, Bhoori S, Castelli C et al. Hepatocellular carcinoma is associated with gut microbiota profile and inflammation in nonalcoholic fatty liver disease. *Hepatology* 2019;69(1):107–120.

16. He LH, Yao DH, Wang LY, Zhang L, Bai XL. Gut microbiome-mediated alteration of immunity, inflammation, and metabolism involved in the regulation of non-alcoholic fatty liver disease. *Front Microbiol* 2021;12:761836.

17. Sookoian S, Pirola CJ. Liver tissue microbiota in nonalcoholic liver disease: a change in the paradigm of host-bacterial interactions. *Hepatobiliary Surg Nutr* 2021;10(3):337–349.

18. Heeg K, Sparwasser T, Lipford GB, Hacker H, Zimmermann S, Wagner H. Bacterial DNA as an evolutionary conserved ligand signalling danger of infection to immune cells. *Eur J Clin Microbiol Infect Dis* 1998;17(7):464–469.

19. Fujieda S, Iho S, Kimura Y et al. DNA from Mycobacterium bovis bacillus Calmette-Guerin (MY-1) inhibits immunoglobulin E production by human lymphocytes. *Am J Respir Crit Care Med* 1999;160(6):2056–2061.

20. De VF, Kovatcheva-Datchary P, Goncalves D et al. Microbiota-generated metabolites promote metabolic benefits via gut-brain neural circuits. *Cell* 2014;156(1–2):84–96.

21. Ren Z, Li A, Jiang J et al. Gut microbiome analysis as a tool towards targeted non-invasive biomarkers for early hepatocellular carcinoma. *Gut* 2019;68(6):1014–1023.

22. Yoshimoto S, Loo TM, Atarashi K et al. Obesity-induced gut microbial metabolite promotes liver cancer through senescence secretome. *Nature* 2013;499(7456):97–101.

23. Demir M, Lang S, Hartmann P et al. The fecal mycobiome in non-alcoholic fatty liver disease. *J Hepatol* 2021.

24. Hoffmann C, Dollive S, Grunberg S et al. Archaea and fungi of the human gut microbiome: correlations with diet and bacterial residents. *PLoS ONE* 2013;8(6):e66019.

25. Manrique P, Bolduc B, Walk ST, van der Oost J, de Vos WM, Young MJ. Healthy human gut phageome. *Proc Natl Acad Sci U S A* 2016;113(37):10400–10405.

26. Hsu CL, Duan Y, Fouts DE, Schnabl B. Intestinal virome and therapeutic potential of bacteriophages in liver disease. *J Hepatol* 2021;75(6):1465–1475.

27. Manrique P, Zhu Y, van der Oost J et al. Gut bacteriophage dynamics during fecal microbial transplantation in subjects with metabolic syndrome. *Gut Microbes* 2021;13(1):1–15.

28. Lang S, Demir M, Martin A et al. Intestinal virome signature associated with severity of nonalcoholic fatty liver disease. *Gastroenterology* 2020;159(5):1839–1852.

29. Duan Y, Llorente C, Lang S et al. Bacteriophage targeting of gut bacterium attenuates alcoholic liver disease. *Nature* 2019;575(7783):505–511.

30. Amar J, Lange C, Payros G et al. Blood microbiota dysbiosis is associated with the onset of cardiovascular events in a large general population: the D.E.S.I.R. study. *PLoS ONE* 2013;8(1):e54461.

31. Koren O, Spor A, Felin J et al. Human oral, gut, and plaque microbiota in patients with atherosclerosis. *Proc Natl Acad Sci U S A* 2011;108(Suppl 1):4592–4598.

32. Lelouvier B, Servant F, Paisse S et al. Changes in blood microbiota profiles associated with liver fibrosis in obese patients: A pilot analysis. *Hepatology* 2016;64(6):2015–2027.

33. Puri P, Liangpunsakul S, Christensen JE et al. The circulating microbiome signature and inferred functional metagenomics in alcoholic hepatitis. *Hepatology* 2018;67(4):1284–1302.

34. Cho EJ, Leem S, Kim SA et al. Circulating microbiota-based metagenomic signature for detection of hepatocellular carcinoma. *Sci Rep* 2019;9(1):7536.

35. Kajihara M, Koido S, Kanai T et al. Characterisation of blood microbiota in patients with liver cirrhosis. *Eur J Gastroenterol Hepatol* 2019;31(12):1577–1583.

36. Bajaj JS, Betrapally NS, Hylemon PB et al. Salivary microbiota reflects changes in gut microbiota in cirrhosis with hepatic encephalopathy. *Hepatology* 2015;62(4):1260–1271.

37. Sookoian S, Salatino A, Castano GO et al. Intrahepatic bacterial metataxonomic signature in non-alcoholic fatty liver disease. *Gut* 2020;69(8):1483–1491.

38. Costello EK, Lauber CL, Hamady M, Fierer N, Gordon JI, Knight R. Bacterial community variation in human body habitats across space and time. *Science* 2009;326(5960):1694–1697.

39. Pirola CJ, Sookoian S. The lipidome in nonalcoholic fatty liver disease: actionable targets. *J Lipid Res* 2021;62:100073.

40. Postler TS, Ghosh S. Understanding the holobiont: How microbial metabolites affect human health and shape the immune system. *Cell Metab* 2017;26(1):110–130.

41. Willemsen LE, Koetsier MA, van Deventer SJ, van Tol EA. Short chain fatty acids stimulate epithelial mucin 2 expression through differential effects on prostaglandin E(1) and E(2) production by intestinal myofibroblasts. *Gut* 2003;52(10):1442–1447.

42. Ridlon JM, Kang DJ, Hylemon PB, Bajaj JS. Bile acids and the gut microbiome. *Curr Opin Gastroenterol* 2014;30(3):332–338.

43. Sookoian S, Flichman D, Castano GO, Pirola CJ. Mendelian randomisation suggests no beneficial effect of moderate alcohol consumption on the severity of nonalcoholic fatty liver disease. *Aliment Pharmacol Ther* 2016;44(11–12):1224–1234.

44. Vilar-Gomez E, Sookoian S, Pirola CJ et al. ADH1B *2 is associated with reduced severity of nonalcoholic fatty liver disease in adults, independent of alcohol consumption. *Gastroenterology* 2020;159(3):929–943.

45. Cope K, Risby T, Diehl AM. Increased gastrointestinal ethanol production in obese mice: implications

for fatty liver disease pathogenesis. *Gastroenterology* 2000;119(5):1340–1347.

46. Nair S, Cope K, Risby TH, Diehl AM. Obesity and female gender increase breath ethanol concentration: potential implications for the pathogenesis of nonalcoholic steatohepatitis. *Am J Gastroenterol* 2001;96(4):1200–1204.

47. Yuan J, Chen C, Cui J et al. Fatty liver disease caused by high-alcohol-producing klebsiella pneumoniae. *Cell Metab* 2019;30(4):675–688.

48. Li NN, Li W, Feng JX et al. High alcohol-producing Klebsiella pneumoniae causes fatty liver disease through 2,3-butanediol fermentation pathway in vivo. *Gut Microbes* 2021;13(1):1979883.

49. Elshaghabee FM, Bockelmann W, Meske D et al. Ethanol production by selected intestinal microorganisms and lactic acid bacteria growing under different nutritional conditions. *Front Microbiol* 2016;7:47.

50. Fouts DE, Torralba M, Nelson KE, Brenner DA, Schnabl B. Bacterial translocation and changes in the intestinal microbiome in mouse models of liver disease. *J Hepatol* 2012;56(6):1283–1292.

51. Yan AW, Fouts DE, Brandl J et al. Enteric dysbiosis associated with a mouse model of alcoholic liver disease. *Hepatology* 2011;53(1):96–105.

52. Henao-Mejia J, Elinav E, Jin C et al. Inflammasome-mediated dysbiosis regulates progression of NAFLD and obesity. *Nature* 2012;482(7384):179–185.

53. Guo S, Nighot M, Al-Sadi R, Alhmoud T, Nighot P, Ma TY. Lipopolysaccharide regulation of intestinal tight junction permeability is mediated by TLR4 signal transduction pathway activation of FAK and MyD88. *J Immunol* 2015;195(10):4999–5010.

54. Goodrich JK, Waters JL, Poole AC et al. Human genetics shape the gut microbiome. *Cell* 2014;159(4):789–799.

55. Goodrich JK, Davenport ER, Beaumont M et al. Genetic determinants of the gut microbiome in UK twins. *Cell Host Microbe* 2016;19(5):731–743.

56. Romeo S, Kozlitina J, Xing C et al. Genetic variation in PNPLA3 confers susceptibility to nonalcoholic fatty liver disease. *Nat Genet* 2008;40(12):1461–1465.

57. Sookoian S, Castano GO, Burgueno AL, Gianotti TF, Rosselli MS, Pirola CJ. A nonsynonymous gene variant in the adiponutrin gene is associated with nonalcoholic fatty liver disease severity. *J Lipid Res* 2009;50(10):2111–2116.

58. Sookoian S, Pirola CJ. Meta-analysis of the influence of I148M variant of patatin-like phospholipase domain containing 3 gene (PNPLA3) on the susceptibility and histological severity of nonalcoholic fatty liver disease. *Hepatology* 2011;53(6):1883–1894.

59. Monga KA, Testerman T, Galuppo B et al. Effect of Gut Microbiota and PNPLA3 rs738409 variant on nonalcoholic fatty liver disease (NAFLD) in obese youth. *J Clin Endocrinol Metab* 2020;105(10).

60. Kozlitina J, Smagris E, Stender S et al. Exome-wide association study identifies a TM6SF2 variant that confers susceptibility to nonalcoholic fatty liver disease. *Nat Genet* 2014;46(4):352–356.

61. Milano M, Aghemo A, Mancina RM et al. Transmembrane 6 superfamily member 2 gene E167K variant impacts on steatosis and liver damage in chronic hepatitis C patients. *Hepatology* 2015;62(1):111–117.

62. Pirola CJ, Sookoian S. The dual and opposite role of the TM6SF2-rs58542926 variant in protecting against cardiovascular disease and conferring risk for nonalcoholic fatty liver: a meta-analysis. *Hepatology* 2015;62(6):1742–1756.

63. Sookoian S, Castano GO, Scian R et al. Genetic variation in transmembrane 6 superfamily member 2 and the risk of nonalcoholic fatty liver disease and histological disease severity. *Hepatology* 2015;61(2):515–525.

64. Mancina RM, Dongiovanni P, Petta S et al. The MBOAT7-TMC4 variant rs641738 increases risk of nonalcoholic fatty liver disease in individuals of European descent. *Gastroenterology* 2016;150(5):1219–1230.

65. Abul-Husn NS, Cheng X, Li AH et al. A protein-truncating HSD17B13 variant and protection from chronic liver disease. *N Engl J Med* 2018;378(12):1096–1106.

66. Ma Y, Belyaeva OV, Brown PM et al. 17-beta hydroxysteroid dehydrogenase 13 is a hepatic retinol dehydrogenase associated with histological features of nonalcoholic fatty liver disease. *Hepatology* 2019;69(4):1504–1519.

67. Pirola CJ, Garaycoechea M, Flichman D et al. Splice variant rs72613567 prevents worst histologic outcomes in patients with nonalcoholic fatty liver disease. *J Lipid Res* 2019;60(1):176–185.

68. Chu AY, Workalemahu T, Paynter NP et al. Novel locus including FGF21 is associated with dietary macronutrient intake. *Hum Mol Genet* 2013;22(9):1895–1902.

69. Pirola CJ, Salatino A, Quintanilla MF, Castano GO, Garaycoechea M, Sookoian S. The influence of host genetics on liver microbiome composition in patients with NAFLD. *EBioMed* 2022. In press.

SECTION II
DIAGNOSTIC TESTS

6 Simple Algorithms in Primary Care

Xixi Xu and Michelle T. Long

CONTENTS

6.1 INTRODUCTION

The global pandemic of obesity impacts an estimated 650 million adults worldwide, and the prevalence is rising[1]. By 2030, approximately 50% of adults in the US will have obesity, and 25% of adults are expected to develop severe obesity[2]. Along with the rise in obesity, associated conditions, including nonalcoholic steatohepatitis (NASH) and nonalcoholic fatty liver disease (NAFLD), will also increase. At present, the prevalence of NAFLD and NASH are high, with an estimated US prevalence of 37% for NAFLD and 14% for NASH[3,4].

Despite the high prevalence of NAFLD and NASH in the population, the guidance on screening for NAFLD or NASH is unclear. Early identification coupled with appropriate clinical intervention may result in improved outcomes and lower mortality for individuals with NAFLD and NASH[5]. Given the high prevalence of disease, it is prudent that primary care providers are well-versed in the diagnosis, risk stratification and management of NAFLD and related cardiometabolic diseases. In this chapter, we present a step-to-step guide for primary care providers to build a knowledge base about identifying and risk-stratifying patients for NAFLD.

6.2 WHO IS AT RISK FOR NAFLD?

NAFLD encompasses a constellation of disease phenotypes based on different histological features. The most common and benign NAFLD phenotype is simple hepatic steatosis, which accounts for 75% of those with NAFLD[6]. However, about 25% of persons with NAFLD have NASH, a progressive NAFLD phenotype associated with hepatic fibrosis, which can lead to end-stage liver disease, hepatocellular carcinoma (HCC) and liver-related death.

So who is at risk for NAFLD? Family aggregation studies and twin studies suggest that the development of NAFLD may, in part, be related to genetic susceptibility[7,8]. Multiple genetic loci associate with NAFLD in the general population, including *PNPLA3* (encoding patatinlike phospholipase domaincontaining protein 3) and *TM6SF2* (encoding transmembrane 6 superfamily member 2)[9]. In addition, epigenetic factors, such as DNA methylation remodeling of fibrosis modifier genes, may contribute to gene–environment interactions in the risk of developing fibrosis in NAFLD[10,11]. From an environmental perspective, an unhealthy lifestyle with low physical activity levels and consuming an unhealthy diet, including diets high in sugar, sodium, and fat and low in fresh fruits and vegetables associate with a high prevalence of NAFLD[12–15].

Obesity, specifically abdominal or visceral adiposity, is a major risk factor for NAFLD[16]. Even a modest weight increase of 2 kg can increase an individual's risk of developing NAFLD[17]. Yu et al. (2015) has shown that increased visceral adipose tissue is independently associated with NASH and development of fibrosis[17]. Type 2 diabetes mellitus (T2DM) is also strongly associated with NAFLD, which has a disease prevalence of over 50% among persons with T2DM with an even higher prevalence for those with poor T2DM control[18].

Metabolic syndrome is another risk factor associated with NAFLD. In a study with a cohort of 11,647 people, the prevalence of NAFLD was significantly higher in individuals with metabolic syndrome, and the prevalence increased as the burden of metabolic risk factors increased[19]. The presence of metabolic syndrome is also seen in more individuals with advanced hepatic fibrosis[19]. In addition, the risk of developing cirrhosis or hepatocellular carcinoma (HCC) also increases with each additional metabolic syndrome factor. For example, in patients with NAFLD, having both hypertension and dyslipidemia would result in 1.8-fold increase in the risk of developing cirrhosis or HCC[20].

Though strongly associated with obesity, NAFLD can also exist in persons with normal weight BMI. Lean NAFLD was first described in Asian populations; however, subsequent studies have observed that between 10 and 20% of Americans and Europeans with NAFLD are lean[21,22]. Lean individuals with NAFLD often have a higher burden of cardiometabolic disease risk factors compared to lean individuals without NAFLD[23]. Additionally, the risk of cardiovascular disease events may be similar or higher for lean persons with NAFLD compared to overweight and obese persons with NAFLD[24,25]. Having normal weight does not reduce the risk of fibrosis progression or mortality from NAFLD[26].

6.3 SCREENING FOR NAFLD: GENERAL POPULATION AND HIGH-RISK GROUPS

As the presence of NAFLD in the population increases, the morbidity and mortality due to disease progression and complication, including cirrhosis, liver failure and HCC, will rapidly rise. At present, NAFLD is the second most common etiology of chronic liver disease among patients listed

DOI: 10.1201/9781003386698-8

for liver transplant in the United States[27]. The prevalence of NAFLD as an indication for liver transplant has almost doubled between 2004 and 2013[28]. The cost associated with diagnosing and treating NAFLD is expected to take up a significant portion of total health care spending. In 2016, the annual economic burden of NAFLD in the US was estimated to be $103 billion[29], and costs are expected to increase with the rising prevalence. Therefore, early detection and early intervention for patients who are at risk for progressive NAFLD are critical to prevent morbidity and mortality.

Whereas it is reasonable to assume that routine screening may improve early detection and intervention, there is no consensus on routine screening for NAFLD. The US Preventive Services Task Force (USPSTF) and National Institute for Health and Care Excellence (NICE) make no recommendations for or against general screening for NAFLD. The American Association for the Study of Liver Diseases (AASLD) practice guidelines do not recommend routine screening for NAFLD, citing the lack of evidence on cost-effectiveness and effective treatments[30], though data on cost-effectiveness are now available since the publication of the guidelines. The European Association for the Study of the Liver (EASL), on the contrary, has recommended screening for every person with persistently abnormal liver biochemical tests[31].

With the emerging of more effective medications, screening for NAFLD among high-risk patient populations is likely to be cost-effective. It is well-established that patients with T2DM and metabolic syndrome are at increased risk of developing NAFLD[32]. Particularly, T2DM is a significant risk factor for the development of NAFLD, liver fibrosis and HCC[33–35]. The AASLD guidelines recommend that clinicians should have a high index of suspicion for NAFLD and NASH in patients with T2DM and encourage the use of clinical tools, such as the NAFLD Fibrosis Score (NFS), the Fibrosis-4 index (FIB-4) or vibration-controlled transient elastography, to further risk-stratify[30]. The American Diabetes Association (ADA) also recognizes the close association of T2DM with the development of NAFLD; thus the 2020 ADA guidelines propose to screen all patients with T2DM, prediabetes, elevated liver aminotransferase levels or fatty liver on ultrasound for NAFLD[36]. Noureddin et al. (2020) have demonstrated that screening for NAFLD in patients with T2DM with ultrasound and liver biochemical tests, followed by noninvasive testing for fibrosis is cost-effective[37].

Although further research is necessary to uncover additional risk factors for NAFLD, it is reasonable to identify patients with T2DM, multiple metabolic risk factors, abnormal liver aminotransferases, or incidental hepatic steatosis on imaging in the primary care setting as patients at high risk for NAFLD. Thus American Gastroenterology Association (AGA) published an NAFLD/NASH Clinical Care Pathway for this purpose through a multidisciplinary task force with the ADA, American Osteopathic Association, Endocrine Society and the Obesity Society[3].

6.4 NONINVASIVE SCREENING MODALITIES FOR NAFLD

Liver biopsy, the gold standard for diagnosis NAFLD, is not an appropriate screening test for NAFLD given the highly invasive nature of the test, risk for complications, and high cost. An ideal screening test should be inexpensive, easy to perform, and have relatively high sensitivity. Given the high prevalence of NAFLD in patients with T2DM,

metabolic risk factors, elevated aminotransferases and incidental findings of steatosis as mentioned in the previous section, the best screening method for primary care providers may be a high clinical suspicion for NAFLD in patients who are at risk. The very initial screening strategy should include detailed history, comprehensive physical exam, focused laboratory tests and abdominal ultrasound.

For patients who have risk factors for NAFLD, a detailed history and full physical examination are obtained. Specifically, clinicians should assess the patients' alcohol consumption, drug use, sexual history, medication history, herbal or alternative medication use, occupational exposure, BMI, past medical history (particularly history of diabetes, hyperlipidemia and hypertension) and family history of liver diseases such as Wilson's disease, hemochromatosis, autoimmune disease and alpha-1 antitrypsin deficiency[38].

If elevated liver biochemical tests are detected, clinicians should consider other causes of liver disease as possible contributing factors (Table 6.1). Depending on the pattern of liver biochemical test elevation, liver diseases that should be considered include viral hepatitis, autoimmune hepatitis, Wilson disease, hemochromatosis, alpha-1 antitrypsin deficiency, drug-induced liver injury and alcohol-related liver disease. The most common blood-based screening test for NAFLD are liver biochemical tests, specifically the serum aminotransferases (alanine aminotransferase [ALT]) and aspartate aminotransferase [AST]). Elevations of ALT or AST may be an indicator of NAFLD with a usual pattern of ALT greater than AST. Along with this pattern of transaminases elevation, γ glutamyltransferase (GGT) may also be elevated[39].

Many patients with NAFLD or NASH are found to have abnormal ALT[40]. Thus patients with incidental findings of abnormal liver biochemical tests warrant further workup. However, AST and ALT can be normal in up to 78% of patients with NAFLD[22]; thus serum aminotansferases may not be sensitive for NAFLD. It is important to keep in mind that normal liver biochemical tests do not rule out possible underlying NAFLD in an asymptomatic patient with risk factors. For patients with chronically elevated liver biochemical tests as well as metabolic risk factors such as obesity, diabetes, hyperlipidemia, and hypertension, the most common cause to consider is NAFLD.

Contrary to the nomenclature often used, ALT, AST, ALP, GGT and bilirubin are markers of liver injury rather than liver function. The markers for hepatocellular function are albumin, bilirubin and prothrombin time. In order to identify abnormal liver biochemical tests, true healthy normal levels are needed. Establishing a normal range for AST and ALT has been problematic given that reference standards were established in a general population, many of whom likely had undiagnosed NAFLD. In the past, abnormal ALT levels were based on multiples of upper limits of normal to avoid specifically defining the normal level of ALT[41]. This method often runs into the issue of different definitions of upper limits of normal by laboratories, making comparison of liver blood tests from different laboratories challenging.

To define a unified lower threshold for ALT, patient factors, such as age, sex, medication and supplement use, alcohol use, BMI, and underlying conditions, such as NAFLD and viral hepatitis status, should be taken into consideration when selecting healthy reference populations. The American College of Gastroenterology currently recommends a true healthy normal ALT level to be 29–33 IU/l for men and 19–25 IU/l for women. However, a recent

Table 6.1: Patterns of Abnormal Liver Function Tests for Diseases

Pattern Type	Causes	ALT	AST	Alkaline Phosphatase	Total Bilirubin	Special Tests
Hepatocellular (↑ALT & AST)	NAFLD	Borderline -4× ULN	Borderline -4× ULN	Normal	Normal	Liver ultrasound and FibroScan
	Alcohol-related liver disease	Borderline -4× ULN	Borderline -4× ULN	Normal	Normal	AST: ALT>2
	Viral infections	Borderline -5× ULN (acute infection >1,000)	Borderline -5× ULN (acute infection >1,000)	Normal	Normal	Check HBsAg, HBsAb, HBcAb, HCV Ab and PCR, HAV IgG/IgM, HSV, EBV, and CMV
	Congestive hepatopathy	Borderline -3× ULN	Borderline -3× ULN	Normal—mildly elevated	Normal	Elevated indirect bilirubin
	Autoimmune hepatitis	Borderline -5× ULN (acute presentation >10–20× ULN)	Borderline -5× ULN (acute presentation >10–20× ULN)	ALK: AST (or ALT) <2 Acute presentation: ALK: AST (or ALT) <5	Normal	ANA, AMA, ASMA, LKM-1, IgG
	Wilson's disease	Borderline -5× ULN	Borderline -5× ULN	Normal to ↓	ALK: Tbili <4	↓ Serum Ceruloplasmin and ↑ urine copper
	Ischemia	Elevated >50× ULN	Elevated >50× ULN	Normal	↑ but lag behind peak 1 week later	Abdominal ultrasound with doppler
	Medication and toxins	Variable	Variable	Normal	Normal	
Cholesteric (↑ALK and direct bilirubin)	Biliary obstruction Intrahepatic cholestasis Biliary epithelial damage	Normal—mildly elevated	Normal—mildly elevated	≥4× ULN	Normal—elevated	GGT to confirm hepatic origin, Abdominal ultrasound, MRCP/ERCP if has obstruction. ANA, AMA, ASMA if no obstruction

ANA: Antinuclear antibodies; ASMA: Anti-smooth muscle antibodies; AMA: Anti-mitochondrial antibodies; LKM-1: Liver kidney microsome type 1; MRCP: Magnetic resonance cholangiopancreatography; ERCP: Endoscopic retrograde cholangiopancreatography; GGT: gamma-glutamyl transferase.

study suggests that age-specific cutoffs may be more appropriate as 10% of healthy men under the age of 45 years had an elevated ALT[42]. Clinical judgement remains to be the foremost important factor when interpretations liver biochemical tests of an individual patient.

The most common imaging-based screening test for NAFLD is abdominal ultrasound (US). US is an easily accessible, noninvasive way to identify hepatic steatosis qualitatively. The criteria to assess hepatic steatosis via US include hepatorenal echo contrast, liver brightness, deep attenuation and vascular blurring[38]. The sensitivity for US to detect small amounts of hepatic steatosis is limited; the sensitivity for detection of steatosis is 64% in the general population[43], though in higher-risk groups with a higher prevalence of steatosis, the sensitivity of US for steatosis improves to 90%[43,44]. The specificity of US in detecting hepatic steatosis remains excellent at >95% regardless of the degree of hepatic steatosis[43]. However, it is important to clarify that hepatic steatosis does not directly translate to a diagnosis of NAFLD as many other liver or systemic diseases can also show hepatic steatosis on US (Table 6.2).

6.5 WHAT TO DO WHEN A PATIENT IS SUSPECTED OF HAVING NAFLD?

To help primary care providers decide on the urgency of management and referral when patients are suspected of having NAFLD, it is critical to review the natural history of NAFLD. In a retrospective study that followed individuals for up to 10 years, the annual incidence of compensated cirrhosis, decompensated cirrhosis and death in patients with NAFLD were 0.28, 0.31 and 0.63%, respectively[45]. A recent prospective study that followed patients with NAFLD for a period of approximately 4 years showed similar findings of slow disease progression, low incidence of decompensated cirrhosis and low incidence of HCC in NASH with cirrhosis[46]. Overall, these studies suggested that NAFLD is a slowly progressive disease, and most people with NAFLD do not have NASH or fibrosis. Individuals with NASH, particularly those with associated hepatic fibrosis, are at increased risk of liver-related events and worsened overall mortality[46,47]. Primary care providers play a frontline role in the identification and risk stratification of patients with NAFLD in order to identify those with hepatic fibrosis and most in need of liver-directed care.

6.6 RISK STRATIFICATION IN NAFLD

6.6.1 Blood-Based Risk Stratification Scores

Some of the commonly used serology tests to assess the risk of disease progression to NASH and advanced fibrosis are FIB-4, NAFLD fibrosis score (NFS) and enhanced liver fibrosis (ELF) (Table 6.3).

Originally used to predict level of fibrosis for patients with Hepatitis C, FIB-4 index is a simple scoring system that combines patient age with AST, ALT and platelet count[48]. FIB-4 was subsequently validated to predict risk for advanced fibrosis in NAFLD for both obese and nonobese patient populations[49,50]. As one of the earliest and most well-studied noninvasive tests for detecting fibrosis, FIB-4 is endorsed by the American College of Gastroenterology as a risk stratification tool in clinical practice[51]. A FIB-4 value less than 1.3, summarized from various studies, showed >90% of negative predictive value to rule out advanced fibrosis[52]. Greater than 90% of positive predictive value for detecting cirrhosis is achieved with a FIB-4 value > 2.68[53]. It is important to note that FIB-4 is unable to accurately diagnose advance fibrosis in patients who are younger than 35 or older than 65 years of age[53]. Patients who are older than 65 years old may require a different cutoff (FIB-4 > 2.0) from the aforementioned values[53].

NFS is another scoring system that is widely validated for predicting advanced fibrosis from NAFLD. NFS includes patient characteristics such as age, BMI, fasting blood glucose, AST, ALT, albumin and platelet count. With a threshold of −1.455, the NFS has a negative predictive value of about 90%, a sensitivity of 72% and a specificity of 73%, which suggests that this test can be useful to rule out advanced fibrosis in persons with NAFLD. NFS has modest to high accuracy to diagnose advance fibrosis with a cutoff value of 0.676 with positive predictive value of around 80%[52,54].

ELF was validated in 2017 as a serology-based scoring system to detect liver fibrosis and NASH. Different from FIB-4 and NFS, the ELF score is based on specialized tests that may not be commonly utilized in the primary care setting. The scoring test is based on the level of hyaluronic acid, procollagen III amino-terminal peptide and tissue inhibitor of matrix metalloproteinase I. For the cutoff value 9.0, the ELF test has a sensitivity of 85.7%, a specificity of 83.3%,

Table 6.2: Common Differential Diagnosis of Hepatic Steatosis on Imaging

Liver-Specific Disease	Endocrine	Inborn Errors of Metabolism	Acquired Metabolic Disorder	Drug and Toxin
• NAFLD • Alcoholic fatty liver disease • Acute fatty liver of pregnancy • Chronic hepatitis C (especially genotype 3) • HIV • Wilson's disease • Hemochromatosis • α1- antitrypsin deficiency	• Hypothyroidism • Hypopituitarism • Polycystic ovary syndrome • Growth hormone insufficiency	• Lysosomal acid lipase deficiency (LAL-D) • Familial hypobetalipoprotein B • Abetalipoproteinemia • Urea cycle disorders • Hereditary fructose intolerance • Glycogen storage disease • Fatty acid oxidation disorders • Autosomal recessive carbamoylphosphate synthetase I (CPSI) deficiency	• Inflammatory bowel disease • Celiac disease • Jejunoileal bypass • Malnutrition/ Kwashiorkor disease • Acute weight loss • Short bowel syndrome • Total parenteral nutrition	• Methotrexate • Amiodarone • Corticosteroids • Valproic acid • Tetracycline • Amphetamines • Older generation of NRTI: didanosine, stavudine and zidovudine • Heavy metal: lead, cadmium and mercury • Herbicide and pesticide

Table 6.3: Comparison of Different Noninvasive Tests for Detecting Advanced Fibrosis in NAFLD

Test	Cutoff	Sensitivity (%)	Specificity (%)	PPV (%)	NPV (%)	Advantages and Disadvantages
ALT[1]	< 35	68.9	22.6			Easily accessible test, and most patients would have ALT measured from annual physical checkup at some point. Poor sensitivity and specificity to detect NASH and advance fibrosis
	> 70	40	57.6			
AST/ALT ratio[2]	< 0.8	74	78	44	93	Both AST and ALT can be easily obtained. Positive predictive value remains low and will miss patients with advance fibrosis
	> 1.0	52	90	55	89	
AST to platelet ratio (APRI)[2]	1	27	89	37	84	
FIB-4 index[2,3]	< 1.3	85	65	36	95	Easily calculated from platelet count, patient's age, AST and ALT. FIB-4 index has been well-validated as a noninvasive test for advanced fibrosis in NAFLD. The test is limited to patients who are between the ages of 35 and 65
	> 2.67	33	98	80	83	
NFS[2]	< −1.455	78	58	30	92	More complex calculation from patient's age, BMI, presence of diabetes, AST, ALT, platelets and albumin. NFS has been well-validated as a noninvasive test for advance fibrosis in NAFLD.
	> 0.676	33	98	76	86	
VCTE[4,5]	< 7.9 kPa	77.3	68.8	44	90.5	Relatively easy and fast test that can be performed in office with lower cost. The test accuracy is limited by patient's BMI, and results may be invalid in patients with BMI > 35.
	> 12.1 kPa	52	90	71	80	
MRE[6]	< 3.02 kPa	55.4	90.7	91.1	54.2	Better accuracy compared to VCTE and provides comprehensive evaluation of the whole liver. Very limited availability given high cost. Requires specialized technician and radiologist to conduct and interpret the study.
	> 3.64 kPa	86.4	90.5	67.9	96.6	

PPV: Positive predictive value; NPV: Negative predictive value; ALT: Alanine aminotransferase; AST: Aspartate aminotransferase; NFS: NAFLD fibrosis score; BMI: body mass index.

1. Verma S, Jensen D, Hart J, Mohanty SR. Predictive value of ALT levels for non-alcoholic steatohepatitis (NASH) and advanced fibrosis in non-alcoholic fatty liver disease (NAFLD). *Liver Int*. Oct 2013;33(9):1398–1405. doi:10.1111/liv.12226
2. McPherson S, Stewart SF, Henderson E, Burt AD, Day CP. Simple non-invasive fibrosis scoring systems can reliably exclude advanced fibrosis in patients with non-alcoholic fatty liver disease. *Gut*. Sep 2010;59(9):1265–1269. doi:10.1136/gut.2010.216077
3. Rikhi R, Singh T, Modaresi Esfeh J. Work up of fatty liver by primary care physicians, review. *Ann Med Surg (Lond)*. Feb 2020;50:41–48. doi:10.1016/j.amsu.2020.01.001
4. Wong VW, Vergniol J, Wong GL, et al. Diagnosis of fibrosis and cirrhosis using liver stiffness measurement in nonalcoholic fatty liver disease. *Hepatology*. Feb 2010;51(2):454–462. doi:10.1002/hep.23312
5. Siddiqui MS, Yamada G, Vuppalanchi R, et al. Diagnostic accuracy of noninvasive fibrosis models to detect change in fibrosis stage. *Clin Gastroenterol Hepatol*. Aug 2019;17(9):1877–1885.e5. doi:10.1016/j.cgh.2018.12.031
6. Loomba R, Wolfson T, Ang B, et al. Magnetic resonance elastography predicts advanced fibrosis in patients with nonalcoholic fatty liver disease: a prospective study. *Hepatology*. Dec 2014;60(6):1920–1928. doi:10.1002/hep.27362

a positive predictive value of 60.0% and negative predictive value of 95.2%. This test can reliably differentiate mild fibrosis (F0/F1) from advanced fibrosis (F2/F3) in patients with NAFLD[55]. A high ELF score (>11.3) may predict a higher risk of developing liver-related outcomes at 1 year, better than FIB-4 or the Model for End-Stage Liver Disease (MELD) score[56]. The ELF test was approved by the FDA in 2021; however, the specific cutoff value that applies to the real-world clinical practice in the US remains to be determined.

However, these noninvasive serology tests can be limited as they might not be applicable to certain populations. For example, FIB-4 has been shown to be inaccurate for older individuals (>65 years old) or those with chronic kidney diseases[53,57]. In addition, NFS and FIB-4 both use lower and upper thresholds to maximize sensitivity or specificity when ruling in or ruling out advanced fibrosis. However, many individuals may fall between the cutoffs into an indeterminate zone, which may still require additional testing to rule out advanced disease. Therefore, a second test may be necessary to further risk-stratify the patients in the indeterminate group.

6.6.2 Imaging-Based Risk Stratification Scores

Supplementing the serology tests, several imaging modalities are validated to assess liver stiffness, a surrogate measure of liver fibrosis. Common imaging modalities include vibration-controlled transient elastography (VCTE), magnetic resonance elastography (MRE) and ultrasound-based 2D shear wave elastography (2D-SWE).

VCTE measures liver stiffness by measuring shear wave velocity of a low-frequency elastic wave directed into the liver from an ultrasound probe. It is a relatively simple and fast test that can be performed in the office. Liver stiffness measurements have been shown to correlate with the degree of liver fibrosis in NAFLD[58,59]. Wong et al. (2010) demonstrated that the area under the receiver-operating characteristic curve of VCTE is significantly better compared to that of serology-based test for liver fibrosis such as FIB-4, NFS and AST-to-platelet ratio index. For a cutoff value of 7.9 kPa, the negative predictive value for advanced fibrosis is 96%; however, the positive predictive value is only at 52%. With liver stiffness measurement less than 7.9 kPa, the VCTE is best used to rule out advanced fibrosis[59]. Other studies have shown that for a cutoff value of 8.2 kPa for fibrosis stage ≥ 2, the negative predictive value is 97% in the general population and 78% among those with T2DM[60]. An upper cutoff threshold of 15 kPa has a positive predictive value and negative predictive value for advanced fibrosis of 77.8 and 100%, respectively[61]. Based on the actual prevalence of NAFLD in the population, with the top threshold of 12.1 kPa, the positive predictive value to include patients with fibrosis stage ≥ 2 is 88%. Individuals with a liver stiffness >12.1 kPa on VCTE are likely to have some degree of hepatic fibrosis[60].

Magnetic resonance elastography (MRE) is another clinically useful tool for evaluating the stage of fibrosis. Similar to VCTE, MRE utilizes MRI to propagate acoustic shear waves into the liver, and the liver stiffness measurements can be calculated based on the propagation of the shear waves. For patients with liver stiffness measurements greater than 3.63 kPa, MRE is an accurate test to diagnose advance fibrosis with the sensitivity, specificity, positive predictive value and negative predictive value of 86, 91, 68 and 97%, respectively[62]. MRE is a superior test compared to VCTE not only because of better accuracy, but also MRE provides a comprehensive evaluation of the whole liver instead of the limited area evaluated by VCTE[63]. For patients with severe abdominal obesity, MRE is also a better test compared to other noninvasive imaging modalities for liver fibrosis[64]. At this time, MRE is not widely used as a point-of-care imaging test due to its high cost and requirement for specialists to interpret the images.

Ultrasound-based 2D-SWE is a novel imaging modality that utilizes a focused ultrasound beam to pass shear waves through an area of liver tissue of interest. 2D-SWE is performed using a conventional ultrasound probe, so it shares the same benefit of ultrasound to obtain real-time and quantitative measures of different areas of the liver. 2D-SWE has been shown to have comparably good diagnostic accuracy for advanced fibrosis as MRE and VCTE, but it is more accessible and easier to operate compared to MRE[65].

6.7 SUGGESTED RISK STRATIFICATION ALGORITHM FOR PRIMARY CARE

Studies have shown that noninvasive tests such as serology and imaging tests are adequate to risk-stratify patients in the primary care setting and to monitor for NAFLD progression. Utilizing two-step algorithms, unnecessary referrals can be reduced by up to 80% while increasing detection of advanced fibrosis and cirrhosis by approximately 5 times[66,67]. Using a simulation model of American patients with NAFLD, Tapper et al. (2016) showed that using NFS alone or the combination of NFS and VCTE in the primary care clinic is the most cost-effective strategy to risk-stratify NAFLD[68]. Other studies based on the US and

European populations have also confirmed that the combination of FIB-4 or NFS with VCTE has diagnostic accuracy and is cost-effective[69–71]. Based the multiple proposed algorithms in the literatures, we proposed an algorithm for primary care providers in identifying, screening and fibrosis risk-assessing patients for NAFLD[3,72,73] (Figure 6.1).

The algorithms to use in the primary care office that are currently published in major guidelines generally follow a two-step model. Clinical practice guideline from the European Association for the Study of the Liver (EASL), European Association for the Study of Diabetes (EASD) and European Association for the Study of Obesity (EASO) suggested a diagnostic flowchart to assess and monitor disease severity in patients with suspected NAFLD or metabolic risk factors. The first diagnostic step recommended by this guideline is liver blood tests (ALT, AST and GGT) and ultrasound. When imaging modalities are not available, then serum biomarkers and scores are acceptable alternatives for diagnosing NAFLD[72].

If there are signs of fatty liver on ultrasound and normal liver blood tests, the second step of the algorithm is to check serum fibrosis markers such as NFS, FIB-4 or ELF. Based on the risk suggested by the serum fibrosis marker, patients with low risk should have a follow-up in 2 years with repeated liver blood tests and serum fibrosis markers. For patients with medium/high risk based on serum fibrosis markers, referral to Hepatology is necessary for a more thorough assessment of disease severity and evaluation for liver biopsy. Similarly, patients with abnormal liver blood tests and signs of fatty liver disease on ultrasound will also require evaluation from specialists. For patients with normal liver ultrasound and liver blood tests, repeated ultrasound and liver blood tests should be done in 3–5 years[72].

Multiple publications have also suggested similar algorithms to screen patients who are at risk for NAFLD. The first step is to identify patients who at risk of NAFLD, which is defined as patient with more than 2 metabolic risk factors (central obesity, hyperlipidemia, hypertension, pre-diabetes or insulin resistance), type 2 diabetes, signs of fatty liver on any imaging modalities, or elevated aminotransferases. Once patients at risk are identified, step 2 is to rule out other pathology that can lead to liver diseases. Extensive past medical history, social history, medication history and physical exams are necessary for all patients with suspected NAFLD[3,73–76].

The next step is risk stratification for the risk of hepatic fibrosis in patients who are at risk of NAFLD with noninvasive testing such as FIB-4, NFS, or ELF. Most of the established algorithms utilize FIB-4 and NFS. ELF is a relatively new serum score test that requires specialized serum tests, and it is mostly utilized in European guidelines. ELF was recently approved in the US to monitor fibrosis in chronic liver disease but not to screen for hepatic fibrosis. More research on ELF is needed before it can be recommended as a tool in primary clinic to evaluate for fibrosis.

FIB-4 and NFS have been shown to have superior diagnostic accuracy to differentiate no fibrosis (F0 and F1) from advanced fibrosis (F3 and F4) compared to other noninvasive fibrosis scores[77,78]. FIB-4 may also be slightly more accurate than NFS[49,79]. In addition, the combinations of noninvasive fibrosis scores such as FIB-4 and aspartate transaminase-to-platelet ratio index or FIB-4 and ELF can also be used together to further increase the diagnostic accuracy[77,80]. Nevertheless, moderate fibrosis is difficult to

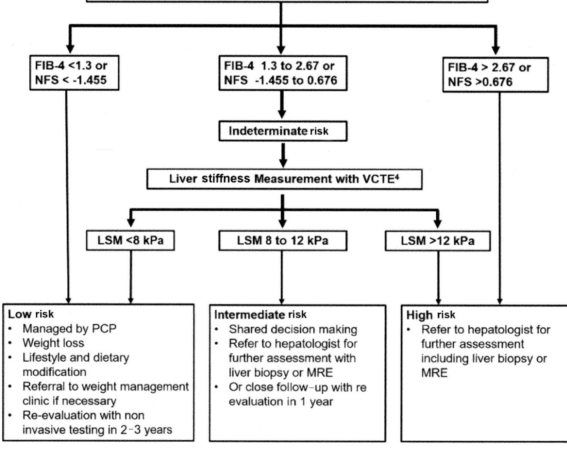

Figure 6.1 Algorithm for identifying, screening and fibrosis risk-assessing patients for NAFLD

determine with any accuracy, and it may not be correctly differentiated by noninvasive fibrosis tests.

Multiple studies have shown that setting a lower threshold of 1.3 for FIB-4 has a negative protective value of greater than 90%, which could reliably rule out advanced fibrosis[50,53,77,78]. Thus, for patients who have FIB-4 score <1.3, no further investigation is necessary. But patients should be followed up closely in primary care with intensive counseling on lifestyle and diet modification to lose weight. And this group of patients should have repeated testing with FIB-4 in 2–3 years[3]. With an upper threshold of 2.67, the positive predictive value of FIB-4 is around 60–80% which suggests a very high possibility of advanced fibrosis[50,52,77,81]. When patients have a FIB-4 score>2.67, they are very likely to have advanced fibrosis and require evaluation by a hepatologist and possibly a liver biopsy[3]. Nevertheless, it should be emphasized that the FIB-4 index is validated in patients aged between 35 and 65 years of age. Different cutoff values, such as FIB-4 >2 as suggested by some studies, may be necessary for patients who are older than 65 years of age[53]. The remaining group of patients who fall into the intermediate risk group with FIB-4 score between 1.3 and 2.67 make up to 40% of patients with suspected NAFLD[35]. The intermediate risk group requires secondary evaluation with liver stiffness measurement to differentiate the risk of fibrosis in this group.

Another study has suggested a combination of NFS and FIB-4 score as the initial step to categorize patients' risk of developing advanced fibrosis. NFS by itself already has good diagnostic accuracy for advanced fibrosis. NFS less than −1.455 can safely exclude patients with advanced fibrosis with a negative predictive value >90%. Using an NFS greater than 0.676, the positive predictive value is around 80–90% which can adequately rule in patients with advanced fibrosis[52,54]. Pandyarajan et al. (2019) proposed a model to combine both NFS and FIB-4 scores together for the initial step of risk stratification. For patients with NFS <−1.455 and FIB-4 < 1.30, the risk of advanced fibrosis is likely to be low, and these patients can be followed by the primary care provider with counseling on lifestyle modification, diet changes and weight loss. The primary care provider can also repeat the NFS and FIB-4 in 1 year to reassess the risk for advanced fibrosis. If patients have NFS >0.676 and FIB-4 >2.67, the risk of advanced fibrosis is likely to be very high, and the patient would benefit from further evaluation and management by Hepatology. The intermediate group refers to patients who have NFS between −1.455 and 0.676 or FIB-4 between 1.30 and 2.67. Patients in the intermediate group should undergo further risk stratification with imaging, such as VCTE for the measurement of the liver stiffness, in order to elucidate the risk of advanced fibrosis[73].

VCTE, MRE and 2D-SWE are all imaging modalities that can be used to measure liver stiffness. Patients with liver stiffness measurement less than 8.0 kPa on VCTE are less likely to have significant hepatic fibrosis[59,60], and this low-fibrosis-risk population can be managed by primary care providers with referral to nutrition, counseling on diet, weight loss and repeated noninvasive testing in 2–3 years[3]. With a liver stiffness measurement >12.0 kPa, the risk of liver fibrosis is very high[60,82]. The high-risk population warrants referral to Hepatology for further evaluation with liver biopsy or MRE. With further evaluation by Hepatology, patients with high risk may be appropriate for medication

and secondary prevention strategies[3]. In addition, it is also helpful for primary care providers to be aware that a high liver stiffness measure of >20 kPa suggests high risk of cirrhosis with esophageal varices[83]. Therefore, patients with a FIB-4 score of > 2.67 and a liver stiffness measure of >20kPa should be promptly referred to Hepatology.

Unfortunately, a proportion of patients still fall into the intermediate range of liver stiffness measurement (i.e., 8.0–12.0 kPa). There is no clear guideline on additional testing or management. The decision largely relies on shared decision making between the patient and the primary care provider or specialist. Given that the patient is at risk for NAFLD and has two indeterminate noninvasive testing results, it is reasonable to refer the patient to Hepatology for MRE or liver biopsy for further evaluation. However, if the patient prefers to wait, individual preferences should also be taken into consideration. Primary care providers can discuss with patient about close follow-up and repeating measurement of liver stiffness in 1 year[3].

6.8 SUMMARY

An increasing evidence base supports the cost-effectiveness of screening for NAFLD, particularly among high-risk groups and as new medications and treatments evolve. Primary care providers play a critical role in the identification and initial risk stratification of persons at risk for NAFLD. With success, earlier detection and risk stratification will prompt early interventions to prevent advanced fibrosis and improve the lives of patients living with NAFLD.

REFERENCES

1. The Lancet Gastroenterology H. Obesity: another ongoing pandemic. *Lancet Gastroenterol Hepatol.* 2021;6(6):411. doi:10.1016/s2468-1253(21)00143-6
2. Ward ZJ, Bleich SN, Cradock AL, et al. Projected U.S. state-level prevalence of adult obesity and severe obesity. *N Engl J Med.* 2019;381(25):2440–2450. doi:10.1056/NEJMsa1909301
3. Kanwal F, Shubrook JH, Adams LA, et al. Clinical care pathway for the risk stratification and management of patients with nonalcoholic fatty liver disease. *Gastroenterology.* 2021;161(5):1657–1669. doi:10.1053/j.gastro.2021.07.049
4. Harrison SA, Gawrieh S, Roberts K, et al. Prospective evaluation of the prevalence of non-alcoholic fatty liver disease and steatohepatitis in a large middle-aged US cohort. *J Hepatol.* 2021;75(2):284–291. doi:10.1016/j.jhep.2021.02.034
5. Vilar-Gomez E, Martinez-Perez Y, Calzadilla-Bertot L, et al. Weight loss through lifestyle modification significantly reduces features of nonalcoholic steatohepatitis. *Gastroenterology.* 2015;149(2):367–378.e5; quiz e14–15. doi:10.1053/j.gastro.2015.04.005
6. Rinella ME. Nonalcoholic fatty liver disease: a systematic review. *Jama.* 9 2015;313(22):2263–2273. doi:10.1001/jama.2015.5370
7. Schwimmer JB, Celedon MA, Lavine JE, et al. Heritability of nonalcoholic fatty liver disease. *Gastroenterology.* 2009;136(5):1585–1592. doi:10.1053/j.gastro.2009.01.050
8. Loomba R, Schork N, Chen CH, et al. Heritability of hepatic fibrosis and steatosis based on a prospective twin study. *Gastroenterology.* 2015;149(7):1784–1793. doi:10.1053/j.gastro.2015.08.011

9. Anstee QM, Day CP. The genetics of nonalcoholic fatty liver disease: spotlight on PNPLA3 and TM6SF2. *Semin Liver Dis*. 2015;35(3):270–290. doi:10.1055/s-0035-1562947

10. Zarrinpar A, Gupta S, Maurya MR, Subramaniam S, Loomba R. Serum microRNAs explain discordance of non-alcoholic fatty liver disease in monozygotic and dizygotic twins: a prospective study. *Gut*. 2016;65(9):1546–1554. doi:10.1136/gutjnl-2015-309456

11. Hardy T, Zeybel M, Day CP, et al. Plasma DNA methylation: a potential biomarker for stratification of liver fibrosis in non-alcoholic fatty liver disease. *Gut*. 2017;66(7):1321–1328. doi:10.1136/gutjnl-2016-311526

12. Kim CH, Kallman JB, Bai C, et al. Nutritional assessments of patients with non-alcoholic fatty liver disease. *Obes Surg*. 2010;20(2):154–160. doi:10.1007/s11695-008-9549-0

13. McCarthy EM, Rinella ME. The role of diet and nutrient composition in nonalcoholic Fatty liver disease. *J Acad Nutr Diet*. 2012;112(3):401–409. doi:10.1016/j.jada.2011.10.007

14. Gerber L, Otgonsuren M, Mishra A, et al. Non-alcoholic fatty liver disease (NAFLD) is associated with low level of physical activity: a population-based study. *Aliment Pharmacol Ther*. 2012;36(8):772–781. doi:10.1111/apt.12038

15. Hallsworth K, Thoma C, Moore S, et al. Non-alcoholic fatty liver disease is associated with higher levels of objectively measured sedentary behaviour and lower levels of physical activity than matched healthy controls. *Frontline Gastroenterol*. 2015;6(1):44–51. doi:10.1136/flgastro-2014-100432

16. Farrell GC. The liver and the waistline: fifty years of growth. *J Gastroenterol Hepatol*. 2009;24(Suppl 3):S105–118. doi:10.1111/j.1440-1746.2009.06080.x

17. Chang Y, Ryu S, Sung E, et al. Weight gain within the normal weight range predicts ultrasonographically detected fatty liver in healthy Korean men. *Gut*. 2009;58(10):1419–1425. doi:10.1136/gut.2008.161885

18. Portillo-Sanchez P, Bril F, Maximos M, et al. High prevalence of nonalcoholic fatty liver disease in patients with type 2 diabetes mellitus and normal plasma aminotransferase levels. *J Clin Endocrinol Metab*. 2015;100(6):2231–2238. doi:10.1210/jc.2015-1966

19. Jinjuvadia R, Antaki F, Lohia P, Liangpunsakul S. The association between nonalcoholic fatty liver disease and metabolic abnormalities in the United States population. *J Clin Gastroenterol*. 2017;51(2):160–166. doi:10.1097/mcg.0000000000000666

20. Kanwal F, Kramer JR, Li L, et al. Effect of metabolic traits on the risk of cirrhosis and hepatocellular cancer in nonalcoholic fatty liver disease. *Hepatology*. 2020;71(3):808–819. doi:10.1002/hep.31014

21. Sherif ZA, Saeed A, Ghavimi S, et al. Global epidemiology of nonalcoholic fatty liver disease and perspectives on US minority populations. *Dig Dis Sci*. 2016;61(5):1214–1225. doi:10.1007/s10620-016-4143-0

22. Browning JD, Szczepaniak LS, Dobbins R, et al. Prevalence of hepatic steatosis in an urban population in the United States: impact of ethnicity. *Hepatology*. 2004;40(6):1387–1395. doi:10.1002/hep.20466

23. Semmler G, Wernly S, Bachmayer S, et al. Nonalcoholic fatty liver disease in lean subjects: associations with metabolic dysregulation and cardiovascular risk-a single-center cross-sectional study. *Clin Transl Gastroenterol*. 2021;12(4):e00326. doi:10.14309/ctg.0000000000000326

24. Hagström H, Nasr P, Ekstedt M, et al. Risk for development of severe liver disease in lean patients with nonalcoholic fatty liver disease: a long-term follow-up study. *Hepatol Commun*. 2018;2(1):48–57. doi:10.1002/hep4.1124

25. Leung JC, Loong TC, Wei JL, et al. Histological severity and clinical outcomes of nonalcoholic fatty liver disease in nonobese patients. *Hepatology*. 2017;65(1):54–64. doi:10.1002/hep.28697

26. Younossi Z, Anstee QM, Marietti M, et al. Global burden of NAFLD and NASH: trends, predictions, risk factors and prevention. *Nat Rev Gastroenterol Hepatol*. 2018;15(1):11–20. doi:10.1038/nrgastro.2017.109

27. Wong RJ, Singal AK. Trends in liver disease etiology among adults awaiting liver transplantation in the United States, 2014–2019. *JAMA Netw Open*. 2020;3(2):e1920294. doi:10.1001/jamanetworkopen.2019.20294

28. Wong RJ, Aguilar M, Cheung R, et al. Nonalcoholic steatohepatitis is the second leading etiology of liver disease among adults awaiting liver transplantation in the United States. *Gastroenterology*. 2015;148(3):547–555. doi:10.1053/j.gastro.2014.11.039

29. Younossi ZM, Blissett D, Blissett R, et al. The economic and clinical burden of nonalcoholic fatty liver disease in the United States and Europe. *Hepatology*. 2016;64(5):1577–1586. doi:10.1002/hep.28785

30. Chalasani N, Younossi Z, Lavine JE, et al. The diagnosis and management of nonalcoholic fatty liver disease: practice guidance from the American association for the study of liver diseases. *Hepatology*. 2018;67(1):328–357. doi:10.1002/hep.29367

31. EASL-EASD-EASO clinical practice guidelines for the management of non-alcoholic fatty liver disease. *Diabetologia*. 2016;59(6):1121–1140. doi:10.1007/s00125-016-3902-y

32. National Guideline C. National institute for health and care excellence: guidance. *Non-alcoholic fatty liver disease: Assessment and management*. National Institute for Health and Care Excellence (UK) Copyright © National Institute for Health and Care Excellence 2016; 2016.

33. Angulo P, Keach JC, Batts KP, Lindor KD. Independent predictors of liver fibrosis in patients with nonalcoholic steatohepatitis. *Hepatology*. 1999;30(6):1356–1362. doi:10.1002/hep.510300604

34. Yang JD, Ahmed F, Mara KC, et al. Diabetes is associated with increased risk of hepatocellular carcinoma in patients with cirrhosis from nonalcoholic fatty liver disease. *Hepatology*. 2020;71(3):907–916. doi:10.1002/hep.30858

35. Lomonaco R, Godinez Leiva E, Bril F, et al. Advanced liver fibrosis is common in patients with type 2 diabetes followed in the outpatient setting: the need for systematic screening. *Diabetes Care*. 2021;44(2):399–406. doi:10.2337/dc20-1997

36. Draznin B, Aroda VR, Bakris G, et al. 4. Comprehensive medical evaluation and assessment of comorbidities: standards of medical care in diabetes-2022. *Diabetes Care*. 2022;45(Suppl 1):S46–s59. doi:10.2337/dc22-S004

37. Noureddin M, Jones C, Alkhouri N, Gomez EV, Dieterich DT, Rinella ME. Screening for nonalcoholic fatty liver disease in persons with type 2 diabetes in the United States is cost-effective: a comprehensive cost-utility

analysis. *Gastroenterology.* 2020;159(5):1985–1987.e4. doi:10.1053/j.gastro.2020.07.050

38. Torres DM, Harrison SA. Diagnosis and therapy of nonalcoholic steatohepatitis. *Gastroenterology.* 2008;134(6):1682–1698. doi:10.1053/j.gastro.2008.02.077

39. Sattar N, Forrest E, Preiss D. Non-alcoholic fatty liver disease. *BMJ.* 2014;349:g4596. doi:10.1136/bmj.g4596

40. Ma X, Liu S, Zhang J, et al. Proportion of NAFLD patients with normal ALT value in overall NAFLD patients: a systematic review and meta-analysis. *BMC Gastroenterology.* 2020;20(1):1–8.

41. Green RM, Flamm S. AGA technical review on the evaluation of liver chemistry tests. *Gastroenterology.* 2002;123(4):1367–1384. doi:10.1053/gast.2002.36061

42. Petroff D, Bätz O, Jedrysiak K, Kramer J, Berg T, Wiegand J. Age dependence of liver enzymes: an analysis of over 1,300,000 consecutive blood samples. *Clin Gastroenterol Hepatol.* 2022;20(3):641–650. doi:10.1016/j.cgh.2021.01.039

43. Palmentieri B, de Sio I, La Mura V, et al. The role of bright liver echo pattern on ultrasound B-mode examination in the diagnosis of liver steatosis. *Dig Liver Dis.* 2006;38(7):485–489. doi:10.1016/j.dld.2006.03.021

44. Saadeh S, Younossi ZM, Remer EM, et al. The utility of radiological imaging in nonalcoholic fatty liver disease. *Gastroenterology.* 2002;123(3):745–750. doi:10.1053/gast.2002.35354

45. Nyberg LM, Cheetham TC, Patton HM, et al. The natural history of NAFLD, a community-based study at a large health care delivery system in the United States. *Hepatol Commun.* 2021;5(1):83–96. doi:10.1002/hep4.1625

46. Sanyal AJ, Van Natta ML, Clark J, et al. Prospective study of outcomes in adults with nonalcoholic fatty liver disease. *N Engl J Med.* 2021;385(17):1559–1569. doi:10.1056/NEJMoa2029349

47. Angulo P, Kleiner DE, Dam-Larsen S, et al. Liver fibrosis, but no other histologic features, is associated with long-term outcomes of patients with nonalcoholic fatty liver disease. *Gastroenterology.* 2015;149(2):389–397.e10. doi:10.1053/j.gastro.2015.04.043

48. Sterling RK, Lissen E, Clumeck N, et al. Development of a simple noninvasive index to predict significant fibrosis in patients with HIV/HCV coinfection. *Hepatology.* 2006;43(6):1317–1325. doi:10.1002/hep.21178

49. Drolz A, Wolter S, Wehmeyer MH, et al. Performance of non-invasive fibrosis scores in non-alcoholic fatty liver disease with and without morbid obesity. *Int J Obes (Lond).* 2021;45(10):2197–2204. doi:10.1038/s41366-021-00881-8

50. Shah AG, Lydecker A, Murray K, Tetri BN, Contos MJ, Sanyal AJ. Comparison of noninvasive markers of fibrosis in patients with nonalcoholic fatty liver disease. *Clin Gastroenterol Hepatol.* 2009;7(10):1104–1112. doi:10.1016/j.cgh.2009.05.033

51. Younossi ZM, Noureddin M, Bernstein D, et al. Role of noninvasive tests in clinical gastroenterology practices to identify patients with nonalcoholic steatohepatitis at high risk of adverse outcomes: expert panel recommendations. *Am J Gastroenterol.* 2021;116(2):254–262. doi:10.14309/ajg.0000000000001054

52. Xiao G, Zhu S, Xiao X, Yan L, Yang J, Wu G. Comparison of laboratory tests, ultrasound, or magnetic resonance elastography to detect fibrosis in patients with nonalcoholic fatty liver disease: a meta-analysis. *Hepatology.* 2017;66(5):1486–1501. doi:10.1002/hep.29302

53. McPherson S, Hardy T, Dufour JF, et al. Age as a confounding factor for the accurate non-invasive diagnosis of advanced NAFLD fibrosis. *Am J Gastroenterol.* 2017;112(5):740–751. doi:10.1038/ajg.2016.453

54. Angulo P, Hui JM, Marchesini G, et al. The NAFLD fibrosis score: a noninvasive system that identifies liver fibrosis in patients with NAFLD. *Hepatology.* 2007;45(4):846–854. doi:10.1002/hep.21496

55. Polyzos SA, Slavakis A, Koumerkeridis G, Katsinelos P, Kountouras J. Noninvasive liver fibrosis tests in patients with nonalcoholic fatty liver disease: an external validation cohort. *Horm Metab Res.* 2019;51(2):134–140. doi:10.1055/a-0713-1330

56. Are VS, Vuppalanchi R, Vilar-Gomez E, Chalasani N. Enhanced liver fibrosis score can be used to predict liver-related events in patients with nonalcoholic steatohepatitis and compensated cirrhosis. *Clin Gastroenterol Hepatol.* 2021;19(6):1292–1293.e3. doi:10.1016/j.cgh.2020.06.070

57. Mikolasevic I, Orlic L, Zaputovic L, et al. Usefulness of liver test and controlled attenuation parameter in detection of nonalcoholic fatty liver disease in patients with chronic renal failure and coronary heart disease. *Wien Klin Wochenschr.* 2015;127(11–12):451–458. doi:10.1007/s00508-015-0757-z

58. Foucher J, Chanteloup E, Vergniol J, et al. Diagnosis of cirrhosis by transient elastography (FibroScan): a prospective study. *Gut.* 2006;55(3):403–408. doi:10.1136/gut.2005.069153

59. Wong VW, Vergniol J, Wong GL, et al. Diagnosis of fibrosis and cirrhosis using liver stiffness measurement in nonalcoholic fatty liver disease. *Hepatology.* 2010;51(2):454–462. doi:10.1002/hep.23312

60. Eddowes PJ, Sasso M, Allison M, et al. Accuracy of FibroScan controlled attenuation parameter and liver stiffness measurement in assessing steatosis and fibrosis in patients with nonalcoholic fatty liver disease. *Gastroenterology.* 2019;156(6):1717–1730. doi:10.1053/j.gastro.2019.01.042

61. Takemoto R, Nakamuta M, Aoyagi Y, et al. Validity of FibroScan values for predicting hepatic fibrosis stage in patients with chronic HCV infection. *J Dig Dis.* 2009;10(2):145–148. doi:10.1111/j.1751-2980.2009.00377.x

62. Loomba R, Wolfson T, Ang B, et al. Magnetic resonance elastography predicts advanced fibrosis in patients with nonalcoholic fatty liver disease: a prospective study. *Hepatology.* 2014;60(6):1920–1928. doi:10.1002/hep.27362

63. Xiao H, Shi M, Xie Y, Chi X. Comparison of diagnostic accuracy of magnetic resonance elastography and Fibroscan for detecting liver fibrosis in chronic hepatitis B patients: a systematic review and meta-analysis. *PLoS ONE.* 2017;12(11):e0186660. doi:10.1371/journal.pone.0186660

64. Wentworth BJ, Caldwell SH. Pearls and pitfalls in nonalcoholic fatty liver disease: tricky results are common. *Metabolism and Target Organ Damage.* 2021;1(1):2.

65. Furlan A, Tublin ME, Yu L, Chopra KB, Lippello A, Behari J. Comparison of 2D shear wave elastography, transient elastography, and MR elastography for the

diagnosis of fibrosis in patients with nonalcoholic fatty liver disease. *AJR Am J Roentgenol.* 2020;214(1):W20–26. doi:10.2214/ajr.19.21267

66. Davyduke T, Tandon P, Al-Karaghouli M, Abraldes JG, Ma MM. Impact of Implementing a "FIB-4 first" strategy on a pathway for patients with NAFLD referred from primary care. *Hepatol Commun.* 2019;3(10):1322–1333. doi:10.1002/hep4.1411

67. Srivastava A, Gailer R, Tanwar S, et al. Prospective evaluation of a primary care referral pathway for patients with non-alcoholic fatty liver disease. *J Hepatol.* 2019;71(2):371–378. doi:10.1016/j.jhep.2019.03.033

68. Tapper EB, Hunink MG, Afdhal NH, Lai M, Sengupta N. Cost-effectiveness analysis: risk stratification of nonalcoholic fatty liver disease (NAFLD) by the primary care physician using the NAFLD fibrosis score. *PLoS ONE.* 2016;11(2):e0147237. doi:10.1371/journal.pone.0147237

69. Vilar-Gomez E, Lou Z, Kong N, Vuppalanchi R, Imperiale TF, Chalasani N. Cost effectiveness of different strategies for detecting cirrhosis in patients with nonalcoholic fatty liver disease based on United States health care system. *Clin Gastroenterol Hepatol.* 2020;18(10):2305–2314.e12. doi:10.1016/j.cgh.2020.04.017

70. Congly SE, Shaheen AA, Swain MG. Modelling the cost effectiveness of non-alcoholic fatty liver disease risk stratification strategies in the community setting. *PLoS ONE.* 2021;16(5):e0251741. doi:10.1371/journal.pone.0251741

71. Asphaug L, Thiele M, Krag A, Melberg HO. Cost-effectiveness of noninvasive screening for alcohol-related liver fibrosis. *Hepatology.* 2020;71(6):2093–2104. doi:10.1002/hep.30979

72. EASL-EASD-EASO clinical practice guidelines for the management of non-alcoholic fatty liver disease. *J Hepatol.* 2016;64(6):1388–1402. doi:10.1016/j.jhep.2015.11.004

73. Pandyarajan V, Gish RG, Alkhouri N, Noureddin M. Screening for nonalcoholic fatty liver disease in the primary care clinic. *Gastroenterol Hepatol (NY).* 2019;15(7):357–365.

74. Newsome PN, Cramb R, Davison SM, et al. Guidelines on the management of abnormal liver blood tests. *Gut.* 2018;67(1):6–19. doi:10.1136/gutjnl-2017-314924

75. Dokmak A, Lizaola-Mayo B, Trivedi HD. The impact of nonalcoholic fatty liver disease in primary care: a population health perspective. *Am J Med.* 2021;134(1):23–29. doi:10.1016/j.amjmed.2020.08.010

76. Ando Y, Jou JH. Nonalcoholic fatty liver disease and recent guideline updates. *Clin Liver Dis (Hoboken).* 2021;17(1):23–28. doi:10.1002/cld.1045

77. Siddiqui MS, Yamada G, Vuppalanchi R, et al. Diagnostic accuracy of noninvasive fibrosis models to detect change in fibrosis stage. *Clin Gastroenterol Hepatol.* 2019;17(9):1877–1885.e5. doi:10.1016/j.cgh.2018.12.031

78. McPherson S, Stewart SF, Henderson E, Burt AD, Day CP. Simple non-invasive fibrosis scoring systems can reliably exclude advanced fibrosis in patients with non-alcoholic fatty liver disease. *Gut.* 2010;59(9):1265–1269. doi:10.1136/gut.2010.216077

79. Sun W, Cui H, Li N, et al. Comparison of FIB-4 index, NAFLD fibrosis score and BARD score for prediction of advanced fibrosis in adult patients with non-alcoholic fatty liver disease: a meta-analysis study. *Hepatol Res.* 2016;46(9):862–870. doi:10.1111/hepr.12647

80. Younossi ZM, Felix S, Jeffers T, et al. Performance of the enhanced liver fibrosis test to estimate advanced fibrosis among patients with nonalcoholic fatty liver disease. *JAMA Netw Open.* 2021;4(9):e2123923. doi:10.1001/jamanetworkopen.2021.23923

81. Mózes FE, Lee JA, Selvaraj EA, et al. Diagnostic accuracy of non-invasive tests for advanced fibrosis in patients with NAFLD: an individual patient data meta-analysis. *Gut.* 2021. doi:10.1136/gutjnl-2021-324243

82. Papatheodoridi M, Hiriart JB, Lupsor-Platon M, et al. Refining the Baveno VI elastography criteria for the definition of compensated advanced chronic liver disease. *J Hepatol.* 2021;74(5):1109–1116. doi:10.1016/j.jhep.2020.11.050

83. de Franchis R. Expanding consensus in portal hypertension: report of the Baveno VI consensus workshop: stratifying risk and individualizing care for portal hypertension. *J Hepatol.* 2015;63(3):743–752. doi:10.1016/j.jhep.2015.05.022

7 Ultrasound-Based Techniques in NAFLD

Vikas Taneja, Nezam H. Afdhal and Michelle J. Lai

CONTENTS

Abbreviations

ARFI:	acoustic radiation force impulse
CAP:	controlled attenuation parameter
CSPH:	clinically significant portal hypertension
HVPG:	hepatic venous pressure gradient
LSM:	liver stiffness measurement
NAFLD:	nonalcoholic fatty liver disease
NASH:	nonalcoholic steatohepatitis
VCTE:	vibration-controlled transient elastography
ROI:	region of interest
SWE:	shear wave elastography

7.1 INTRODUCTION

While liver biopsy has remained the gold standard for evaluation of NAFLD, its use is limited by invasive risk, sampling error, cost and low patient acceptance.[1] Consequently, the use of noninvasive modalities, such as ultrasound- (US-) based techniques for diagnosis of NAFLD has evolved rapidly in the last few years to become the standard of care.[2] Abdominal US, which is commonly utilized as a screening test for elevated liver enzymes was one of the earliest diagnostic modality to be used for noninvasive evaluation of NAFLD. It is widely available, well-tolerated and relatively inexpensive. However, US is not sensitive (cannot detect mild steatosis), can be confounded by other factors that increase hepatic echogenicity and does not offer quantitative assessment or assessment of inflammation or fibrosis. These limitations have resulted in the development of ultrasound-based elastographic techniques to better quantify hepatic fibrosis and fat and more recently to try to differentiate simple steatosis from nonalcoholic steatohepatitis (NASH). Initially the use of elastography was developed for the diagnosis of fibrosis in viral hepatitis C but now has emerged as one of the most accurate noninvasive methods of assessment of both fibrosis and steatosis in patients with NAFLD.[3] Subsequently, current guidelines recommend utilizing transient elastography for noninvasive evaluation of fibrosis in patients with NAFLD.[2]

In this chapter, we will examine the current use of elastographic techniques for diagnosing liver steatosis and fibrosis in NAFLD and differentiating simple steatosis from NASH.

7.2 DESCRIPTION OF ULTRASOUND-BASED TECHNOLOGIES

In addition to standard 3D ultrasound, currently several newer elastographic technologies are available for the evaluation of fat and fibrosis in NAFLD, including vibration-controlled transient elastography (VCTE), shear wave elastography (SWE) and acoustic radiation force impulse (ARFI) elastography. All three techniques share the same principle of estimating liver stiffness through measurement of elastic modulus; i.e., the stiffer the tissue is, the faster the shear wave velocity will be. While VCTE has been extensively studied in the setting of well-designed studies with paired histology leading to established cutoffs and quality criteria, the choice of technique is also influenced by local availability and expertise (Table 7.1).

7.2.1 Vibration-Controlled Transient Elastography

Ultrasound propagation through liver parenchyma is attenuated to varying degrees in the presence of steatosis. Controlled attenuation parameter (CAP) is a measure that estimates hepatic steatosis by capturing the extent of such attenuation. Vibration-controlled transient elastography (VCTE) (FibroScan®, Echosens, Paris, France) was approved by the United States Food and Drug Administration (FDA) in 2013. The device can measure CAP and liver stiffness (a surrogate for fibrosis, measured in kPa) simultaneously. The machine was initially introduced with a standard-sized probe (M) (3.5 MHz, 2 mm vibration amplitude). The performance of the M probe was limited by high rates of failure in obese patients of about 20%,[4] but subsequently, with the introduction of an XL probe (2.5 MHz, 3 mm vibration amplitude) and introduction of a software to automatically determine the choice of probe, the failure rates have improved to less than 5%.[5]

DOI: 10.1201/9781003386698-9

Table 7.1: Characteristics of Elastography Techniques for Evaluation of Fibrosis in NAFLD

Technique	Strength of Evidence	Cost	Performance	Quality Criteria	Limitations
VCTE	+++	++	+++	Standardized	Requires a dedicated device.
SWE	++	++	+++ (F4) ++ (F1, F2 and F3)	Individual operator dependent	Elimination of artifacts during ROI placement requires attention/optimal technique.
ARFI	++	++	+++	Individual operator dependent	Not enough evidence to establish intraobserver agreement.[1]

+: Low; ++: Moderate; +++: High

[1] Ferraioli G, Filice C, Castera L, et al. WFUMB Guidelines and Recommendations for Clinical Use of Ultrasound Elastography: Part 3: Liver. *Ultrasound in Medicine & Biology*. 2015;41(5):1161–1179. doi:10.1016/j.ultrasmedbio.2015.03.007

VCTE utilizes an automated movement of the ultrasound transducer to generate a brief push ("thump"), which propagates a shear wave. The probe is placed within the 9th–11th intercostal space, and the shear wave is evaluated by the receiver at a fixed distance.[6] CAP values are expressed as dB/m and range from 100 dB/m to 400 dB/m. As compared to a liver biopsy, CAP is much more convenient as it provides immediate result and is less prone to sampling error.[7] Additionally, CAP has good interobserver agreement, which makes it a valuable tool for longitudinal follow-up of patients.[8] TE values in a healthy population range from 4.4 kPa to 5.5 kPa,[9,10] with higher values in males as compared to females.[11] Values are not affected by age.[12] The following criteria are utilized to establish the validity of a result:[13] (1) at least 10 valid measurements; (2) a success rate (the ratio of valid measurements to the total number of measurements) above 60%; and (3) an interquartile range (IQR) less than 30% of the median LS measurements.[14] The mechanical impulse is aborted if the probe fails to detect liver parenchyma (e.g., if the probe lies over the rib).

7.2.2 Shear Wave Elastography

SWE targets a region of interest (ROI) in the liver using acoustic impulses, and the shear wave speed is measured to generate liver stiffness measurement (LSM) in kPa. The operator defines a vessel-free region using conventional B mode ultrasound, and a series of push pulses are utilized to create a plane of shear waves. After generating the shear wave, the device switches to radio frequency imaging mode to capture the shear wave velocity.[15] Subsequently, tissue stiffness is calculated by the formula $E = pc^2$, where E is the tissue elasticity (in kPa), p is the tissue density and c is the shear wave speed.[16] The technique has an advantage of being an existing feature on some of the US machines.

7.2.3 Acoustic Radiation Force Imaging (ARFI)

ARFI is a technique that utilizes focused acoustic energy to provide mechanical excitation directly to the tissue of interest and subsequently generating shear waves in vivo. The tissue in the region of interest is excited mechanically using short duration acoustic pulses with a frequency of 2.67 MHz to generate tissue displacement, which results in shear wave propagation away from the area of excitation. The speed of the shear wave away from the region of excitation (ROE) is used to estimate shear moduli (measured in kPa).[17] This unique mechanism circumvents the challenge associated with propagation of external mechanical excitation into the liver tissue. Notably, quality criteria for 2D SWE and ARFI remain to be established in large-scale

studies, and most studies on their use have utilized quality criteria similar to the criteria for VCTE.[18–21]

7.3 STEATOSIS MEASUREMENT

7.3.1 Performance of Conventional Ultrasound

Steatosis leads to increased echogenicity of the hepatic parenchyma due to closely spaced, fine echoes. The echogenicity of normal hepatic parenchyma is equal to or slightly greater than that of the renal cortex.[22] In the presence of enough fat (>30%), the echogenicity of the liver may exceed that of the kidney and spleen, a feature called "bright liver," which is a commonly used diagnostic feature. Additionally, the presence of liver fat reduces the ability of the US beam to penetrate the hepatic parenchyma.[22] This leads to loss of definition of diaphragm and posterior darkness, described as "posterior beam attenuation."[23] Focal fat deposition or focal fat sparing may be challenging to identify with US; however, it can be identified by the localized presence of the preceding imaging characteristics. Features such as poorly delineated margins and absence of mass effect are helpful in distinguishing focal fat deposition or sparing from mass lesions, but frequently an MRI is necessary.[22] The extent of steatosis is commonly reported as mild, moderate or severe; some studies have utilized scoring systems to mirror the histological classification.[24]

The sensitivity and specificity of US for detection of steatosis are dependent on the severity of steatosis, with higher accuracy for moderate (25–50%) to severe (>50%) steatosis. A meta-analysis based on 19 studies noted a sensitivity of 73.3% (95% CI 62.2–82.1%) and specificity of 84.4 (76.2–90.1) for any steatosis (>0% steatosis on biopsy).[26] However, the performance of US was improved in patients with higher grades of steatosis. The sensitivity and specificity in patients with moderate steatosis (25–50% steatosis) were 85.7% (95% CI 78.4–90.8%) and 85.2% (95% CI 76.9–90.9%), and in those with severe steatosis (>50% steatosis), they were 91.1% (95% CI 63.0–98.4%) and 91.9% (95% CI 74.3–97.8%), respectively. The overall sensitivity and specificity for detecting moderate-severe steatosis on US was reported to be 84.8% (95% CI 79.5–88.9%) and 93.6% (95% CI 87.2–97.0%), respectively, in a meta-analysis that included 49 studies (4,720 participants).[25] Positive likelihood ratio and negative likelihood ratio were 13.3 (6.4–27.6), and 0.16 (0.12–0.22), respectively. Area under the receiver operating characteristic curve (AUROC) was 0.931 (95% CI: 0.91–0.95%). For detection of milder steatosis (≥10% steatosis), the specificity was reduced to 88% (95% CI 63–97%); however, sensitivity was maintained at 93% (88–97%). (Additionally, this study compared sensitivity and specificity of various parameters such as liver to kidney contrast, vessel wall brightness, and deep beam attenuation for detection of steatosis. However, it included NAFLD and non-NAFLD patients.)

A few studies have evaluated the use of US for quantitative estimation of steatosis, such as hepatorenal index[27] and far-field slope (FFS) algorithm,[28] which estimates the extent of deep beam attenuation to quantify steatosis. However, such methods have not yet been validated in larger cohorts. Limitations of US include operator dependency, inability to detect <30% steatosis or to differentiate steatosis from NASH or to quantify fibrosis. Furthermore, the performance of US for detection of steatosis is reduced in patients with obesity and coexistent renal disease. In a study of 187 morbidly obese patients with 91.4% steatosis on liver biopsy who underwent bariatric surgery (BMI 35–40), the sensitivity was reduced to around 49% with a specificity of 75%.[29]

In conclusion, US has a limited sensitivity, specificity and reliability in the diagnosis and evaluation of severity of steatosis.[30]

7.3.2 Performance of VCTE

In an individual patient data meta-analysis, Karlas et al. reported optimal cutoffs of 248 dB/m (95% CI 237–261 dB/m), 268 dB/m (95% CI 257–284 dB/m) and 280 dB/m (95% CI 268–294 dB/m) for identifying steatosis grades >S0, >S1 and >S2, respectively.[31] However, this study included a high proportion of patients (80.4%) with other liver diseases such as chronic viral hepatitis, who may have undergone liver biopsy for indications other than NAFLD. Additionally, the study was conducted prior to the introduction of the XL probe and consequently only included

data from the M probe (BMI ≥35 was an exclusion criterion). The AUCROC for the presence of hepatic steatosis as compared to liver biopsy as a reference was 0.82.

A more recent meta-analysis by Petroff et al.[32] (930 patients: XL probe, 1,274 patients: M probe) reported the overall cutoffs of 294 dB/m (95% CI 286–313 dB/m), 310 dB/m (95% CI 305–321 dB/m) and 331 dB/m (95% CI 319–340 dB/m) for diagnosing steatosis grades >S0, >S1 and >S2, respectively. The corresponding cutoffs for the XL probe were 297 dB/m (95% CI 287–323 dB/m), 317 dB/m (95% CI 306–334 dB/m) and 333 dB/m (95% CI 320–340 dB/m), respectively. Notably, in order to optimize the sensitivity and specificity of the estimates, the authors used the Youden approach to determine the cutoffs. If instead of the Youden approach, the sensitivity was set at 90%, the overall cutoffs (M and XL probes) were 263 dB/m (95% CI 256–270 dB/m), 286 dB/m (95% CI 282–292 dB/m) and 297 dB/m (95% CI 286–307 dB/m) for steatosis grades >S0, >S1 and >S2, respectively. The AUC for diagnosing steatosis grades >S0, >S1 and >S2 were 0.82, 0.75 and 0.71, respectively (Table 7.2). In our clinical practice, we use a cutoff of 285 dB/m for steatosis and 330 dB/m for severe steatosis.

7.4 DIFFERENTIATION OF SIMPLE STEATOSIS FROM NASH

The biopsy characteristics of NASH include inflammation, apoptosis (balloon degeneration) and fibrosis, and a key component of NAFLD management lies in identification of the subgroup of patients who develop NASH and fibrosis. Few studies have reported the diagnostic utility of TE in detecting NASH. The largest such study included 183 patients undergoing liver biopsy and concomitant TE for suspected NAFLD. A scoring system that incorporated

Table 7.2: Performance of Controlled Attenuation Parameter in Studies among Patients with NAFLD Using Histology as Reference

Stage of Steatosis	Cutoff (dB/m)	Sensitivity (%)	Specificity (%)	Positive Predictive Value (%)	Negative Predictive Value (%)	References
≥S1	236	82	91	99	67	Imajo[1]
	261	72	86	98	23	Park[2]
	270	84	82	NR	NR	Enooku[3]
	285	80	77	99	16	Siddiqui[4]
≥S2	270	78	81	73	76	Imajo[1]
	305	63	69	56	75	Park[2]
	310	79	71	86	59	De Ledinghen[5]
S3	301	76	68	NR	NR	Friedrich-Rust[6]
	306	80	40	32	85	Siddiqui[4]
	311	87	47	43	88	De Ledinghen[5]
	312	64	70	26	92	Park[2]

[1] Imajo K, Kessoku T, Honda Y, et al. Magnetic resonance imaging more accurately classifies steatosis and fibrosis in patients with nonalcoholic fatty liver disease than transient elastography. *Gastroenterology*. 2016;150(3):626–637.e7. doi:10.1053/j.gastro.2015.11.048

[2] Park CC, Nguyen P, Hernandez C, et al. Magnetic resonance elastography vs transient elastography in detection of fibrosis and noninvasive measurement of steatosis in patients with biopsy-proven nonalcoholic fatty liver disease. *Gastroenterology*. 2017;152(3):598–607.e2. doi:10.1053/j.gastro.2016.10.026

[3] Enooku K, Tateishi R, Fujiwara N, et al. 1330 Non-invasive measurement of liver steatosis by controlled attenuation parameter (CAP) using FibroScan® in patients with nonalcoholic fatty liver disease (NAFLD). *Journal of Hepatology*. 2013; Supplement 1(58):S536–S537. doi:10.1016/S0168–8278(13)61330–6

[4] Siddiqui MS, Vuppalanchi R, Van Natta ML, et al. Vibration-controlled transient elastography to assess fibrosis and steatosis in patients with nonalcoholic fatty liver disease. *Clin Gastroenterol Hepatol*. 2019;17(1):156–163.e2. doi:10.1016/j.cgh.2018.04.043

[5] de Lédinghen V, Wong GLH, Vergniol J, et al. Controlled attenuation parameter for the diagnosis of steatosis in non-alcoholic fatty liver disease. *J Gastroenterol Hepatol*. 2016;31(4):848–855. doi:10.1111/jgh.13219

[6] Friedrich-Rust M, Romen D, Vermehren J, et al. Acoustic radiation force impulse-imaging and transient elastography for non-invasive assessment of liver fibrosis and steatosis in NAFLD. *Eur J Radiol*. 2012;81(3):e325–331. doi:10.1016/j.ejrad.2011.10.029

CAP and LSM in addition to ALT values was able to identify patients with NASH with AUROC of 0.812 (95% CI 0.724–0.880%).[33] The prevalence of NASH in this study was 51.6%. In another study of 47 patients that underwent transient elastography withing 2 weeks of liver biopsy, TE was noted to have an AUC of 0.82 (0.70–0.94) for diagnosis of NASH vs. simple steatosis.[34]

The role of SWE and ARFI in diagnosing NASH also remains unclear owing to a paucity of large-scale studies. In a single-center study of prospectively enrolled 102 patients with biopsy-proven NAFLD, AUC for diagnosis of lobular inflammatory activity, as assessed by a shear wave dispersion slope, for grades >I0, >I1, >I2, were 0.89, 0.85 and 0.78, respectively.[35] However, only about 8% of the patients had advanced fibrosis or cirrhosis. Similarly, only one study has evaluated the use of ARFI in NASH.[36] Among 64 biopsy-proven NAFLD, ARFI had AUC of 0.86 in discriminating NASH from simple steatosis. At a cutoff of ARFI velocity >1.1 m/s, the sensitivity and specificity of identifying NASH were 77 and 72%, respectively (positive predictive value 85%, negative predictive value 60%). The study was limited by a small sample size, and some of the patients in the study underwent liver biopsy as long as 6 months before ARFI elastography, thus limiting the validity of the findings.

7.5 FIBROSIS

Fibrosis in the liver alters liver stiffness, which can be measured by elastography. Elastography utilizes US to measure tissue shear deformations resulting from an externally applied force, such as acoustic vibration or probe palpation.[40] Three techniques as just described are available: TE, SWE and ARFI. The importance of staging fibrosis in NAFLD cannot be underestimated since fibrosis has the strongest correlation with clinical liver outcomes including morbidity and mortality.[41–43] Fibrosis is also one of the hallmarks of progressive NASH, and therefore diagnosing fibrosis greater than F2 is diagnostic of probable NASH when combined with clinical risk factors such as obesity and diabetes and elevated ALT.

7.5.1 Performance of VCTE

In a systematic review involving 1,047 patients across 9 studies, the diagnostic accuracy of TE was satisfactory for F3 (85% sensitivity, 82% specificity) and cirrhosis (92% sensitivity, 92% specificity), respectively. However, the accuracy dropped to 79% sensitivity, 75% specificity for F2 fibrosis.[44] In a recent meta-analysis that included up to 4,219 patients who underwent VCTE (both M and XL probes) and liver biopsy, the AUC, sensitivity and specificity of VCTE in diagnosing any fibrosis (≥F1) was 0.82 (95% CI 0.78–0.85%), 78% (95% CI 73–82%), 72% (95% CI 65–79%). The performance of VCTE improved for the diagnosis of advanced fibrosis (≥F3) and cirrhosis (F = 4), with AUC, sensitivity and specificity of 0.85 (95% CI 0.83–0.87%), 80% (95% CI 77–83%), 77% (95% CI 74–80%) for advanced fibrosis and 0.89 (95% CI 0.84–0.93%), 76% (95% CI 70–82%), 88% (95% CI 85–91%) for cirrhosis, respectively.[45]

Estimates of optimal cutoffs for LSM by VCTE for the diagnosis of various stages of fibrosis for maximal sensitivity and specificity vary from 7.2 to 11.4 kPa (Table 7.3). In a study involving 246 patients who underwent liver stiffness measurement and liver biopsy, at a cutoff value of 7.9 kPa, the sensitivity, specificity, and positive and negative predictive values for F3 or greater disease were 91, 75, 52, and 97, respectively.[46] The negative predictive value of LSM <7.2 kPa to exclude F3 or greater disease was 89% (95% CI 84–95%). In a recent meta-analysis that included data from 53 studies on VCTE, the sensitivity and specificity of VCTE for the diagnosis of advanced fibrosis (F0–2 vs. F3–4) at a cutoff of 8.9 kPa and 9.5 kPa were 80, 77 and 76, 80% respectively. AUC, sensitivity and specificity for the diagnosis of cirrhosis were 0.89, 76% (95% CI 70–82%) and 88% (95% CI 85–91%).[45]

7.5.2 Comparison among M and XL Probes

Few studies have compared the performance of XL-probe vs. M-probe in the same cohort of patients and reported similar results for both types of probes. The largest such study recruited 496 patients with biopsy-proven NAFLD and noted that the XL probe generated lower LSM than the M probe in obese (≥30 kg/m²) and nonobese (<30 kg/m²) patients.[47] However, for the same fibrosis stage, patients with obesity (≥30 kg/m²) were noted to have higher LSM than those with BMI <30 kg/m². When compared with liver histology, which was utilized as the reference, the authors noted that these factors partially cancelled each other and that the median LSM at each fibrosis stage was almost identical for M and XL probes when used in patients with BMI <30 and ≥30 kg/m², respectively. The study concluded that when used according to the appropriate body size, the same LSM cutoffs may be applied for both M and XL probes. In a Japanese cohort of prospectively enrolled 122 patients, median LSM values measured with the XL probe were lower as compared to M probe (7.40 kPa vs. 9.35 kPa, $p < 0.001$); however, there was a strong correlation among the LSM values from M and XL probes ($\rho = 0.8876$, $p < 0.001$).[48] No significant differences in the AUROC for LSM and CAP were noted between the two probes in patients with BMIs of < 30 and ≥ 30 kg/m². Similarly, CAP measurement through the M and XL probes were strongly corelated ($\rho = 0.7708$, $p < 0.001$). While CAP measurement was higher with the XL probe as compared to the M probe (315 vs. 303 dB/m, $p < 0.001$), there were no significant differences in the AUROC between CAP-M and CAP-XL (CAP-M vs. CAP-XL for steatosis score of ≥ 2, 0.638 vs. 0.680, $p = 0.290$; steatosis score of 3, 0.687 vs. 0.713, $p = 0.489$). In a cross-sectional Brazilian cohort of 81 patients with NAFLD (biopsy-proven) that underwent FibroScan® with M and XL probes on the same day, the performances of both the probes for the detection of moderate/severe (S1 vs. S2/S3) and severe steatosis (S1/S2 vs. S3) were similar.[49] None of the included patients in the sample had an absence of steatosis to evaluate the performance of CAP for the diagnosis of mild steatosis. Notably, 92.6% of the participants had BMI ≥25 kg/m². Similarly, AUROCs of M and XL probes for assessment of fibrosis (≥F2) were comparable at 0.82 (0.71–0.93) and 0.80 (0.69–0.92) ($P = 0.66$), respectively.

7.5.3 Performance of SWE and ARFI

The performance of SWE in diagnosing fibrosis was most recently reported by Selvaraj et al. Among 4 studies with 488 patients, AUC, sensitivity and specificity for diagnosing >F1 fibrosis were relatively low at 0.75 (0.58–0.87), 71% (56–83%), 67% (43–84%). The diagnostic performance was higher for diagnosing >F2 and >F3 fibrosis with AUC, sensitivity and specificity of 0.72 (0.60–0.84), 72% (65–78%),

Table 7.3: Performance of VCTE in Studies among Patients with NAFLD Using Histology as Reference

Stage of Fibrosis	Cutoff (kPa)	Sensitivity (%)	Specificity (%)	Positive Predictive Value (%)	Negative Predictive Value (%)	References
≥F1	6.1	78	68	87	53	Kumar[4]
	6.1	67	65	69	62	Park[2]
	6.7	66	85	88	63	Lee[5]
	7.0	62	100	100	87	Imajo[1]
≥F2	7.0	77	78	75	81	Kumar[4]
	7.3	70	59	53	76	Garg[6]
	8.0	83	85	64	94	Lee[5]
	8.6	66	80	78	70	Siddiqui[3]
≥F3	8.6	80	74	59	89	Siddiqui[3]
	9.0	96	86	55	99	Lee[5]
	9.3	82	75	NR	NR	Cassinotto 2016[7]
	9.7	71	75	63	81	Eddowes[8]
	10.2	100	97	71	100	Lupsor[9]
F4	10.3	92	88	46	99	Wong 2010[10]
	10.6	100	82	33	100	Kumar[4]
	11.0	100	90	45	100	Lee[5]
	14.0	100	76	73	100	Imajo[1]

[1] Imajo K, Kessoku T, Honda Y, et al. Magnetic resonance imaging more accurately classifies steatosis and fibrosis in patients with nonalcoholic fatty liver disease than transient elastography. *Gastroenterology*. 2016;150(3):626–637.e7. doi:10.1053/j.gastro.2015.11.048

[2] Park CC, Nguyen P, Hernandez C, et al. Magnetic resonance elastography vs transient elastography in detection of fibrosis and noninvasive measurement of steatosis in patients with biopsy-proven nonalcoholic fatty liver disease. *Gastroenterology*. 2017;152(3):598–607.e2. doi:10.1053/j.gastro.2016.10.026

[3] Siddiqui MS, Vuppalanchi R, Van Natta ML, et al. Vibration-controlled transient elastography to assess fibrosis and steatosis in patients with nonalcoholic fatty liver disease. *Clin Gastroenterol Hepatol*. 2019;17(1):156–163.e2. doi:10.1016/j.cgh.2018.04.043

[4] Kumar R, Rastogi A, Sharma MK, et al. Liver stiffness measurements in patients with different stages of nonalcoholic fatty liver disease: diagnostic performance and clinicopathological correlation. *Dig Dis Sci*. 2013;58(1):265–274. doi:10.1007/s10620-012-2306-1

[5] Lee MS, Bae JM, Joo SK, et al. Prospective comparison among transient elastography, supersonic shear imaging, and ARFI imaging for predicting fibrosis in nonalcoholic fatty liver disease. *PLoS One*. 2017;12(11):e0188321. doi:10.1371/journal.pone.0188321

[6] Garg H, Aggarwal S, Shalimar null, et al. Utility of transient elastography (fibroscan) and impact of bariatric surgery on nonalcoholic fatty liver disease (NAFLD) in morbidly obese patients. *Surg Obes Relat Dis*. 2018;14(1):81–91. doi:10.1016/j.soard.2017.09.005

[7] Cassinotto C, Boursier J, de Lédinghen V, et al. Liver stiffness in nonalcoholic fatty liver disease: A comparison of supersonic shear imaging, FibroScan, and ARFI with liver biopsy. *Hepatology*. 2016;63(6):1817–1827. doi:10.1002/hep.28394

[8] Eddowes PJ, McDonald N, Davies N, et al. Utility and cost evaluation of multiparametric magnetic resonance imaging for the assessment of non-alcoholic fatty liver disease. *Aliment Pharmacol Ther*. 2018;47(5):631–644. doi:10.1111/apt.14469

[9] Lupsor M, Badea R, Stefanescu H, et al. Performance of unidimensional transient elastography in staging non-alcoholic steatohepatitis. *J Gastrointestin Liver Dis*. 2010;19(1):53–60.

[10] Wong VWS, Vergniol J, Wong GLH, et al. Diagnosis of fibrosis and cirrhosis using liver stiffness measurement in nonalcoholic fatty liver disease. *Hepatology*. 2010;51(2):454–462. doi:10.1002/hep.23312

72% (52–86%) and 0.88 (0.81–0.91), 78% (50–93%), 84% (–90%), respectively. The same study also reported the performance of ARFI among 11 studies with 1,209 patients and the overall performance was noted to be better than that of SWE. The AUC, sensitivity and specificity for diagnosing >F1 fibrosis were 0.86 (0.78–0.90), 69% (59–77%), 85% (80–88%); for diagnosing >F2 fibrosis were 0.89 (0.83–0.95), 80% (70–88%), 86% (82–92%); and for diagnosing >F3 fibrosis were 0.90 (0.82–0.95), 76% (59–87%), 88% (82–92%), respectively (Tables 7.4 and 7.5).

7.5.4 Comparison among VCTE, SWE and ARFI

Few studies have compared TE, SWE and ARFI in the same cohort of patients. In a French cohort of prospectively enrolled 291 patients with biopsy proven NAFLD, Cassinotto et al. noted comparable performance among TE, ARFI and 2D SWE.[19] The AUC for SWE, FibroScan®, and ARFI were 0.86, 0.82, and 0.77 for diagnoses of F2; 0.89,

0.86, and 0.84 for F3; and 0.88, 0.87, and 0.84 for F4, respectively. Obesity (BMI ≥ 30 kg/m², waist circumference ≥ 102 cm or increased parietal wall thickness) was associated with unreliable results in ARFI and with LSM failures in TE and SWE. However, overall, there were no differences in the reliability of results, with 79.7% reliable results produced by SWE, 76.6% by FibroScan®, and 81% by ARFI (*p* values for all comparisons were nonsignificant).

7.5.5 Combination of VCTE with Serum Markers

In a study of 139 biopsy-proven NAFLD patients, a combination of LSM with Fib-4 or NFS increased the accuracy of fibrosis detection in NAFLD, yielding a positive predictive value of 0.735 at a sensitivity of 89% and a negative predictive value of 0.932 at a specificity of 82%.[50] A combination of LSM by VCTE, platelet count, diabetes, ALT-to-AST ratio, gender and age (AGILE 3+) has demonstrated a more optimal positive predictive value compared to

Table 7.4: Performance of SWE in Studies among Patients with NAFLD Using Histology as Reference

Stage of Fibrosis	Cutoff (kPa)	Sensitivity (%)	Specificity (%)	References
≥F2	8.3	87	55	Lee[1]
	8.4	77	66	Ozturk[3]
	8.7	71	90	Cassinotto 2016[2]
≥F3	9.3	84	70	Ozturk[3]
	10.7	90	61	Lee[1]
F4	14.4	59	90	Cassinotto 2016[2]
	15.1	90	78	Lee[1]
	15.7	100	82	Takeuchi[4]

[1] Lee MS, Bae JM, Joo SK, et al. Prospective comparison among transient elastography, supersonic shear imaging, and ARFI imaging for predicting fibrosis in nonalcoholic fatty liver disease. *PLOS ONE.* 2017;12(11):e0188321. doi:10.1371/journal.pone.0188321

[2] Cassinotto C, Boursier J, de Lédinghen V, et al. Liver stiffness in nonalcoholic fatty liver disease: A comparison of supersonic shear imaging, FibroScan, and ARFI with liver biopsy. *Hepatology.* 2016;63(6):1817–1827. doi:10.1002/hep.28394

[3] Ozturk A, Mohammadi R, Pierce TT, et al. diagnostic accuracy of shear wave elastography as a non-invasive biomarker of high-risk non-alcoholic steatohepatitis in patients with non-alcoholic fatty liver disease. *Ultrasound in Medicine & Biology.* 2020;46(4):972–980. doi:10.1016/j.ultrasmedbio.2019.12.020

[4] Takeuchi H, Sugimoto K, Oshiro H, et al. Liver fibrosis: noninvasive assessment using supersonic shear imaging and FIB4 index in patients with non-alcoholic fatty liver disease. *J Med Ultrason (2001).* 2018;45(2):243–249. doi:10.1007/s10396-017-0840-3

Table 7.5: Performance of ARFI in Studies among Patients with NAFLD Using Histology as Reference

Stage of Fibrosis	Cutoff (m/s)	Sensitivity (%)	Specificity (%)	AUC	References
≥F1	1.105	77	71	NR	Fierbinteau[2]
	1.29	54	77	0.66	Cui[4]
≥F2	1.165	85	90	0.94	Fierbinteau[3]
	1.17	86	87	0.90	Attia[5]
	1.32	56	91	0.77	Cassinotto 2016[2]
≥F3	1.42	97	97	0.99	Attia[5]
	1.45	76	68	91	Friedrich-Rust[1]
	1.48	86	95	0.98	Fierbinteau[3]
F4	1.635	92	92	0.98	Fierbinteau[3]
	1.75	74	67	0.91	Friedrich-Rust[1]
	1.89	90	95	0.98	Attia[5]

[1] Friedrich-Rust M, Romen D, Vermehren J, et al. Acoustic radiation force impulse imaging and transient elastography for non-invasive assessment of liver fibrosis and steatosis in NAFLD. *Eur J Radiol.* 2012;81(3):e325–331. doi:10.1016/j.ejrad.2011.10.029

[2] Cassinotto C, Boursier J, de Lédinghen V, et al. Liver stiffness in nonalcoholic fatty liver disease: a comparison of supersonic shear imaging, FibroScan, and ARFI with liver biopsy. *Hepatology.* 2016;63(6):1817–1827. doi:10.1002/hep.28394

[3] Fierbinteanu Braticevici C, Sporea I, Panaitescu E, Tribus L. Value of acoustic radiation force impulse imaging elastography for non-invasive evaluation of patients with nonalcoholic fatty liver disease. *Ultrasound in Medicine & Biology.* 2013;39(11):1942–1950. doi:10.1016/j.ultrasmedbio.2013.04.019

[4] Cui J, Heba E, Hernandez C, et al. Magnetic resonance elastography is superior to acoustic radiation force impulse for the diagnosis of fibrosis in patients with biopsy-proven nonalcoholic fatty liver disease: a prospective study. *Hepatology.* 2016;63(2):453–461. doi:10.1002/hep.28337

[5] Attia D, Bantel H, Lenzen H, Manns MP, Gebel MJ, Potthoff A. Liver stiffness measurement using acoustic radiation force impulse elastography in overweight and obese patients. *Alimentary Pharmacology & Therapeutics.* 2016;44(4):366–379. doi:10.1111/apt.13710

LSM alone. More recently, an improved version of this combination (AGILE 4)[51] was shown to reduce the percentage of patients with indeterminate results to 13%, as compared to 21% for VCTE. The AGILE4 score achieved an AUC of 0.93 (95% CI 0.91–0.96%) and outperformed LSM alone (AUC 0.89, 95% CI 0.86–0.93%) and FIB4 score (AUC 0.83, 95% CI 0.79–0.88%).

In order to address the challenge of identifying patients that are at the greatest risk of NAFLD progression, a combination of LSM by VCTE, CAP and AST, called the FibroScan® aspartate aminotransferase (FAST) score, has been developed.[52] The score has demonstrated satisfactory performance for diagnosis of NASH (using the FLIP definition) with NAS 4 or higher and fibrosis stage 2 or higher with a PPV of 0·83 NPV of 0·85. The score was initially derived from a cohort of

350 prospectively enrolled patients and subsequently validated in seven cohorts of a total of 1,026 patients.

7.5.6 Comparisons with Other Modalities

In a meta-analysis of 13,294 patients, CAP-TE, SWE and MRE were superior than lab tests (NFS, BARD, FIB-4, APRI) in diagnosing fibrosis.[53] SWE was similar in accuracy to MRE for detection of the following stages of fibrosis– significant fibrosis (F2–F4), advanced fibrosis (F3–F4) and cirrhosis (F4). The sensitivities and specificities of the FibroScan® M (threshold of 8.7–9), SWE and MRE for detecting advanced fibrosis were 0.87 and 0.79, 0.90 and 0.93, and 0.84 and 0.90, respectively. The summary AUROC values using the FibroScan® M probe, XL probe, SWE, and MRE for diagnosing advanced fibrosis were 0.88, 0.85, 0.95, and

0.96, respectively. The authors noted that SWE and MRE were statistically better than VCTE in identifying advanced fibrosis. However, in the meta-analysis by Selvaraj et al., which included studies on ARFI in addition, the authors concluded that in the setting of a reliable LSM, all three US-based modalities (VCTE, SWE and ARFI) had acceptable diagnostic accuracy for advanced fibrosis and cirrhosis. When minimum acceptable criteria were defined as greater than 80% for both sensitivity and specificity, ARFI and MRE met these criteria for diagnosis of advanced fibrosis, and only MRE met these criteria for diagnosis of cirrhosis.

7.6 LIMITATIONS OF ELASTOGRAPHY

Since all three techniques are based on the principle of measuring tissue elasticity through shear wave propagation, they share a majority of limitations that have been most extensively studied in VCTE. The propagation of shear wave across fluid is inconsistent, and subsequently LSM values in patients with ascites are unreliable. Although the failure rates in patients with obesity have been largely mitigated by the introduction of the XL probe, extreme obesity with skin-to-liver capsule distance > 3.4 cm (BMI > 40 kg/m^2) may still be associated with unreliable estimates up to 15%.[54] Liver stiffness is also increased with hepatic inflammation (ALT/AST >5 ULN), obstructive cholestasis, alcoholic hepatitis, amyloidosis, lymphomas and extramedullary hematopoiesis. Furthermore, enlarged veins damp shear stress, thus affecting the accuracy of LSM measurement in hepatic congestion (CHF).

7.7 PORTAL HYPERTENSION

LSM as measured by VCTE has been shown to corelate with hepatic venous pressure gradient (HVPG). In a study of 150 patients who underwent liver biopsy with hemodynamic measurements, LSM had AUC of 0.94 (95% CI 0.90–0.98%) for diagnosing clinically significant portal hypertension (CSPH), defined as HVPG ≥10 mmHg.[55] At a cutoff value of >21 kPa, the sensitivity and specificity for identifying CSPH were 89.9 and 93.2%, respectively. The role of spleen stiffness has also been evaluated in identifying patients with PHT. The increased spleen stiffness in advanced chronic liver disease is hypothesized to be due to increased splenic congestion and, to some extent, splenic fibrosis.[56] Subsequently, while LSM identifies liver fibrosis burden, SS may be more reflective of downstream hemodynamic consequences.[57] In a study of 113 patients with cirrhosis due to hepatitis C, Colecchia et al.[58] noted a good correlation between SS and HVPG. Patients with PHT had higher SS than patients without PHT (59kPa vs. 39 kPa) when CSPH was defined as HVPG> 10 mmHg, and a model that incorporated LSM and SS achieved a robust R^2 of 0.82 for prediction of HVPG.

While CSPH is a hemodynamic measure related to HVPG, due to a sufficiently large body of evidence demonstrating the accuracy of LSM in the assessment of hepatic fibrosis which is the primary driver of HVPG, recent guidelines recommend utilizing LSM to identify patients that are at high or low risk of CSPH as outlined in the Baveno VII criteria.[59] Whereas LSM by TE ≤15 kPa plus platelet count ≥150×109/L rules out CSPH (sensitivity and negative predictive value >90%) (LOE B, weak recommendation), identification of patients at high risk of CSPH may be accomplished by utilizing the ANTICIPATE model for nonobese NASH-related cACLD[60] (LOE B, weak recommendation) or the ANTICIPATE-NASH model for NASH-related cACLD[61] (LOE C, weak recommendation).

In conclusion, ultrasound-based technologies that utilize elastography has become the standard of care for noninvasive diagnosis and staging of liver fibrosis in NAFLD. While VCTE is the best characterized modality, there is growing literature to support the use of SWE and ARFI, which have demonstrated comparable diagnostic accuracy and reliability. However, quality criteria and prespecified thresholds remain to be established for SWE and ARFI. Additionally, the role of elastography in the evaluation of NASH remains an area of active research to identify patients for enrollment in clinical trials for treatment of NASH without needing a liver biopsy. Future studies to evaluate the longitudinal association of change in fibrosis severity on elastography and risk of development of hepatic decompensation (increase in LSM) or improvement in fibrosis (reduction in LSM) would be crucial to assess the treatment response when pharmacological therapy becomes available.

REFERENCES

1. Ratziu V, Charlotte F, Heurtier A, et al. Sampling variability of liver biopsy in nonalcoholic fatty liver disease. *Gastroenterology.* 2005;128(7):1898–1906.
2. European Association for the Study of the Liver. Electronic address: easloffice@easloffice.eu, Clinical Practice Guideline Panel, Chair: EASL Governing Board representative: Panel members: EASL Clinical Practice Guidelines on non-invasive tests for evaluation of liver disease severity and prognosis—2021 update. *J Hepatol.* 2021;75(3):659–689. doi:10.1016/j.jhep.2021.05.025
3. Tapper EB, Loomba R. Noninvasive imaging biomarker assessment of liver fibrosis by elastography in NAFLD. *Nat Rev Gastroenterol Hepatol.* 2018;15(5):274–282. doi:10.1038/nrgastro.2018.10
4. Castéra L, Foucher J, Bernard PH, et al. Pitfalls of liver stiffness measurement: a 5-year prospective study of 13,369 examinations. *Hepatology.* 2010;51(3):828–835.
5. Vuppalanchi R, Siddiqui MS, Van Natta ML, et al. Performance characteristics of vibration-controlled transient elastography for evaluation of nonalcoholic fatty liver disease. *Hepatology.* 2018;67(1):134–144.
6. Sandrin L, Fourquet B, Hasquenoph JM, et al. Transient elastography: a new noninvasive method for assessment of hepatic fibrosis. *Ultrasound Med Biol.* 2003;29(12):1705–1713. doi:10.1016/j.ultrasmedbio.2003.07.001
7. Lédinghen V de, Wong GLH, Vergniol J, et al. Controlled attenuation parameter for the diagnosis of steatosis in non-alcoholic fatty liver disease. *J Gastroenterol Hepatol.* 2016;31(4):848–855.
8. Ferraioli G, Tinelli C, Lissandrin R, et al. Interobserver reproducibility of the controlled attenuation parameter (CAP) for quantifying liver steatosis. *Hepatol Int.* 2014;8(4):576–581.
9. Colombo S, Belloli L, Zaccanelli M, et al. Normal liver stiffness and its determinants in healthy blood donors. *Dig Liver Dis.* 2011;43(3):231–236. doi:10.1016/j.dld.2010.07.008
10. Roulot D, Costes JL, Buyck JF, et al. Transient elastography as a screening tool for liver fibrosis and cirrhosis in a community-based population aged over 45 years. *Gut.* 2011;60(7):977–984. doi:10.1136/gut.2010.221382
11. Corpechot C, El Naggar A, Poupon R. Gender and liver: is the liver stiffness weaker in weaker sex? *Hepatology.* 2006;44(2):513–514. doi:10.1002/hep.21306

12. Sirli R, Sporea I, Tudora A, Deleanu A, Popescu A. Transient elastographic evaluation of subjects without known hepatic pathology: does age change the liver stiffness? *J Gastrointestin Liver Dis.* 2009;18(1):57–60.

13. Zhang X, Wong GLH, Wong VWS. Application of transient elastography in nonalcoholic fatty liver disease. *Clin Mol Hepatol.* 2020;26(2):128.

14. Castera L, Forns X, Alberti A. Non-invasive evaluation of liver fibrosis using transient elastography. *J Hepatol.* 2008;48(5):835–847. doi:10.1016/j.jhep.2008.02.008

15. Muller M, Gennisson JL, Deffieux T, Tanter M, Fink M. Quantitative viscoelasticity mapping of human liver using supersonic shear imaging: preliminary in vivo feasability study. *Ultrasound Med Biol.* 2009;35(2):219–229. doi:10.1016/j.ultrasmedbio.2008.08.018

16. Ferraioli G, Tinelli C, Dal Bello B, et al. Accuracy of real-time shear wave elastography for assessing liver fibrosis in chronic hepatitis C: a pilot study. *Hepatology.* 2012;56(6):2125–2133. doi:10.1002/hep.25936

17. Palmeri ML, Wang MH, Dahl JJ, Frinkley KD, Nightingale KR. Quantifying hepatic shear modulus in vivo using acoustic radiation force. *Ultrasound Med Biol.* 2008;34(4):546–558. doi:10.1016/j. ultrasmedbio.2007.10.009

18. Cassinotto C, Lapuyade B, Aït-Ali A, et al. Liver fibrosis: Noninvasive assessment with acoustic radiation force impulse elastography—Comparison with FibroScan M and XL probes and FibroTest in patients with chronic liver disease. *Radiology.* 2013;269(1):283–292. doi:10.1148/radiol.13122208

19. Cassinotto C, Boursier J, de Lédinghen V, et al. Liver stiffness in nonalcoholic fatty liver disease: a comparison of supersonic shear imaging, FibroScan, and ARFI with liver biopsy. *Hepatology.* 2016;63(6):1817–1827. doi:10.1002/hep.28394

20. Attia D, Bantel H, Lenzen H, Manns MP, Gebel MJ, Potthoff A. Liver stiffness measurement using acoustic radiation force impulse elastography in overweight and obese patients. *Aliment Pharmacol Ther.* 2016;44(4):366–379. doi:10.1111/apt.13710

21. Ozturk A, Mohammadi R, Pierce TT, et al. Diagnostic accuracy of shear wave elastography as a non-invasive biomarker of high-risk non-alcoholic Steatohepatitis in patients with non-alcoholic fatty liver disease. *Ultrasound Med Biol.* 2020;46(4):972–980. doi:10.1016/j. ultrasmedbio.2019.12.020

22. Hamer OW, Aguirre DA, Casola G, Lavine JE, Woenckhaus M, Sirlin CB. Fatty liver: imaging patterns and pitfalls. *Radiographics.* 2006;26(6):1637–1653. doi:10.1148/rg.266065004

23. Mishra P, Younossi ZM. Abdominal ultrasound for diagnosis of nonalcoholic fatty liver disease (NAFLD). *Am J Gastroenterol.* 2007;102(12):2716–2717. doi:10.1111/j.1572-0241.2007.01520.x

24. Ballestri S, Lonardo A, Romagnoli D, et al. Ultrasonographic fatty liver indicator, a novel score which rules out NASH and is correlated with metabolic parameters in NAFLD. *Liver International.* 2012;32(8):1242–1252.

25. Hernaez R, Lazo M, Bonekamp S, et al. Diagnostic accuracy and reliability of ultrasonography for the detection of fatty liver: a meta-analysis. *Hepatology.* 2011;54(3):1082–1090. doi:10.1002/hep.24452

26. Bohte AE, van Werven JR, Bipat S, Stoker J. The diagnostic accuracy of US, CT, MRI and 1H-MRS for the evaluation of hepatic steatosis compared with liver biopsy: a meta-analysis. *Eur Radiol.* 2011;21(1):87–97. doi:10.1007/s00330-010-1905-5

27. Webb M, Yeshua H, Zelber-Sagi S, et al. Diagnostic value of a computerized hepatorenal index for sonographic quantification of liver steatosis. *AJR Am J Roentgenol.* 2009;192(4):909–914. doi:10.2214/AJR.07.4016

28. Graif M, Yanuka M, Baraz M, et al. Quantitative estimation of attenuation in ultrasound video images: correlation with histology in diffuse liver disease. *Invest Radiol.* 2000;35(5):319–324. doi:10.1097/00004424-200005000-00006

29. Mottin CC, Moretto M, Padoin AV, et al. The role of ultrasound in the diagnosis of hepatic steatosis in morbidly obese patients. *Obes Surg.* 2004;14(5):635–637. doi:10.1381/096089204323093408

30. Loomba R. Role of imaging-based biomarkers in NAFLD: recent advances in clinical application and future research directions. *J Hepatol.* 2018;68(2):296–304.

31. Karlas T, Petroff D, Sasso M, et al. Individual patient data meta-analysis of controlled attenuation parameter (CAP) technology for assessing steatosis. *J Hepatol.* 2017;66(5):1022–1030. doi:10.1016/j.jhep.2016.12.022

32. Petroff D, Blank V, Newsome PN, et al. Assessment of hepatic steatosis by controlled attenuation parameter using the M and XL probes: an individual patient data meta-analysis. *Lancet Gastroenterol Hepatol.* 2021;6(3):185–198.

33. Lee HW, Park SY, Kim SU, et al. Discrimination of nonalcoholic steatohepatitis using transient elastography in patients with nonalcoholic fatty liver disease. *PLoS ONE.* 2016;11(6):e0157358. doi:10.1371/journal. pone.0157358

34. Eddowes PJ, McDonald N, Davies N, et al. Utility and cost evaluation of multiparametric magnetic resonance imaging for the assessment of non-alcoholic fatty liver disease. *Aliment Pharmacol Ther.* 2018;47(5):631–644. doi:10.1111/apt.14469

35. Lee DH, Cho EJ, Bae JS, et al. Accuracy of two-dimensional shear wave elastography and attenuation imaging for evaluation of patients with nonalcoholic steatohepatitis. *Clin Gastroenterol Hepatol.* 2021;19(4):797–805.e7. doi:10.1016/j.cgh.2020.05.034

36. Fierbinteanu Braticevici C, Sporea I, Panaitescu E, Tribus L. Value of acoustic radiation force impulse imaging elastography for non-invasive evaluation of patients with nonalcoholic fatty liver disease. *Ultrasound Med Biol.* 2013;39(11):1942–1950. doi:10.1016/j. ultrasmedbio.2013.04.019

37. Imajo K, Kessoku T, Honda Y, et al. Magnetic resonance imaging more accurately classifies steatosis and fibrosis in patients with nonalcoholic fatty liver disease than transient elastography. *Gastroenterology.* 2016;150(3):626–637.e7. doi:10.1053/j.gastro.2015.11.048

38. Park CC, Nguyen P, Hernandez C, et al. Magnetic resonance elastography vs transient elastography in detection of fibrosis and noninvasive measurement of steatosis in patients with biopsy-proven nonalcoholic fatty liver disease. *Gastroenterology.* 2017;152(3):598–607. e2. doi:10.1053/j.gastro.2016.10.026

39. Lee YS, Yoo YJ, Jung YK, et al. Multiparametric MR is a valuable modality for evaluating disease severity of nonalcoholic fatty liver disease. *Clin Transl Gastroenterol.* 2020;11(4):e00157. doi:10.14309/ctg.0000000000000157

40. Bamber J, Cosgrove D, Dietrich CF, et al. EFSUMB guidelines and recommendations on the clinical use of ultrasound elastography. Part 1: Basic principles

and technology. *Ultraschall Med*. 2013;34(2):169–184. doi:10.1055/s-0033-1335205

41. Tada T, Kumada T, Toyoda H, et al. Progression of liver fibrosis is associated with non-liver-related mortality in patients with nonalcoholic fatty liver disease. *Hepatol Commun*. 2017;1(9):899–910. doi:10.1002/hep4.1105

42. Unalp-Arida A, Ruhl CE. Liver fibrosis scores predict liver disease mortality in the United States population. *Hepatology*. 2017;66(1):84–95. doi:10.1002/hep.29113

43. Schonmann Y, Yeshua H, Bentov I, Zelber-Sagi S. Liver fibrosis marker is an independent predictor of cardiovascular morbidity and mortality in the general population. *Dig Liver Dis*. 2021;53(1):79–85. doi:10.1016/j.dld.2020.10.014

44. Kwok R, Tse YK, Wong GLH, et al. Systematic review with meta-analysis: non-invasive assessment of non-alcoholic fatty liver disease-the role of transient elastography and plasma cytokeratin-18 fragments. *Aliment Pharmacol Ther*. 2014;39(3):254–269. doi:10.1111/apt.12569

45. Selvaraj EA, Mózes FE, Jayaswal ANA, et al. Diagnostic accuracy of elastography and magnetic resonance imaging in patients with NAFLD: a systematic review and meta-analysis. *J Hepatol*. 2021;75(4):770–785. doi:10.1016/j.jhep.2021.04.044

46. Wong VWS, Vergniol J, Wong GLH, et al. Diagnosis of fibrosis and cirrhosis using liver stiffness measurement in nonalcoholic fatty liver disease. *Hepatology*. 2010;51(2):454–462. doi:10.1002/hep.23312

47. Wong VWS, Irles M, Wong GLH, et al. Unified interpretation of liver stiffness measurement by M and XL probes in non-alcoholic fatty liver disease. *Gut*. 2019;68(11):2057–2064.

48. Oeda S, Takahashi H, Imajo K, et al. Accuracy of liver stiffness measurement and controlled attenuation parameter using FibroScan® M/XL probes to diagnose liver fibrosis and steatosis in patients with nonalcoholic fatty liver disease: a multicenter prospective study. *J Gastroenterol*. 2020;55(4):428–440.

49. Cardoso AC, Cravo C, Calçado FL, et al. The performance of M and XL probes of FibroScan for the diagnosis of steatosis and fibrosis on a Brazilian nonalcoholic fatty liver disease cohort. *Eur J Gastroenterol Hepatol*. 2020;32(2):231–238.

50. Jafarov F, Kaya E, Bakir A, Eren F, Yilmaz Y. The diagnostic utility of fibrosis-4 or nonalcoholic fatty liver disease fibrosis score combined with liver stiffness measurement by fibroscan in assessment of advanced liver fibrosis: a biopsy-proven nonalcoholic fatty liver disease study. *Eur J Gastroenterol Hepatol*. 2020;32(5):642–649. doi:10.1097/MEG.0000000000001573

51. Younossi ZM, Harrison SA, Newsome PN, et al. Improving diagnosis of cirrhosis in patients with NAFLD by combining liver stiffness measurement by vibration-controlled transient elastography and routine biomarkers: a global derivation and validation study. In: *The Liver Meeting Digital Experience™*. AASLD.

52. Newsome PN, Sasso M, Deeks JJ, et al. FibroScan-AST (FAST) score for the non-invasive identification of patients with non-alcoholic steatohepatitis with significant activity and fibrosis: a prospective derivation and global validation study. *Lancet Gastroenterol Hepatol*. 2020;5(4):362–373. doi:10.1016/S2468-1253(19)30383-8

53. Xiao G, Zhu S, Xiao X, Yan L, Yang J, Wu G. Comparison of laboratory tests, ultrasound, or magnetic resonance elastography to detect fibrosis in patients with nonalcoholic fatty liver disease: a meta-analysis. *Hepatology*. 2017;66(5):1486–1501. doi:10.1002/hep.29302

54. Chen J, Yin M, Talwalkar JA, et al. Diagnostic performance of MR elastography and vibration-controlled transient elastography in the detection of hepatic fibrosis in patients with severe to morbid obesity. *Radiology*. 2017;283(2):418–428. doi:10.1148/radiol.2016160685

55. Bureau C, Metivier S, Peron JM, et al. Transient elastography accurately predicts presence of significant portal hypertension in patients with chronic liver disease. *Aliment Pharmacol Ther*. 2008;27(12):1261–1268. doi:10.1111/j.1365-2036.2008.03701.x

56. Bolognesi M, Merkel C, Sacerdoti D, Nava V, Gatta A. Role of spleen enlargement in cirrhosis with portal hypertension. *Digestive and Liver Disease*. 2002;34(2):144–150. doi:10.1016/S1590-8658(02)80246-8

57. Abraldes JG, Reverter E, Berzigotti A. Spleen stiffness: toward a noninvasive portal sphygmomanometer? *Hepatology*. 2013;57(3):1278–1280. doi:10.1002/hep.26239

58. Colecchia A, Montrone L, Scaioli E, et al. Measurement of spleen stiffness to evaluate portal hypertension and the presence of esophageal varices in patients with HCV-related cirrhosis. *Gastroenterology*. 2012;143(3):646–654. doi:10.1053/j.gastro.2012.05.035

59. Franchis R de, Bosch J, Garcia-Tsao G, et al. Baveno VII—Renewing consensus in portal hypertension. *J Hepatol*. 2022;76(4):959–974. doi:10.1016/j.jhep.2021.12.022

60. Abraldes JG, Bureau C, Stefanescu H, et al. Noninvasive tools and risk of clinically significant portal hypertension and varices in compensated cirrhosis: the "Anticipate" study. *Hepatology*. 2016;64(6):2173–2184. doi:10.1002/hep.28824

61. Pons M, Augustin S, Scheiner B, et al. Noninvasive diagnosis of portal hypertension in patients with compensated advanced chronic liver disease. *Off J Am Coll Gastroenterol | ACG*. 2021;116(4):723–732. doi:10.14309/ajg.0000000000000994

8 MRI-Based Technologies

Victor de Lédinghen

CONTENTS

Key Points

- MRI-PDFF is a useful surrogate for liver biopsy in the diagnosis of steatosis and assessment of treatment response.

- MRE has several advantages over ultrasound-based elastography, as it samples a much larger volume of the liver, is not affected by body mass index or degree of steatosis, is not operator-dependent, has favorable test-retest repeatability, and has a high success rate.

- MRE is the most accurate noninvasive method for staging liver fibrosis.

- MRE is an accurate prognostic noninvasive imaging biomarker that can risk-stratify patients with NAFLD.

8.1 INTRODUCTION

Magnetic resonance imaging (MRI) is an imaging method with contrast mechanisms capable of enabling the detection and quantification of liver fat. Liver MR elastography (MRE) is an imaging technique used to measure liver stiffness in the evaluation for possible fibrosis or cirrhosis. In this chapter, we will mainly discuss MRI and MRE, which have revolutionized the noninvasive diagnosis of steatosis and liver fibrosis, respectively. However, we need to keep in mind that MRI cannot be performed in patients who have contraindications including metallic implants and severe claustrophobia.

8.2 MRI FOR STEATOSIS ASSESSMENT

Quantitative imaging methods are increasingly used for the diagnosis and management of steatosis, including treatment monitoring. Despite the high accuracy of MRI for detecting and grading steatosis, cost and limited availability restrict its use in clinical practice.

8.2.1 Technique

MRI is an imaging method with contrast mechanisms capable of enabling the detection and quantification of liver fat content by means of the direct measurement of proton signal in water and fat (1). Magnetic resonance proton density fat fraction (MRI-PDFF) is an accurate, reproducible, quantitative imaging-based technique that has the ability to quantify liver fat in its entire dynamic range.

MRI-PDFF is increasingly accepted as the most optimal method, among the invasive or noninvasive methods, for quantifying liver fat content—even overperforming biopsy. Currently, there is no consensus on a standardized approach to measuring liver fat with manually drawn regions of interest (ROIs). Because a heterogeneous pattern of steatosis has been reported in up to 60% of patients with NAFLD, the placement of a single ROI is unlikely to be sufficient to correctly estimate the true severity of liver fat. Although placement of largest-fit-possible ROIs in all liver segments was shown to be the most reproducible and repeatable method, it is time-consuming and thus difficult for clinical practice. Therefore, placement of one large single-section ROI in the anterior, posterior, medial and lateral segments of the liver, avoiding bigger vessels and bile ducts, has been proposed as an acceptable alternative.

8.2.2 MRI-PDFF for the Diagnosis of Steatosis

The utility of imaging methods used for the assessment of steatosis is crucial. Moreover, given the high prevalence of steatosis, it is a common incidental finding at

DOI: 10.1201/9781003386698-10

cross-sectional imaging. This provides a unique opportunity to report and grade the severity of steatosis to initiate lifestyle modifications or other interventions. Table 8.1 reports some studies that evaluated the performance of MRI-PDFF for the diagnosis of steatosis.

In a recent meta-analysis (2), the areas under the ROC curve (AUROCs) of MRI-PDFF for detecting steatosis >−5%, >−33% and >−66% were 0.98, 0.91 and 0.90, respectively.

MRI-PDFF could be also a valuable biomarker for pre-operative risk assessment in donor candidates for living donor liver transplant (3). At last, MRI-PDFF has high diagnostic accuracy to classify steatosis grade in histological steatosis grade in children with NAFLD (4).

Practice guidance statements from the American Association for the Study of Liver Diseases recommend the following for incidentally detected steatosis at imaging:

1. Patients with abnormal liver function tests or signs attributable to liver disease should be evaluated as suspected for NAFLD and approached accordingly.

2. Patients with normal liver function tests should be assessed for metabolic risk factors such as obesity, dyslipidemia or diabetes mellitus or for other alternative causes for steatosis such as excessive alcohol consumption or possibly medication induced. In patients with abnormal liver function tests or incidental findings of hepatic steatosis at imaging and high clinical suspicion for NAFLD, a rapid MRI protocol targeted for liver fat quantification is the method of choice for estimating the severity of steatosis.

8.2.3 Evaluation of Steatosis over Time with or without Treatment

A major obstacle in NASH therapeutic trials is the need for repeated liver biopsies to assess the longitudinal treatment response, and these are invasive and subject to sampling error and variability in interpretation. In this context, MRI-PDFF has emerged as a noninvasive and reproducible alternative in assessing NASH and monitoring the treatment response, as well as in aiding the initial NASH diagnosis. MRI-PDFF is one of the leading imaging-based biomarkers of assessing antisteatotic benefits of a drug therapy in NASH. MRI-PDFF is frequently used as an endpoint in early-phase NASH trials. Because of its increased utilization in NASH clinical trials, there is a need for standardization of criteria for assessing treatment response in NASH trials. The optimal cut-point that was associated with histologic response was noted to be ≥30% relative reduction in MRI-PDFF. Subsequently, a recent meta-analysis has been published that provides pooled estimates on the association between MRI-PDFF responders, defined as ≥30% reduction in MRI-PDFF relative to baseline and histologic response. Seven studies were examined

in this meta-analysis, including 346 subjects. The rate of histologic response as defined as ≥2-point improvement in NAS in MRI-PDFF responders vs. nonresponders was 51 vs. 14% (P value < 0.01), respectively, and the rate of NASH resolution as defined as 0 ballooning and 0–1 in lobular inflammation in MRI-PDFF responders vs. nonresponders was 41 vs. 7% (P value < 0.01), respectively (9).

In a secondary analysis of a prospective phase Ib clinical trial evaluating a candidate treatment (MET409, a farnesoid X receptor agonist) for NASH, 48 participants were analyzed at baseline and at 4 and 12 weeks after active treatment with either MET409 (n=30) or placebo (n=18) treatment (10). An at least 19.3% relative MRI-PDFF reduction at W4 yielded an AUROC of 0.98 (sensitivity, 89%; specificity, 95%) for predicting an at least 30% relative MRI-PDFF reduction at W12. Therefore, early MRI-PDFF measurements may serve as early indicators of the treatment effect, as early indicators of the treatment response, and as potential early endpoints in NASH trials.

Finally, MRI-PDFF has high diagnostic accuracy to predict histological steatosis change in histological steatosis grade in children with NAFLD (4).

In conclusion, MRI-PDFF responder is defined as a ≥30% relative reduction in MRI-PDFF between baseline and end of treatment. Super-responder on MRI-PDFF is defined as a ≥50% relative reduction in MRI-PDFF between baseline and end of treatment. This is associated with significantly higher rates of NASH resolution. However, MRI-PDFF may not be useful for therapeutic agents that target primarily either inflammation or fibrosis and do not have any metabolic effects.

8.2.4 Guidelines

Recently, EASL published its guidelines about noninvasive tests for the evaluation of liver disease severity and prognosis (11). First, they indicated that noninvasive scores are not recommended for the diagnosis of steatosis in clinical practice (LoE 2; strong recommendation). But they added that MRI-PDFF is the most accurate noninvasive method for detecting and quantifying steatosis. However, it is not recommended as a first-line tool given its cost and limited availability. Therefore, it is more suited to clinical trials (LoE 2; strong recommendation). MRI-PDFF can be used to assess steatosis evolution under treatment (LoE 2; weak recommendation). However, the minimal decrease in MRI-PDFF that defines a clinically relevant change or treatment response needs to be better defined.

8.3 MRE FOR LIVER FIBROSIS ASSESSMENT

8.3.1 Introduction

Elastography is an imaging technique used to evaluate the mechanical properties of tissue according to the propagation of mechanical waves. MRI is coupled with a device

Table 8.1: Diagnosis of Steatosis Using MRI-PDFF

Author	Year	N	Steatosis Grades 2 and 3	Steatosis Grade 3
Gu J (2)	2019	635 meta-analysis	0.91	0.90
Middleton MS (4)	2018	110 Children	0.87 (0.80, 0.94)	0.79 (0.70, 0.87)
Park CC (5)	2017	104	0.90 (0.82–0.97)	0.92 (0.84–0.99)
Imajo K(6)	2016	142	0.90 (0.82–0.97	
Tang A (7)	2013	77	0.825 (0.734, 0.915)	0.893 (0.809, 0.977)
Idilman I (8)	2013	70	0.95 (0.91, 1.00)	

that generates mechanical waves, typically shear waves within the tissue(s) of interest. The shear wave velocity is then measured to calculate quantitative results. The shear wave velocity in tissue is directly related to the stiffness of the tissue. Propagation of shear waves is faster in stiff or hard tissues and slower in soft tissues. Liver MRE is an imaging technique used to measure liver stiffness in the evaluation for possible fibrosis or cirrhosis.

MRE has several advantages over ultrasound-based elastography, as it samples a much larger volume of the liver, is not affected by body mass index or degree of steatosis, is not operator dependent, has favorable test-retest repeatability, and has a high success rate (Table 8.2).

8.3.2 MRE Technique and Image Interpretation

MRE estimates liver stiffness, which correlates to the amount of collagen deposition in the extracellular matrix, but liver stiffness is also influenced by other factors, such as inflammation, vascular congestion, and cholestasis. Consequently, in early NASH when inflammation and cellular injury prevail over mild fibrosis, conventional MRE detects increased liver stiffness but cannot distinguish whether the increase is due to viscoelastic changes of inflammation or due to mild fibrosis.

In a typical liver MRE configuration, an active pneumatic mechanical wave driver is located outside the MRE room and is connected to a passive driver that is fastened onto the abdominal wall over the liver. The passive driver generates a continuous acoustic vibration that is transmitted through the entire abdomen, including the liver, at a fixed frequency, which is typically 60 Hz.

The most commonly used clinical MRE pulse sequence approved by the US Food and Drug Administration is a two-dimensional gradient-recalled-echo MR elastography sequence. After the magnitude and phase images are created, an inversion algorithm installed in the MRI unit automatically processes these raw data images to create several additional images and maps. The most common output images generated by MRI units are a color wave image depicting the propagation of shear waves through the abdomen, a grayscale elastogram without a superimposed 95% confidence map, a grayscale elastogram with a superimposed 95% confidence map, a color elastogram without a superimposed 95% confidence map, and a color elastogram with a superimposed 95% confidence map. The confidence map is a statistical derivation used to overlay a "checkerboard" on the stiffness map to exclude regions in the liver that have less reliable (i.e., noisy and discontinuous) stiffness data, so that a high-quality liver stiffness measurement can be obtained. The grayscale elastogram is commonly used to obtain quantitative liver stiffness measurements in kilopascals (kPa). The color elastogram is generally used for qualitative liver stiffness evaluation. However, the color elastograms created by MRI units from some vendors can also be used to obtain quantitative measurements. The color elastogram used clinically has a stiffness range of 0–8 kPa.

Liver stiffness measurement are obtained in the largest measurable portion of the liver on each of the four elastograms. On each image, a mean liver stiffness measurement, in kilopascals, along with the ROI size, in square centimeters (cm²), is obtained. Then the overall mean liver stiffness is obtained by calculating the weighted arithmetic mean, which reflects the relative contribution of the area of the liver measured on each image.

On the magnitude images, which provide the best anatomic detail of the liver, it is important to avoid the liver edge (≥1 cm from liver edge), nonhepatic tissues, fissures, gallbladder fossa, and large blood vessels. The left hepatic lobe can have a significant motion artifact due to cardiac pulsations and thus should be avoided as well, unless no motion artifact is identified. On the wave images, areas

Table 8.2: Comparison of Elastography Techniques (11)

	Transient Elastography	pSWE	2D-SWE	MRE
Advantages	Most widely used and validated technique Point-of-care (bedside, rapid, easy to learn) Quality criteria well-defined Good reproducibility High performance for cirrhosis (AUROC >0.9) Prognostic value in compensated cirrhosis well-validated	Can be performed in combination with regular ultrasound if the device is provided with adequate software ROI smaller than TE and location chosen by the operator Higher applicability than TE (ascites and obesity) Performance equivalent to that of TE and advanced fibrosis and cirrhosis High applicability for spleen stiffness measurement	Can be performed in combination with regular ultrasound if the device is provided with adequate software Large ROI that can be adjusted in size and location chosen by the operator Measures liver stiffness in real time Good applicability High performance for the diagnosis of significant fibrosis and cirrhosis Prognostic value in compensated cirrhosis	Can be implemented on a regular MRI machine Examination of the whole liver Higher applicability than TE (ascites, obesity) High performance for the earlier fibrosis stage and for diagnosis of cirrhosis Used in clinical trials for the assessment of fibrosis regression
Disadvantages	Requires a dedicated device ROI cannot be chosen	No clear cutoffs for the diagnosis of advanced fibrosis or cirrhosis No strong evaluation of liver fibrosis evolution over time	No clear cutoffs for the diagnosis of advanced fibrosis or cirrhosis No strong evaluation of liver fibrosis evolution over time	Requires an MRI facility Time-consuming Costly No strong data on prognostic value

2D-SWE: Bidimensional shear wave elastography; MRE: Magnetic resonance elastography; MRI: Magnetic resonance imaging; pSWE: Point-shear wave elastography; ROI: Region of interest; TE: Transient elastography.

of poor wave propagation, wave distortion and low-amplitude waves should be avoided. On the grayscale and color elastograms, the crosshatched regions on the superimposed 95% confidence map must be excluded from measurements. Finally, on the color elastogram, hot spots need to be recognized and excluded from measurements.

Obtaining and reporting accurate and reliable liver stiffness measurements with MRE requires an understanding of the three core components of liver MRE: optimization of imaging technique, prompt quality control of images, and proper interpretation and reporting of elastogram findings. When performing MRE, six technical parameters should be optimized:

- Patient fasting before the examination
- Proper passive driver placement
- Proper MRE section positioning over the largest area of the liver
- Use of MRE-related sequences at end expiration
- Choosing the best timing of the MRE sequence
- Optimization of several essential pulse sequence parameters

As soon as the MRE examination is performed, the elastograms should be reviewed to ensure that they are of diagnostic quality so that corrective steps can be taken, if needed, and the MRE can be repeated before the diagnostic portion of the examination concludes.

8.3.3 MRE for the Diagnosis of Liver Fibrosis

Several studies demonstrated the value of MRE for a noninvasive detection of liver fibrosis and the potential of MRE for distinguishing different fibrosis stages in NAFLD. The main results of different studies are indicated in Table 8.3.

8.3.4 Clinical Interpretation

As with all diagnostic studies, the choice of a cutoff value for the diagnosis of advanced fibrosis or cirrhosis is crucial. The choice of this value depends on the practitioner's wish: preference for better sensitivity or better specificity?

In a meta-analysis including 9 studies and 232 patients with NAFLD, liver stiffness measurement cutoffs of 3.77 and 4.09 kPa discriminated advanced fibrosis and cirrhosis, respectively (18). In another recent meta-analysis, the cutoff values of 3.62–4.8 kPa and 4.15–6.7 kPa were proposed for the diagnosis of advanced fibrosis and cirrhosis,

respectively (14). Loomba et al. proposed that a MRE liver stiffness cutoff of 4.67 kPa could predict cirrhosis. In another study from the same center, Park et al. reported that an MRE liver stiffness cutoff of 3.35 kPa could detect cirrhosis. Cui et al. found that a cutoff of 4.15 kPa distinguished cirrhosis from other stages. Imajo et al. found that a slightly higher MRE liver stiffness cutoff 6.7 kPa detected cirrhosis (19). In a recent study, MRE liver stiffness of 4.7 and 5.5 kPa was suggested as detecting advanced fibrosis and cirrhosis, respectively. A pooled analysis of 230 NAFLD patients suggested that the optimal cutoff for cirrhosis was 4.7 kPa. At last, Hsu et al. proposed 3.62 kPa and 4.7 kPa for the diagnosis of advanced fibrosis and cirrhosis, respectively (20). At this time, there is no guidelines for any cutoff value for the diagnosis of advanced fibrosis and cirrhosis.

8.3.5 MRE for the Diagnosis of NASH

Liver biopsy remains the reference standard for the diagnosis of NASH because none of the available noninvasive tests has acceptable accuracy (LoE 2) (11).

But, recently, a meta-analysis of 224 patients (4 studies) reported an AUROC of 0.83 (0.69–0.91) for the diagnosis of NASH using MRE with a sensitivity of 0.65 (0.46–0.80), and a specificity of 0.83 (0.69–0.91) (12). Loomba et al. suggested that a cutoff value of 3.26 kPa could discriminate NASH from NAFL, which was similar to another study by Costa-Silva et al., who reported a cutoff of 3.2 kPa (21) (13).

8.3.6 Evaluation of Liver Fibrosis Overtime with or without Treatment

In NAFLD, the severity of histological features, such as steatohepatitis without fibrosis, does not predict the prognosis of patients, whereas only fibrosis predicts a long-term prognosis (22). There are limited longitudinal data on the association between changes in MRE and liver fibrosis on paired liver biopsies.

A prospective cohort study included 102 patients with biopsy-proven NAFLD who underwent contemporaneous MRE and liver biopsy at baseline followed by a repeat paired liver biopsy and MRE assessment (23). The median time interval between the two paired assessments was 1.4 years. In unadjusted analysis, a 15% increase in MRE was associated with increased odds of histologic fibrosis progression (OR 3.56; 95% CI, 1.17–10.76; $P = 0.0248$). These findings remained clinically and statistically significant even after multivariable adjustment for age, sex and BMI (adjusted OR, 3.36; 95% CI, 1.10–10.31; $P = 0.0339$). A 15%

Table 8.3: Performance of MRE for the Diagnosis of Liver Fibrosis in NAFLD

	Year	N	AUROC F2F3F4 (95% CI)	AUROC F3F4 (95% CI)	AUROC F4 (95% CI)
Selvaraj E. A. (12)	2021	Meta-analysis 14,609	0.91 (0.80–0.97)	0.92 (0.88–0.95)	0.90 (0.81–0.95)
Costa Silva L. (13)	2018	49	0.932 (0.823–0.984)	0.928 (0.817–0.982)	0.964 (0.867–0.996)
Xiao G. (14)	2017	Meta-analysis 384	0.92	0.96	0.97
Park C. C. (5)	2017	94	0.89 (0.85–0.96)	0.87 (0.78–0.96)	0.87 (0.71–1.00)
Imajo K. (6)	2016	142	0.89 (0.85–0.94)	0.89 (0.83–0.95)	0.97 (0.94–1.00)
Cui J. (15)	2016	125	0.885 (0.816–0.953)	0.934 (0.863–1.000)	0.882 (0.729–1.000)
Kim D. (16)	2014	142		0.954 (0.905, 0.982)	
Lomba R. (17)	2014	117	0.856	0.924	0.894

AUROC: Area under the ROC curve; CI: Confidence interval.

increase in MRE was the strongest predictor of progression to advanced fibrosis (OR, 4.90; 95% CI, 1.35–17.84; $P = 0.0159$). Therefore, a 15% increase in liver stiffness on MRE may be associated with histologic fibrosis progression and progression from early fibrosis to advanced fibrosis (23). However, these results should be confirmed in ongoing clinical trials.

8.3.7 Comparison of Different Methods

MRE and transient elastography (FibroScan®) have been compared head to head in patients with biopsy-proven NAFLD in a small number of studies. These studies found that MRE is equal or more accurate than FibroScan® in identification of liver fibrosis, using liver biopsy analysis as the standard (Table 8.4).

A study evaluated the performances of MRE vs. ARFI for diagnosing fibrosis in NAFLD patients (15). For diagnosing any fibrosis (>stage 1), the MRE AUROC was 0.799 (95% CI 0.723–0.875), significantly higher than the ARFI AUROC of 0.664 (95% CI 0.568–0.760). In a recent meta-analysis, it was shown that MRE and shear wave elastography have the highest diagnostic accuracy for staging fibrosis in NAFLD patients (12).

The American Gastroenterological Association published clinical guidelines on the role of FibroScan® and MRE for the diagnosis of liver fibrosis in NAFLD (25). They conclude that MRE has little to no increased diagnostic accuracy in identifying cirrhosis in patients who truly have cirrhosis over FibroScan® but has considerably higher diagnostic accuracy in ruling out cirrhosis in patients who do not have cirrhosis, over FibroScan® (very low quality of evidence). EASL guidelines conclude that MRE is the most accurate noninvasive method for staging liver fibrosis (11). However, it is only marginally better than other noninvasive tests for F3–F4 fibrosis, and it is not recommended as a first-line given its cost and limited availability (LoE 2; strong recommendation). Therefore, it is more suited to clinical trials.

AASLD guidelines conclude that FibroScan® and MRE are clinically useful tools for identifying advanced fibrosis in patients with NAFLD (26).

At last, French guidelines indicate that the measurement of liver stiffness by MR could be useful (27).

8.3.8 MRE for the Evaluation of the Severity of the Liver Disease

8.3.8.1 Portal Hypertension

That liver stiffness correlates with the degree of portal hypertension has been shown in many studies using FibroScan® or ultrasound devices. It is also the case with MRE. Recently, 52 patients with cirrhosis underwent hepatic vein catheterization and 2D-MRE on separate days (28). Thirty-six of the patients had a hepatic venous pressure gradient (HVPG) of ≥12 mmHg and were tested prior to and after intravenous infusion of nonselective beta-blockers (NSBB) using HVPG measurement and MRE. HVPG showed a strong, positive, linear relationship with liver stiffness ($r^2 = 0.92$; $P < 0.001$) and spleen stiffness ($r^2 = 0.94$; $P < 0.001$). The cutoff points for identifying patients with a HVPG ≥ 12 mmHg were 7.7 kPa for liver stiffness (sensitivity, 0.78; specificity, 0.64) and 10.5 kPa for spleen stiffness (sensitivity, 0.8; specificity, 0.79). Intravenous administration of NSBB significantly decreased spleen stiffness by 6.9% (CI: 3.5–10.4, $P < 0.001$), but NSBB had no consistent effect on liver stiffness. However, changes in spleen stiffness were not related to the HVPG response ($P = 0.75$). An estimation by 2D-MRE of liver or spleen stiffness could reflect the degree of portal hypertension in patients with liver cirrhosis, but changes in stiffness after NSBB do not predict the effect on HVPG.

8.3.8.2 Liver Events

Fibrosis stage on histology has been shown to be a strong predictor of liver-associated outcomes (29). Liver stiffness measurement with FibroScan® is associated with liver events and prognosis in chronic liver diseases, especially NAFLD (30,31). The same results were published about liver stiffness measurement with MRE.

A recent retrospective cohort study of 829 adults with NAFLD who underwent MRE showed that baseline liver stiffness measurement was predictive of future cirrhosis development (32). Moreover, baseline liver stiffness measurement was predictive of future decompensation or death. The 1-year probability of future decompensation or death in cirrhosis with baseline LSM of 5 kPa vs. 8 kPa was 9% vs. 20%, respectively.

Table 8.4: Comparison of Different Methods for the Diagnosis of Advanced Liver Fibrosis and Cirrhosis

Author	Year	N	AUROC MRE	AUROC TE	AUROC 2D-SWE	AUROC MRE	AUROC TE	AUROC 2D-SWE	p
			Advanced fibrosis			Cirrhosis			
Sevaraj E. A. (12)	2021	14,609 meta-analysis	0.92 (0.88–0.95)	0.85 (0.83–0.87)	0.72 (0.60–0.84)	0.90 (0.81–0.95)	0.89 (0.84–0.93)	0.88 (0.81–0.91)	
Imajo K. (19)	2020	231	0.937 (0.882–0.958)	0.924 (0.867–0.947)	0.920 (0.865–0.953)	0.923 (0.871–0.955) *	0.872 (0.807–0.917)	0.886 (0.836–0.925)	<0.05 vs. TE and SWE
Furlan A. (24)	2019	59	0.95 (0.89–1.00)	0.86 (0.77–0.95)	0.89 (0.80–0.98)				NS
Hsu C. (20)	2019	230	0.93 (0.89–0.96)	0.84 (0.78–0.90)		0.94 (0.89–0.99)	0.84 (0.73–0.94)		<0.01
Park C. C. (5)	2017	104	0.87 (0.78–0.96)	0.80 (0.67–0.93)		0.87 (0.71–1.00)	0.69 (0.45–0.94)		

TE: Transient elastography; SWE: Shear wave elastography; MRE: Magnetic resonance elastography; AUROC: Area under the ROC curve.

Another multicenter retrospective study of 320 NAFLD patients who underwent MRE between 2016 and 2019 was reported (33). The best threshold for distinguishing cirrhosis from noncirrhosis was 4.39 kPa (AUROC 0.92), and from decompensated cirrhosis it was 6.48 kPa (AUROC 0.71). Odds of decompensation increased as liver stiffness increased (OR 3.28) ($P < 0.001$). Increased liver stiffness was associated with ascites, hepatic encephalopathy, esophageal variceal bleeding and mortality (median 7.10, 10.15 and 10.15 kPa, respectively).

These data expand the role of MRE from an accurate diagnostic method to a prognostic noninvasive imaging biomarker that can risk-stratify patients with NAFLD.

8.3.8.3 MRE and Cardiovascular Disease

Many epidemiological studies have reported the association between NAFLD and cardiovascular disease. The evaluation of liver stiffness by MRE could be an independent predictor for the presence of CAC (defined as a coronary artery calcium score > 0) in patients with NAFLD. In a recent study, 105 NAFLD patients with contemporaneous cardiac computed tomography and MRE were evaluated (34). In multivariable-adjusted analysis, liver stiffness was independently associated with the presence of CAC in a sex- and age-adjusted model (adjusted odd ratios = 2.23, 95% confidence interval = 1.31–4.34, $P = 0.007$). Moreover, CAC was more prevalent in patients with significant fibrosis than in those without, as determined by MRE (67.6% vs. 39.7%, $P = 0.012$). According to this study, patients with MRE ≥ 2.97 kPa should be considered for cardiovascular risk assessment.

8.3.9 MRE in Pediatric NAFLD

Normal range for MRE measured liver stiffness in children without liver disease could be around 2.45 ± 0.35 kPa (35). More attention has recently been paid to the diagnosis of pediatric NAFLD due to the increased obesity and high prevalence of fatty liver in children and adolescents. Considering that the histopathologic patterns in pediatric NAFLD patient differ from those of the adult cohort, a few MRE studies were conducted in order to evaluate the diagnostic performance of MRE for the detection of fibrosis and steatosis in children with NAFLD. However, MRE is limited in children due to a lack of cooperation, motion artifacts and inconsistent breathing encountered.

8.4 3D MR ELASTOGRAPHY

This is a more advanced version of MRE technology that acquires wave data throughout a 3D volume and that can also acquire wave data with sensitization to motion in all three directions. The more complete dataset provided by 3D MRE allows more sophisticated processing to be performed, permitting reliable calculation of new markers (36). Recent preclinical studies have shown that varying the frequency of mechanical waves and using 3D-MRE software enables identification of MR parameters that are sensitive to early viscoelastic alterations in NASH before fibrosis onset. Compared with 2D-MRE, 3D-MRE allows a more comprehensive analysis of the steady-state dynamic shear wave propagation in the entire liver. If multifrequency 3D-MRE (mf3D-MRE) can be used to discriminate NASH from simple steatosis, it is conceivable that an imaging biomarker that combines the mf3D-MRE for assessment of inflammation and ballooning with the MRI-PDFF for assessment of steatosis could predict the histologic parameters of NASH and estimate disease activity by the histologic NAFLD activity score (NAS) without the need for a liver biopsy. Moreover, the mf3D-MRE might be considered for use as a surrogate endpoint in interventional clinical trials because it offers the advantage of predicting not only NAS (the most commonly used surrogate endpoint in NASH trials) but also separate estimations of the three components of NAS (steatosis, inflammation/ballooning and fibrosis), which are individually targeted in certain experimental monotherapies.

For example, recently, the diagnostic accuracy of 3D-MRE and MRI-PDFF was evaluated in the detection of NASH in 175 individuals undergoing bariatric surgery (37). These parameters were fit into a logistic regression model that predicted NASH with a cross-validated AUROC of 0.73 (sensitivity, 0.67; specificity, 0.80; positive predictive value, 0.73; and negative predictive value, 0.74) and disease activity by NAS with a cross-validated AUROC of 0.82.

8.5. UNRESOLVED ISSUES TO BE ADDRESSED IN THE FUTURE

Further advances are needed to identify patients at risk of fibrosis progression and of complications. The evolution of liver stiffness (increase/decrease) over time needs to be more evaluated and better understood. The diagnosis of NASH is a key point in the management of patients with NAFLD. The usefulness of liver stiffness for the diagnosis of NASH is a challenge for the coming years. The cost-effectiveness of utilizing MRE vs. FibroScan® vs. other methods and/or biopsy must also be evaluated to develop optimal diagnostic strategies for diagnosing NAFLD-associated fibrosis.

8.6 CONCLUSION

MRI-PDFF is a useful surrogate for liver biopsy in the diagnosis of steatosis and assessment of treatment response. As a result, MRI-PDFF has been increasingly implemented in clinical and drug discovery trials and will likely have increasing impact on future clinical trial design.

For equipped centers, ultrasound-based elastography such as FibroScan® and SWE has moderate to high accuracy in diagnosing advanced fibrosis or cirrhosis and can be used in routine clinical practice.

As indicated in the recent EASL guidelines, MRE is the most accurate noninvasive method for staging liver fibrosis (11). However, it is not recommended as a first-line noninvasive test given its cost and limited availability (LoE 2; strong recommendation). In 2022, the usefulness of MRE is mainly for the follow-up of patients included in clinical trials.

REFERENCES

1. Starekova J, Hernando D, Pickhardt PJ, Reeder SB. Quantification of liver fat content with CT and MRI: state of the art. *Radiology*. 2021;301(2):250–262.
2. Gu J, Liu S, Du S, Zhang Q, Xiao J, Dong Q, et al. Diagnostic value of MRI-PDFF for hepatic steatosis in patients with non-alcoholic fatty liver disease: a meta-analysis. *Eur Radiol*. 2019;29(7):3564–3573.
3. Kim B, Kim SY, Kim KW, Jang HY, Jang JK, Song GW, et al. MRI in donor candidates for living donor liver transplant: technical and practical considerations. *J Magn Reson Imaging*. 2018;48(6):1453–1467.
4. Middleton MS, Van Natta ML, Heba ER, Alazraki A, Trout AT, Masand P, et al. Diagnostic accuracy of magnetic resonance imaging hepatic proton density fat fraction in pediatric nonalcoholic fatty liver disease. *Hepatology*. 2018;67(3):858–872.

5. Park CC, Nguyen P, Hernandez C, Bettencourt R, Ramirez K, Fortney L, et al. Magnetic resonance elastography vs transient elastography in detection of fibrosis and noninvasive measurement of steatosis in patients with biopsy-proven nonalcoholic fatty liver disease. *Gastroenterology*. 2017;152(3):598–607 e2.

6. Imajo K, Kessoku T, Honda Y, Tomeno W, Ogawa Y, Mawatari H, et al. Magnetic resonance imaging more accurately classifies steatosis and fibrosis in patients with nonalcoholic fatty liver disease than transient elastography. *Gastroenterology*. 2016;150(3):626–637 e7.

7. Tang A, Tan J, Sun M, Hamilton G, Bydder M, Wolfson T, et al. Nonalcoholic fatty liver disease: MR imaging of liver proton density fat fraction to assess hepatic steatosis. *Radiology*. 2013;267(2):422–431.

8. Idilman IS, Aniktar H, Idilman R, Kabacam G, Savas B, Elhan A, et al. Hepatic steatosis: quantification by proton density fat fraction with MR imaging vs. liver biopsy. *Radiology*. 2013;267(3):767–775.

9. Stine JG, Munaganuru N, Barnard A, Wang JL, Kaulback K, Argo CK, et al. Change in MRI-PDFF and histologic response in patients with nonalcoholic steatohepatitis: a systematic review and meta-analysis. *Clin Gastroenterol Hepatol*. 2021;19(11):2274–2283 e5.

10. Jiang H, Chen HC, Lafata KJ, Bashir MR. Week 4 liver fat reduction on MRI as an early predictor of treatment response in participants with nonalcoholic steatohepatitis. *Radiology*. 2021;300(2):361–368.

11. European Association for the Study of the Liver. Electronic address eee, Clinical Practice Guideline P, Chair, representative EGB, Panel M. EASL Clinical Practice Guidelines on non-invasive tests for evaluation of liver disease severity and prognosis—2021 update. *J Hepatol*. 2021;75(3):659–689.

12. Selvaraj EA, Mozes FE, Jayaswal ANA, Zafarmand MH, Vali Y, Lee JA, et al. Diagnostic accuracy of elastography and magnetic resonance imaging in patients with NAFLD: a systematic review and meta-analysis. *J Hepatol*. 2021;75(4):770–785.

13. Costa-Silva L, Ferolla SM, Lima AS, Vidigal PVT, Ferrari TCA. MR elastography is effective for the non-invasive evaluation of fibrosis and necroinflammatory activity in patients with nonalcoholic fatty liver disease. *Eur J Radiol*. 2018;98:82–89.

14. Xiao G, Zhu S, Xiao X, Yan L, Yang J, Wu G. Comparison of laboratory tests, ultrasound, or magnetic resonance elastography to detect fibrosis in patients with nonalcoholic fatty liver disease: a meta-analysis. *Hepatology*. 2017;66(5):1486–1501.

15. Cui J, Heba E, Hernandez C, Haufe W, Hooker J, Andre MP, et al. Magnetic resonance elastography is superior to acoustic radiation force impulse for the Diagnosis of fibrosis in patients with biopsy-proven nonalcoholic fatty liver disease: a prospective study. *Hepatology*. 2016;63(2):453–461.

16. Kim D, Kim WR, Talwalkar JA, Kim HJ, Ehman RL. Advanced fibrosis in nonalcoholic fatty liver disease: noninvasive assessment with MR elastography. *Radiology*. 2013;268(2):411–419.

17. Loomba R. Rationale for conducting a randomized trial to examine the efficacy of metformin in improving survival in cirrhosis: pleiotropic effects hypothesis. *Hepatology*. 2014;60(6):1818–1822.

18. Singh S, Venkatesh SK, Loomba R, Wang Z, Sirlin C, Chen J, et al. Magnetic resonance elastography for staging liver fibrosis in non-alcoholic fatty liver disease: a diagnostic accuracy systematic review and individual participant data pooled analysis. *Eur Radiol*. 2016;26(5):1431–1440.

19. Imajo K, Honda Y, Kobayashi T, Nagai K, Ozaki A, Iwaki M, et al. Direct comparison of US and MR elastography for staging liver fibrosis in patients with non-alcoholic fatty liver disease. *Clin Gastroenterol Hepatol*. 2022;20(4):908-917.

20. Hsu C, Caussy C, Imajo K, Chen J, Singh S, Kaulback K, et al. Magnetic resonance vs transient elastography analysis of patients with nonalcoholic fatty liver disease: a systematic review and pooled analysis of individual participants. *Clin Gastroenterol Hepatol*. 2019;17(4):630–637 e8.

21. Loomba R, Wolfson T, Ang B, Hooker J, Behling C, Peterson M, et al. Magnetic resonance elastography predicts advanced fibrosis in patients with nonalcoholic fatty liver disease: a prospective study. *Hepatology*. 2014;60(6):1920–1928.

22. Hagstrom H, Nasr P, Ekstedt M, Hammar U, Stal P, Hultcrantz R, et al. Fibrosis stage but not NASH predicts mortality and time to development of severe liver disease in biopsy-proven NAFLD. *J Hepatol*. 2017;67(6):1265–1273.

23. Ajmera VH, Liu A, Singh S, Yachoa G, Ramey M, Bhargava M, et al. Clinical utility of an increase in magnetic resonance elastography in predicting fibrosis progression in nonalcoholic fatty liver disease. *Hepatology*. 2020;71(3):849–860.

24. Furlan A, Tublin ME, Yu L, Chopra KB, Lippello A, Behari J. Comparison of 2D shear wave elastography, transient elastography, and MR elastography for the diagnosis of fibrosis in patients with non-alcoholic fatty liver disease. *AJR Am J Roentgenol*. 2020;214(1):W20–W6.

25. Singh S, Muir AJ, Dieterich DT, Falck-Ytter YT. American gastroenterological association institute technical review on the role of elastography in chronic liver diseases. *Gastroenterology*. 2017;152(6):1544–1577.

26. Chalasani N, Younossi Z, Lavine JE, Charlton M, Cusi K, Rinella M, et al. The diagnosis and management of nonalcoholic fatty liver disease: practice guidance from the American association for the study of liver diseases. *Hepatology*. 2018;67(1):328–357.

27. Boursier J, Guillaume M, Bouzbib C, Lannes A, Pais R, Smatti S, et al. Non-invasive diagnosis and follow-up of non-alcoholic fatty liver disease. *Clin Res Hepatol Gastroenterol*. 2021;46(1):101769.

28. Danielsen KV, Hove JD, Nabilou P, Yin M, Chen J, Zhao M, et al. Using MR elastography to assess portal hypertension and response to beta-blockers in patients with cirrhosis. *Liver Int*. 2021;41(9):2149–2158.

29. Ekstedt M, Hagstrom H, Nasr P, Fredrikson M, Stal P, Kechagias S, et al. Fibrosis stage is the strongest predictor for disease-specific mortality in NAFLD after up to 33 years of follow-up. *Hepatology*. 2015;61(5):1547–1554.

30. Shili-Masmoudi S, Wong GL, Hiriart JB, Liu K, Chermak F, Shu SS, et al. Liver stiffness measurement predicts long-term survival and complications in non-alcoholic fatty liver disease. *Liver Int*. 2020;40(3):581–589.

31. Decraecker M, Dutartre D, Hiriart JB, Irles-Depe M, Marraud des Grottes H, Chermak F, et al. Long-term prognosis of patients with alcohol-related liver disease or non-alcoholic fatty liver disease according to metabolic syndrome or alcohol use. *Liver Int*. 2022;42(2):350-362.

32. Gidener T, Yin M, Dierkhising RA, Allen AM, Ehman RL, Venkatesh SK. MRE for prediction of long-term progression and outcome in chronic liver disease: a retrospective study. *Hepatology*. 2022;75(2):379-390.

33. Han MAT, Vipani A, Noureddin N, Ramirez K, Gornbein J, Saouaf R, et al. MR elastography-based liver fibrosis correlates with liver events in nonalcoholic fatty liver patients: a multicenter study. *Liver Int*. 2020;40(9):2242–2251.

34. Park JG, Jung J, Verma KK, Kang MK, Madamba E, Lopez S, et al. Liver stiffness by magnetic resonance elastography is associated with increased risk of cardiovascular disease in patients with non-alcoholic fatty liver disease. *Aliment Pharmacol Ther*. 2021;53(9):1030–1037.

35. Sawh MC, Newton KP, Goyal NP, Angeles JE, Harlow K, Bross C, et al. Normal range for MR elastography measured liver stiffness in children without liver disease. *J Magn Reson Imaging*. 2020;51(3):919–927.

36. Reeder SB. Emergence of 3D MR elastography-based quantitative markers for diffuse liver disease. *Radiology*. 2021;301(1):163–165.

37. Allen AM, Shah VH, Therneau TM, Venkatesh SK, Mounajjed T, Larson JJ, et al. The role of three-dimensional magnetic resonance elastography in the diagnosis of nonalcoholic steatohepatitis in obese patients undergoing bariatric surgery. *Hepatology*. 2020;71(2):510–521.

9 Artificial Intelligence in NAFLD Diagnosis

Joseph C. Ahn and Samer Gawrieh

CONTENTS

Key Points

■ Artificial intelligence (AI), interchangeably used with machine learning (ML), refers to algorithms and statistical models that can learn from and interpret datasets from which they are able to detect patterns in the same or other datasets.

■ AI models demonstrate good diagnostic performance for detecting NAFLD and NASH in large electronic health records databases or in radiographic imaging studies.

■ AI models can help find NAFLD or NASH signatures in enormous amounts of complex molecular information generated by multiple "omics" datasets.

■ While a remarkable progress has been made using different AI models to generate reproducible and continuous measures of NAFLD histological lesions, the accuracy of automated detection of lobular inflammation and hepatocellular ballooning remain suboptimal.

■ Prediction of clinical outcomes is an emerging area for AI in NAFLD.

■ The intense interest and research in various AI applications in NAFLD are very likely to lead to further improvements in performance and more routine use in clinical practice and clinical trials.

9.1 INTRODUCTION

Health care systems throughout the world must serve a large and growing number of patients with nonalcoholic fatty liver disease (NAFLD) who make up approximately 25% of the global population. (1) Currently, there are areas of unmet need in early detection, risk stratification and prediction of complications and outcomes for patients with NAFLD. Patients with NAFLD generate an enormous volume of multimodal data from various sources, including clinical documents, laboratory tests, radiologic and histopathologic images and multiomics studies. While such an abundance of information holds great promise to enhance care for patients with NAFLD, turning it into actionable knowledge remains a major challenge. (2) Recently, revolutionary breakthroughs in the field of artificial intelligence (AI) fueled by state-of-the-art machine learning algorithms including deep learning have enabled computers to synthesize and analyze large volumes of complex, high-dimensional data with superhuman performances and speed. Now, AI is being applied across almost all fields of medicine with hepatology, with the study of NAFLD being no exception. (3) There are AI models that help identify individuals with NAFLD among the general population, distinguish patients with nonalcoholic steatohepatitis (NASH) among patients with NAFLD, estimate the degree of hepatic fibrosis and predict clinical outcomes in patients with NAFLD (Table 9.1). This chapter will provide an overview of AI and highlight some important and up-to-date applications of AI in NAFLD.

9.2 ARTIFICIAL INTELLIGENCE, MACHINE LEARNING AND DEEP LEARNING

9.2.1 Artificial Intelligence

While commonly regarded as a recent invention, the concept of AI is in fact nearly a century old—first described in 1937 by Alan Turing, who proposed the idea of a "universal computing machine." (4) In 1956, the term "artificial intelligence" was coined by John McCarthy at the historic Dartmouth Summer Research Project on Artificial Intelligence. (5) Today, AI is broadly defined as "a system's ability to interpret external data correctly, to learn from such data, and to use those learnings to achieve specific goals and tasks through flexible adaptation." (6) AI is an all-encompassing term that covers many other methods such as different techniques of machine learning and natural language processing (Figure 9.1).

9.2.2 Machine Learning

"Machine learning" is a field of AI that involves training computer algorithms on sample data to make predictions or decisions based on the learned relationships

DOI: 10.1201/9781003386698-11

Table 9.1: Artificial Intelligence Applications in NAFLD

Data Type	Potential Applications
Structured clinical data: • Demographics • Vital signs • Laboratory values • Billing codes Natural language processing: • Physician documentation • Test reports in text format • Patient messages Multiomics: • Genomics • Epigenomics • Transcriptomics • Proteomics • Metabolomics Radiologic imaging: • Ultrasound • CT • MRI Histopathologic imaging: • Liver biopsy slides	• Screening for NAFLD • Prediction of NASH • Prediction of fibrosis • Prediction of clinical outcomes and response to therapy • Discovery of novel biomarkers • Discovery of novel patient clusters • Automated quantification of hepatic steatosis and fibrosis on imaging • Automated quantification of hepatic steatosis, inflammation, ballooning and fibrosis on histology

CT: Computerized tomography; MRI: Magnetic resonance imaging; NAFLD: Nonalcoholic fatty liver disease; NASH: Nonalcoholic steatohepatitis

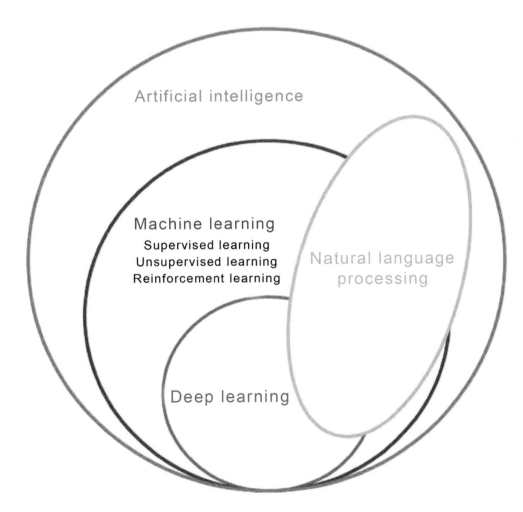

Figure 9.1 Artificial intelligence different techniques (Used with permission from Ahn J. et. *Hepatology* 2021.)

between different variables. (7) Machine learning is broadly divided into supervised learning and unsupervised learning. The key difference between the two is the presence or absence of labeled outputs in the sample data. Supervised learning algorithms train on sample input data with labeled output, with the goal of accurately predicting the output when faced with a new set of input data. An example of supervised learning would be using a dataset of patients with labeled outputs of NAFLD vs. no NAFLD, along with various input variables including age, gender, body mass index (BMI), lipid profile, liver enzymes, etc. The machine learning algorithm will learn the relationship between the input variables and the outputs of NAFLD vs. no NAFLD, and its performance will be evaluated based on how well it can make the determination of NAFLD vs. no NAFLD when provided with a new set of input data. On the other hand, unsupervised learning algorithms train on sample data with input variables alone and no labeled outputs. In a process called "clustering," the unsupervised machine learning algorithm analyzes inherent structure or patterns within the data to divide the sample into new clusters. For example, the application of an unsupervised machine learning algorithm to whole genome sequencing data from a large group of patients with NAFLD may lead to identification of new clusters of patients with distinct genotypes and clinical trajectory. Another use of unsupervised learning is in dimensionality reduction. When tasked with processing high-dimensional data with thousands of input variables, dimensionality reduction techniques can help simplify the data down to a smaller number of input variables that are more relevant.

9.2.3 Artificial Neural Networks and Deep Learning

Artificial neural networks (ANNs) are a subset of machine learning algorithms that consist of layers of interconnected mathematical formulas, loosely modeling the neurons of the brain. (8) "Deep learning" refers to AI models that utilize deep neural networks, or ANNs with multiple layers of mathematical functions that are capable of analyzing complex, nonlinear, high-dimensional data. Over the past decade, deep learning has emerged as the state-of-the-art AI technique in speech recognition, visual object recognition and many other domains such as drug discovery and genomics. (9) Deep learning can be divided into different forms based on the architecture, or the connectivity patterns within the deep neural network. Convolutional neural networks (CNNs) have connectivity patterns that resemble the animal visual cortex and facilitate the recognition of inherent spatial features of high-dimensional images. (10) Consequently, CNNs are highly useful AI tools in medical image processing. On the other hand, recurrent neural networks (RNNs) have neural connections that form a directed graph along a temporal sequence, as well as loops that preserve the memory of previous inputs. (11) These features make RNNs ideal for analysis of sequential time-series data within electronic health records (EHR).

9.3 AI MODELS FOR NAFLD PREDICTION USING CLINICAL DATA

9.3.1 Screening for Presence or Absence of NAFLD

Patients with NAFLD tend to remain asymptomatic until the development of advanced fibrosis and portal hypertension. Given the high prevalence of NAFLD in the general population, a simple, inexpensive and easily accessible screening tool that can be used by primary care providers is necessary for early diagnosis of NAFLD and prevention of its complications. As no single laboratory test can diagnose NAFLD, noninvasive scoring systems such as the fatty liver index, (12) NAFLD liver fat score, (13) hepatic steatosis index, (14) SteatoTest, (15) lipid accumulation product (16) and NAFL screening score (17) have been developed to help identify NAFLD using a combination of routinely available clinical and laboratory variables. However, their performances are not perfect, and many recent studies have attempted to develop novel screening tools for NAFLD using machine learning techniques. In most instances, supervised machine learning approaches were used for training a binary classifier, with the outcome of interest being the presence or absence of NAFLD.

In 2017, the NAFLD ridge score was developed using routine clinical and laboratory parameters from 922 subjects in a population-based screening study. (18) The ridge regression model—using six predictors including alanine aminotransferase (ALT), high-density lipoprotein (HDL) cholesterol, triglyceride, hemoglobin A1c, white blood cell count and the presence of hypertension—achieved an area under a receiver-operating characteristic curve (AUROC) of 0.88 in the validation group with 92% sensitivity, 90% specificity, 96% negative predictive value (NPV) and 69% positive predictive value (PPV). Several other machine learning models constructed using clinical and laboratory variables within large, population-based EHR data from different countries demonstrated moderate to good discriminative performances for NAFLD with AUROCs ranging between 0.73 and 0.87. (19–22) In 2021, a deep learning model based on 11 clinical variables (age, sex, height, weight, waist circumference, AST, ALT, GGT, cholesterol, triglyceride and platelet count) demonstrated a remarkable performance of classifying patients with or without NAFLD, with an AUROC of 0.95, 97.2% sensitivity, 97.8% specificity, 98.6% PPV, and 95.7% NPV. (23) In addition, a neural network-based web application trained on sex, age, abdominal volume index, fasting serum glucose and GGT from 2,970 patients was effective at predicting the absence of NAFLD, with 73% sensitivity and 100% specificity. (24)

9.3.2 Prediction of NASH or Fibrosis

In addition to screening for NAFLD among the general population, it is also important to identify those with more advanced disease such as NASH and hepatic fibrosis who are at higher risk of liver-related complications. (25) While the NAFLD fibrosis score (NFS) (26) and the fibrosis-4 index (FIB-4) (27) are widely accepted and have a high diagnostic ability for advanced fibrosis, they have limited ability to identify NASH patients with a lesser extent of fibrosis. (28) In 2018, four supervised machine learning algorithms trained on longitudinal laboratory parameters from a large US claims database exhibited AUROCs between 0.84 and 0.88 for distinguishing patients with NASH. (29) In another study, an XGBoost algorithm called the NASHmap model was trained on 14 clinical variables from a cohort of 704 patients with biopsy-proven NASH. When applied to a large external real-world database of around 3 million patients, the NASHmap had satisfactory performances with an AUROC of 0.82, 81% sensitivity and 81% PPV. (30) A single-center study from Spain developed random forest algorithms that correctly classified patients with NASH with 87% accuracy, and identified insulin resistance, ferritin, insulin levels, and triglycerides to be important predictors of NASH. (31) Additional single-center studies using supervised machine learning algorithms also showed promising ability for predicting fibrotic NASH and outperformed conventional scoring systems. (32,33)

9.4 AI MODELS FOR NAFLD PREDICTION USING MULTI-OMICS

As previously discussed, there is a major unmet need for novel biomarkers in the diagnosis of NAFLD and NASH. Recent advances in high-throughput multiomics in basic and translational research may be able to address this problem. Multiomics refers to the study of datasets from multiple "omics," such as genomics, epigenomics, transcriptomics, proteomics, metabolomics, lipidomics, etc. Multiomics research generates an enormous amount of complex molecular information beyond human analytic capacities, and advanced machine learning algorithms can handle the computational burden of such high-dimensional data.

As NAFLD is a disorder of metabolism, many studies have investigated metabolomic signatures associated with NAFLD, which may also provide insights on the disease pathophysiology. In 2017, Chiappini et al. performed a comprehensive lipidomic analysis on liver biopsies from patients with normal liver, NAFLD and NASH. Using a random forest-based machine learning approach, they identified a set of 32 lipids that discriminated NASH with 100% sensitivity and specificity. (34) In 2019, a support vector machine (SVM) model trained using lipidomic, glycomic and free fatty acid data from NAFLD, NASH and healthy subjects differentiated the three conditions with up to 90% accuracy and discriminated the presence of liver fibrosis with 98% accuracy. (35) Another metabolomic study using an ensemble learning approach identified glycocholic acid, taurocholic acid, phenylalanine and branched chain amino acid levels as markers of disease severity from NAFLD to NASH and NASH-cirrhosis and accurately predicted the different clinical stages. (36) Proteomic studies utilizing a machine learning approach have identified novel protein biomarkers associated with liver fibrosis in patients with NASH. (37,38)

Data from different omics can also be combined and analyzed together by machine learning algorithms. Wood et al. trained a multicomponent classifier for NAFLD based on phenotypic, genomic and proteomic variables from 576 adults. The final model consisted of PNPLA3 rs738409 genotype, 8 proteins and 19 phenotypic variables and exhibited an AUROC of 0.913. (39) Another study analyzed genetic, transcriptomic, proteomic and metabolomic data from a large multicenter cohort of high-risk European adults and applied LASSO and random forest algorithms to predict NAFLD with an AUROC of 0.84, which outperformed existing noninvasive NAFLD prediction tools. (40) Beyond the diagnosis of NAFLD or NASH, multiomics may also help predict the development of complications such as hepatocellular carcinoma (HCC). A recent study used machine learning to build a diagnostic model for NAFLD-related HCC using 1,295 metabolites, which discriminated the three groups of NAFLD, HCC and healthy controls with AUROCs between 0.87 and 0.93 and discovered the unique metabolomic profile of patients with NAFLD-HCC. (41)

9.5 AI MODELS FOR NAFLD PREDICTION USING RADIOLOGIC IMAGING

One of the most impressive breakthroughs in the real-life application of AI has been computer vision, a field of AI

that trains computers to interpret, understand and react to the visual world. Deep learning algorithms using the CNN architecture have shown outstanding capabilities to process and interpret digitized medical images from radiologic studies. In NAFLD, various deep learning models have shown promising results for the assessment of hepatic steatosis and disease severity on ultrasound, computerized tomography (CT) and magnetic resonance imaging (MRI) studies. Using MRI-derived proton density fat fraction (PDFF) as the gold standard, Han et al. developed a deep learning algorithm using radio frequency ultrasound data from 140 patients with NAFLD and 64 controls, which provided 96% accuracy, 97% sensitivity, 94% specificity, 97% PPV, and 94% NPV for NAFLD diagnosis. (42) Another study used ultrasound images acquired from four different liver views to develop a deep learning model for NAFLD diagnosis and created an ensemble model based on all four views that achieved an AUROC of 0.91. (43) Another ultrasound-based deep learning model based on two-dimensional hepatic ultrasound images showed an ability to distinguish moderate and severe NAFLD with an AUROC of 0.96. (44)

Deep learning has also enabled automated assessment of liver fat using CT liver Hounsfield unit values and MRI-PDFF maps. (45) A fully automated liver segmentation algorithm using noncontrast CT scan images from 9,552 adults was able to quantify liver fat with excellent correlation between manual and automated measurements ($r^2 = 0.92$). (46) Deep learning algorithms have repeatedly demonstrated a high correlation of automated and manual quantification in CT Houndsfield units and MRI-PDFF measurements. (47) Furthermore, deep learning was able to accurately estimate liver attenuation even in noncontrast, low-dose chest CT images with incomplete coverage of the liver and to identify patients with moderate to severe hepatic steatosis. (48)

9.6 NATURAL LANGUAGE PROCESSING

Natural language processing (NLP) is a branch of AI that strives to teach computers how to process and analyze large amounts of natural language data in the form of text and spoken words. (3) Every day, a large amount of data about patients and their care is generated in an unstructured format as narrative note entries or textual reports. While these data are not suited for analysis by traditional methods, NLP can be used to extract meaningful diagnostic and prognostic information from them. A recent study sought to establish an NAFLD cohort in primary care by identifying patients with evidence of hepatic steatosis on imaging. (49) Using NLP to search for specific terms associated with hepatic steatosis, the authors were able to quickly identify 1,237 patients with NAFLD out of over 8,000 unique patients in their primary care cohort. In another study from Israel, the use of NLP in 1 million imaging reports combined with laboratory data allowed the investigators to double the NAFLD detection rate compared to using diagnosis codes. (50)

9.7 AI MODELS FOR NAFLD PREDICTION USING HISTOPATHOLOGIC IMAGING

The gold standard for the diagnosis and staging of NAFLD is manual histological assessment of liver biopsy specimens by pathologists and documentation of findings such as steatosis, ballooning, inflammation and fibrosis. (51) However, interpretation of liver biopsy can be highly time-consuming, and significant intra- and interobserver variations among pathologists have been reported. (52,53) Further, it offers only semiquantitative assessment of each of the NAFLD lesions with limited ranges for quantifying lesions' severity and abundance. Machine learning techniques including deep learning are emerging as highly promising tools for accurate and efficient interpretation of digitized liver biopsy images in patients with NAFLD. In addition to being reproducible, AI-based methods offer continuous and precise measurements of each of the NAFLD lesions, which are advantages over manual semiquantification of these lesions when assessing response to therapeutic interventions in clinical trials of NAFLD and NASH.

It is important to emphasize that AI-based methods for the detection and quantification of NAFLD lesions in digital images of liver biopsy only address factors related to human interpretation (intra- and interobserver variability) and replaces semiquantitative scores with continuous measures of NAFLD lesions. However, AI-based methods do not address other factors that affect the diagnostic yield of a liver biopsy sample such as adequacy of sample size, length and processing.

In 2014, investigators used digital images of hematoxylin and eosin (H&E)-stained slides of 47 liver biopsies to train an SVM algorithm to classify white regions on the images into macrosteatosis, central veins, portal veins, portal arteries, sinusoids and bile ducts. (54) The model had an overall accuracy of 89% and over 95% precision and sensitivity for detection of macrosteatosis. The classifier was further trained to automatically identify and quantify lobular inflammation and hepatocyte ballooning (Figure 9.2) but demonstrated weak to moderate correlation with pathologists' grading (R^2 0.17 and 0.49, respectively). (55) In 2020, the same group developed another SVM model for the automated estimation of collagen proportionate area as well as classification of six different architectural patterns of fibrosis distribution in NAFLD liver biopsies. (56) Using a different approach, another group used digitized liver biopsy specimens from 246 consecutive patients with biopsy-proven NAFLD to train a K-means algorithm that automatically computes percentages of fat, inflammation, ballooning, fibrosis and collagen proportionate area. (57)

The results from the software exhibited weak to moderate degrees of correlation with human pathologists and validated in a separate group of patients (correlation [rho] with pathologists: steatosis: 0.66; inflammation: 0.36; ballooning: 0.52; fibrosis: 0.57).

In the largest study of using AI for interpretation of liver histology, thousands of liver biopsy samples from three randomized controlled trials of therapies for patients with NASH were used to develop a CNN-based deep learning model for quantitative histologic grading and assessment of disease severity. (58) The deep learning model predictions were significantly correlated with expert pathologists' estimates of the NAFLD activity score (NAS) and fibrosis. The correlation of detection and quantification of lesions were strong for fibrosis using the Ishak scoring system (rho, 0.71) but weak to moderate for lobular inflammation, ballooning, steatosis and fibrosis using the NASH Clinical Research Network scoring system (rho, 035, 0.41, 0.60 and 0.56, respectively). (58) Several additional studies utilizing deep learning demonstrated good performances for quantifying and grading histologic features in NAFLD and NASH. (59–61)

Consistently across these studies, different AI methods at the present offer less than optimal accuracy and precision in the identification and quantification of hepatocyte ballooning and lobular inflammation, two cardinal lesions of NASH. (55,57,58,62) A recent study highlighted the challenges of defining ballooning by expert hepatopathologists, which resulted in poor agreement among pathologist on detecting ballooning (kappa, 0.197) and poor concordance between the trained AI model and pathologists (19–42%). Creating a consensus atlas by expert liver pathologists, as in that study for agreed-upon labels for specific NAFLD lesions, can be a useful but challenging task to provide a reliable training set to develop AI models. How representative and comprehensive such a classic labels atlas of the entire spectrum of NAFLD, including milder cases seen in a community and with lower severity of each of the lesions, would require further studies. The use of various supervised and unsupervised AI methods to detect these lesions based on reliable training datasets may be another approach to address these challenges.

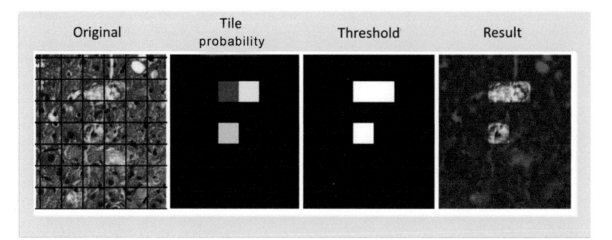

Figure 9.2 Process of identifying hepatocyte ballooning (Used with permission from Vanderbeck S. et al. *Human Pathology* 2015.)

Original digitally scanned images of H&E-stained liver biopsy are first divided into tiles. Each tile is assigned a probability of containing hepatocyte ballooning (black is a probability of 0, middle gray is 50%, and white is 100%). Last, a threshold is determined for what probability is required for a tile to be automatically classified as hepatocyte ballooning.

9.8 AI MODELS FOR PREDICATION OF NAFLD CLINICAL OUTCOMES

Beyond screening and diagnosis, prediction of clinical outcomes is an emerging area for AI in NAFLD. In a single-center study using the electronic health records from 38,575 patients, NLP significantly outperformed ICD and a text search in NAFLD identification and also was able to identify patients with NAFLD at risk for disease progression to NASH or cirrhosis. (63) Another study used 198 machine learning-based histological features from their deep learning model to perform Cox proportional hazards regression for the prediction of two clinical outcomes of interest: progression to cirrhosis in patients with bridging fibrosis at baseline and liver-related clinical events in those with cirrhosis. (58) Among the 198 histological features, 99 and 61 predicted progression to cirrhosis and liver-related clinical events, respectively, and the machine learning-based features were slightly more prognostic than the parameters from central pathologists' review. (58) Finally, Bosch et al. conducted another interesting study to predict the hepatic venous pressure gradient (HVPG) from liver histology. (64) The authors used HVPG measurements and liver histology from 218 subjects enrolled in a randomized, placebo-controlled phase 2b study of simtuzumab in patients with compensated cirrhosis due to NASH, and they trained an end-to-end convolutional neural network model to classify patients' HVPG into 6 categories (0–5; 5.5–9.5; 10–11.5; 12–15.5; 16–19.5; ≥20 mmHg) based on histological findings. The ML-HVPG score was significantly correlated with true HVPG in the test set (rho, 0.47; P < 0.001) and predicted the presence of clinically significant portal hypertension (HVPG ≥10 mmHg) with an AUROC of 0.76, 85% sensitivity, 62% specificity, 81% PPV, and 68% NPV. (64)

9.9 CURRENT PROMISES AND CHALLENGES

It is evident that the application of AI for the care of patients with NAFLD is not a futuristic idea but is rapidly becoming a reality. There has been an exponential increase in the number of published studies applying AI to NAFLD, and this trend will likely continue to accelerate. Integration of AI-based tools into the EHR as clinical decision aids may enable independent flagging of patients with suspected NAFLD, NASH or advanced liver fibrosis and help identify patients at risk of poor outcomes, allowing clinicians to take the necessary steps for early diagnosis and appropriate management.

However, several key issues must be addressed before AI can be universally implemented in everyday clinical practice. The first limitation is the generalizability of the AI models. Most AI models are developed by single-center studies using historical datasets from highly specialized academic institutions, whose patient populations may not represent patients who receive care in rural/community settings. This has raised concerns that AI models may overrepresents individuals with higher income, of younger age, and of the white race category and may not be as applicable to low-income, minority patients presenting to community hospitals. AI-based histology

Table 9.2: AI Studies in NAFLD with External Validation Cohorts

Study	Development Cohort	Validation Cohort	AI Method	Input	Output	Model Performance in External Validation
Sorino et al. 2021	MICOL III trial $n = 2,860$	NUTRIHEP $n = 100$	Neural network	Age, sex, AVI, glucose, GGT	NAFLD diagnosis	AUROC 0.82, 73% sensitivity, 100% specificity, 77% accuracy
Docherty et al. 2021	NIDDK NAFLD database $n = 704$	Optum database $n = 3,902$	XGBoost	HbA1c, AST, ALT, TP, AST/ALT, BMI, TG, height, Plt, WBC, Hct, Alb	NASH vs. non-NASH NAFLD	AUROC 0.82, 81% sensitivity, 81% precision, 75% accuracy
Chiappini et al. 2017	Brousse Hospital $n = 61$	L'Archet Hospital $n = 7$	Random forest	32 lipids from lipidomic analysis	NASH diagnosis	100% accuracy
Luo Y et al. 2021	VCU $n = 113$	NCT02413372 $n = 71$	Elastic-Net	12 proteins from proteomic analysis	Liver fibrosis in NASH	AUROC 0.78 for stage 0–1; 0.43 for stage 2; 0.78 for stage 3–4 fibrosis
Atabaki-Pasdar et al. 2020	IMI DIRECT $n = 1514$	UK Biobank $n = 4,609$	Random forest	Genetic, transcriptomic, proteomic, metabolomic variables	Early stage NAFLD	AUROC 0.79, 67% sensitivity, 74% specificity, 71% accuracy
Lewinska et al. 2021	Spain and France $n = 196$	Chile, Spain, Brazil, Denmark $n = 53$	SVM	Metabolomic variables	NAFLD-HCC	AUROC 0.87 vs. healthy controls; 0.93 vs. morbidly obese NAFLD; 0.87 vs. alcohol/viral HCC
Wang et al. 2019	UCSD $n = 530$	7 institutions $n = 298$	CNN	CT and MRI	Liver segmentation	Segmentation accuracy, 0.92–0.95
Taylor-Weiner et al. 2021	STELLAR-3 STELLAR-4 $n = 644$	STELLAR-3 STELLAR-4 ATLAS $n = 3034$	CNN	Liver biopsy slides	Histologic features of NAFLD	Correlation with central pathologists Steatosis: 0.66; lobular inflammation: 0.36; hepatocyte ballooning: 0.52; fibrosis stage: 0.57

Alb: Albumin; ALT: Alanine aminotransferase; AST: Aspartate aminotransferase; AUROC: Area under receiver operating characteristics curve; AVI: Abdominal volume index; BMI: Body mass index; CNN: Convolutional neural network; CT: Computerized tomography; GGT: Gamma-glutamyl transferase; HbA1c: Hemoglobin A1c; HCC: Hepatocellular carcinoma; Hct: Hematocrit; MRI: Magnetic resonance imaging; NAFLD: Nonalcoholic fatty liver disease; NASH: Nonalcoholic steatohepatitis; Plt: Platelet count; SVM: Support vector machines; TG: Triglycerides; UCSD: University of California–San Diego; VCU: Virginia Commonwealth University; WBC: White blood cell count.

models may be biased by training on patients seen at academic centers who tend to have more severe disease severity and who may not have the same degree of performance when applied to patients seen in the community hospitals. Therefore, large-scale, prospective, multisite validation of AI models using diverse populations of patients will be essential for universal implementation of AI models. (65) Table 9.2 lists a selection of AI-NAFLD studies to date that have included external validation for their AI algorithms.

Another limitation is the interpretability of AI models. Complex AI algorithms such as deep learning are considered "black-box," which means that humans cannot understand how AI is making its decisions. It has been argued that clinicians may feel uncomfortable with using black-box AI models for patient care and that AI should be explainable in a way that clinical users can understand. (66) This concern is being addressed by the recent development of various "explainable AI," or XAI techniques. However, there also have been arguments that explainability methods do not guarantee performance and that rigorous internal and external validation of AI models is a better and more direct means of ensuring their utility. (67)

9.10 CONCLUSIONS AND FUTURE DIRECTIONS

This chapter has provided a comprehensive overview of the current landscape of AI research in NAFLD. State-of-the-art machine learning algorithms can be trained using various forms of multimodal data from patients with NAFLD. Machine learning algorithms can help make highly accurate diagnostic and prognostic predictions using structured and unstructured clinical data and complex molecular data from multiomics. In the era of rapid drug development for NAFLD, AI tools may help identify patients who are more likely to be responders to therapeutic interventions and assist in the delivery of more personalized effective therapies. Furthermore, sophisticated machine learning algorithms including deep learning can accurately automate the interpretation of radiologic and histopathologic images with extremely fast speed and also lead to the discovery of new biologic pathways and disease subgroups by analyzing complex high-dimensional data in ways impossible for the human brain. Despite the challenges of generalizability and explainability, AI will soon play a major role in the diagnosis, prognostication and management of patients with NAFLD.

REFERENCES

1. Younossi ZM, Koenig AB, Abdelatif D, Fazel Y, Henry L, Wymer M. Global epidemiology of nonalcoholic fatty liver disease-Meta-analytic assessment of prevalence, incidence, and outcomes. *Hepatology* 2016;64:73–84.
2. Pastorino R, De Vito C, Migliara G, Glocker K, Binenbaum I, Ricciardi W, Boccia S. Benefits and challenges of Big Data in healthcare: an overview of the European initiatives. *Eur J Public Health* 2019;29:23–27.
3. Ahn JC, Connell A, Simonetto DA, Hughes C, Shah VH. Application of artificial intelligence for the diagnosis and treatment of liver diseases. *Hepatology* 2021;73:2546–2563.
4. Church A, Turing AM. On computable numbers, with an application to the Entscheidungs problem. Proceedings of the London Mathematical Society, 2 s. vol. 42 (1936–1937), pp. 230–265. *J Symb Log* 1937;2:42–43.
5. McCarthy J. What is artificial intelligence? 2004.
6. Haenlein M, Kaplan A. A brief history of artificial intelligence: on the past, present, and future of artificial intelligence. *Calif Manag Rev* 2019;61:5–14.
7. Rajkomar A, Dean J, Kohane I. Machine learning in medicine. *N Engl J Med* 2019;380:1347–1358.
8. Esteva A, Robicquet A, Ramsundar B, Kuleshov V, DePristo M, Chou K, Cui C, et al. A guide to deep learning in healthcare. *Nat Med* 2019;25:24–29.
9. LeCun Y, Bengio Y, Hinton G. Deep learning. *Nature* 2015;521:436–444.
10. Shen D, Wu G, Suk H-I. Deep learning in medical image analysis. *Ann Rev Biomed Eng* 2017;19:221–248.
11. Al-Askar H, Radi N, MacDermott A. Chapter 7 – Recurrent neural networks in medical data analysis and classifications. In: Al-Jumeily D, Hussain A, Mallucci C, Oliver C, eds. *Applied Computing in Medicine and Health*. Boston: Morgan Kaufmann, 2016; 147–165.
12. Bedogni G, Bellentani S, Miglioli L, Masutti F, Passalacqua M, Castiglione A, Tiribelli C. The Fatty Liver index: a simple and accurate predictor of hepatic steatosis in the general population. *BMC Gastroenterol* 2006;6:33.
13. Kotronen A, Peltonen M, Hakkarainen A, Sevastianova K, Bergholm R, Johansson LM, Lundbom N, et al. Prediction of non-alcoholic fatty liver disease and liver fat using metabolic and genetic factors. *Gastroenterology* 2009;137:865–872.
14. Sviklāne L, Olmane E, Dzērve Z, Kupčs K, Pīrāgs V, Sokolovska J. Fatty liver index and hepatic steatosis index for prediction of non-alcoholic fatty liver disease in type 1 diabetes. *J Gastroenterol Hepatol* 2018;33:270–276.
15. Poynard T, Ratziu V, Naveau S, Thabut D, Charlotte F, Messous D, Capron D, et al. The diagnostic value of biomarkers (SteatoTest) for the prediction of liver steatosis. *Comp Hepatol* 2005;4:10.
16. Bedogni G, Kahn HS, Bellentani S, Tiribelli C. A simple index of lipid overaccumulation is a good marker of liver steatosis. *BMC Gastroenterol* 2010;10:98.
17. Zhou YJ, Zhou YF, Zheng JN, Liu WY, Van Poucke S, Zou TT, Zhang DC, et al. NAFL screening score: a basic score identifying ultrasound-diagnosed non-alcoholic fatty liver. *Clin Chim Acta* 2017;475:44–50.
18. Yip TC, Ma AJ, Wong VW, Tse YK, Chan HL, Yuen PC, Wong GL. Laboratory parameter-based machine learning model for excluding non-alcoholic fatty liver disease (NAFLD) in the general population. *Aliment Pharmacol Ther* 2017;46:447–456.
19. Perveen S, Shahbaz M, Keshavjee K, Guergachi A. A systematic machine learning based approach for the diagnosis of Non-alcoholic fatty liver disease risk and progression. *Sci Rep* 2018;8:2112.
20. Ma H, Xu CF, Shen Z, Yu CH, Li YM. Application of machine learning techniques for clinical predictive modeling: a cross-sectional study on nonalcoholic fatty liver disease in China. *Biomed Res Int* 2018;2018:4304376.
21. Liu YX, Liu X, Cen C, Li X, Liu JM, Ming ZY, Yu SF, et al. Comparison and development of advanced machine learning tools to predict nonalcoholic fatty liver disease: an extended study. *Hepatobiliary Pancreat Dis Int* 2021;20:409–415.
22. Atsawarungruangkit A, Laoveeravat P, Promrat K. Machine learning models for predicting nonalcoholic fatty liver disease in the general United States population: NHANES database. *World J Hepatol* 2021;13:1417–1427.

23. Okanoue T, Shima T, Mitsumoto Y, Umemura A, Yamaguchi K, Itoh Y, Yoneda M, et al. Artificial intelligence/neural network system for the screening of nonalcoholic fatty liver disease and nonalcoholic steatohepatitis. *Hepatol Res* 2021;51:554–569.

24. Sorino P, Campanella A, Bonfiglio C, Mirizzi A, Franco I, Bianco A, Caruso MG, et al. Development and validation of a neural network for NAFLD diagnosis. *Sci Rep* 2021;11:20240.

25. Diehl AM, Day C. Cause, pathogenesis, and treatment of nonalcoholic steatohepatitis. *N Engl J Med* 2017;377:2063–2072.

26. Angulo P, Hui JM, Marchesini G, Bugianesi E, George J, Farrell GC, Enders F, et al. The NAFLD fibrosis score: a noninvasive system that identifies liver fibrosis in patients with NAFLD. *Hepatology* 2007;45:846–854.

27. Sterling RK, Lissen E, Clumeck N, Sola R, Correa MC, Montaner J, Sulkowski M, et al. Development of a simple noninvasive index to predict significant fibrosis in patients with HIV/HCV coinfection. *Hepatology* 2006;43:1317–1325.

28. Cheah MC, McCullough AJ, Goh GB. Current modalities of fibrosis assessment in non-alcoholic fatty liver disease. *J Clin Transl Hepatol* 2017;5:261–271.

29. Fialoke S, Malarstig A, Miller MR, Dumitriu A. Application of machine learning methods to predict non-alcoholic steatohepatitis (NASH) in non-alcoholic fatty liver (NAFL) patients. *AMIA Annu Symp Proc* 2018;2018:430–439.

30. Docherty M, Regnier SA, Capkun G, Balp MM, Ye Q, Janssens N, Tietz A, et al. Development of a novel machine learning model to predict presence of nonalcoholic steatohepatitis. *J Am Med Inform Assoc* 2021;28:1235–1241.

31. García-Carretero R, Holgado-Cuadrado R, Barquero-Pérez Ó. Assessment of classification models and relevant features on nonalcoholic steatohepatitis using random forest. *Entropy (Basel)* 2021;23.

32. Feng G, Zheng KI, Li YY, Rios RS, Zhu PW, Pan XY, Li G, et al. Machine learning algorithm outperforms fibrosis markers in predicting significant fibrosis in biopsy-confirmed NAFLD. *J Hepatobiliary Pancreat Sci* 2021;28:593–603.

33. Aggarwal M, Rozenbaum D, Bansal A, Garg R, Bansal P, McCullough A. Development of machine learning model to detect fibrotic non-alcoholic steatohepatitis in patients with non-alcoholic fatty liver disease. *Digestive and Liver Disease* 2021;53:1669–1672.

34. Chiappini F, Coilly A, Kadar H, Gual P, Tran A, Desterke C, Samuel D, et al. Metabolism dysregulation induces a specific lipid signature of nonalcoholic steatohepatitis in patients. *Sci Rep* 2017;7:46658.

35. Perakakis N, Polyzos SA, Yazdani A, Sala-Vila A, Kountouras J, Anastasilakis AD, Mantzoros CS. Non-invasive diagnosis of non-alcoholic steatohepatitis and fibrosis with the use of omics and supervised learning: a proof of concept study. *Metabolism* 2019;101:154005.

36. Masarone M, Troisi J, Aglitti A, Torre P, Colucci A, Dallio M, Federico A, et al. Untargeted metabolomics as a diagnostic tool in NAFLD: discrimination of steatosis, steatohepatitis and cirrhosis. *Metabolomics* 2021;17:12.

37. Hou W, Janech MG, Sobolesky PM, Bland AM, Samsuddin S, Alazawi W, Syn WK. Proteomic screening of plasma identifies potential noninvasive biomarkers associated with significant/advanced fibrosis in patients with nonalcoholic fatty liver disease. *Biosci Rep* 2020;40.

38. Luo Y, Wadhawan S, Greenfield A, Decato BE, Oseini AM, Collen R, Shevell DE, et al. SOMAscan proteomics identifies serum biomarkers associated with liver fibrosis in patients with NASH. *Hepatol Commun* 2021;5:760–773.

39. Wood GC, Chu X, Argyropoulos G, Benotti P, Rolston D, Mirshahi T, Petrick A, et al. A multi-component classifier for nonalcoholic fatty liver disease (NAFLD) based on genomic, proteomic, and phenomic data domains. *Sci Rep* 2017;7:43238.

40. Atabaki-Pasdar N, Ohlsson M, Viñuela A, Frau F, Pomares-Millan H, Haid M, Jones AG, et al. Predicting and elucidating the etiology of fatty liver disease: a machine learning modeling and validation study in the IMI DIRECT cohorts. *PLoS Med* 2020;17:e1003149.

41. Lewinska M, Santos-Laso A, Arretxe E, Alonso C, Zhuravleva E, Jimenez-Agüero R, Eizaguirre E, et al. The altered serum lipidome and its diagnostic potential for Non-Alcoholic Fatty Liver (NAFL)-associated hepatocellular carcinoma. *EBioMedicine* 2021;73:103661.

42. Han A, Byra M, Heba E, Andre MP, Erdman JW, Jr., Loomba R, Sirlin CB, et al. Noninvasive diagnosis of nonalcoholic fatty liver disease and quantification of liver fat with radiofrequency ultrasound data using one-dimensional convolutional neural networks. *Radiology* 2020;295:342–350.

43. Byra M, Han A, Boehringer AS, Zhang YN, O'Brien WD, Jr., Erdman JW, Jr., Loomba R, et al. Liver fat assessment in multiview sonography using transfer learning with convolutional neural networks. *J Ultrasound Med* 2022;41:175–184.

44. Cao W, An X, Cong L, Lyu C, Zhou Q, Guo R. Application of deep learning in quantitative analysis of 2-dimensional ultrasound imaging of nonalcoholic fatty liver disease. *J Ultrasound Med* 2020;39:51–59.

45. Starekova J, Hernando D, Pickhardt PJ, Reeder SB. Quantification of liver fat content with CT and MRI: state of the Art. *Radiology* 2021;301:250–262.

46. Graffy PM, Sandfort V, Summers RM, Pickhardt PJ. Automated liver fat quantification at nonenhanced abdominal CT for population-based steatosis assessment. *Radiology* 2019;293:334–342.

47. Wang K, Mamidipalli A, Retson T, Bahrami N, Hasenstab K, Blansit K, Bass E, et al. Automated CT and MRI liver segmentation and biometry using a generalized convolutional neural network. *Radiol: Artif Intell* 2019;1:180022.

48. Jirapatnakul A, Reeves AP, Lewis S, Chen X, Ma T, Yip R, Chin X, et al. Automated measurement of liver attenuation to identify moderate-to-severe hepatic steatosis from chest CT scans. *Eur J Radiol* 2020;122:108723.

49. Schreiner AD, Livingston S, Zhang J, Gebregziabher M, Marsden J, Koch DG, Petz CA, et al. Identifying patients at risk for fibrosis in a primary care NAFLD cohort. *J Clin Gastroenterol* 2023;57(1):89–96.

50. Goldshtein I, Chodick G, Kochba I, Gal N, Webb M, Shibolet O. Identification and characterization of non-alcoholic fatty liver disease. *Clin Gastroenterol Hepatol* 2020;18:1887–1889.

51. Chalasani N, Younossi Z, Lavine JE, Charlton M, Cusi K, Rinella M, Harrison SA, et al. The diagnosis and management of nonalcoholic fatty liver disease: practice guidance from the American Association for the Study of Liver Diseases. *Hepatology* 2018;67:328–357.

52. Theodossi A, Skene AM, Portmann B, Knill-Jones RP, Patrick RS, Tate RA, Kealey W, et al. Observer variation in assessment of liver biopsies including analysis by kappa statistics. *Gastroenterology* 1980;79:232–241.

53. Gawrieh S, Knoedler DM, Saeian K, Wallace JR, Komorowski RA. Effects of interventions on intra- and interobserver agreement on interpretation of nonalcoholic fatty liver disease histology. *Ann Diagn Pathol* 2011;15:19–24.

54. Vanderbeck S, Bockhorst J, Komorowski R, Kleiner DE, Gawrieh S. Automatic classification of white regions in liver biopsies by supervised machine learning. *Hum Pathol* 2014;45:785–792.

55. Vanderbeck S, Bockhorst J, Kleiner D, Komorowski R, Chalasani N, Gawrieh S. Automatic quantification of lobular inflammation and hepatocyte ballooning in nonalcoholic fatty liver disease liver biopsies. *Hum Pathol* 2015;46:767–775.

56. Gawrieh S, Sethunath D, Cummings OW, Kleiner DE, Vuppalanchi R, Chalasani N, Tuceryan M. Automated quantification and architectural pattern detection of hepatic fibrosis in NAFLD. *Ann Diag Pathol* 2020;47:151518.

57. Forlano R, Mullish BH, Giannakeas N, Maurice JB, Angkathunyakul N, Lloyd J, Tzallas AT, et al. High-throughput, machine learning-based quantification of steatosis, inflammation, ballooning, and fibrosis in biopsies from patients with nonalcoholic fatty liver disease. *Clin Gastroenterol Hepatol* 2020;18:2081–2090.e2089.

58. Taylor-Weiner A, Pokkalla H, Han L, Jia C, Huss R, Chung C, Elliott H, et al. A machine learning approach enables quantitative measurement of liver histology and disease monitoring in NASH. *Hepatology* 2021;74:133–147.

59. Arjmand A, Angelis CT, Christou V, Tzallas AT, Tsipouras MG, Glavas E, Forlano R, et al. Training of deep convolutional neural networks to identify critical liver alterations in histopathology image samples. *Appl Sci* 2020;10.

60. Roy M, Wang F, Vo H, Teng D, Teodoro G, Farris AB, Castillo-Leon E, et al. Deep-learning-based accurate hepatic steatosis quantification for histological assessment of liver biopsies. *Lab Invest* 2020;100:1367–1383.

61. Salvi M, Molinaro L, Metovic J, Patrono D, Romagnoli R, Papotti M, Molinari F. Fully automated quantitative assessment of hepatic steatosis in liver transplants. *Comput Biol Med* 2020;123:103836.

62. Brunt EM, Clouston AD, Goodman Z, Guy C, Kleiner DE, Lackner C, Tiniakos DG, et al. Complexity of ballooned hepatocyte feature recognition: defining a training atlas for artificial intelligence-based imaging in NAFLD. *J Hepatol* 2022.

63. Van Vleck TT, Chan L, Coca SG, Craven CK, Do R, Ellis SB, Kannry JL, et al. Augmented intelligence with natural language processing applied to electronic health records for identifying patients with non-alcoholic fatty liver disease at risk for disease progression. *Int J Med Inform* 2019;129:334–341.

64. Bosch J, Chung C, Carrasco-Zevallos OM, Harrison SA, Abdelmalek MF, Shiffman ML, Rockey DC, et al. A Machine learning approach to liver histological evaluation predicts clinically significant portal hypertension in NASH cirrhosis. *Hepatology* 2021;74:3146–3160.

65. Gianfrancesco MA, Tamang S, Yazdany J, Schmajuk G. Potential biases in machine learning algorithms using electronic health record data. *JAMA Int Med* 2018;178:1544–1547.

66. Cutillo CM, Sharma KR, Foschini L, Kundu S, Mackintosh M, Mandl KD. Machine intelligence in healthcare-perspectives on trustworthiness, explainability, usability, and transparency. *NPJ Digit Med* 2020;3:47.

67. Ghassemi M, Oakden-Rayner L, Beam AL. The false hope of current approaches to explainable artificial intelligence in health care. *Lancet Digit Health* 2021;3:e745–e750.

SECTION III
MANAGEMENT

10 Dietary Interventions

Monica Tincopa

CONTENTS

Key Points

- Healthy nutrition is a key component of the management and treatment of nonalcoholic fatty liver disease (NAFLD) and nonalcoholic steatohepatitis (NASH). The comparative effectiveness of different dietary patterns to resolve different histologic components of NAFLD/NASH remains unclear due to limitations in study design and available data.

- Current society guidelines focus on reduction in total calorie restriction/day (500–1000 kcal/day) targeted toward total body weight reduction (7–10%) to direct nutritional guidance in NAFLD/NASH.

- Emerging data have highlighted the importance of the composition of macro- and micronutrients on the impact of hepatic steatosis and metabolic health irrespective of weight loss. Reduction of refined carbohydrates (in particular high-fructose corn syrup), trans- and saturated fats and red and processed meats and increased amounts of omega-3 fatty acids, monounsaturated fats and plant-based proteins have beneficial associations with NAFLD specific outcomes.

- A growing body of evidence has supported the use of a Mediterranean Diet specifically in NAFLD given its associations with reduction in intrahepatic triglycerides and beneficial cardiovascular outcomes.

- A key component to any nutritional plan must take into account individual nutritional preferences and feasibility of implementing nutritional changes in order to optimize effectiveness and long-term sustainability.

10.1 INTRODUCTION

Nutrition is a key component of management of nonalcoholic fatty liver disease NAFLD) and nonalcoholic steatohepatitis (NASH) given the underlying pathophysiology of the condition. The average diet consumed by adults in the United States (US) consists of high amounts of refined and high glycemic index (GI) carbohydrates (CHO), red and processed meats and fructose including high-fructose corn syrup (HFCS). The average diet is also low in beneficial nutrients like polyunsaturated fatty acids (PUFA),

monounsaturated fatty acids (MUFA) and plant-based proteins. Longitudinal studies have demonstrated that improvements in macro- and micronutrients are associated with histologic improvement of NAFLD and NASH. These benefits have been seen even in the absence of weight loss and without concomitant exercise. There have been conflicting data regarding the comparative effectiveness of different diets for patients with NAFLD/NASH, though there is strong epidemiologic data outlining the association between macro- and micronutrient intake and the prevalence of NAFLD. Difficulty in outlining evidence-based guidelines for nutrition in NAFLD stems from the limitations and biases of existing data of clinical trials evaluating nutritional interventions in NAFLD and NASH. Many of the existing studies have small sample sizes and are nonrandomized or noncontrolled trials. There is also significant heterogeneity in inclusion and exclusion criteria, assessment of adherence to the dietary intervention, outcomes assessed and method of outcome assessment. Lastly, there is a paucity of randomized controlled trials (RCTs) with head-to-head comparisons of different diets on hepatic outcomes. In this chapter, we have focused on data from studies specifically enrolling NAFLD/NASH patients that include a dietary-only intervention in order to optimally evaluate the isolated impact of nutrition on hepatic outcomes. Studies evaluating the association of nutrition with NAFLD focus either on total energy consumption/calories per day, specific intake of macro- and micronutrients or different "diets." We highlight the evidence in support of beneficial or adverse effects of these nutritional patterns and outline the areas where there is currently a paucity of data to draw meaningful conclusions to direct clinical care.

10.2 MACRONUTRIENTS

There is a strong body of evidence documenting the importance of intake of specific types of both macro- and micronutrients in NAFLD. In general, effective dietary assessments focus on not only the breakdown of carbohydrate intake, protein intake and percentage of fats but the specific subtypes within each category in order to direct effective individualized nutritional recommendations. The recommended dietary allowances (RDA) provide a

DOI: 10.1201/9781003386698-13

Table 10.1: Macro- and Micronutrients and Their Associated Impact on NAFLD

CHO		Fats		Protein		Other	
+	−	+	−	+	−	+	−
Whole	Refined	UFA	TFA	Plant-based	Red meats	Black coffee	Heavy ETOH
	HFCS		SFA	Poultry	Processed meats		
				Fish			

Table 10.2: Dietary Patterns Evaluated as Treatment for NAFLD

Type	Calorie/Energy Restriction	Low CHO	Low Fat	MD	DASH	IF
Definition	500–1,000 kcal/d deficit	<40% or 130 g CHO/day	<30% fat/d	40% CHO, 40% fats (MUFA and omega-3 FA), lean plant-based proteins	Daily servings: —Grains: 6–8 —Meats/poultry/ fish: </= 6 —Vegetables: 4–5 —Fruit:4–5 —LF dairy: 2–3 —Fats/oils: 2–3 —Sodium: 2,300 mg —Nuts/seeds/ beans/peas: 4–5 —Sweets: 5 or less	TRF: Restrict to one 6–8 hour period/day ADF: Limit to one 500–600 calorie meal/ day alternating with baseline diet
Recommendations	Personalized calculation of daily energy requirements with relative reduction	Remove HFCS, refined CHO and high GI foods. Replace CHO with lean protein (plant based, fish/ poultry) PUFA, MUFA.	Remove trans-FA and SFA. Replace fats with lean protein (plant based, fish/poultry), low GI and unrefined CHO.	As above	Remove SFA, SSB and refined sugars. Replace with vegetables, fruits and whole grains, fat-free or low-fat dairy, lean protein (fish and poultry) and plant based protein (beans, nuts, vegetable oils).	As above
Studies showing benefit in NAFLD/ NASH	Fontana (30) Haufe (31) Kirk (32) Elias (33) Arefhosseini (34) Vilar-Gomez (35) Viljanen (36)	Jang (9) Browning (11) Tendler (13)	Ahn (10) Properzi (46)	Misciagna (42) Katsagoni (43) Trovato (44) Abenavoli (45) Ryan (47)	Razavi (51)	Johari (52) Cai (53)

frame of reference for levels of intake of essential nutrients that are judged to be adequate to provide the nutritional needs of healthy adults. (1) Above is a summary of the key subtypes of each macronutrient and the association with these subtypes and development or resolution of NAFLD and NASH (Tables 10.1 and 10.2).

10.2.1 Carbohydrates

When assessing nutritional intake, it is critical to evaluate not only total percentage or grams of each macronutrient but the proportion of subtype of each macronutrient as there are differential impacts on hepatic steatosis, inflammation and fibrosis based on what subtype comprises the overall intake. Categorizing a diet as "high CHO" vs. "low CHO" alone is insufficient to meaningfully assess the benefit on liver health. Carbohydrates (CHO) are categorized as simple or complex and whole vs. refined. A CHO is categorized as simple vs. complex based on its chemical structure and how quickly it is digested or absorbed. Simple CHO include monosaccharides (glucose, fructose, galactose) and disaccharides (sucrose, lactose, maltose and cellobiose). Simple CHO are quickly digested and therefore result in a quick but short-lasting burst of energy. Refined CHO are processed to remove protein, fat-rich germ and fiber-rich bran and thus do not provide valuable micronutrients but add to calories. Refined sugars can be found in white rice, bread, sweets, cereals and sugary drinks. Simple CHO can also be naturally found in nutritious foods like fruit and dairy. As unprocessed CHO, these types of simple sugars do provide vitamins, minerals and fiber. Individual foods can be categorized according to their GI which indicates how quickly and by how much that food can cause increases in blood sugar. Low-GI foods release glucose slowly, whereas high-GI foods provide a rapid burst of glucose. Complex CHO are digested more slowly and thus often make individuals feel full longer.

Whole grain, fiber, legumes and starchy vegetables are some examples of complex CHO. Similar to simple CHO, refined complex CHO have less nutritional value due to the processing.

There is no standard definition for a "low CHO" (LC) diet, which makes the interpretation of dietary interventions challenging. The RDA for CHO is set at 130 g/day for adults, though the estimated median intake for men is 220–330 g/day and 180–230 g/day for women. (1) On average, most LC diets have 40–60 g of CHO/day and comprise <40% of daily calories compared to a standard US diet that typically has 45–65% of calories from CHO. The percentage of CHO included across diets categorized as "low CHO" varies considerably, however. Many LC diets consist of only 10–25% of calories from CHO a day. Ketogenic diets (KD) restrict only 5–10% of calories/day from CHO, with 15–30% from protein and 70–80% from fat.

High CHO intake, particularly sucrose and fructose, has been shown to promote de novo lipogenesis. (2) Individuals with excess CHO intake develop significant increases in hepatic steatosis and serum triglyceride (TG) levels. (3) These impacts have been shown to occur even in the absence of total body weight gain. HFCS in particular has a significant association with development of hepatic steatosis and in some studies also with hepatic fibrosis. (4) A cross-sectional study of 427 individuals with biopsy-proven NAFLD demonstrated that >/=7 sugar-sweetened beverages (SSB)/week was associated with significantly higher fibrosis and inflammation when controlling for age, body mass index (BMI) and total calorie intake. (4) HFCS is commonly found in regular sodas, sweetened juices, processed desserts, prepackaged meals, breads and pastas and many fast food items. Pathophysiologically HFCS promotes visceral adiposity, insulin resistance and hepatic inflammation. The impact of processed and high-fructose foods is thought to potentially be mediated through advanced glycation end products (AGEs). High levels of AGEs have been linked to NASH (compared to NAFLD) and insulin resistance. Soluble receptors of AGEs (sRAGE) prevent the binding of AGEs, and levels of sRAGE have been inversely correlated to amount of liver fat. (5,6). Several studies have not found the same association of diet soda with increased liver fat, though there remains ongoing controversy about the overall health benefits/harms to diet sodas and artificial sweeteners. (7,8)

The comparative effectiveness of a low-CHO diet is difficult to discern given available data and study heterogeneity. When compared to a low-fat (LF) diet, several studies have shown more pronounced reduction in hepatic steatosis with a low-CHO diet. A study by Jang et al. evaluated 106 NAFLD patients and randomized them to 8 weeks of either a low-CHO (25 kcal/kg ideal body weight; 50–60% CHO, 20–25% protein, 20–25% fats) or LF (25 kcal/kg ideal body weight; 60–70% CHO, 15–20% protein, 15–20% fats) and found that the low-CHO diet was more effective in reducing intrahepatic fat accumulation (0.85 vs. 0.92 liver/spleen, p <0.05). (9) In contrast, a meta-analysis of 11 clinical trials assessing the impact of a low-CHO vs. LF diet, there was not a statistically significant difference in improvement in hepatic fat content between low-CHO and LF or low-calorie (LC) diets in NAFLD. (10) There are similarly conflicting data regarding the comparative effectiveness of a low-CHO vs. calorie-restricted diet in NAFLD. A small study by Browning et al. had individuals with NAFLD follow a low-CHO (<20 g/day)

or calorie-restricted (1,200–1,500 kcal/day with 50% CHO, 34% fat and 16% protein) diet for 2 weeks. Intrahepatic TG significantly decreased by magnetic resonance spectroscopy (MRS) in both groups, but there was a more pronounced reduction in the low-CHO group (−55% +/−14% vs. −28% +/−23%).(11) This enhanced reduction in hepatic steatosis of a low-CHO diet to a calorie-restricted diet (5:2 diet with 2 days limited to 500 kcal/day for women and 600 kcal/day men with 5 days of 2,000 or 2,400 kcal/day, respectively) was not seen in a 12-week study of 74 patients with NAFLD. Liver stiffness did improve in the calorie-restricted diet, however. (12)

Ketogenic diets (KD) require significant restriction of CHO (<20 g CHO/day) and traditionally have unrestricted fat and total calorie intake and a relative increase in protein (0.8–1.2 g/kg/day). There have been concerns regarding the impact of a KD on NAFLD given the increased fat content in this diet. Despite this, several studies have shown improvement in the amount of hepatic steatosis. Tendler et al. evaluated the impact of a KD (<20 g CHO/day) for 6 months among 5 patients with biopsy-proven NAFLD and showed histologic improvement in steatosis and inflammatory grade. (13) A 2-week study of a HFKD among 18 NAFLD patients with obesity also demonstrated an improvement in hepatic steatosis via MRS. (11) KD can be very challenging for individuals to implement and maintain in the long term, making this option less feasible for many patients.

10.2.2 Fats

The nutritional value of fats is heavily weighted by subtype. Trans-fatty acids (TFA) do not provide nutritional value, and individuals should be counseled to remove TFA from their diet. TFA are commonly found in fast and fried food, cakes and pastries. Most commonly this is found in hydrogenated vegetable oil that is used to create longer shelf life or certain consistency. TFA are also found in ruminant animal fat. The Food and Drug Administration (FDA) has required that TFA be phased out of foods. Saturated fatty acids (SFA) also do not add nutritional value to diets, and the recommendation is to limit SFA to <7% of total daily calorie as they have been linked to heart disease risk and weight gain. They predominantly come from animal sources and are commonly found in high-fat cheeses, cuts of meat, butter, whole-fat dairy products and tropical oils. Unsaturated fatty acids (UFA) have the most nutritional value and are usually plant based and come in the form of liquid oils and nuts.

When evaluating the impact of high or LF diets in NAFLD, it is important to consider what subtype of fat is being consumed as they have differential impacts on propensity for hepatic steatosis and visceral adiposity, though overall weight gain may not be significantly different. Within the different subtypes of PUFA, omega-3 appears to be more beneficial than omega-6 in relation to development of hepatic steatosis. (14, 15) Diets enriched in omega-3 PUFA also appear to improve insulin sensitivity. (16, 17) In studies evaluating patients with NASH and normal BMI, compared to age, sex and BMI matched controls, NASH patients had higher intake of saturated fat and cholesterol and low intake of PUFA. (18,19) In another study, 39 normal weight individuals were overfed SFA or omega-6 PUFA, and those in the SFA had markedly increased steatosis and a 2 times larger increase in visceral fat compared to the PUFA arm. (20) A number of studies have evaluated whether using omega-3 supplements have a beneficial effect on hepatic steatosis, though results have been conflicting and hard to compare given variations in study design. (21)

There is not a set RDA for total fat, given the lack of sufficient data to identify what level of fat intake is associated with prevention of disease or risk of inadequate intake. The acceptable macronutrient distribution range (AMDR) for total fat is 20–35% of total daily energy intake. (1) LF diets generally consist of <30% of calories coming from fat. For comparison, the average diet of adults in the United States has approximately 35–40% of calories from fat. The comparative effectiveness of LF vs. Low-CHO diets is summarized in the preceding CHO section.

10.2.3 Proteins

The RDA of high-quality protein (with an emphasis on plant-based protein) is 0.8 g/kg body weight per day. The upper range for total protein in the diet is 35% to decrease risk of chronic disease. (1) To date, little data have been generated evaluating the impact of varying amounts and sources of protein as a primary treatment for NAFLD. A study of 48 patients with NAFLD who underwent a 75-day trial of a hypocaloric high-protein diet (1,299 kcal/d women, 1,400kcal/day men 25% fat, 35% protein, 40% CHO) demonstrated improvement in lipid profile and liver enzymes. (22) The source rather than the percentage of protein appears to be most important in impacting hepatic outcomes. Proteins from animal sources tend to be of higher fat and are associated with a higher risk of diabetes and cardiac disease. (23) Several studies have highlighted the relationship between high consumption of red and processed meats and NAFLD. (24, 25) This association is thought to be related to higher SFA and cholesterol in these items. In addition, cooking methods to prepare these foods are associated with the formation of heterocyclic amines (HCA) that have been linked to certain types of cancer and increased oxidative stress. In contrast, protein sources from plants, low-fat dairy, poultry, fish and nuts have favorable associations with weight loss, lower cardiovascular risk, as well as reductions in liver enzymes and hepatic steatosis. (26)

10.3 TOTAL CALORIES/ENERGY RESTRICTION

Excess calorie consumption has been strongly linked with prevalence of obesity and its associated metabolic conditions. (27) The American Association for the Study of Liver Diseases (AASLD) guidelines and the European Association for the Study of the Liver (EASL) recommend a hypocaloric diet, specifically a daily reduction by 500–1,000 kcal a day as part of a lifestyle intervention for NAFLD/NASH. (28, 29) Calorie restriction has been associated with mobilization of hepatic fat. (30) Studies have been most supportive of a reduction in total daily caloric intake by at least 30% or approximately 750–1,000 kcal/day to see a reduction in the amount of hepatic steatosis. (31–33) Even at less dramatic reductions of total calories for a short duration (500 kcal/day for 6 weeks), reductions in the amount of hepatic steatosis were noted by ultrasound. (34)

A paired biopsy study of 261 patients with biopsy-proven NASH who followed a 750-kcal/day diet noted a dose response relationship between weight loss and improvement in liver biopsy findings over the course of one year. (35) Of note, participants in this study were also counseled to walk 200 minutes/week. A very-low-calorie diet (550 kcal/day with 50% CHO, 7% fat, 43% protein) over 7 weeks in 34 individuals (only 50% of whom had NAFLD) noted an 11% reduction in body weight and 60% reduction in intrahepatic TG. (36)

10.4 OTHER DIETS

10.4.1 Mediterranean Diet

A Mediterranean diet (MD) consists of a large proportion of minimally processed plant-based food rich in monounsaturated fat (like olive oil) and low in saturated fats, meats and dairy. Lean proteins, like seafood and poultry, are included in moderation. Importantly, there is a reduced carbohydrate intake (only 40%), particularly refined sugars. Fats consist of 40% of the calories, with composition to be focused on monounsaturated and omega-3 fatty acids. Of note, many standard MD plans recommend consumption of wine as part of the regular diet, and therefore this caveat requires attention in patients with liver disease, particularly those with advanced fibrosis and cirrhosis. (37) Complete abstinence is recommended for all patients with cirrhosis. Alcohol consumption in NASH cirrhosis has been associated with a higher risk of hepatocellular carcinoma (HCC). There is conflicting data regarding whether moderate amounts of alcohol consumption (30 g in men and 20 g in women), wine in particular, may confer any protective effect in NAFLD and NASH among individuals without cirrhosis. (38, 39) The MD differs from a paleo diet in the percentage of fat (35% paleo vs. 40% MD) and percentage of carbohydrates (45–65% in paleo vs. 40% in MD). The paleo diet also has a decreased intake of grains. Data is lacking to specifically evaluate the impact of a paleo diet on NAFLD.

There is strong evidence in support of an MD to promote cardiovascular health. A meta-analysis of 45 prospective studies concluded that adherence to an MD is associated with clinically meaningfully reductions in rates of coronary heart disease, ischemic stroke and total cardiovascular disease. (40) A number of recent studies have evaluated the impact of an MD on NAFLD, which lead to the EASL clinical practice guidelines recommending a Mediterranean-based diet for NAFLD. (29,41) An RCT of 98 individuals with NAFLD given a low-GI MD compared to a control diet over 6 months noted a significant negative interaction between time and the low-GI MD and NAFLD score on ultrasound. (42) Similar findings were noted in an RCT of 63 patients with NAFLD who were randomized to a usual diet, MD or MD with exercise and sleep counseling over 6 months. The MD group showed significant improvement in liver stiffness assessed via shear-wave elastography compared to the control diet. (43) A single arm study of 90 NAFLD patients following an MD for 6 months noted a significant decrease in steatosis, as did an RCT of 50 overweight patients with NAFLD randomized to control or MD for 6 months. (44,45)

The comparative effectiveness of the MD compared to low-CHO and LF diets have also been studied. An RCT compared an ad libitum MD to a LF diet among 56 individuals with NAFLD over 12 weeks and compared the amount of hepatic steatosis via MRS. Individuals in both groups had significant reductions in hepatic steatosis with minimal weight loss. Adherence was higher among the MD compared to LF diets. (46) The impact of an MD on hepatic steatosis and insulin resistance was evaluated compared to a LF/high-CHO diet among 12 individuals without diabetes. All subjects followed a control diet, MD and LF/HC diet in random order with 6-week washout periods. Hepatic steatosis was evaluated via MRS and insulin sensitivity via clamp study. This study found that even in the absence of weight loss, there was a significant relative reduction in hepatic steatosis after the MD compared to the LF/HC diet. Insulin sensitivity also improved with the MD but not in the LF/HC diet. (47) An RCT of 45 adults with type 2 diabetes randomized to 8 weeks of a LF/high-CHO vs. a diet high in MUFA as used in the MD noted clinically relevant reduction in hepatic fat content (25–29% vs. 4–6%) independently of exercise. (48)

A subtype of the MD was developed by Marin-Alejandre, the Fatty Liver in Obesity (FLiO) Diet. The FLiO diet was compared to an American Heart Association (AHA) diet among 98 NAFLD patients who were overweight or obese over 26 weeks. The FLiO diet consisted of 7 meals/day with 40–45% CHO with low GI, 25% protein primarily from vegetable sources and 30–35% lipids overall. The AHA diet consisted of 3–5 meals per day with 50–55% CHO, 15% protein and 30% lipids. No significant differences between group findings were noted, though there were significant reductions in weight (–10.1% vs. –9.7%), TG and steatosis within each group. (49)

10.4.2 DASH DIET

There are limited data available to assess the impact of the Dietary Approaches to Stop Hypertension (DASH) diet as treatment for NAFLD. A cross-sectional study of 11,888 participants noted an inverse correlation between adherence to a DASH diet and risk of NAFLD. (50) Razavi et al. compared the effect of the DASH diet to a calorie-restricted diet with 52–55% CHO, 16–18% proteins and 30% total fat. Individuals on the DASH diet lost 3.8 +/–2.2 kg compared to 2.3 +/–1.7 kg, and those in the intervention arm had significant improvements in alanine aminotransferase (ALT) and TG. (51)

10.4.3 Intermittent Fasting

There have been a limited number of studies evaluating the impact of varying forms of intermittent fasting (IF) as a treatment for NAFLD. Johari et al. evaluated the impact of modified alternate day calorie restriction (MADCR), a form of IF, compared to usual dietary patterns among 43 patients with NAFLD. Over 8 weeks, participants restricted 70% of their baseline calories and consumed meals only between 2 and 8 p.m. on fasting days, alternating with normal ad libitum diet on the other days. Individuals in the MADCR group had a mean reduction of 3.06 (1.14–4.63) kg and also had significant reduction in steatosis and fibrosis scores using two-dimensional shear wave elastography (SWE). (52) IF in the form of alternate day fasting (ADF) and time-restricted feeding (TRF) were compared to the usual diet among 271 patients over 12 weeks among patients with NAFLD. The ADF group had a fasting day with 25% of baseline energy needs alternating with baseline diet. TRF group had meals restricted to an 8-hour window, and the control group had a calorie-restricted diet with 80% of energy needs. In this study, there were no significant improvements between groups, though there were within-group pre-/post improvements in weight and fat mass. (53)

The timing of calorie intake, aside from IF, has been shown to impact hepatic steatosis. A study of 46 lean men randomized to either a eucaloric or 40% hypercaloric (high-fat, high-sugar or high-sugar only) diet for 6 weeks. The excess calories were consumed either with 3 main meals or between meals. While all types of hypercaloric diets increased BMI, the increased meal frequency significantly increased intrahepatic fat compared to increased meal size, suggesting that not only total calories but timing of calories impact hepatic fat deposition. (54)

10.5 OTHER DIETARY ASSOCIATIONS

Coffee consumption has been associated with protective effects in liver disease. There appears to be an inverse relationship with coffee consumption and hepatic fibrosis, though the data regarding the relationship to steatosis is conflicting. (55,56) These effects were seen with both caffeinated and decaffeinated coffee. Importantly, much of the data focused on studies of black coffee, and it is important to highlight this, as many times coffee is consumed with high-calorie components like dairy and sugar.

10.6 CAVEATS FOR NUTRITION IN NASH CIRRHOSIS

Individuals with NASH and cirrhosis have unique nutritional needs compared to individuals without cirrhosis, though an extended discussion about nutrition in cirrhosis is beyond the scope of this chapter. Key differences in cirrhosis include the presence of protein calorie malnutrition and sarcopenia and the potential for volume overload and thus attention to salt and fluid intake. (57) Protein intake is a key area of focus given that cirrhosis is associated with muscle wasting and creates a protein-deficient state. In general, 1.0–1.5 g/kg of protein is recommended. A high protein bedtime snack has also been shown to be beneficial given that muscle breakdown is pronounced while in the fasting state during sleep. (58) Individuals with ascites and or hyponatremia also require management of sodium intake (2 g/d) and fluid (1.5 L/day) if serum sodium </=125 mmol/L. (59)

10.7 CONCLUSION/SUMMARY POINTS

Until the advent of adjunctive pharmacotherapy for the treatment of NAFLD and NASH, healthy nutrition will remain the key component of management. Healthy nutrition plays a critical role in reducing hepatic steatosis and promoting overall metabolic health given the direct role that the intake of different macro- and micronutrients has in the pathophysiology of this condition. In addition, nutrition accounts for approximately 80–90% of weight loss. (60) Clinical guidelines recommend a reduction in total energy/calorie intake targeted toward reduction in total body weight as these reductions have been shown to have a dose response in relation to improvements in histologic outcomes in NASH. Diets that minimize intake in trans- and SFA, refined/processed CHO (in particular HFCS) and animal-based proteins have been efficacious in reducing hepatic steatosis even in the absence of weight loss. Dietary plans with a heavy focus on MUFA and PUFA, low CHO and lean plant-based proteins, such as the MD, represent ideal options for individuals with NAFLD and NASH (Figure 10.1). Future studies will add to our understanding of the comparative effectiveness of total calorie reduction, different balances of micro- and macronutrients, and the timing of nutrient consumption.

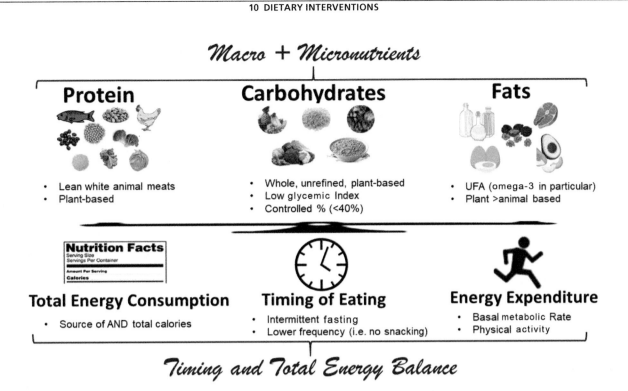

Figure 10.1 Relevant Factors When Assessing Impact of Diet in NAFLD/NASH

REFERENCES

1. National Research Council Subcommittee on the Tenth Edition of the Recommended Dietary A. *The National Academies Collection: Reports funded by National Institutes of Health*. Recommended Dietary Allowances: 10th Edition. Washington, DC: National Academies Press (US) Copyright © 1989 by the National Academy of Sciences; 1989.
2. Poulsom R. Morphological changes of organs after sucrose or fructose feeding. *Prog Biochem Pharmacol*. 1986;21:104–134.
3. Sevastianova K, Santos A, Kotronen A, Hakkarainen A, Makkonen J, Silander K, et al. Effect of short-term carbohydrate overfeeding and long-term weight loss on liver fat in overweight humans. *Am J Clin Nutr*. 2012;96(4):727–734.
4. Abdelmalek MF, Suzuki A, Guy C, Unalp-Arida A, Colvin R, Johnson RJ, et al. Increased fructose consumption is associated with fibrosis severity in patients with nonalcoholic fatty liver disease. *Hepatology*. 2010;51(6):1961–1971.
5. Hyogo H, Yamagishi S, Iwamoto K, Arihiro K, Takeuchi M, Sato T, et al. Elevated levels of serum advanced glycation end products in patients with non-alcoholic steatohepatitis. *J Gastroenterol Hepatol*. 2007;22(7):1112–1119.
6. Zelber-Sagi S, Salomone F, Kolodkin-Gal I, Erez N, Buch A, Yeshua H, et al. Protective role of soluble receptor for advanced glycation end-products in patients with non-alcoholic fatty liver disease. *Dig Liver Dis*. 2017;49(5):523–529.
7. Ma J, Fox CS, Jacques PF, Speliotes EK, Hoffmann U, Smith CE, et al. Sugar-sweetened beverage, diet soda, and fatty liver disease in the Framingham Heart Study cohorts. *J Hepatol*. 2015;63(2):462–469.

8. Maersk M, Belza A, Stødkilde-Jørgensen H, Ringgaard S, Chabanova E, Thomsen H, et al. Sucrose-sweetened beverages increase fat storage in the liver, muscle, and visceral fat depot: a 6-mo randomized intervention study. *Am J Clin Nutr*. 2012;95(2):283–289.
9. Jang EC, Jun DW, Lee SM, Cho YK, Ahn SB. Comparison of efficacy of low-carbohydrate and low-fat diet education programs in non-alcoholic fatty liver disease: a randomized controlled study. *Hepatol Res*. 2018;48(3):E22–E9.
10. Ahn J, Jun DW, Lee HY, Moon JH. Critical appraisal for low-carbohydrate diet in nonalcoholic fatty liver disease: review and meta-analyses. *Clin Nutr*. 2019;38(5):2023–2030.
11. Browning JD, Baker JA, Rogers T, Davis J, Satapati S, Burgess SC. Short-term weight loss and hepatic triglyceride reduction: evidence of a metabolic advantage with dietary carbohydrate restriction. *Am J Clin Nutr*. 2011;93(5):1048–1052.
12. Holmer M, Lindqvist C, Petersson S, Moshtaghi-Svensson J, Tillander V, Brismar TB, et al. Treatment of NAFLD with intermittent calorie restriction or low-carb high-fat diet—a randomised controlled trial. *JHEP Rep*. 2021;3(3):100256.
13. Tendler D, Lin S, Yancy WS, Jr., Mavropoulos J, Sylvestre P, Rockey DC, et al. The effect of a low-carbohydrate, ketogenic diet on nonalcoholic fatty liver disease: a pilot study. *Dig Dis Sci*. 2007;52(2):589–593.
14. Cortez-Pinto H, Jesus L, Barros H, Lopes C, Moura MC, Camilo ME. How different is the dietary pattern in non-alcoholic steatohepatitis patients? *Clin Nutr*. 2006;25(5):816–823.
15. Zelber-Sagi S, Nitzan-Kaluski D, Goldsmith R, Webb M, Blendis L, Halpern Z, et al. Long term nutritional intake and the risk for non-alcoholic fatty liver disease (NAFLD): a population based study. *J Hepatol*. 2007;47(5):711–717.

16. Storlien LH, Kraegen EW, Chisholm DJ, Ford GL, Bruce DG, Pascoe WS. Fish oil prevents insulin resistance induced by high-fat feeding in rats. *Science*. 1987;237(4817):885–888.

17. Levy JR, Clore JN, Stevens W. Dietary n-3 polyunsaturated fatty acids decrease hepatic triglycerides in Fischer 344 rats. *Hepatology*. 2004;39(3):608–616.

18. Musso G, Gambino R, De Michieli F, Cassader M, Rizzetto M, Durazzo M, et al. Dietary habits and their relations to insulin resistance and postprandial lipemia in nonalcoholic steatohepatitis. *Hepatology*. 2003;37(4):909–916.

19. Toshimitsu K, Matsuura B, Ohkubo I, Niiya T, Furukawa S, Hiasa Y, et al. Dietary habits and nutrient intake in non-alcoholic steatohepatitis. *Nutrition*. 2007;23(1):46–52.

20. Rosqvist F, Kullberg J, Ståhlman M, Cedernaes J, Heurling K, Johansson HE, et al. Overeating saturated fat promotes fatty liver and ceramides compared with polyunsaturated fat: a randomized trial. *J Clin Endocrinol Metab*. 2019;104(12):6207–6219.

21. Parker HM, Johnson NA, Burdon CA, Cohn JS, O'Connor HT, George J. Omega-3 supplementation and non-alcoholic fatty liver disease: a systematic review and meta-analysis. *J Hepatol*. 2012;56(4):944–951.

22. Bezerra Duarte SM, Faintuch J, Stefano JT, Sobral de Oliveira MB, de Campos Mazo DF, Rabelo F, et al. Hypocaloric high-protein diet improves clinical and biochemical markers in patients with nonalcoholic fatty liver disease (NAFLD). *Nutr Hosp*. 2014;29(1):94–101.

23. Campmans-Kuijpers MJ, Sluijs I, Nöthlings U, Freisling H, Overvad K, Weiderpass E, et al. Isocaloric substitution of carbohydrates with protein: the association with weight change and mortality among patients with type 2 diabetes. *Cardiovasc Diabetol*. 2015;14:39.

24. Zelber-Sagi S, Ivancovsky-Wajcman D, Fliss Isakov N, Webb M, Orenstein D, Shibolet O, et al. High red and processed meat consumption is associated with non-alcoholic fatty liver disease and insulin resistance. *J Hepatol*. 2018;68(6):1239–1246.

25. Rahimi-Sakak F, Maroofi M, Emamat H, Hekmatdoost A. Red and processed meat intake in relation to non-alcoholic fatty liver disease risk: results from a case-control study. *Clin Nutr Res*. 2022;11(1):42–49.

26. Mazidi M, Kengne AP. Higher adherence to plant-based diets are associated with lower likelihood of fatty liver. *Clin Nutr*. 2019;38(4):1672–1677.

27. Younossi ZM, Koenig AB, Abdelatif D, Fazel Y, Henry L, Wymer M. Global epidemiology of nonalcoholic fatty liver disease-meta-analytic assessment of prevalence, incidence, and outcomes. *Hepatology*. 2016;64(1):73–84.

28. Chalasani N, Younossi Z, Lavine JE, Charlton M, Cusi K, Rinella M, et al. The diagnosis and management of nonalcoholic fatty liver disease: practice guidance from the American Association for the Study of Liver Diseases. *Hepatology*. 2018;67(1):328–357.

29. EASL-EASD-EASO clinical practice guidelines for the management of non-alcoholic fatty liver disease. *J Hepatol*. 2016;64(6):1388–1402.

30. Fontana L, Meyer TE, Klein S, Holloszy JO. Long-term calorie restriction is highly effective in reducing the risk for atherosclerosis in humans. *Proc Natl Acad Sci U S A*. 2004;101(17):6659–6663.

31. Haufe S, Engeli S, Kast P, Bohnke J, Utz W, Haas V, et al. Randomized comparison of reduced fat and reduced carbohydrate hypocaloric diets on intrahepatic fat in overweight and obese human subjects. *Hepatology*. 2011;53(5):1504–1514.

32. Kirk E, Reeds DN, Finck BN, Mayurranjan SM, Patterson BW, Klein S. Dietary fat and carbohydrates differentially alter insulin sensitivity during caloric restriction. *Gastroenterology*. 2009;136(5):1552–1560.

33. Elias MC, Parise ER, de Carvalho L, Szejnfeld D, Netto JP. Effect of 6-month nutritional intervention on non-alcoholic fatty liver disease. *Nutrition*. 2010;26(11–12):1094–1099.

34. Arefhosseini SR, Ebrahimi-Mameghani M, Farsad Naeimi A, Khoshbaten M, Rashid J. Lifestyle modification through dietary intervention: health promotion of patients with non-alcoholic fatty liver disease. *Health Promot Perspect*. 2011;1(2):147–154.

35. Vilar-Gomez E, Martinez-Perez Y, Calzadilla-Bertot L, Torres-Gonzalez A, Gra-Oramas B, Gonzalez-Fabian L, et al. Weight loss through lifestyle modification significantly reduces features of nonalcoholic steatohepatitis. *Gastroenterology*. 2015;149(2):367–378.e5; quiz e14–15.

36. Viljanen AP, Iozzo P, Borra R, Kankaanpää M, Karmi A, Lautamäki R, et al. Effect of weight loss on liver free fatty acid uptake and hepatic insulin resistance. *J Clin Endocrinol Metab*. 2009;94(1):50–55.

37. Ascha MS, Hanouneh IA, Lopez R, Tamimi TA, Feldstein AF, Zein NN. The incidence and risk factors of hepatocellular carcinoma in patients with nonalcoholic steatohepatitis. *Hepatology*. 2010;51(6):1972–1978.

38. Dunn W, Sanyal AJ, Brunt EM, Unalp-Arida A, Donohue M, McCullough AJ, et al. Modest alcohol consumption is associated with decreased prevalence of steatohepatitis in patients with non-alcoholic fatty liver disease (NAFLD). *J Hepatol*. 2012;57(2):384–391.

39. Dunn W, Xu R, Schwimmer JB. Modest wine drinking and decreased prevalence of suspected nonalcoholic fatty liver disease. *Hepatology*. 2008;47(6):1947–1954.

40. Martínez-González MA, Gea A, Ruiz-Canela M. The Mediterranean diet and cardiovascular health. *Circ Res*. 2019;124(5):779–798.

41. Saeed N, Nadeau B, Shannon C, Tincopa M. Evaluation of dietary approaches for the treatment of non-alcoholic fatty liver disease: a systematic review. *Nutrients*. 2019;11(12).

42. Misciagna G, Del Pilar Díaz M, Caramia DV, Bonfiglio C, Franco I, Noviello MR, et al. Effect of a low glycemic index Mediterranean diet on non-alcoholic fatty liver disease. A randomized controlled clinical trial. *J Nutr Health Aging*. 2017;21(4):404–412.

43. Katsagoni CN, Papatheodoridis GV, Ioannidou P, Deutsch M, Alexopoulou A, Papadopoulos N, et al. Improvements in clinical characteristics of patients with non-alcoholic fatty liver disease, after an intervention based on the Mediterranean lifestyle: a randomised controlled clinical trial. *Br J Nutr*. 2018;120(2):164–175.

44. Trovato FM, Catalano D, Martines GF, Pace P, Trovato GM. Mediterranean diet and non-alcoholic fatty liver disease: the need of extended and comprehensive interventions. *Clin Nutr*. 2015;34(1):86–88.

45. Abenavoli L, Greco M, Milic N, Accattato F, Foti D, Gulletta E, et al. Effect of Mediterranean diet and antioxidant formulation in non-alcoholic fatty liver disease: a randomized study. *Nutrients*. 2017;9(8).

46. Properzi C, O'Sullivan TA, Sherriff JL, Ching HL, Jeffrey GP, Buckley RF, et al. Ad libitum mediterranean

and low-fat diets both significantly reduce hepatic steatosis: a randomized controlled trial. *Hepatology.* 2018;68(5):1741–1754.

47. Ryan MC, Itsiopoulos C, Thodis T, Ward G, Trost N, Hofferberth S, et al. The Mediterranean diet improves hepatic steatosis and insulin sensitivity in individuals with non-alcoholic fatty liver disease. *J Hepatol.* 2013;59(1):138–143.

48. Bozzetto L, Prinster A, Annuzzi G, Costagliola L, Mangione A, Vitelli A, et al. Liver fat is reduced by an isoenergetic MUFA diet in a controlled randomized study in type 2 diabetic patients. *Diabetes Care.* 2012;35(7):1429–1435.

49. Marin-Alejandre BA, Abete I, Cantero I, Monreal JI, Elorz M, Herrero JI, et al. The metabolic and hepatic impact of two personalized dietary strategies in subjects with obesity and nonalcoholic fatty liver disease: the fatty liver in obesity (FLiO) randomized controlled trial. *Nutrients.* 2019;11(10).

50. Sun Y, Chen S, Zhao X, Wang Y, Lan Y, Jiang X, et al. Adherence to the dietary approaches to stop hypertension diet and non-alcoholic fatty liver disease. *Liver Int.* 2022.

51. Razavi Zade M, Telkabadi MH, Bahmani F, Salehi B, Farshbaf S, Asemi Z. The effects of DASH diet on weight loss and metabolic status in adults with non-alcoholic fatty liver disease: a randomized clinical trial. *Liver Int.* 2016;36(4):563–571.

52. Johari MI, Yusoff K, Haron J, Nadarajan C, Ibrahim KN, Wong MS, et al. A randomised controlled trial on the effectiveness and adherence of modified alternate-day calorie restriction in improving activity of non-alcoholic fatty liver disease. *Sci Rep.* 2019;9(1):11232.

53. Cai H, Qin YL, Shi ZY, Chen JH, Zeng MJ, Zhou W, et al. Effects of alternate-day fasting on body weight and dyslipidaemia in patients with non-alcoholic fatty liver disease: a randomised controlled trial. *BMC Gastroenterol.* 2019;19(1):219.

54. Koopman KE, Caan MW, Nederveen AJ, Pels A, Ackermans MT, Fliers E, et al. Hypercaloric diets with increased meal frequency, but not meal size, increase intrahepatic triglycerides: a randomized controlled trial. *Hepatology.* 2014;60(2):545–553.

55. Bambha K, Wilson LA, Unalp A, Loomba R, Neuschwander-Tetri BA, Brunt EM, et al. Coffee consumption in NAFLD patients with lower insulin resistance is associated with lower risk of severe fibrosis. *Liver Int.* 2014;34(8):1250–1258.

56. Birerdinc A, Stepanova M, Pawloski L, Younossi ZM. Caffeine is protective in patients with non-alcoholic fatty liver disease. *Aliment Pharmacol Ther.* 2012;35(1):76–82.

57. Moss O. Nutrition priorities: diet recommendations in liver cirrhosis. *Clin Liver Dis (Hoboken).* 2019;14(4):146–148.

58. Amodio P, Bemeur C, Butterworth R, Cordoba J, Kato A, Montagnese S, et al. The nutritional management of hepatic encephalopathy in patients with cirrhosis: international society for hepatic encephalopathy and nitrogen metabolism consensus. *Hepatology.* 2013;58(1):325–336.

59. Biggins SW, Angeli P, Garcia-Tsao G, Ginès P, Ling SC, Nadim MK, et al. Diagnosis, evaluation, and management of ascites, spontaneous bacterial peritonitis and hepatorenal syndrome: 2021 practice guidance by the American association for the study of liver diseases. *Hepatology.* 2021;74(2):1014–1048.

60. Kawahara T, Oniyama K, Tominaga N. Which is more important diet or exercise for obese patients? *Curr Dev Nutr.* 2020;4(Supplement_2):1647.

11 Weight Loss Medications

Mohammad Qasim Khan, Manhal Izzy and Kymberly D. Watt

CONTENTS

11.1 INTRODUCTION

The rising incidence and prevalence of nonalcoholic fatty liver disease (NAFLD) in tandem with the obesity pandemic has highlighted the importance of developing safe and effective weight loss strategies in at-risk patients. Weight loss has been associated with histological improvement of nonalcoholic fatty liver (NAFL) and nonalcoholic steatohepatitis (NASH) in a dose-dependent fashion. Weight loss ≥5% of total body weight decreases hepatic steatosis, and weight loss ≥7% promotes steatohepatitis resolution, whereas weight loss ≥10% facilitates fibrosis regression and stability[1,2]. Weight loss additionally confers improved insulin sensitivity, quality of life and reduction in portal pressures in patients with cirrhotic-stage NASH[3–5].

Weight loss achieved through a combination of dietary interventions and aerobic exercise, with or without resistance training, represents the initial management of choice in NAFLD[6]. However, compliance with calorie-restricted diets and exercise regimens are often difficult to sustain. Up to 50% of patients with NAFLD will not readily accept or implement dietary interventions for the management of their disease[7]. While NAFLD patients may understand the benefits of exercise, factors such as lack of confidence, fear of falling and associated difficulty in performing physical activity are major barriers against compliance[8]. Considering these limitations, the need to develop and explore additional weight loss tools in the management of NAFLD is being increasingly recognized. To this end, pharmacotherapy as well as endoscopic and surgical bariatric procedures are additional weight loss strategies that need to be considered. Bariatric procedures may not be clinically feasible for most patients with NAFLD/NASH, and thus weight loss medications can be effectively utilized to augment weight loss through lifestyle interventions[9].

Currently, five weight loss medications have been approved by the US Food and Drug Administration (FDA)—orlistat, phentermine-topiramate, naltrexone-bupropion, liraglutide and semaglutide[10,11]. The use of these weight loss medications can seamlessly be incorporated in the management of NAFLD, for two reasons. (1) Weight loss medications can facilitate weight loss of 7–10% total body weight, coinciding with losses needed to reverse hepatic steatosis and inflammation, and (2) most patients with NAFLD already meet the criteria for the use of weight loss medications, i.e., BMI > 27 kg/m² and a weight-related comorbidity[10].

In this chapter, we review the mechanisms of the action, efficacy, utility and safety of these FDA-approved weight loss medications, as they pertain to the management of NAFLD. Furthermore, in light of rising public interest, we will also discuss the role and safety of over-the-counter, alternative weight loss therapies in patients with NAFLD.

11.2 FDA-APPROVED WEIGHT LOSS MEDICATIONS

11.2.1 Orlistat

11.2.1.1 Overview

In 1999, Davidson et al. published data from their randomized control trial evaluating orlistat in obese patients. They revealed

DOI: 10.1201/9781003386698-14

significant weight loss and less weight regain over a 2-year period of use, with concurrent improvements in low-density lipoprotein and insulin levels[12]. Later that year, after a review of 6 placebo-controlled trials, the FDA approved orlistat (120 mg) as a prescription product to manage obesity and minimize weight regain, *in conjunction with a hypocaloric diet*[13]. In 2007, a lower dose of orlistat (60 mg) was approved for over-the-counter (OTC) use to promote weight loss in overweight adults, in combination with a hypocaloric, low-fat diet[14]. This was the first over-the-counter weight loss pill to be approved by the FDA.

11.2.1.2 Mechanism of Action

Orlistat is a minimally absorbed medication that covalently binds to serine sites on pancreatic and gastric lipases, rendering them inactive. As a result, ingested fats are not hydrolyzed into their constituent free fatty acids and monoglycerides and subsequently are not absorbed into the portal circulation. These unabsorbed fats are ultimately excreted in the feces. Orlistat blocks the gastrointestinal absorption of ~30% of calories ingested as fats, thus promoting weight loss[13]. The recommended prescription dose of orlistat is 120 mg 3 times daily with each fat-containing meal, whereas the over-the-counter dose is 60 mg three times daily.

11.2.1.3 Efficacy and Utility Appertaining to NAFLD

The efficacy of orlistat in promoting weight loss has been demonstrated in numerous clinical trials. In a meta-analysis of 12 trials evaluating outcomes at 1 year in patients randomly assigned to either orlistat plus a behavioral intervention or placebo plus a behavioral intervention, those in the intervention group lost 5–10 kg of body weight (corresponding to approximately 8% of baseline body weight), whereas the control group lost 3–6 kg, resulting in a mean difference of 3 kg (95% CI −3.9 to −2.0 kg)[15]. One of the longest randomized, double-blinded trials evaluating orlistat in over 3,305 patients revealed that while weight loss was greater in orlistat-treated patients compared to placebo at 1 year (11% weight loss vs. 6% weight loss from baseline), patients in both groups gained weight in the following three years, such that weight loss at the end of the 4-year evaluation period was 6.9% below baseline in the orlistat-treated group compared to 4.1% in the placebo group. Orlistat-treated patients also had a lower cumulative incidence of diabetes[16].

The efficacy of orlistat in patients with NAFL and NASH has been evaluated in three randomized controlled trials. Zelber-Sagi et al. evaluated orlistat (120 mg 3 times daily) vs. placebo in 52 patients with ultrasound- and biopsy-proven NAFLD for a duration of 6 months. Of note, only patients in the orlistat group had evidence of impaired glycemic control. In addition, the orlistat group had a higher degree of fibrosis compared to placebo with 27.3% having stage 4 fibrosis and 9% having stage 0, whereas none of the patients in the placebo group had stage 4 fibrosis and ~55% had stage 0 fibrosis. On average, patients on orlistat lost 8% of their baseline body weight compared to 6% in the placebo group (p = 0.26). The orlistat group achieved greater reductions in ALT (48% vs. 26.4%) and had a higher rate of reversal of steatosis on ultrasound (24% vs. 17.4%). Improvement in fibrosis staging was comparable between the groups[17]. Harrison et al. evaluated weight loss and liver histology in 50 overweight patients with biopsy-proven NASH on a 1400 kCal diet and vitamin E (800 IU daily) with or without orlistat. Patients in the orlistat group achieved a mean weight loss of 8.3% compared to 6.0% in

the diet and vitamin E-only group (p = 0.86). Improvements in insulin resistance, cholesterol, liver transaminases, hepatic steatosis, inflammation, ballooning, and fibrosis were also comparable between the groups[18]. In comparison, in NAFLD patients without advanced fibrosis randomized to a hypocaloric diet with or without orlistat, Ali Khan et al. illustrated that patients on orlistat achieved significantly greater reductions in body weight, waist circumference and insulin resistance, with more favorable lipid profiles[19]. Overall, these trials revealed that improvement of steatosis in patients with NAFLD is weight loss dependent, irrespective of orlistat use. While discrepancies exist between the studies with regard to weight loss achieved and histological improvement of NAFLD, a meta-analysis of 7 studies, including the aforementioned trials, revealed that orlistat use in patients with NAFL or NASH was associated with a significant reduction in BMI (standard mean difference of −1.97, p = 0.02), insulin resistance (mean difference in HOMA-IR of −1.05, p = 0.04), triglycerides (mean difference of −0.93, p = 0.01) and liver chemistries (standard mean reduction in ALT of −1.41, p = 0.01), but not fibrosis scores[20].

11.2.1.4 Safety & Adverse Reactions

The major side effects of orlistat are gastrointestinal, varying in pattern and severity, including nausea, abdominal cramps, flatulence, fecal urgency and fecal incontinence. In trials evaluating orlistat in patients with NAFLD, these side effects infrequently resulted in subject withdrawal[17,21].

By virtue of its inhibition of gastric and pancreatic lipases, orlistat can lower levels of fat-soluble vitamins (A, D, E, K) and beta-carotene, and thus monitoring patients on therapy with appropriate supplementation should be considered[22]. Similarly, due to the resultant fat malabsorption, patients on orlistat are also at risk of developing calcium oxalate stones and oxalate-induced acute kidney injury[23].

While a causal relationship has not been well-established, severe liver injury has very rarely been reported with the use of orlistat. The FDA announced concerns regarding hepatotoxicity after a review identified 13 cases of severe liver injury, over a 10-year period of use, in 40 million users worldwide. The pattern of injury was hepatocellular, developing within the first 2–12 weeks of use. A few cases of liver failure were also reported, progressing to death or liver transplantation. While it has been posited that the likely mechanism of injury is a hypersensitivity reaction, typical features of hypersensitivity have not been noted in published case reports[24].

11.2.2 Phentermine-Topiramate
11.2.2.1 Overview

A combination preparation of phentermine and extended-release topiramate was approved by the FDA in 2012 for patients with obesity, preferentially in those with no history of cardiovascular disease. It is administered once daily in the morning, to avoid insomnia, at a starting dose of phentermine 3.75 mg/topiramate 23 mg. This is titrated up after 2 weeks to 7.5 mg/46 mg once daily. If at least 3% weight loss is not achieved after 14 weeks of therapy, up-titrations can be considered in patients without moderate renal or hepatic impairment (i.e., Child–Pugh score < 7), to a maximum of 15 mg/92 mg once daily[25].

11.2.2.2 Mechanism of Action

Phentermine is a sympathomimetic agent with pharmacological activity like amphetamine. It is an anorectic, reducing appetite by stimulating the release of catecholamines in the hypothalamus[25].

Topiramate is an anticonvulsant whose mechanism of action in chronic weight management is not exactly known. Its appetite suppression and satiety-enhancing effects are postulated to be due to blocking neuronal voltage-dependent sodium channels, enhancing GABA(A) activity, antagonizing AMPA/kainite glutamate receptors and weakly inhibiting carbonic anhydrase[25].

11.2.2.3 Efficacy and Utility Appertaining to NAFLD

The efficacy of phentermine-topiramate in chronic weight management has been illustrated in two trials, CONQUER and EQUIP. The CONQUER trial assigned 2,487 adults to either phentermine-topiramate 7.5/46 mg, phentermine-topiramate 15/92 mg or placebo over a course of 1 year. After 1 year, mean weight loss was greater in patients assigned to treatment compared to those on placebo (−8–10% vs. −1.2%, $p < 0.0001$)[26]. A 1-year extension of this trial (SEQUEL) showed that phentermine-topiramate was less effective for weight loss in the second year of use, although most patients maintained the weight they had lost in year 1[27]. In addition, patients on treatment (particularly those on the 15/92 mg dose) had more significant improvements in lipid profiles (i.e., lower triglycerides, lower LDL cholesterol and higher HDL cholesterol) and decreased incident rates of diabetes, compared to placebo. The EQUIP trial exclusively evaluated phentermine-topiramate in patients with BMI≥ 35 kg/m^2 for 56 weeks. Patients were randomly assigned to either receive phentermine-topiramate 3.75/23 mg, phentermine-topiramate 15/92 mg or placebo. Similar to the CONQUER trial, patients on active treatment showed greater weight loss compared to placebo (−5.1–10.9% vs. −1.6%, $p < 0.0001$). Notably, of the patients on active treatment, 45–67% achieved at least 5% weight loss[28]. Overall, phentermine-topiramate offers a significant, dose-dependent reduction in body weight in addition to favorable lipid and glycemic profiles, particularly at the higher 15/92 mg dose.

To date, no trials have investigated the efficacy of phentermine-topiramate in patients with NAFLD.

11.2.2.4 Safety & Adverse Reactions

In both the CONQUER and EQUIP trials, the most common adverse effects were dry mouth, paresthesias, constipation, insomnia, dizziness, and dysgeusia[26,27]. A dose-dependent increase in the incidence of psychiatric (depression, anxiety) and cognitive (attention disturbances) adverse events was also noted in the active treatment groups[26].

In patients with moderate hepatic impairment (Child–Pugh B; score 7–9), dosing should not exceed 7.5mg/46mg once daily, and the drug should be avoided in patients with severe hepatic impairment (Child–Pugh C; score 10–15)[25].

Phentermine-topiramate is contraindicated in pregnancy due to risk of orofacial clefts in infants exposed to the drug combination in the first trimester of pregnancy. It is also contraindicated in patients with hyperthyroidism, glaucoma and those who have taken monoamine oxidase inhibitors within 14 days[25].

11.2.3 Naltrexone-Bupropion

11.2.3.1 Overview

Combination naltrexone-bupropion was approved by the FDA for chronic obesity management in September 2014[29]. While it is not favored as a first-line therapy, the combination is particularly useful in obese patients who smoke or those with alcohol use disorder, given that bupropion and naltrexone are approved therapies for smoking cessation and alcohol use disorder, respectively. The combination comes in 8 mg/90 mg tablets administered as one tablet, once daily, up-titrated to two tablets, twice daily.

11.2.3.2 Mechanism of Action

Naltrexone is an opioid antagonist, and bupropion is a weak inhibitor of neuronal reuptake of dopamine and norepinephrine. Nonclinical studies suggest that naltrexone and bupropion affect activity in the hypothalamus and mesolimbic dopamine circuit—important regulators of food intake. The specific neurochemical effects that drive weight loss with this combination are not well-understood although naltrexone has been postulated to augment bupropion's activation of hypothalamic neurons[29,30].

11.2.3.3 Efficacy and Utility Appertaining to NAFLD

The original drug trials evaluating efficacy of naltrexone-bupropion excluded patients with history of liver disease, alcohol use disorder and those with AST/ALT > 2.5 times the upper limit of normal[29]. However, a pooled, post hoc analysis of 4 randomized controlled trials ($n = 2,073$) evaluating naltrexone-bupropion over 56 weeks illustrated significantly greater reductions in body weight (−8.7 kg (−8.8%) vs. −3.2 kg (−3.1%), $p < 0.001$) in naltrexone-bupropion-treated patients vs. placebo[31]. In addition, weight loss, independent of treatment, was associated with improved ALT and FIB-4 scores ($p < 0.001$). Furthermore, naltrexone-bupropion displayed a significant, independent change in FIB-4 scores from baseline ($p < 0.001$). While the results of this analysis provide reassurance of the safety of this regimen with regard to liver health, further dedicated, prospective studies are needed to investigate the safety and efficacy of naltrexone-bupropion in patients with NAFLD[31]. In addition to weight loss and transaminase improvements, improved insulin resistance and lipid profiles have been noted with naltrexone-bupropion use in obese and overweight patients[32].

11.2.3.4 Safety & Adverse Reactions

Common adverse effects of naltrexone-bupropion include nausea, vomiting, constipation, diarrhea, headaches, insomnia, dizziness and dry mouth[32,33].

Naltrexone is contraindicated in patients with decompensated cirrhosis. Dosing in patients with NAFLD should not exceed 8/90 mg daily[30].

Other contraindications of naltrexone-bupropion include pregnancy, uncontrolled hypertension, seizure disorders, eating disorders, chronic opioid use and concurrent use of other bupropion-containing products or MAO inhibitors[29].

11.2.4 GLP-1 Receptor Agonists

11.2.4.1 Overview

Two glucagon-like peptide-1 (GLP-1) receptor agonists, liraglutide and semaglutide, initially approved for the management of diabetes in 2010 and 2017, respectively, have since been approved for the management of obesity in light of promising results in drug trials[34,35]. While various formulations (including oral tablets) and doses exist for these agents, for obesity management indications, both medications are administered via subcutaneous injection with semaglutide being administered once weekly and liraglutide once daily. Liraglutide is initiated at 0.6 mg daily with a dose increase by 0.6 mg/day each week up to a target dose of 3 mg once daily. If this target dose cannot be achieved due to intolerance, there may be benefit in continuing the maximum tolerated dose[34]. Recommended dosing for semaglutide in obese patients follows a structured schedule that involves dose up-titration over 17 weeks:

Weeks 1–4: 0.25 mg once weekly
Weeks 5–8: 0.5 mg once weekly
Weeks 9–12: 1 mg once weekly
Weeks 13–16: 1.7 mg once weekly
Week 17 and thereafter (maintenance): 2.4 mg once weekly

If the goal maintenance dose is not tolerated initially, a temporary reduction in dose to 1.7 mg can be considered for an additional month before reattempting up-titration to 2.4 mg once weekly.

11.2.4.2 Mechanism of Action

GLP-1 is a gastrointestinal peptide that induces glucose-dependent insulin secretion. In addition, it inhibits glucagon release and delays gastric emptying. As a result, agonist activity on the GLP-1 receptor improves glycemia, promotes satiety and appetite suppression, with subsequent weight loss[30]. In addition to weight loss, GLP-1 receptor agonists have been shown to directly reduce hepatic de novo lipogenesis and decrease lipolysis-induced free fatty acid levels and levels of triglyceride-derived toxic metabolites[36].

11.2.4.3 Efficacy and Utility Appertaining to NAFLD

A 56-week trial of liraglutide administered at a dose of 3 mg daily vs. placebo in 3,731 patients with a BMI ≥ 30 kg/m² or ≥ 27 kg/m² with dyslipidemia and/or hypertension revealed significantly greater weight loss in the liraglutide group (−8.0 kg vs. −2.6 kg with placebo, $p < 0.001$). A total of 63.2% of patients in the liraglutide group vs. 27.1% of patients in the placebo group lost at least 5% of their baseline body weight ($p < 0.001$). Furthermore, 33.1% and 10.6% of patients, respectively, achieved >10% weight loss ($p < 0.001$). Liver-related outcomes were not reported. However, modest improvements in cardiometabolic risk factors, including HgbA1c, and quality of life were noted in the liraglutide group[37].

The LEAN study evaluated the safety and efficacy of a lower dose of liraglutide, i.e., 1.8 mg daily, compared with placebo in 52 patients who were overweight and who had clinical evidence of NASH (F3–F4 fibrosis). Patients with Child–Pugh B or C cirrhosis were excluded. The primary outcome was histological resolution of NASH with no worsening fibrosis from baseline to the end of treatment at 48 weeks. Thirty-nine percent of liraglutide-treated patients vs. 9% of placebo-treated patients achieved resolution of NASH ($p = 0.019$). Furthermore, 9% of patients in the liraglutide group and 36% of patients in the placebo group had progression of fibrosis ($p = 0.04$). Expectedly, patients in the liraglutide group also had significantly greater improvements in metabolic covariates including HgbA1c, BMI and HDL, as well as in quality of life scores[38].

More recently, Khoo et al. evaluated the efficacy of the higher, chronic weight management dose of liraglutide, 3 mg daily, in patients with NAFLD, compared to a structured diet-exercise program. Over 26 weeks, patients on liraglutide achieved significant reduction of weight (−3.0 ± 2.2 kg), liver fat fraction (−7.0 ± 7.1%) and serum alanine aminotransferase (ALT) (−26 ± 33 IU/L)[39].

The landmark STEP trials demonstrated exceptional efficacy of semaglutide in promoting weight loss in overweight and obese patients with or without diabetes. In STEP 1, which compared once-weekly subcutaneous semaglutide 2.4 mg to placebo, mean weight loss in the semaglutide group was greater than placebo (−15.3 kg [−14.9%] vs. −2.6 kg [−2.4%], $p < 0.001$). In addition, a significantly greater proportion of patients achieved ≥10% body weight loss (69.1% vs. 12.0%) and ≥15% weight loss (50.5% vs. 4.9%) in the semaglutide group. Patients on semaglutide also had significantly greater reductions in waist circumference and systolic blood pressures as well as higher quality of life scores, compared to placebo[40]. Similar favorable results were noted in the STEP 2 trials, which evaluated the efficacy of semaglutide 1 mg, 2.4 mg and placebo in patients with type 2 diabetes mellitus and obesity (−6.9 kg, −9.7 kg and −3.5 kg, respectively)[41]. While the STEP 3 trials included 45 patients with known NAFLD at baseline, liver-related outcomes were not reported and subgroup analyses in the NAFLD patients were not carried out[42]. The STEP 8 trial made a head-to-head comparison of semaglutide 2.4 mg weekly with liraglutide 3.0 mg daily in 338 adults, over 68 weeks. At the end of treatment, patients in the semaglutide arm achieved significantly greater weight loss compared to those in the liraglutide arm (−15.8% vs. −6.4%; treatment difference −9.4% [95% CI −12.0 to −6.8])[43].

A phase II study evaluating lower-dose, daily semaglutide use (0.1 mg, 0.2 mg and 0.4 mg) in NASH patients showed greater propensity for NASH resolution in treated patients vs. placebo. However, no between-group differences in improvement in fibrosis stage were noted[44]. Phase III trials evaluating semaglutide use in NASH patients are underway.

11.2.4.4 Safety & Adverse Reactions

Gastrointestinal side effects, including nausea (liraglutide: 14.7–80%, semaglutide: 44.2–61.1%), vomiting (liraglutide: 4.1–20.5%, semaglutide: up to 25.4%) and diarrhea (liraglutide: 9.3–38%, semaglutide: up to 31.5%), are very common with liraglutide and semaglutide[37–40,43]. Fortunately, these are mild and transient in nature. In the STEP 8 trial, 84.1% of patients on semaglutide and 82.7% of patients on liraglutide experienced gastrointestinal symptoms. However, this led to discontinuation of the drug in only 8/253 patients (1 in the semaglutide arm; 7 in the liraglutide arm)[43].

Liraglutide has less commonly been associated with pancreatitis, gallbladder disease and kidney injury. Animal studies showed that liraglutide was associated with benign and malignant thyroid C-cell tumors. There is no evidence of these tumors developing in humans[34].

Both liraglutide and semaglutide are contraindicated during pregnancy, in those with a history of pancreatitis, or personal or family history of medullary thyroid cancer or multiple endocrine neoplasia 2A/2B. Caution should be taken, and blood glucose levels closely monitored for hypoglycemic events when these agents are given to patients already on insulin or insulin secretagogues. Angioedema and anaphylaxis have rarely been reported with semaglutide use[34,35].

11.3 ALTERNATIVE THERAPIES

There has been a steady and persistent increase in the use of herbal and dietary supplements by adults in the US[45].

Data from the US suggest that approximately 1/3–1/2 of all Americans use herbal or dietary supplements, and worldwide prevalence may approach 80%[46–48]. While the majority of these agents are multivitamins and minerals, the rising burden of obesity and the inherent challenges faced by consumers to inculcate lifestyle changes has seen many Americans turn to herbal and dietary supplements for weight management[49]. In 2020, the weight loss supplements industry in the US alone was estimated at USD $6.5 billion and is expected to continue growing worldwide[50]. This is due to a combination of aggressive marketing strategies claiming efficacy with minimal effort or data, as well as easy availability, driven by the lenient regulatory framework for herbal and dietary supplements compared to pharmaceuticals.

Several supplements used for weight loss and body-building have been associated with significant hepato-toxicity[49]. OxyELITE Pro's "Super Thermogenic", a weight loss and fat-burning product resulting in over 50 cases of acute hepatitis and multiple instances of acute liver failure, famously brought to light the potential for serious harm imposed by readily available supplements[24]. Similar multi-ingredient nutritional supplements (MINS) such as products by Herbalife, Hydroxycut and SLIMQUICK, have repeatedly been implicated in liver injury, including cases of acute liver failure[24]. Green tea extract, an ingredient in numerous weight loss supplements, advertised as having "fat burning" and "metabolism-supporting" properties, has also been associated with severe hepato-toxicity and acute liver failure[51]. In vivo studies identified (-)-epigallocatechin-3-gallate, a polyphenol found in green tea extract, to be the implicating toxin[52]. *Garcinia cambogia*, derived from the fruit rind of the *G. cambogia* tree, is another common ingredient in commercially available weight loss supplements. The active ingredient, hydroxy-citric acid (HCA), has been linked to hepatotoxicity with underlying mechanisms including oxidative stress, inflammation and fibrosis[53,54]. Usnic acid, derived from lichens, was proposed as a potential weight loss therapy in the 1930s after unintentional weight loss was reported in plant workers exposed to another lichen acid, 2,4-dinitrophenol[55]. LipoKinetix, a supplement containing usnic acid, was linked to several cases of severe acute liver injury and withdrawn by the FDA in 2001[56]. Conjugated linolenic acid, an omega-6 fatty acid mechanistically believed to induce lipid peroxidation and reduce fat storage, has been associated with hepatocellular and cholestatic liver injury[57,58]. One case of fulminant hepatic failure warranting trans-plantation has been reported[59].

Nevertheless, few weight loss supplements with acceptable safety profiles and some evidence of efficacy in patients with underlying chronic liver disease will be discussed here.

11.3.1 Green Cardamom (*Elettaria cardamomum*)

Cardamom is a spice derived from the seeds of various plants in the Zingiberaceae family, of which, *Elettaria carda-moum* is the most cultivated species. Numerous essential oils contained in this spice are believed to exhibit anti-inflammatory, antioxidant, hypolipidemic and antibacterial properties. Emerging data also suggest benefit and utility in lipid metabolism, glycemic control and potential weight loss[30]. A double-blinded randomized placebo-controlled trial ($n = 87$) evaluating the efficacy of green cardamom in NAFLD patients demonstrated improved serum glucose indices, lipid profiles, ALT and hepatic steatosis on ultrasound. However, no significant difference in weight was noted in these patients when compared to placebo (85.2 kg vs. 88.6 kg). Green cardamom was well-tolerated, and no adverse effects were reported[60]. There are no known reports of hepatotoxicity with green cardamom.

11.3.2 Curcumin

Curcumin is a key chemical commonly available as a food additive, cosmetics ingredient and herbal supplement with potential anti-inflammatory, antimicrobial and antioxidant properties. It has been theorized to facilitate weight loss and favorable metabolic profiles by inhibiting proteins necessary for adipogenesis as well as pro-inflammatory cytokines. Numerous trials have aimed to evaluate the effects of curcumin in overweight and obese patients with or without NAFLD. In 2015, Di Pierro et al. evaluated the efficacy of curcumin in patients with the metabolic syndrome who failed to achieve significant weight loss after 30 days of dietary and exercise-based interventions. They revealed significant reduction in weight (−4.91%), waist circumference (−4.14%) and body fat (−8.43%)[61]. A meta-analysis of 9 randomized controlled trials ($n = 588$) investigating short-term curcumin use (2–3 months, 50–1500 mg/day) in patients with NAFLD illustrated significant decrease in ALT, AST, total cholesterol, LDL cholesterol, fasting blood sugars, HOMA-IR and waist circumference, but not body weight, body mass index, serum triglyceride or HgbA1c levels[62]. Given the conflicting results with regard to the weight loss benefit with curcumin and potential favorable effects on lipemic and glycemic indices, clinical trials with larger sample sizes would be reasonable. No adverse effects of curcumin have been reported, although transient elevations of serum aminotransferases have been noted, albeit without clinically significant liver injury[24].

11.3.3 Carnitine

Carnitine is a natural, water-soluble molecule that serves multiple functions in the human body, including trans-port of long-chain fatty acids into the mitochondrial matrix ("carnitine shuttle"), regulation of acetyl Co-A, interorganellar Acyl transfer and reduction of oxidative stress[63]. As a result, carnitine supplementation has been proposed to facilitate β-oxidation of fatty acids, thereby promoting free fatty acid uptake and ultimately reducing hepatic fat accumulation. A meta-analysis of 43 randomized controlled trials studying the weight loss potential of L-carnitine in overweight and obese adults with or without comorbid conditions such as NAFLD, prediabetes, diabetes, polycystic ovarian syndrome, etc. showed a modest but statistically significant reduction in weight following carnitine supplementation (−1.13 kg; 95% CI: −1.590, −0.669, $p < 0.001$). However, this weight loss effect was not seen in patients with a baseline BMI < 25 kg/m^{2,64}. Notably, the two included studies evaluating patients with NAFLD/NASH showed conflicting results. Somi et al. ($n = 80$) demonstrated statistically significant weight reductions in L-carnitine-treated (250 mg BID) patients (88.3 ± 13.1 kg to 85.8 ± 12.6 kg) with sonographic evidence of NAFLD[65]. However, in another trial with 74 patients with biopsy-proven NASH, randomly assigned to 1,000 mg L-carnitine plus dietary intervention vs. placebo plus dietary intervention, L-carnitine did not yield significant reductions in weight/BMI[66]. Most studies have reported significant improvements and even normalization of liver enzymes in

Table 11.1: Summary of FDA-Approved Medications for Chronic Obesity Management

Drug	Mechanism(s) of Action	Weight Loss vs. Placebo	Adverse Effects	Advantages	Disadvantages/Concerns
Orlistat	Inhibition of pancreatic and gastric lipases	• −8% vs. −6% (NS)[17] • −8.3% vs. −6.0% (NS)[18] • −6.31 ± 1.47 kg vs. −4.07 ± 0.69 kg ($p < 0.01$)[19]	Nausea, abdominal cramps, flatulence, fecal urgency, fecal incontinence	• Oral • OTC option available • Minimal drug interactions • Improves AST, ALT, IR, lipid profiles and hepatic steatosis • Can be safely used in cirrhosis (Child–Pugh A–C)	• Modest weight loss benefit • Calcium oxalate renal stones/oxalate-induced nephropathy • Very rarely: severe hepatocellular injury • Contraindicated in pregnancy
Phentermine-Topiramate	Suppresses appetite via hypothalamic adrenergic agonism. Promotes satiety via GABA-ergic agonism, glutamate antagonism, and blockade of voltage-dependent sodium channels.	• −8–10% vs. −1.2% ($p < 0.0001$)[26] • −5.1–10.9% vs. −1.6% ($p < 0.0001$)[28]	Dry mouth, paresthesias, constipation, insomnia, dizziness, dysgeusia Dose-dependent increase in psychiatric and cognitive adverse events	• Oral • Promotes favorable lipid (↓LDL and TAG, ↑HDL) and glycemic profiles • Good weight loss potential after 1-year of use, with sustained weight loss at 2 years[27]	• Avoid in patients with hypertension or coronary artery disease • Contraindicated in Child-Pugh C cirrhosis; Maximum dose in Child–Pugh B cirrhosis of 7.5 mg/46 mg • Contraindicated in pregnancy, hypothyroidism, glaucoma and concurrent MAO-inhibitor use • Teratogenic
Naltrexone-Bupropion	Modulates activity in the hypothalamus and the mesolimbic dopamine circuit via inhibition of neuronal dopamine and norepinephrine reuptake	• −8.8% vs. −3.1% ($p < 0.001$)[31]	Nausea, vomiting, constipation, diarrhea, headaches, insomnia, dizziness, dry mouth	• Oral • Useful option in concurrent nicotine or alcohol use disorder • Moderate weight loss benefit with demonstrated improvement in liver enzymes and FIB-4 scores	• Contraindicated in Child-Pugh C cirrhosis; • Contraindicated in pregnancy, uncontrolled hypertension, seizure disorders, eating disorders, chronic opioid use and with concurrent use of other bupropion-containing products or MAO inhibitors
Liraglutide	Glucagon-like peptide-1 receptor agonist	SCALE[37]: • −8.0 kg vs. −2.6 kg ($p < 0.001$); • 33.1% vs. 10.6% achieve >10% weight loss Khoo et. al. (vs. diet + exercise)[39]: • −3.0 ± 2.2 kg vs. −3.5 ± 3.3 kg (NS)	Transient nausea, vomiting, diarrhea Pancreatitis (rare)	• Good weight loss benefit • Histological improvement of NASH and slower progression of fibrosis has been demonstrated vs. placebo • Improves lipid profiles, glycemic profiles and quality of life	• Subcutaneous injection • Contraindications: pregnancy, history of pancreatitis, personal or family history of medullary thyroid cancer or multiple endocrine neoplasia 2A/2B
Semaglutide	Glucagon-like peptide-1 receptor agonist	• −14.9% vs. −2.4% ($p < 0.001$)[40]	Transient nausea, vomiting, diarrhea	• Robust weight loss benefit and propensity for NASH resolution • Concurrent reductions in waist circumference, systolic blood pressures, glycated hemoglobin; improved quality of life • Weekly administration	• Subcutaneous injection • Contraindications: pregnancy, history of pancreatitis, personal or family history of medullary thyroid cancer or multiple endocrine neoplasia 2A/2B

OTC: Over-the-counter; AST: Aspartate aminotransferase; ALT: Alanine aminotransferase; IR: Insulin resistance; GABA: Gamma-aminobutyric acid; LDL: Low-density lipoprotein; TAG: Triglycerides; HDL: High-density lipoprotein; MAO: Monoamine oxidase.

NAFLD patients receiving L-carnitine[65–70]. Furthermore, in patients with NAFLD and diabetes, improvements in fasting blood glucose, HgbA1c levels, insulin resistance, lipid profile and mitochondrial function have also been reported[66,68,70]. Although generally well-tolerated, the adverse effects of L-carnitine include mild gastrointestinal symptoms such as nausea and abdominal pain. Headaches, musculoskeletal pain, muscle weakness and seizures have also been rarely reported[66,69,71].

11.4. FUTURE DIRECTIONS

Unequivocally, the GLP-1 receptor analogues have transformed the horizon of pharmacotherapeutic management of obesity given their profound weight loss effects as well as additional cardio- and nephro-protective effects. Not surprisingly, emerging drug therapies are looking at newer iterations and combinations of these agents to achieve significant weight loss in overweight and obese patients, with or without NAFLD.

Tirzepatide is an investigational dual glucose-dependent insulinotropic polypeptide (GIP) and GLP-1 receptor agonist that has shown remarkable weight loss benefit and glycemic control in patients with type 2 diabetes. A head-to-head trial of once weekly, subcutaneously administered tirzepatide vs. semaglutide in patients with type 2 diabetes not only showed superior reductions in baseline glycated hemoglobin levels at all investigated doses (5 mg, 10 mg and 15 mg) but also greater reductions in body weight (least-square means estimated treatment difference, −1.9 kg, −3.6 kg and −5.5 kg, respectively) in tirzepatide-treated patients[72]. Phase II trials are currently ongoing, investigating the efficacy of tirzepatide (SYNERGY-NASH) in overweight, biopsy-proven NASH patients, with or without diabetes.

Danuglipron is the first oral, small-molecule GLP-1 receptor agonist found to have comparable efficacy to injectable peptidic GLP-1 receptor agonists in humanized mouse models. The drug was then studied in a placebo-controlled, randomized, double-blinded, multiple ascending dose phase 1 study in 98 patients with type II diabetes, over 28 days. Danuglipron was generally well-tolerated with only mild adverse events being reported. The most frequent adverse events were nausea, vomiting and dyspepsia. Compared to placebo, body weight was significantly reduced in the danuglipron 70 mg BID, 120 mg BID, 120 mg BID slow titration (ST), 120 mg QID and 200 mg QID controlled release (CR) groups. Weight reductions ranged from −7.2 ± 0.7 kg to −2.2 kg ± 0.7 kg, compared with −1.8 ± 0.4 kg for placebo, over 28 days. Phase II studies are currently underway for obesity management. Long-term weight loss and maintenance will need to be evaluated in further studies[73].

Noiiglutide is a GLP-1 analogue currently under development for the management of obesity. A multicenter, randomized, double-blinded, placebo-controlled trial is ongoing to assess the safety and efficacy of three doses of injectable noiiglutide on change in baseline body weight over 24 weeks of therapy[74].

Cotadutide (MEDI0382) is an injectable oxyntomoduline-like peptide with targeted dual GLP-1 and glucagon receptor agonist activity. It is under development for patients with NASH/chronic kidney disease with type 2 diabetes. A 54-week phase IIb study randomized obese and overweight type 2 diabetics to cotadutide 100 μg, 200 μg, 300 μg, placebo or liraglutide 1.8 mg. Significant decreases in body weight from baseline to week 14 were observed with cotadutide 100 μg (LS mean −2.98%, 95% CI: −3.87, −2.09), 200 μg (LS mean −3.67%, 95% CI: −4.22, −3.13), 300 μg (LS mean −5.01%, 95% CI: −5.57, −4.45) and liraglutide 1.8 mg (LS mean −3.44%, 95% CI: −4.20, −2.68), vs. placebo (LS mean −0.74%, 95% CI: −1.56, 0.07; all $p <$ 0.001). At 54 weeks, all three doses of cotadutide showed

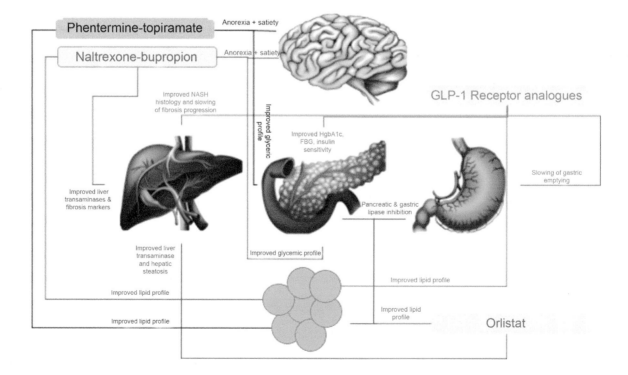

Figure 11.1 Schematic representation of weight loss medications' mechanisms of action and metabolic effects of relevance in patients with NAFLD

significant decreases in % body weight vs. placebo (−3.70%, −3.22% and −5.02%, respectively, vs. −0.68%; all $p < 0.001$). Additionally, significant improvements in AST, ALT, FIB-4 index and NFS were observed with cotadutide 300 μg vs. placebo[75]. (See Table 11.1 and Figure 11.1.)

REFERENCE

1. Musso G, Cassader M, Rosina F, Gambino R. Impact of current treatments on liver disease, glucose metabolism and cardiovascular risk in non-alcoholic fatty liver disease (NAFLD): a systematic review and meta-analysis of randomised trials. *Diabetologia* 2012;55:885–904.

2. Vilar-Gomez E, Martinez-Perez Y, Calzadilla-Bertot L, et al. Weight loss through lifestyle modification significantly reduces features of nonalcoholic steatohepatitis. *Gastroenterology* 2015;149:367–378.e5.

3. Petersen KF, Dufour S, Befroy D, Lehrke M, Hendler RE, Shulman GI. Reversal of nonalcoholic hepatic steatosis, hepatic insulin resistance, and hyperglycemia by moderate weight reduction in patients with type 2 diabetes. *Diabetes* 2005;54:603–608.

4. Tapper EB, Lai M. Weight loss results in significant improvements in quality of life for patients with non-alcoholic fatty liver disease: a prospective cohort study. *Hepatology* 2016;63:1184–1189.

5. Berzigotti A, Albillos A, Villanueva C, et al. Effects of an intensive lifestyle intervention program on portal hypertension in patients with cirrhosis and obesity: the SportDiet study. *Hepatology* 2017;65:1293–1305.

6. European Association for the Study of the L, European Association for the Study of D, European Association for the Study of O. EASL-EASD-EASO clinical practice guidelines for the management of non-alcoholic fatty liver disease. *J Hepatol* 2016;64:1388–1402.

7. Yasutake K, Kohjima M, Kotoh K, Nakashima M, Nakamuta M, Enjoji M. Dietary habits and behaviors associated with nonalcoholic fatty liver disease. *World J Gastroenterol* 2014;20:1756–1767.

8. Frith J, Day CP, Robinson L, Elliott C, Jones DE, Newton JL. Potential strategies to improve uptake of exercise interventions in non-alcoholic fatty liver disease. *J Hepatol* 2010;52:112–116.

9. Jensen MD, Ryan DH, Apovian CM, et al. 2013 AHA/ACC/TOS guideline for the management of overweight and obesity in adults: a report of the American College of Cardiology/American Heart Association task force on practice guidelines and the obesity society. *Circulation* 2014;129:S102–138.

10. Do A, Kuszewski EJ, Langberg KA, Mehal WZ. Incorporating weight loss medications into hepatology practice for nonalcoholic steatohepatitis. *Hepatology* 2019;70:1443–1456.

11. *FDA Approves New Drug Treatment for Chronic Weight Management: First Since*, 2014 (Accessed October 21, 2021, at www.fda.gov/news-events/press-announcements/fda-approves-new-drug-treatment-chronic-weight-management-first-2014).

12. Davidson MH, Hauptman J, DiGirolamo M, et al. Weight control and risk factor reduction in obese subjects treated for 2 years with orlistat: a randomized controlled trial. *JAMA* 1999;281:235–242.

13. Administration USFaD. *Statistical Review and Evaluation—NDA #20–766/Class 1S*. 1997:1–16.

14. Administration USFaD. *Center for Drug Evaluation and Research—Application Number: 21–887*. 2007:1–61.

15. Leblanc ES, O'Connor E, Whitlock EP, Patnode CD, Kapka T. Effectiveness of primary care-relevant treatments for obesity in adults: a systematic evidence review for the U.S. Preventive Services Task Force. *Ann Intern Med* 2011;155:434–447.

16. Torgerson JS, Hauptman J, Boldrin MN, Sjostrom L. XENical in the prevention of diabetes in obese subjects (XENDOS) study: a randomized study of orlistat as an adjunct to lifestyle changes for the prevention of type 2 diabetes in obese patients. *Diabetes Care* 2004;27:155–161.

17. Zelber-Sagi S, Kessler A, Brazowsky E, et al. A double-blind randomized placebo-controlled trial of orlistat for the treatment of nonalcoholic fatty liver disease. *Clin Gastroenterol Hepatol* 2006;4:639–644.

18. Harrison SA, Fecht W, Brunt EM, Neuschwander-Tetri BA. Orlistat for overweight subjects with nonalcoholic steatohepatitis: a randomized, prospective trial. *Hepatology* 2009;49:80–86.

19. Ali Khan R, Kapur P, Jain A, Farah F, Bhandari U. Effect of orlistat on periostin, adiponectin, inflammatory markers and ultrasound grades of fatty liver in obese NAFLD patients. *Ther Clin Risk Manag* 2017;13:139–149.

20. Wang H, Wang L, Cheng Y, Xia Z, Liao Y, Cao J. Efficacy of orlistat in non-alcoholic fatty liver disease: a systematic review and meta-analysis. *Biomed Rep* 2018;9:90–96.

21. Fan ZQD, Xie W, Hu H, Chen Y, Sun Z, Liu S, Zeng MC. Clinical study of obesity associated non-alcoholic fatty liver disease. *Chin Hepatol* 2004:155–158.

22. Padwal R, Li SK, Lau DC. Long-term pharmacotherapy for obesity and overweight. *Cochrane Database Syst Rev* 2003:CD004094.

23. Weir MA, Beyea MM, Gomes T, et al. Orlistat and acute kidney injury: an analysis of 953 patients. *Arch Intern Med* 2011;171:703–704.

24. Diseases NIoDaDaK. *LiverTox: Clinical and Research Information on Drug-Induced Liver Injury*.

25. *Highlights of Prescribing Information—QYSMIA*. 2012 (Accessed January 6, 2022, at www.accessdata.fda.gov/drugsatfda_docs/label/2012/022580s000lbl.pdf).

26. Gadde KM, Allison DB, Ryan DH, et al. Effects of low-dose, controlled-release, phentermine plus topiramate combination on weight and associated comorbidities in overweight and obese adults (CONQUER): a randomised, placebo-controlled, phase 3 trial. *Lancet* 2011;377:1341–1352.

27. Garvey WT, Ryan DH, Look M, et al. Two-year sustained weight loss and metabolic benefits with controlled-release phentermine/topiramate in obese and overweight adults (SEQUEL): a randomized, placebo-controlled, phase 3 extension study. *Am J Clin Nutr* 2012;95:297–308.

28. Allison DB, Gadde KM, Garvey WT, et al. Controlled-release phentermine/topiramate in severely obese adults: a randomized controlled trial (EQUIP). *Obesity (Silver Spring)* 2012;20:330–342.

29. *Highlights of Prescribing Information—CONTRAVE*, 2014 (Accessed January 19, 2022, 2022, at www.accessdata.fda.gov/drugsatfda_docs/label/2014/200063s000lbl.pdf).

30. Brown SA, Izzy M, Watt KD. Pharmacotherapy for weight loss in cirrhosis and liver transplantation: translating the data and underused potential. *Hepatology* 2021;73:2051–2062.

31. Bajaj HS, Burrows M, Blavignac J, et al. Extended-release naltrexone/bupropion and liver health: pooled,

post hoc analysis from four randomized controlled trials. *Diabetes Obes Metab* 2021;23:861–865.

32. Apovian CM, Aronne L, Rubino D, et al. A randomized, phase 3 trial of naltrexone SR/bupropion SR on weight and obesity-related risk factors (COR-II). *Obesity (Silver Spring)* 2013;21:935–943.

33. Greenway FL, Fujioka K, Plodkowski RA, et al. Effect of naltrexone plus bupropion on weight loss in overweight and obese adults (COR-I): a multicentre, randomised, double-blind, placebo-controlled, phase 3 trial. *Lancet* 2010;376:595–605.

34. *Highlights of Prescribing Information—SAXENDA.* 2014 (Accessed January 19, 2022, at www.accessdata.fda.gov/drugsatfda_docs/label/2014/206321Orig1s000lbl.pdf).

35. *Highlights of Prescribing Information—WEGOVY.* 2017. (Accessed January 19, 2022, at www.accessdata.fda.gov/drugsatfda_docs/label/2021/215256s000lbl.pdf).

36. Armstrong MJ, Hull D, Guo K, et al. Glucagon-like peptide 1 decreases lipotoxicity in non-alcoholic steato-hepatitis. *J Hepatol* 2016;64:399–408.

37. Pi-Sunyer X, Astrup A, Fujioka K, et al. A randomized, controlled trial of 3.0 mg of liraglutide in weight management. *N Engl J Med* 2015;373:11–22.

38. Armstrong MJ, Gaunt P, Aithal GP, et al. Liraglutide safety and efficacy in patients with non-alcoholic steatohepatitis (LEAN): a multicentre, double-blind, randomised, placebo-controlled phase 2 study. *Lancet* 2016;387:679–690.

39. Khoo J, Hsiang JC, Taneja R, et al. Randomized trial comparing effects of weight loss by liraglutide with lifestyle modification in non-alcoholic fatty liver disease. *Liver Int* 2019;39:941–949.

40. Wilding JPH, Batterham RL, Calanna S, et al. Once-weekly semaglutide in adults with overweight or obesity. *N Engl J Med* 2021;384:989.

41. Davies M, Faerch L, Jeppesen OK, et al. Semaglutide 2.4 mg once a week in adults with overweight or obesity, and type 2 diabetes (STEP 2): a randomised, double-blind, double-dummy, placebo-controlled, phase 3 trial. *Lancet* 2021;397:971–984.

42. Wadden TA, Bailey TS, Billings LK, et al. Effect of subcutaneous semaglutide vs placebo as an adjunct to intensive behavioral therapy on body weight in adults with overweight or obesity: the STEP 3 randomized clinical trial. *JAMA* 2021;325:1403–1413.

43. Rubino DM, Greenway FL, Khalid U, et al. Effect of weekly subcutaneous semaglutide vs daily liraglutide on body weight in adults with overweight or obesity without diabetes: the STEP 8 randomized clinical trial. *JAMA* 2022;327:138–150.

44. Newsome PN, Buchholtz K, Cusi K, et al. A placebo-controlled trial of subcutaneous semaglutide in nonalcoholic steatohepatitis. *N Engl J Med* 2021;384:1113–1124.

45. Zheng EX, Navarro VJ. Liver injury from herbal, dietary, and weight loss supplements: a review. *J Clin Transl Hepatol* 2015;3:93–98.

46. Bailey RL, Gahche JJ, Lentino CV, et al. Dietary supplement use in the United States, 2003–2006. *J Nutr* 2011;141:261–266.

47. Rashrash M, Schommer JC, Brown LM. Prevalence and predictors of herbal medicine use among adults in the United States. *J Patient Exp* 2017;4:108–113.

48. Ekor M. The growing use of herbal medicines: issues relating to adverse reactions and challenges in monitoring safety. *Front Pharmacol* 2014;4:177.

49. Navarro VJ, Barnhart H, Bonkovsky HL, et al. Liver injury from herbals and dietary supplements in the U.S. drug-induced liver injury network. *Hepatology* 2014;60:1399–1408.

50. Research GV. *Weight Loss Supplements Market Size, Share & Trends Analysis Report By End User, By Distribution Channel, By Type, By Ingredient, and Segment Forecasts, 2021–2028.* 2021.

51. Sarma DN, Barrett ML, Chavez ML, et al. Safety of green tea extracts: a systematic review by the US Pharmacopeia. *Drug Saf* 2008;31:469–484.

52. Lambert JD, Kennett MJ, Sang S, Reuhl KR, Ju J, Yang CS. Hepatotoxicity of high oral dose (-)-epigallocatechin-3-gallate in mice. *Food Chem Toxicol* 2010;48:409–416.

53. Walter J, Navarro V, Rossi S. Drug-induced liver injury associated with weight loss supplements. *Curr Hepatol Rep* 2018;17:245–253.

54. Kim YJ, Choi MS, Park YB, Kim SR, Lee MK, Jung UJ. Garcinia Cambogia attenuates diet-induced adiposity but exacerbates hepatic collagen accumulation and inflammation. *World J Gastroenterol* 2013;19:4689–4701.

55. Colman E. Dinitrophenol and obesity: an early twentieth-century regulatory dilemma. *Regul Toxicol Pharmacol* 2007;48:115–117.

56. Durazo FA, Lassman C, Han SH, et al. Fulminant liver failure due to usnic acid for weight loss. *Am J Gastroenterol* 2004;99:950–952.

57. Ramos R, Mascarenhas J, Duarte P, Vicente C, Casteleiro C. Conjugated linoleic acid-induced toxic hepatitis: first case report. *Dig Dis Sci* 2009;54:1141–1143.

58. Bilal M, Patel Y, Burkitt M, Babich M. Linoleic acid induced acute hepatitis: a case report and review of the literature. *Case Reports Hepatol* 2015;2015:807354.

59. Nortadas R, Barata J. Fulminant hepatitis during self-medication with conjugated linoleic acid. *Ann Hepatol* 2012;11:265–267.

60. Daneshi-Maskooni M, Keshavarz SA, Qorbani M, et al. Green cardamom increases Sirtuin-1 and reduces inflammation in overweight or obese patients with non-alcoholic fatty liver disease: a double-blind randomized placebo-controlled clinical trial. *Nutr Metab (Lond)* 2018;15:63.

61. Di Pierro F, Bressan A, Ranaldi D, Rapacioli G, Giacomelli L, Bertuccioli A. Potential role of bioavailable curcumin in weight loss and omental adipose tissue decrease: preliminary data of a randomized, controlled trial in overweight people with metabolic syndrome. Preliminary study. *Eur Rev Med Pharmacol Sci* 2015;19:4195–4202.

62. Jalali M, Mahmoodi M, Mosallanezhad Z, Jalali R, Imanieh MH, Moosavian SP. The effects of curcumin supplementation on liver function, metabolic profile and body composition in patients with non-alcoholic fatty liver disease: a systematic review and meta-analysis of randomized controlled trials. *Complement Ther Med* 2020;48:102283.

63. Li N, Zhao H. Role of carnitine in non-alcoholic fatty liver disease and other related diseases: an update. *Front Med (Lausanne)* 2021;8:689042.

64. Askarpour M, Hadi A, Miraghajani M, Symonds ME, Sheikhi A, Ghaedi E. Beneficial effects of l-carnitine supplementation for weight management in overweight and obese adults: an updated systematic review and dose-response meta-analysis of randomized controlled trials. *Pharmacol Res* 2020;151:104554.

65. Somi MH, Fatahi E, Panahi J, Havasian MR, Judaki A. Data from a randomized and controlled trial of LCarnitine prescription for the treatment for Non-Alcoholic Fatty Liver Disease. *Bioinformation* 2014;10:575–579.

66. Malaguarnera M, Gargante MP, Russo C, et al. L-carnitine supplementation to diet: a new tool in treatment of nonalcoholic steatohepatitis--a randomized and controlled clinical trial. *Am J Gastroenterol* 2010;105:1338–1345.

67. Abolfathi M, Mohd-Yusof BN, Hanipah ZN, Mohd Redzwan S, Yusof LM, Khosroshahi MZ. The effects of carnitine supplementation on clinical characteristics of patients with non-alcoholic fatty liver disease: a systematic review and meta-analysis of randomized controlled trials. *Complement Ther Med* 2020;48:102273.

68. Lim CY, Jun DW, Jang SS, Cho WK, Chae JD, Jun JH. Effects of carnitine on peripheral blood mitochondrial DNA copy number and liver function in non-alcoholic fatty liver disease. *Korean J Gastroenterol* 2010;55:384–389.

69. Bae JC, Lee WY, Yoon KH, et al. Improvement of nonalcoholic fatty liver disease with carnitine-orotate complex in type 2 diabetes (CORONA): a randomized controlled trial. *Diabetes Care* 2015;38:1245–1252.

70. Hong ES, Kim EK, Kang SM, et al. Effect of carnitine-orotate complex on glucose metabolism and fatty liver: a double-blind, placebo-controlled study. *J Gastroenterol Hepatol* 2014;29:1449–1457.

71. Alavinejad P, Zakerkish M, Hajiani E, Hashemi SJ, Chobineh M, Moghaddam EK. Evaluation of L-carnitine efficacy in the treatment of non-alcoholic fatty liver disease among diabetic patients: a randomized double blind pilot study. *J Gastroenterol Hepatol Res* 2016;5:2191–2195.

72. Frias JP, Davies MJ, Rosenstock J, et al. Tirzepatide versus semaglutide once weekly in patients with type 2 diabetes. *N Engl J Med* 2021;385:503–515.

73. Saxena AR, Gorman DN, Esquejo RM, et al. Danuglipron (PF-06882961) in type 2 diabetes: a randomized, placebo-controlled, multiple ascending-dose phase 1 trial. *Nat Med* 2021;27:1079–1087.

74. *The Effect of SHR20004 (Noiiglutide) on Body Weight in Obese Subjects Without Diabetes* (Accessed January 27, 2022, at https://clinicaltrials.gov/ct2/show/NCT04799327?cond=noiiglutide&draw=2&rank=1).

75. Nahra R, Wang T, Gadde KM, et al. Effects of cotadutide on metabolic and hepatic parameters in adults with overweight or obesity and type 2 diabetes: a 54-week randomized phase 2b study. *Diabetes Care* 2021;44:1433–1442.

12 De Novo Lipogenesis Inhibitors

Brent A. Neuschwander-Tetri

CONTENTS

Key Points

- De novo lipogenesis, or the synthesis of fatty acids from metabolic precursor substrates such as carbohydrates and amino acids, is a necessary metabolic pathway in all cell types to meet the demands for synthesizing cell and organelle membranes and production of molecules with fatty acid components.

- A high level of de novo lipogenesis is also a requisite pathway for tissues that make and secrete triglyceride (e.g., hepatocytes, enterocytes and milk-producing mammary epithelial cells).

- Because excess production or availability of fatty acids in hepatocytes is linked to the generation of lipotoxic species when disposal routes are impaired or overwhelmed, de novo lipogenesis has been identified as a potentially viable target in treating patients with NASH.

- For hepatocytes, the major source of fatty acids is their uptake from the circulation. However, de novo lipogenesis may contribute up to 25–38% of the flux of fatty acids in the liver in patients with NAFLD.

- The enzymes of the de novo lipogenesis pathway have been targeted individually with small molecule inhibitors or globally at the level of gene expression with multiple agents that are now in clinical trials for patients with NASH.

12.1 INTRODUCTION

The ability to synthesize fatty acids from small molecule metabolic substrates, mainly carbohydrates and amino acids derived from the food that we eat, is found in all cell types to meet the universal demands for membrane synthesis as well as more cell-type specific requirements for specific fatty acid species. This process has been called de novo lipogenesis (DNL), or, literally, the synthesis of new fat. Some cell types also use the fatty acids synthesized through DNL to make large amounts of triglyceride for intracellular storage (e.g., adipocytes) or secretion (e.g., hepatocytes, enterocytes and milk-producing mammary epithelial cells). Whether the formation of triglyceride from fatty acids and glycerol can be considered part of DNL is not formally established. For the purpose of this chapter, DNL will be defined as the synthesis of fatty acids that can then be used by diverse metabolic processes that include the synthesis of membrane phospholipids, the synthesis of molecules that contain fatty acids (e.g., cholesterol esters, acyl-sonic hedgehog, acyl-ghrelin), and the synthesis of triglyceride (Figure 12.1). Also, the word "triglyceride" in this chapter will indicate both the singular and plural when referring to both single and many triglyceride molecules.

This chapter reviews fatty acid synthesis by first defining fatty acids, then discussing the steps in their biosynthesis, and finally discussing how these pathways are targeted with pharmacologic inhibitors as potential therapies for NASH.

12.2 FATTY ACIDS—WHAT ARE THEY?

Soap. In our daily lives, we most often encounter free fatty acids outside of our body in the form of soap. In the reverse of what happens when cells make triglyceride from three fatty acid molecules bound covalently to a glycerol molecule, triglyceride from vegetable fat (e.g., olive oil) or animal fat (e.g., tallow) is treated in a factory with a strong base such as sodium hydroxide (lye) to break the covalent ester bonds between the fatty acids and glycerol to generate a mixture of free fatty acids and glycerol in a 3:1 ratio. This process of producing soap has been known to humankind for millennia because of the beneficial

DOI: 10.1201/9781003386698-15

ability of the free fatty acids to be somewhat water soluble and mix with other lipophilic molecules (e.g., skin oil) and solubilize them to act as effective cleansing agents. They also break down bacterial lipid membranes and are thus antiseptic as well.

As wonderful as it is to have something with such valuable properties for removing excess oils from our skin, clothes, cookware and other items needing regular cleaning and disinfecting, these molecules are inherently dangerous to the cells that produce them because they can solubilize cell membranes or facilitate the generation of other damaging lipids if not carefully constrained. The level of that control is the highly regulated process of de novo lipogenesis as well as the production of proteins that avidly bind free fatty acids to take them where they belong and prevent them from acting as soap within our circulation and cells. In the circulation, albumin serves this purpose and in the cytoplasm of cells, a variety of tissue-specific fatty acid binding proteins (FABPs) serve this purpose.

Fatty acids are produced in a wide variety of species with respect to chain length and the number and position of double bonds. Plants also produce branched chain fatty acids. In terms of chain length, they can range from 2 carbons to well over 20 carbons in length. The lone carboxyl group on one end is not enough to keep fatty acids with chain lengths over about 26 carbons in aqueous solution to be useful as soaps. One the other hand, the shortest "fatty" acid is the 2-carbon acetic acid (i.e., vinegar when in an aqueous solution). The shorter fatty acids are not only quite soluble but also volatile. The smell of acetic acid is familiar to anyone who enjoys cooking or dying Easter eggs. Four carbon butyric acid contributes to the characteristically unpleasant smells of rotting food and body odor, whereas the 6 and 8 carbon fatty acids, caproic and caprylic acid, respectively, contribute to the characteristic pungency of goat cheeses.

12.3 SYNTHESIS OF FREE FATTY ACIDS: De Novo Lipogenesis

To make fatty acids, our cells start with citrate (citric acid) to generate acetyl-CoA in the cytoplasm (Figure 12.1). The citrate is generated by the mitochondrial tricarboxylic acid cycle ("Krebs cycle") using products of glucose, fructose and amino acid metabolism, and thus these dietary nutrients are the primary substrates for fat generation in the liver that starts with their conversion to citrate.

Stable isotope studies have been used to assess the relative contribution of DNL to the flux of fatty acids in the liver, and these studies have shown that in the normal liver, DNL contributes only about 5–10% to this flux. The predominant source of fatty acids in hepatocytes is lipolysis of adipocyte triglyceride[1,2] with the release of free fatty acids into the circulation where they are carried by albumin to the liver and other tissues that can take up free fatty acids. In patients with NAFLD, however, DNL provides more fatty acids to the flux, contributing up to 25–38% of the fatty acid flux in the liver.[1,2] The concept of "flux" through the liver is used because the actual amount of free fatty acids in the liver varies within a relatively small range when the supply is increased. A good metaphor may be a garden hose in which the volume of water in the hose does not increase much even as the flow, or flux, increases.

While the focus on inhibiting DNL as a treatment for NASH has been on the role of this pathway in hepatocytes, it should be noted that DNL also appears to be important for hepatic stellate cell activation. Thus it is conceivable or perhaps even likely that inhibiting DNL in stellate cells could have direct antifibrotic effects.[3,4]

A comment about the role of substrate availability for DNL is essential in the context of fatty liver disease. Excessive DNL would generally not occur without excessive substrate availability. While amino acids are a source of precursors to produce citrate, they are a minor source, even with high dietary protein intake. Carbohydrates are the major source. In terms of the typical diet, this comes down to glucose (mostly from starches, e.g., bread, rice, pasta) and the glucose-fructose disaccharide sucrose (table sugar) that is rapidly cleaved to glucose and fructose in the small intestine by enterocyte sucrase-isomaltase. Also fructose itself is commonly mixed with glucose in our foods and drinks as high-fructose corn syrup.[5] Thus an effective approach to curbing the contribution of DNL to NASH is to curtail the dietary intake of excessive carbohydrate substrates for DNL.[6,7]

12.3.1 Measuring DNL

Measuring DNL is important for understanding its role in NAFLD and assessing the impact of pharmacological treatments that target this pathway. The most accurate method is to measure the incorporation of intravenously administered stable isotope-labeled substrates (e.g., ^{13}C-acetate, ^2H_2O) into serum lipids.[2,8,9] Other surrogate methods that are simpler but less accurate include measuring tripalmitin (triglyceride composed of 3 palmitic acid chains and glycerol) in serum lipids[10] or incorporation of palmitoleate (C16:1, i.e., 16 carbon fatty acid with one double bond) into serum triglyceride.[11]

Next is a discussion of each of the sequential steps in DNL that lead to the formation of fatty acids of various chain lengths and degrees of desaturation (i.e., introduction of double bonds between specific carbons; a saturated fatty acid has no carbon–carbon double bonds).

12.3.2 ATP-citrate Lyase (ACLY, ACL)

Although acetyl-Co-enzyme A (acetyl-CoA) is often thought of as the starting metabolic substrate for DNL, one step upstream from acetyl CoA is its formation from citrate. Citrate is a product of the mitochondrial tricarboxylic acid cycle when this cycle is fed by excess pyruvate, itself a product of excess glucose and fructose metabolism. Pyruvate is transported into the mitochondrial by the mitochondrial pyruvate transporter (MPC). Pharmacologically inhibiting this transporter has been evaluated as a treatment for NASH, and it has improved a number of metabolic parameters but has not had significant histological effects on improving NASH in a phase 2 study.[12] Transport of citrate out of the mitochondria is handled by the protein Slc25a1, and inhibition of this carrier has been shown to have benefits in NASH in mouse models[13] but has not been evaluated in clinical trials. Once in the cytosol where DNL occurs, citrate is used by the enzyme ATP-citrate lyase (ACLY or ACL) along with ATP and coenzyme A to make acetyl-CoA and oxaloacetate. Hepatic ACLY is overexpressed in NASH, compared to NAFL, and in the normal liver, which has been attributed to differential epigenetic DNA methylation.[14]

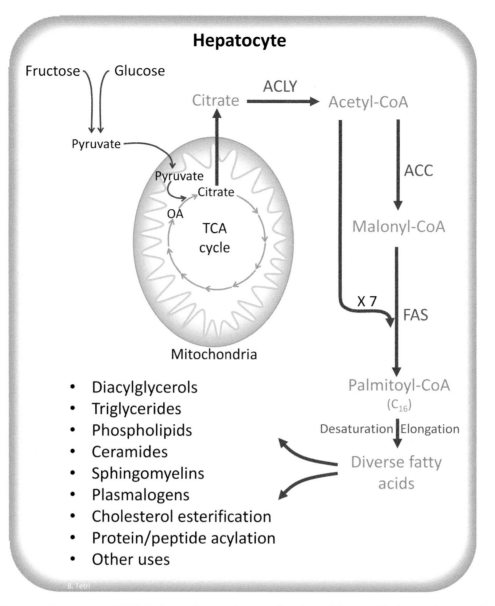

Figure 12.1 De novo lipogenesis (DNL) is the pathway of generating "new" fatty acids from other metabolic substrates, primarily carbohydrates and, to a lesser extent, amino acids.

Glycolysis, fructose metabolism and catabolic pathways that metabolize amino acids generate pyruvate that is taken up by mitochondria to generate citrate via the tricarboxylic acid (Krebs) cycle. Citrate is a substrate for cytosolic ACLY to generate acetyl-CoA, which is then built upon 2 carbons at a time to generate the 16-carbon saturated fatty acid palmitate. At that point, the palmitate can be desaturated and elongated to generate palmitoleate, stearate and oleate. These are the major fatty acids used to form a variety of lipid species that play essential roles in cell signaling (e.g., diacylglycerols, ceramides, sphingolipids), fat storage (e.g., triglyceride), membrane structure (e.g., phospholipids), cholesterol esterification and post-translational modification of protein (e.g., acylation). ACLY: ATP-citrate lyase; ACC: Acetyl-CoA carboxylase; FAS: Fatty acid synthetase; OA: Oxaloacetate; TCA: Tricarboxylic acid.

12.3.3 Acyl-CoA Carboxylase (ACC)

The enzyme ACC creates the metabolic intermediary malonyl-CoA from acetyl-CoA and bicarbonate and is the rate-controlling step in DNL. The product, malonyl-CoA, plays a critical regulatory role in fatty acid oxidation by inhibiting the transport of fatty acids into the mitochondria for beta-oxidation. This is a logical response to a surfeit of acetyl-CoA, which generally occurs when there is an abundance of energy substrates, i.e., glucose and fructose, and the oxidation of fatty acids by the mitochondria is not needed for ATP generation. Malonyl-CoA is also the precursor for cholesterol synthesis, and thus reducing its formation could have hypothetical benefits with respect to cellular and mitochondrial dysfunction caused by excess cholesterol as well as reduced cardiovascular disease risk. Given the central role of ACC in de novo lipogenesis, it is highly regulated by multiple endogenous mechanisms. ACC is inhibited by AMPK-mediated phosphorylation, a logical response to energy deprivation when converting metabolic substrates to an energy storage form (fat) is not warranted. It is also subject to feedback inhibition by palmitate, the primary product of DNL. Animal studies demonstrated that deletion or inhibition of ACC prevents fatty liver, whereas overactivation causes a NASH phenotype.[15] ACC is found in two similar isoforms, ACC1 in the hepatocyte cytoplasm and ACC2, which is predominantly in muscle where it is anchored to mitochondria. A newly discovered regulatory mechanism of ACC is a nonenzymatic protein–protein interaction with arachidonate 12-lipoxygenase (ALOX12) that prevents ACC1 degradation and thus promotes DNL and a NASH phenotype.[16]

12.3.4 Fatty Acid Synthase (FAS)
Using the malonyl-CoA generated by ACC, the aptly named enzyme fatty acid synthetase complex (FAS or FASN, both are used; *FASN* is the gene name) is a multiprotein complex that progressively lengthens the nascent fatty acid chain by using 2 carbon acetate attached to CoA to produce progressively lengthened acyl CoA species with even numbers of carbons up to C_{16} (palmitoyl-CoA).[9]

12.3.5 Further Elongation
ELOVL6 elongates palmitate generated by FAS to stearate, and this conversion was demonstrated to be important in generating lipid species that mediate insulin resistance and inflammation in mice and human liver tissue.[17] Moreover, this study demonstrated that impairing ELOVL6 expression in mice does not reduce steatosis, but it does reduce insulin resistance and cell injury. This adds to the evidence that the accumulation of triglyceride in the liver is not the cause of injury and insulin resistance, but it is a lipid species other than triglyceride that is the mediator of NASH.[18–20] Elongase inhibitors are currently not in development for the treatment of NASH.

12.3.6 Introduction of Double Bonds (Desaturation)
Fatty acid synthase produces fully saturate fatty acids, i.e., fatty acids without any double bonds between carbons. Double bonds in the carbon skeleton of fatty acids are important in increasing membrane fluidity, and the introduction of double bonds is the primary function of the family of stearoyl-CoA desaturases (SCDs).[21] The biological importance of double bonds in fatty acids cannot be overstated. The double bonds put a relatively inflexible bend in the fatty acid chain that creates some disorganization in membranes and makes them less likely to form organized solid structures. The impact of this is readily observed in our foods. When the fatty acids in triglyceride are mostly saturated, the fat is typically solid at room temperature. Vegetable shortening, butter and beef fat are good examples. When triglyceride contains abundant fatty acids that have even one double bond, the result is a reduced propensity to solidify at room temperature. Olive oil is a great example of that. These physicochemical properties are relevant not only to our food characteristics but also to the membrane fluidity of our cells and their organelles. Reduction in the availability of unsaturated fatty acids for membranes increases membrane stiffness and impairs the function of many membrane-bound proteins.[22] In the context of NASH, saturated fatty acids are commonly used in cell culture models to induce cell stress, whereas adding unsaturated fatty acids such as oleic acid to the culture media can prevent cell stress and death induced by the addition of saturated fatty acids.[23]

12.4 REGULATION OF DE NOVO LIPOGENESIS
Because fatty acids are inherently toxic to cells, their production is highly regulated at the substrate level as well as in the transcriptional regulation of the enzymes just described. In recognition of the potential role of DNL in NASH, the enzymes of DNL and their transcriptional regulation have been identified as reasonable targets of therapy.[24]

12.4.1 Substrate Availability
Since glycolysis is a major source of pyruvate, which is used by the mitochondria to make citrate that feed into the DNL, the uptake and fate of glucose in hepatocytes is highly regulated.[25] The handling of dietary fructose is different in that fructose uptake by hepatocytes is not regulated. It is taken up and trapped in the hepatocyte by phosphorylation by hexokinase using ATP as a substrate. Some of it can be converted to glucose which can be stored as glycogen, but much of it is converted into pyruvate, the precursor for DNL. Results of a phase 2a clinical trial of a ketohexokinase inhibitor PF-06835919 demonstrated reduction in liver fat,[26] but the further development of this agent is uncertain.

12.4.2 Transcriptional Regulation
A master regulator controlling the expression of the genes for the enzymes of DNL is the transcription factor sterol regulatory element-binding protein-1c (SREBP-1c).[27] The expression of all of the DNL enzymes is regulated by SREBP-1c. Because if its central role in lipid metabolism is in the liver, the regulation of SREBP-1c is complex and controlled transcriptionally and post-transcriptionally. Insulin is a driver of SREBP-1c expression, but the protein also requires translocation from the ER to the Golgi and then to the nucleus, a process involving multiple regulatory proteins.[28,29]

Other important transcription regulators of the enzymes of DNL include carbohydrate response element binding protein (ChREBP), LXR and PPARα.[30] As its name suggests, ChREBP is activated by increased carbohydrates as a mechanism to convert those carbohydrates to fat for storage. Like SREBP1c, ChREBP is highly regulated transcriptionally and post-transcriptionally to respond dynamically to fluctuating nutritional conditions.[31]

12.5 PHARMACOLOGIC INHIBITION OF DE NOVO LIPOGENESIS AS A TREATMENT OF NASH
Because DNL can contribute up to 25–38% of the fatty acid flux through the liver and these fatty acids contribute to the development of NASH, DNL has been identified as a potential therapy for NASH.[32] Lifestyle modifications with a focus on healthy eating habits is the primary approach to reduce the consumption of excess substrates for DNL such as glucose, fructose, sucrose (glucose-fructose disaccharide), and starches (glucose polymers). Pharmacological approaches include specifically targeting the enzymes of DNL or reducing their expression at the transcriptional level (Figure 12.2). Multiple drugs that target the steps of DNL to improve NASH are in development (Table 12.1).

12.5.1 Inhibition of ACLY
Animal studies of the ACLY inhibitor bempedoic acid have shown beneficial effects in NASH models, but there are currently no major clinical trials of ACLY inhibitors to treat patients with NASH. ACLY inhibitors have been developed primarily for the treatment of hyperlipidemia[33], and bempedoic acid was approved in the US for this purpose in 2021. Bempedoic acid is a prodrug that requires enzymatic activation by thioesterification with coenzyme A. This is achieved by the liver-specific enzyme

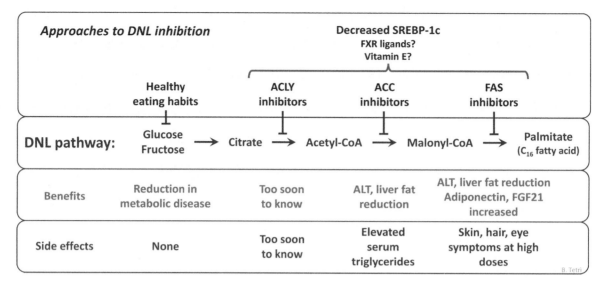

Figure 12.2 Approaches to reducing DNL in patients with NASH.

Reduction in excess dietary sugars limits the substrate for DNL and should always be the first recommendation. Specific inhibitors of the DNL pathway as well as global inhibitors of the expression of the DNL pathway enzymes are in clinical development.

SREBP-1c: Sterol regulatory element binding protein-1c; FXR: Farnesoid X receptor; ACLY: ATP-citrate lyase; ACC: Acetyl-CoA carboxylase; FAS: Fatty acid synthase.

Table 12.1: Drugs That Regulate Hepatic De Novo Lipogenesis in Clinical Trials for NASH

Drug	Patients	Clinical Trials Number(s)	Results
ACC inhibitors			
Fircosostat (GS-0976)	F1–3	NCT02856555	37,41
with FXR ligand cilofexor (ATLAS)	F3–4	NCT03449446	38
with FXR ligand cilofexor and GLP1RA semaglutide	F2–3	NCT03987074	
with FXR ligand cilofexor and GLP1RA semaglutide	F4	NCT04971785	
Clesacostat (PF-05221304)		NCT03248882	44
with DGAT2 inhibitor ervogastat		NCT03776175	44
MK-4074		NCT01431521	39
with DGAT2 inhibitor ervogastat	F2–3	NCT04321031	Ongoing
FAS inhibitors			
TVB-2640 (FASCINATE-1)	F1–3	NCT03938246	10
TVB-2640 (FASCINATE-2)	F2–3	NCT04906421	
FT-4101	F2–3	NCT04004325	46
SCD inhibitors			
Aramchol (ARMOR)	F0–3	NCT04104321	51
Transcriptional regulators of DNL			
FXR ligands			
Obeticholic acid (REGENERATE)	F1–3	NCT02548351	65
Tropifexor (FLIGHT-FXR)		NCT02855164	
EDP-305	F1–3	NCT03421431	66
TERN-101		NCT04328077	
Vitamin E			
DGAT-2 inhibitors			
Ervogastat (PF-06865571)	F2–3	NCT04321031	
IONIS-DGAT2Rx	NAFLD	NCT03334214	64

very-long-chain acyl-CoA synthetase 1, which likely restricts its pharmacologic effects to the liver. The reported side effects in clinical trials were minimal, but the product of ACLY, acetyl-CoA, is used metabolically for so many diverse processes (e.g., histone acetylation, phase 2 detoxifying reactions) that caution may still be warranted during its early clinical use.

12.5.2 Inhibition of ACC

Because ACC is a major regulator of DNL and also as a source of malonyl-CoA for cholesterol synthesis, this enzyme has been identified as a possible target for treating NASH and the metabolic syndrome.[34] The drug in this class furthest along in development is firsocostat (GS-0976, ND-630), a drug designed to induce the same inhibitory conformational change in the enzyme structure as AMPK-mediated phosphorylation, a key endogenous inhibitor of ACC activity[35] while having characteristics that target it for liver-specific uptake.[36] A phase 2a study confirmed reduction in DNL, steatosis and serum ALT levels[37], and a phase 2b study showed histologic improvement when combined with the FXR ligand cilofexor.[38]

Firsocostat was found to increase serum triglycerides in rodents studies,[39,40] and this was also found in the clinical trials where pretreatment of hypertriglyceridemia with firsocostat was predictive of further increases.[39,41] This potentially undesirable effect is thought to be due to the decrease in fatty acid production by DNL leading to decreased formation of polyunsaturated fatty acids causing decreased activation of PPARα leading to increased VLDL secretion.[39] Supporting this explanation was that coadministration of the PPARα ligand fenofibrate was shown to prevent the rise in serum triglycerides caused by ACC inhibitors.[42]

Other inhibitors of ACC that have been in development include clesacostat (PF-05221304), another liver-specific inhibitor that demonstrated beneficial effects in preclinical models.[43] A 16-week phase 2a trial (NCT03248882) demonstrated dose-dependent reduction in liver fat and serum ALT, and it was also evaluated in combination with the DGAT2 inhibitor ervogastat (PF-06865571), which blunted the rise in serum triglycerides (NCT03776175).[44] The ACC inhibitor MK-4074 has also been shown to reduce DNL and liver fat in a phase 1 study[39] but was not in any registered clinical trials in the US as of early 2022. Interestingly, one ACC inhibitor that was not liver-targeted, PF-05175157, was withdrawn from development due to thrombocytopenia in humans but not dogs or rodents. This observation led to the discovery that DNL (but not subsequent triglyceride synthesis) is needed for megakaryocyte maturation, thus highlighting the need for ACC inhibitors that are targeted to the liver.[45]

12.5.3 Inhibition of FAS

Using the malonyl-CoA generated from ACC and sequentially adding an additional seven molecules of acetyl-CoA, FAS generates the 16-carbon fatty acid palmitate. Pharmacologic inhibition of FAS as a means of inhibiting DNL is most advanced with the oral drug TVB-2640. A phase 2a study of 25 or 50 mg daily for 12 weeks demonstrated a dose response in reduction of liver fat measured by MRI-PDFF with a >30% fat reduction of 11%, 23%, 61% in placebo-treated, 25 mg, and 50 mg groups, respectively.[10] Reductions were also observed in serum ALT, LDL cholesterol, Pro-C3, and TIMP levels with favorable increases

in serum FGF21 and adiponectin levels. Higher doses of TVB-2640 have been evaluated in cancer patients as an adjunctive means of reducing tumor growth, and the dose-limiting toxicities found in those studies included reversible skin dryness, hair loss and ocular symptoms. At least one other FAS inhibitor, FT-4101, is in clinical development for NASH with early studies showing dose-dependent reductions in DNL and liver fat content.[46]

12.5.4 Inhibition of SCD

Inhibition of stearoyl-CoA desaturase-1 (SCD-1) is thought to underlie the benefits of the fatty acid-bile salt conjugate Aramchol in animal models of NASH and early human trials.[47,48] While the availability of desaturated fatty acids for the formation of diacylglycerol molecules (DAGs) and triglyceride that contain unsaturated fatty acids has been demonstrated in cell culture models to prevent lipotoxicity from saturated fatty acids,[49] the empirical data from human studies have not validated this concern. It may be that the increased fatty acid partitioning to oxidative disposal pathways promoted by SCD-1 inhibition results in a net benefit.[50] Aramchol was evaluated in a 52-week clinical trial where it did not meet the primary endpoint of liver fat reduction by MRI-PDFF, but potentially beneficial reductions in ALT and other markers were noted.[51] A large phase 3 trial of Aramchol with primary endpoints of NASH resolution without worsening of fibrosis or of fibrosis improvement without worsening of NASH is now underway (ARMOR, NCT04104321).

12.5.5 Targeting Transcriptional Expression of the DNL Pathway Enzymes

Because SREBP-1c transcriptionally induces the expression of all the enzymes responsible for DNL,[52] targeting its expression or activation may be a logical approach to diminishing the contribution of DNL to lipotoxic injury in NASH. One of the many pleiotropic effects of the FXR ligands currently in development of NASH (e.g., obeticholic acid, cilofexor, tropifexor, nidufexor, vonafexor, EDP-305, TERN-101) is the upregulation of small heterodimer partner-1 (SHP-1) expression. SHP-1 interferes with nuclear transcriptional complexes to generally inhibit the expression of many proteins including *CYP7a1* (and thus decrease bile salt synthesis from cholesterol) and *SREPBF1*, the gene encoding SREBP-1c.[53] Whether downregulating SREBP1c expression is the dominant or even relevant mechanism of the benefits of FXR ligands in NASH needs to be further clarified.[54] Preventing the activation of SREBP1c by impairing its translocation from the ER to the nucleus could also be a viable approach to reducing DNL. Interestingly, studies using HepG2 cells and human hepatocytes in culture have demonstrated that the beneficial effects of vitamin E in NASH may be mediated by interfering with oxidant stress-induced SREBP1c translocation/activation.[55] Consistent with these studies, a substantial reduction in liver fat content was found in the placebo-controlled randomized trial of vitamin E in patients with NASH.[56]

12.5.6 Targeting Conversion of Fatty Acids to Triglyceride

Although the formation triglyceride from 3 free fatty acid molecules and 1 glycerol molecule may not be included in the definition of de novo lipogenesis as just discussed, this pathway has also been targeted with the idea that the formation and accumulation of triglyceride contribute to the pathogenesis of NASH and its comorbidities such as insulin resistance.[57] However, mechanistic data have accumulated over the past 2 decades demonstrating that triglyceride is a relatively inert storage form of fat and that thus its formation is a protective adaptation to an oversupply of fatty acids.[18–20,58–60] Early preclinical data suggested that impairing the formation of triglyceride might predispose to lipotoxic liver injury,[61] but further animal studies and human clinical trial data suggest that impairing triglyceride formation promotes disposal of fatty acids through beneficial oxidative pathways.[62,63] Multiple approaches to inhibit the final step in triglyceride synthesis mediated by diacylglycerol acyltransferase-2 (DGAT2) are being explored with a focus in siRNA approaches. One such preliminary trial demonstrated reduction in liver fat,[64] and a larger phase 2b trial is underway examining the effects of ervostastat (PF-06865571) with or without the ACC inhibitor clesacostat (Pfizer PF-05221304) on liver fat content and liver histology (NCT04321031).

12.6 CONCLUSION/SUMMARY POINTS

The endogenous production of free fatty acids in the liver contributes to the development of NASH, and thus inhibiting this de novo lipogenesis pathway is a logical target for reversing NASH. A focus on healthy eating habits with curbing the consumption of glucose, fructose, sucrose and starches limits the substrates for DNL and is thus the primary recommendation for patients with NASH. When that is not successful, limiting the impact of conversion of sugar into fatty acids appears to be a viable option based on limited data from clinical trials of these agents. Because the release of fatty acids from adipose tissue is the major source of fatty acids delivered to the liver, DNL inhibitors might be ideal candidates to be paired with approaches that increase disposal of fatty acids through peripheral and hepatic oxidative pathways or prevent their release from dysfunctional adipose tissue.

REFERENCES

1. Donnelly KL, Smith CI, Schwarzenberg SJ, Jessurun J, Boldt MD, Parks EJ. Sources of fatty acids stored in liver and secreted via lipoproteins in patients with nonalcoholic fatty liver disease. *J Clin Invest.* 2005;115(5):1343–1351.

2. Smith GI, Shankaran M, Yoshino M, et al. Insulin resistance drives hepatic de novo lipogenesis in nonalcoholic fatty liver disease. *J Clin Invest.* 2020;130(3):1453–1460.

3. Bates J, Vijayakumar A, Ghoshal S, et al. Acetyl-CoA carboxylase inhibition disrupts metabolic reprogramming during hepatic stellate cell activation. *J Hepatol.* 2020;73(4):896–905.

4. Trivedi P, Wang S, Friedman SL. The power of plasticity--metabolic regulation of hepatic stellate cells. *Cell Metab.* 2021;33(2):242–257.

5. Tappy L, Lê K-A. Metabolic effects of fructose and the worldwide increase in obesity. *Physiol Rev.* 2010;90(1):23–46.

6. Bray GA, Nielsen SJ, Popkin BM. Consumption of high-fructose corn syrup in beverages may play a role in the epidemic of obesity. *Am J Clin Nutr.* 2004;79(4):537–543.

7. Sullivan S. Implications of diet on nonalcoholic fatty liver disease. *Curr Opin Gastroenterol.* 2010;26(2):160–164.

8. Turner SM, Murphy EJ, Neese RA, et al. Measurement of TG synthesis and turnover in vivo by ^{2}H2O incorporation into the glycerol moiety and application of MIDA. *Am J Physiol Endocrinol Metab.* 2003;285(4):E790–803.

9. Paglialunga S, Dehn CA. Clinical assessment of hepatic de novo lipogenesis in non-alcoholic fatty liver disease. *Lipids Health Dis.* 2016;15(1):159.

10. Loomba R, Mohseni R, Lucas KJ, et al. TVB-2640 (FASN inhibitor) for the treatment of nonalcoholic steatohepatitis: FASCINATE-1, a randomized, placebo-controlled phase 2a trial. *Gastroenterology.* 2021;161(5):1475–1486.

11. Lee JJ, Lambert JE, Hovhannisyan Y, et al. Palmitoleic acid is elevated in fatty liver disease and reflects hepatic lipogenesis. *Am J Clin Nutr.* 2015;101(1):34–43.

12. Harrison SA, Alkhouri N, Davison BA, et al. Insulin sensitizer MSDC-0602K in non-alcoholic steatohepatitis: a randomized, double-blind, placebo-controlled phase IIb study. *J Hepatol.* 2020;72(4):613–626.

13. Tan M, Mosaoa R, Graham GT, et al. Inhibition of the mitochondrial citrate carrier, Slc25a1, reverts steatosis, glucose intolerance, and inflammation in pre-clinical models of NAFLD/NASH. *Cell Death Differ.* 2020;27(7):2143–2157.

14. Ahrens M, Ammerpohl O, von Schonfels W, et al. DNA methylation analysis in nonalcoholic fatty liver disease suggests distinct disease-specific and remodeling signatures after bariatric surgery. *Cell Metab.* 2013;18(2):296–302.

15. Savage DB, Choi CS, Samuel VT, et al. Reversal of diet-induced hepatic steatosis and hepatic insulin resistance by antisense oligonucleotide inhibitors of acetyl-CoA carboxylases 1 and 2. *J Clin Invest.* 2006;116(3):817–824.

16. Zhang X-J, She Z-G, Wang J, et al. Multiple omics study identifies an interspecies conserved driver for nonalcoholic steatohepatitis. *Sci Transl Med.* 2021;13(624):eabg8117.

17. Matsuzaka T, Atsumi A, Matsumori R, et al. Elovl6 promotes nonalcoholic steatohepatitis. *Hepatology.* 2012;56(6):2199–2208.

18. Neuschwander-Tetri BA. Hepatic lipotoxicity and the pathogenesis of nonalcoholic steatohepatitis: the central role of nontriglyceride fatty acid metabolites. *Hepatology.* 2010;52(2):774–788.

19. Musso G, Cassader M, Paschetta E, Gambino R. Bioactive lipid species and metabolic pathways in progression and resolution of nonalcoholic steatohepatitis. *Gastroenterology.* 2018;155(2):282–302.

20. Geng Y, Faber KN, de Meijer VE, Blokzijl H, Moshage H. How does hepatic lipid accumulation lead to lipotoxicity in non-alcoholic fatty liver disease? *Hepatol Int.* 2021;15(1):21–35.

21. Hodson L, Fielding BA. Stearoyl-CoA desaturase: rogue or innocent bystander? *Prog Lipid Res.* 2013;52(1):15–42.

22. Harayama T, Riezman H. Understanding the diversity of membrane lipid composition. *Nat Rev Mol Cell Biol.* 2018;19(5):281–296.

23. Listenberger LL, Han X, Lewis SE, et al. Triglyceride accumulation protects against fatty acid-induced lipotoxicity. *Proc Natl Acad Sci USA.* 2003;100(6):3077–3082.

24. Neuschwander-Tetri BA. Therapeutic landscape for NAFLD in 2020. *Gastroenterology.* 2020;158(7):1984–1998.

25. Petersen MC, Vatner DF, Shulman GI. Regulation of hepatic glucose metabolism in health and disease. *Nat Rev Endocrinol.* 2017;13(10):572–587.

26. Kazierad DJ, Chidsey K, Somayaji VR, Bergman AJ, Birnbaum MJ, Calle RA. Inhibition of ketohexokinase in adults with NAFLD reduces liver fat and inflammatory markers: a randomized phase 2 trial. *Med.* 2021;2(7):800–813.

27. Shimano H. SREBPs: physiology and pathophysiology of the SREBP family. *Febs J.* 2009;276(3):616–621.

28. Brown MS, Radhakrishnan A, Goldstein JL. Retrospective on cholesterol homeostasis: the central role of SCAP. *Annu Rev Biochem.* 2018;87:783–807.

29. Su L, Zhou L, Chen F-J, et al. Cideb controls sterol-regulated ER export of SREBP/SCAP by promoting cargo loading at ER exit sites. *EMBO J.* 2019;38(8):e100156.

30. Jump DB. Fatty acid regulation of hepatic lipid metabolism. *Curr Opin Clin Nutr Metab Care.* 2011;14(2):115–120.

31. Ortega-Prieto P, Postic C. Carbohydrate sensing through the transcription factor ChREBP. *Front Genet.* 2019;10(472).

32. Batchuluun B, Pinkosky SL, Steinberg GR. Lipogenesis inhibitors: therapeutic opportunities and challenges. *Nat Rev Drug Discov.* 2022;21(4):283–305.

33. Pinkosky SL, Groot PHE, Lalwani ND, Steinberg GR. Targeting ATP-citrate lyase in hyperlipidemia and metabolic disorders. *Trends Mol Med.* 2017;23(11):1047–1063.

34. Tong L, Harwood HJ, Jr. Acetyl-coenzyme a carboxylases: versatile targets for drug discovery. *J Cell Biochem.* 2006;99(6):1476–1488.

35. Harriman G, Greenwood J, Bhat S, et al. Acetyl-CoA carboxylase inhibition by ND-630 reduces hepatic steatosis, improves insulin sensitivity, and modulates dyslipidemia in rats. *Proc Natl Acad Sci U S A.* 2016;113(13):E1796–1805.

36. Alkhouri N, Lawitz E, Noureddin M, DeFronzo R, Shulman GI. GS-0976 (Firsocostat): an investigational liver-directed acetyl-CoA carboxylase (ACC) inhibitor for the treatment of non-alcoholic steatohepatitis (NASH). *Expert Opin Investig Drugs.* 2020;29(2):135–141.

37. Lawitz EJ, Coste A, Poordad F, et al. Acetyl-CoA carboxylase inhibitor GS-0976 for 12 weeks reduces hepatic de novo lipogenesis and steatosis in patients with nonalcoholic steatohepatitis. *Clin Gastroenterol Hepatol.* 2018;16(12):1983–1991 e3.

38. Loomba R, Noureddin M, Kowdley KV, et al. Combination therapies including cilofexor and firsocostat for bridging fibrosis and cirrhosis attributable to NASH. *Hepatology.* 2021;73(2):625–643.

39. Kim CW, Addy C, Kusunoki J, et al. Acetyl CoA carboxylase inhibition reduces hepatic steatosis but elevates plasma triglycerides in mice and humans: a bedside to bench investigation. *Cell Metab.* 2017;26(2):394–406.

40. Goedeke L, Bates J, Vatner DF, et al. Acetyl-CoA carboxylase inhibition reverses NAFLD and hepatic insulin resistance but promotes hypertriglyceridemia in rodents. *Hepatology.* 2018;68(6):2197–2211.

41. Loomba R, Kayali Z, Noureddin M, et al. GS-0976 reduces hepatic steatosis and fibrosis markers in patients with nonalcoholic fatty liver disease. *Gastroenterology.* 2018;155(5):1463–1473.

42. Lawitz EJ, Bhandari BR, Ruane PJ, et al. Fenofibrate mitigates hypertriglyceridemia in nonalcoholic steatohepatitis patients treated with cilofexor/firsocostat. *Clin Gastroenterol Hepatol.* 2022;10. doi:1016/j.cgh.2021.12.044

43. Ross TT, Crowley C, Kelly KL, et al. Acetyl-CoA carboxylase inhibition improves multiple dimensions of NASH pathogenesis in model systems. *Cell Mol Gastroenterol Hepatol.* 2020;10(4):829–851.

44. Calle RA, Amin NB, Carvajal-Gonzalez S, et al. ACC inhibitor alone or co-administered with a DGAT2 inhibitor in patients with non-alcoholic fatty liver disease: two parallel, placebo-controlled, randomized phase 2a trials. *Nat Med.* 2021;27(10):1836–1848.

45. Kelly KL, Reagan WJ, Sonnenberg GE, et al. De novo lipogenesis is essential for platelet production in humans. *Nature Metabolism.* 2020;2(10):1163–1178.

46. Beysen C, Schroeder P, Wu E, et al. Inhibition of fatty acid synthase with FT-4101 safely reduces hepatic de novo lipogenesis and steatosis in obese subjects with non-alcoholic fatty liver disease: results from two early-phase randomized trials. *Diabetes Obes Metab.* 2021;23(3):700–710.

47. Leikin-Frenkel A, Gonen A, Shaish A, et al. Fatty acid bile acid conjugate inhibits hepatic stearoyl coenzyme a desaturase and is non-atherogenic. *Arch Med Res.* 2010;41(6):397–404.

48. Safadi R, Konikoff FM, Mahamid M, et al. The fatty acid-bile acid conjugate Aramchol reduces liver fat content in patients with nonalcoholic fatty liver disease. *Clin Gastroenterol Hepatol.* 2014;12(12):2085–2091.

49. Li ZZ, Berk M, McIntyre TM, Feldstein AE. Hepatic lipid partitioning and liver damage in nonalcoholic fatty liver disease: role of stearoyl-CoA desaturease. *J Biol Chem.* 2009;284(9):5637–5644.

50. Dobrzyn A, Ntambi JM. Stearoyl-CoA desaturase as a new drug target for obesity treatment. *Obes Rev.* 2005;6(2):169–174.

51. Ratziu V, de Guevara L, Safadi R, et al. Aramchol in patients with nonalcoholic steatohepatitis: a randomized, double-blind, placebo-controlled phase 2b trial. *Nat Med.* 2021;27(10):1825–1835.

52. Shimomura I, Shimano H, Korn BS, Bashmakov Y, Horton JD. Nuclear sterol regulatory element-binding proteins activate genes responsible for the entire program of unsaturated fatty acid biosynthesis in transgenic mouse liver. *J Biol Chem.* 1998;273(52):35299–35306.

53. Watanabe M, Houten SM, Wang L, et al. Bile acids lower triglyceride levels via a pathway involving FXR, SHP, and SREBP-1c. *J Clin Invest.* 2004;113(10):1408–1418.

54. Cariou B. The farnesoid X receptor (FXR) as a new target in non-alcoholic steatohepatitis. *Diabetes Metab.* 2008;34(6 Pt 2):685–691.

55. Podszun MC, Alawad AS, Lingala S, et al. Vitamin E treatment in NAFLD patients demonstrates that oxidative stress drives steatosis through upregulation of de-novo lipogenesis. *Redox Biol.* 2020;37:101710.

56. Sanyal AJ, Chalasani N, Kowdley KV, et al. Pioglitazone, vitamin E, or placebo for nonalcoholic steatohepatitis. *N Engl J Med.* 2010;362(18):1675–1685.

57. Targher G, Corey KE, Byrne CD, Roden M. The complex link between NAFLD and type 2 diabetes mellitus—mechanisms and treatments. *Nat Rev Gastroenterol Hepatol.* 2021;18(9):599–612.

58. Malhi H, Gores GJ. Molecular mechanisms of lipotoxicity in nonalcoholic fatty liver disease. *Semin Liver Dis.* 2008;28(4):360–369.

59. Trauner M, Arrese M, Wagner M. Fatty liver and lipotoxicity. *Biochim Biophys Acta.* 2010;1801(3):299–310.

60. Marra F, Svegliati-Baroni G. Lipotoxicity and the gut-liver axis in NASH pathogenesis. *J Hepatol.* 2018;68(2):280–295.

61. Yamaguchi K, Yang L, McCall S, et al. Inhibiting triglyceride synthesis improves hepatic steatosis but exacerbates liver damage and fibrosis in obese mice with nonalcoholic steatohepatitis. *Hepatology.* 2007;45(6):1366–1374.

62. Yu XX, Murray SF, Pandey SK, et al. Antisense oligonucleotide reduction of DGAT2 expression improves hepatic steatosis and hyperlipidemia in obese mice. *Hepatology.* 2005;42(2):362–371.

63. Yen C-LE, Stone SJ, Koliwad S, Harris C, Farese RV, Jr. Thematic review series: glycerolipids. DGAT enzymes and triacylglycerol biosynthesis. *J Lipid Res.* 2008;49(11):2283–2301.

64. Loomba R, Morgan E, Watts L, et al. Novel antisense inhibition of diacylglycerol *O*-acyltransferase 2 for treatment of non-alcoholic fatty liver disease: a multicentre, double-blind, randomised, placebo-controlled phase 2 trial. *Lancet Gastroenterol Hepatol.* 2020;5(9):829–838.

65. Younossi ZM, Ratziu V, Loomba R, et al. Obeticholic acid for the treatment of non-alcoholic steatohepatitis: interim analysis from a multicentre, randomised, placebo-controlled phase 3 trial. *Lancet.* 2019;394(10215):2184–2196.

66. Ratziu V, Rinella ME, Neuschwander-Tetri BA, et al. EDP-305 in patients with NASH: a phase II double-blind placebo-controlled dose-ranging study. *J Hepatol.* 2022;76(3):506–517.

13 Targeting Bile Acids (FXRs and FGF19)

Daniel Garrido, Rukaiya Bashir Hamidu and Dina Halegoua-DeMarzio

CONTENTS

13.1 INTRODUCTION

Nonalcoholic steatohepatitis (NASH) has been linked to several conditions including metabolic syndrome, obesity and type 2 diabetes.[1,2] Although the mechanism of progression from steatosis to NASH is poorly understood, it is thought that insulin resistance, cytokines and oxidative stress play a role.[3] Current modalities aiming to improve outcomes and regress fibrosis in NASH include lifestyle modification, as well as off-label use of vitamin E, thiazolidinediones and glucagon-like peptide-1 (GLP-1) analogues.[4–6] Despite global efforts, there are no Food and Drug Administration (FDA)-approved medications to directly treat NASH. However, evidence supporting a role for bile acids (BAs) in the pathogenesis of liver inflammation and fibrosis is emerging, leading to new investigations on targeting BAs.[7]

BA homeostasis occurs through the binding and activation of hepatic and extrahepatic nuclear hormone receptors such as farsenoid receptor X (FXR), which upon activation promotes a cascade of events resulting in its regulation.[8,9] However, hepatic injury may cause reduced bile flow, resulting in cholestatic states.[9] Elevated BA levels have been reported in patients with NASH.[10,11] These elevations may promote an inflammatory response resulting in further hepatic injury.[12] Consequently, efforts are underway to develop medications to treat NASH by targeting BAs. In this chapter, we will review the current knowledge of the role of BAs in the development of NASH and novel therapies in development for treatment.

13.2 OVERVIEW OF BILE ACIDS, SYNTHESIS AND ENTEROHEPATIC CIRCULATION

BAs are synthesized from cholesterol in the liver and secreted into bile as one of its main components.[13] BAs are synthesized through two main pathways: the classical pathway and the alternative pathway[14] (Figure 13.1). The majority of bile acids are generated through the classical pathway, accounting for over 90% of BA synthesis, whereas the alternative pathway is responsible for about 10% of BA production.[15]

In the classical pathway, cholesterol first passes through the rate-limiting enzyme cholesterol 7α-hydroxylase (CYP7A1). It then goes through the enzyme sterol-27-hydroxylase (CYP27A1), producing cholic acid (CA) and chenodeoxycholic acid (CDCA), which are termed "primary bile acids." However, generation of CA also requires 12α-hydroxylase (CYP8B1) to determine the ratio of CA to CDCA. The alternative pathway is initiated by CYP27A1 and ultimately leads to the formation of CDCA. These newly generated primary BAs are then conjugated with either glycine or taurine. After conjugation, the primary bile acids and their metabolites are secreted by hepatocytes into the canaliculus through the bile salt export pumps (BSEP), producing bile. This bile is then stored in the gallbladder along with cholesterol and phospholipids. Upon consumption of food, the gallbladder is triggered to excrete its contents into the intestine. The excreted conjugated BAs interact with intestinal microbiota where the primary BAs are deconjugated and dehydroxylated creating secondary BAs, such as deoxycholic acid (DCA) and lithocholic acid (LCA) from CA and CDCA, respectfully. Unconjugated BAs are passively absorbed into enterocytes in the jejunum and colon. However, in the terminal ileum, about 95% of conjugated BAs are reabsorbed through active uptake in enterocytes by the apical sodium-dependent bile acid transporter (ASBT) with the remainder of BAs excreted in feces. However, the fecal loss of bile acids is compensated by the synthesis of daily BAs. This repeated process is termed "enterohepatic circulation."[16–19]

In addition to their role in the emulsification of fats and absorption of fat-soluble nutrients, BAs also serve as key players in the regulation of glucose, lipid, energy and

DOI: 10.1201/9781003386698-16

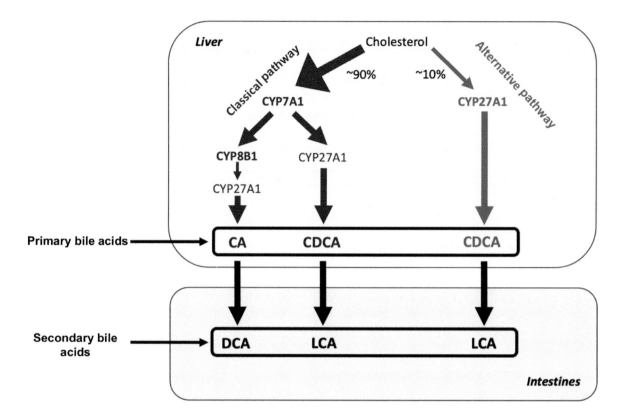

Figure 13.1 Bile acid synthesis begins in the liver. Cholesterol is converted into cholic acid (CA) and chenodeoxycholic acid (CDCA) through two main pathways: the classical pathway and the alternative pathway. The classical pathway produces the majority of bile acids (approximately 90%) and is catalyzed by the rate-limiting enzyme, cholesterol 7α-hydroxylase (CYP7A1). It then produces CA and CDCA through the enzyme sterol-27-hydroxylase hydroxylase (CYP27A1); however, the enzyme 12α-hydroxylase (CYP8B1) is specific only for the production of CA. The alternative pathway is initiated through CYP27A1 and produces CDCA. These primary acids undergo a process of conjugation and are excreted into the intestine, where they are then deconjugated and produce the secondary bile acids deoxycholic acid (DCA) and lithocholic acid (LCA).

inflammation.[20–23] These functions are performed through BA activation of nuclear FXR and membrane-bound Takeda G protein-couple receptor 5 (TGR5, also known as G protein-coupled bile acid receptor-1 [GPBAR1]).[24] A summary by which these ligands function is summarized in Figure 13.2, and will be detailed further later in this chapter.

In addition to their established role in the absorption of fat and fat-soluble vitamins in the intestines, bile acids have emerged as relevant signaling molecules that act, through specific bile acid-activated receptors, at both hepatic and extrahepatic tissues, to regulate various metabolic processes. Dysregulation of bile acid homeostasis affects these various functions of bile acids and is thought to play a role in the pathogenesis NAFLD as well as its progression to NASH.

13.3 ROLE ON BILE ACIDS IN DEVELOPMENT OF NASH

13.3.1 Regulation of Bile Acids

The FXR receptor was first described in 1995 by Forman et al. as a nuclear hormone receptor that was activated by farnesyl pyrophysophate, a farsenol derivative and precursor in the mevalonate pathway (a pathway that synthesizes bile acids and cholesterol).[25,26] BAs were found to be activators of this receptor with CDCA being the greatest activator, followed by DCA and LCA.[27] It was revealed that

activation of FXR had multiple critical functions, one of which was the regulation of BA homeostasis.[28]

Expression of the FXR receptor is seen in both the liver and intestines.[25] Hepatic activation of FXR by BAs induces expression of small heterodimer protein (SHP), which leads to inhibition of both CYP7A1 and CYP8B1 (enzymes critical for BA synthesis). Although SHP does lead to inhibition of both synthetic BA enzymes, repression is seen greatly in CYP8B1 and to a lesser degree in CYP7A1. However, BAs also lead to activation of intestinal FXR-inducing gene expression of the fibroblast growth factor 19 (FGF19). This hormone is then secreted into portal circulation and returns to the liver, whereupon it binds to the fibroblast growth factor receptor 4 (FGFR4) in hepatocytes. Activation of this FGFR4/ß-klotho (KLB) complex leads to the downregulation and inhibition of CYP7A1 and CYP8B1.[29–31] While activation of FXR by BAs in both the liver and intestine provide feedback repression of CYP7A1, this effect is seen most acutely through intestinal FXR.[32] BA activation of FXR in the intestine can also induce genes to express BSEP and organic solute transporter (OST) α and β at the basolateral domain of enterocytes, while also repressing ASBT, thereby inhibiting bile acid uptake and promoting secretion.[33–36] Additionally, bile acid transporters such as NTCP are downregulated, limiting bile acid uptake[37] (see Figure 13.3).

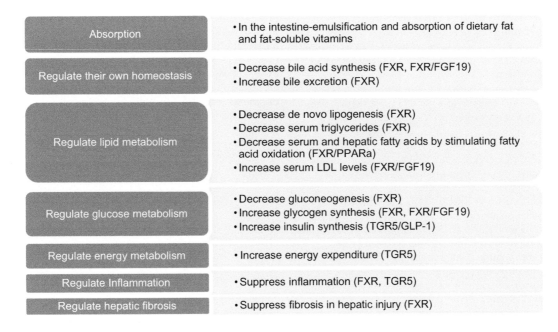

Figure 13.2 Summary of regulatory mechanisms of bile acids

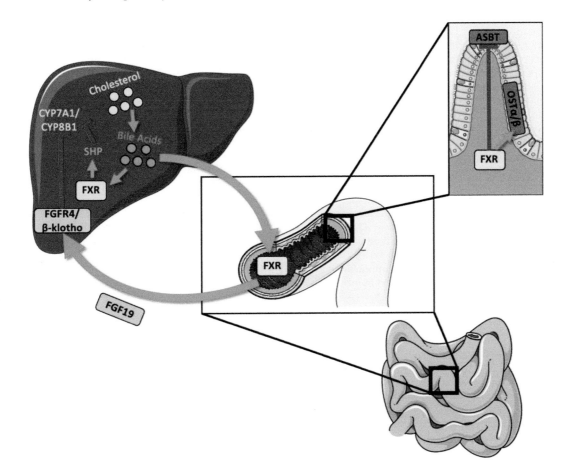

Figure 13.3 Bile acid-FXR-FGF19 pathway (Images courtesy of smart.servier.com). Cholesterol is synthesized into bile acids, which then activate FXR in both the liver and intestines. Liver FXR activation leads to induction of small heterodimer protein (SHP), which then inhibits both CYP7A1 and CYP8B1. Intestinal activation of FXR leads to the expression of FGF19. FGF19 travels back to the liver through portal circulation, whereupon it binds to the FGFR4/β-klotho complex. This results in feedback regression of CYP7A1/CYP8B1. Additionally, intestinal FXR activation may inhibit bile acid uptake and promote secretion through induction of organic solute transporter α and β (OSTα/β) and inhibition of apical sodium-dependent bile acid transporter (ASBT) at the basolateral and apical sides of enterocytes, respectively.

13.3.2 Regulation of Lipid Metabolism

The initial role of bile acids in lipid homeostasis was first described in the 1970s when patients afflicted with gallstones were treated with CDCA to increase bile acid concentration and reduce the cholesterol-stone burden. However, it was later found that treatment with CDCA in these patients led to decreased levels of triglycerides.[38,39] This observation was similarly seen in a study where Fxr-/- mice demonstrated elevated serum levels of triglycerides and cholesterol.[40] However, treatment of mice with FXR agonists resulted in decreased serum triglyceride levels.[41,42] A postulated mechanism for these findings revolves around the activation of FXR-inducing SHP, which then represses the sterol regulatory element binding protein 1c (SREBP-1c)—a key transcription factor in the synthesis of triglycerides.[43,44] Additionally, FXR promotes clearance of very-low-density lipoprotein (VLDL).[45]

FXR activation also functions in the reduction and breakdown of fatty acids (FAs) known as FA β-oxidation. This is promoted through several mechanisms. Much like the regulation of triglyceride, repression of SREBP-1c has been shown to promote FA oxidation. Upregulation of peroxisome-activated receptor alpha (PPARα) by FXR achieved similar results.[43,46]

In addition, the sequence of events whereby intestinal FXR inhibits CYP7A1 through FGF19 and subsequent activation of FGFR4 in hepatocytes may influence cholesterol levels. With the inhibition of CYP7A1, hepatocytes accumulate cholesterol, resulting in downregulation of low-density lipoprotein receptors (LDLR) and thus elevated levels of low-density lipoprotein (LDL).[47]

13.3.3 Regulation of Glucose Homeostasis

FXR appears to have a prominent role in regulation of glucose metabolism. This has been elucidated by the presence of hepatic steatosis, elevated glucose levels and increased insulin resistance in FXR-null mice.[48] Studies have demonstrated that BAs inhibit critical enzymes necessary for gluconeogenesis and glucose homeostasis, including phosphoenolpyruvate carboxykinase (PEPCK), fructose 1,6-bis phosphatase and glucose-6-phosphatase. This is in part due to their activation of FXR, which induces an SHP-mediated mechanism whereby transcriptional factors necessary for the development of these enzymes are inhibited.[49,50] This has also been described in diabetic *db/db* mouse models where mice given GW4064, an FXR agonist, resulted in inhibition of gluconeogenesis.[51] Additionally, BA activation of FXR has been shown to stimulate glycogen synthesis.[52]

In 2002, a new transmembrane receptor influenced by BAs was identified called TGR5 (also known as G protein-coupled bile acid receptor 1 [GBPAR1]).[53] This receptor is expressed in multiple organs including the gallbladder, intestine, and colon, as well as brown and white adipose tissue, and is most potently activated by LCA and DCA.[53–55] In particular, expression of TGR5 has been seen in enteroendocrine L-cells.[56] An investigation of obese mice showed that TGR5 signaling contributed to glucose homeostasis by inducing the release of glucagon-like peptide-1 (GLP-1) and incretin hormone. This resulted in improved glucose tolerance, as well as improved liver and pancreatic function.[57]

13.3.4 Energy Metabolism

Obesity is a condition that results from an energy imbalance whereby the energy intake exceeds the energy expenditure. Energy expenditure is be determined by various means including brown adipose tissue (BAT), where heat is dissipated in the form of energy, known as thermogenesis,

and skeletal muscle metabolism.[58,59] TGR5 has been found in both BAT and skeletal muscle indicating it may serve a prominent role in the regulation of energy expenditure. Upon activation of this receptor by BAs, a cascade of events takes place whereby there are increased levels of cAMP. This subsequently results in activation of a thyroid hormone-activating enzyme known as type 2 iodothyronine deiodinase (D2). D2 then converts inactive thyroid hormone (T_4) to active thyroid hormone (T_3), leading to increased energy expenditure and thermogenesis.[60]

13.3.5 Inflammation and Fibrosis

As mentioned earlier, the development of hepatic steatosis causes stress on the liver that may lead to the development of NASH and cirrhosis. This is a result of an inflammatory response regulated by Kupffer cells (the resident macrophage of the liver) and inflammatory cytokines. BAs regulate this response through its interactions with both FXR and TGR5.[61]

13.3.5.1 FXR

Activation of FXR plays a role in the regulation of hepatic inflammation and fibrosis. One study investigating this role was performed on mice fed a methionine- and choline-deficient (MCD) diet, which served as a nutritional model for NASH. Mice were given WAY-362450, a synthetic agonist of FXR, which resulted in a reduction of liver fibrosis, as well as a reduction in the expression of genes for hepatic fibrosis.[62] Another study performed on FXR-null mice revealed mice treated with lipopolysaccharide (LPS) exhibited hepatic inflammation and necrosis, which was marked by an increase in inflammatory cytokines. However, mouse hepatocytes treated with FXR agonists suppressed nuclear factor kappa B (NF-κB), a transcription factor necessary for the induction of the inflammatory response.[63,64] It has also been suggested that FXR's role in suppressing the inflammatory response may be indirect by means of reduction of cholestasis and accumulation of toxic bile acids within the liver.[65]

The development of hepatic fibrosis results from increased extracellular deposition by hepatic stellate cells (HSCs).[66,67] FXR has been identified within HSCs and is thought to play a role in the regulation of the fibrotic response.[68,69] After FXR activation, SHP mediates a response that increases expression of peroxismal peroliferator-activated receptor γ (PPARγ) in HSCs. Rat models have shown that elevation of PPARγ mRNA levels results in HSC inhibition and improvement in the fibrotic response.[70,71]

13.3.5.2 TGR5

The expression of TGR5 in monocytes, macrophages and Kupffer cells also regulates hepatic inflammation.[72,73] Studies investigating this role found that activation of TGR5 by BAs in human monocytic leukemia THP-1 cells and Kupffer cells inhibited production of LPS-induced cytokines and its subsequent inflammatory response.[72,73] These findings were suggestive that TGR5 serves as a mediator in sequestering inflammation.

13.4 TARGETING BILE ACIDS TO TREAT NASH AND FIBROSIS

13.4.1 FXR as a Drug Target—FXR Agonists

As the potential therapeutic benefit of FXR regulation was shown in prior studies, clinical drug trials have further investigated the benefit of FXR agonists for the treatment of NASH. Investigational drugs have included therapies such as obeticholic acid (OCA), tropifexor, cilofexor and ED-305. Broadly, these drugs can be further categorized

Table 13.1: Summary of Clinical Trial FXR Agonists in NASH Treatment

Drug	Trial	Phase	Population	Intervention	Findings	Adverse Effect	Ongoing
Steroidal							
Obeticholic acid (OCA)	FLINT	2	• NASH with NAS ≥ 4	• 25 mg OCA vs. placebo	• Improvement in NAS (−1.7 in OCA vs. −0.7 in placebo, $p = <0.0001$) • Improved fibrosis (35% in OCA vs. 19% in placebo, $p = 0.004$) • No significance in NASH resolution (22% in OCA vs. 13% in placebo, $p = 0.08$)	• ↑ LDL • ↓ HDL • 33% pruritus	No
	REGENERATE	3	• F2–F3 NASH	• 10 mg OCA vs. 25 mg OCA vs. placebo	• Improved fibrosis (23% in 25 mg OCA, $p = 0.0002$ vs. placebo; 18% in 10 mg OCA, $p = 0.045$ vs. placebo; 12 % placebo) • No NASH resolution (12% in 25 mg OCA group, $p = 0.13$ vs. placebo; 11% in 10 mg OCA group, $p = 0.18$ vs. placebo; 8% in placebo)	• ↑ LDL • Pruritus (51% in 25 mg OCA, 28 % in 10mg OCA, 19 % placebo)	Yes
	REVERSE	3	• Compensated NASH cirrhosis	• 10 mg OCA vs 10-to-25 mg OCA vs placebo	• No significant difference in ≥1-stage improvement in fibrosis without worsening NASH (10 mg OCA at 11.1% vs 10-to-25 mg at 11.9% vs placebo at 9.9%) • Improvement in liver stiffness via transient elastography in both 10 mg and 10-to-25 mg OCA arm	• Pruritus (57% in 10-to-25 mg OCA, 41% in 10 mg OCA, and 31% in placebo) • Serious gallbladder-related events (1.0% 10-to-25 mg OCA, 1.0% in 10 mg OCA, and 0.6% in placebo) • ↑ in gallstones in 10-to-25 mg OCA arm	No
Nonsteroidal							
Cilofexor	ClinicalTrials.gov No. NCT02854605	2	• Noncirrhotic NASH	• Cilofexor 100 mg vs. 30 mg cilofexor vs. placebo	• ↓ in MRI-PDFF in 100 mg cilofexor group (−22.7% median relative decrease in 100 mg cilofexor vs. 1.9% in placebo, $p = 0.003$)	• Pruritus (14% in 100 mg cilofexor, 4% in 30 mg cilofexor, 4% in placebo)	No
	ATLAS	2b	• F3–F4 NASH	• Placebo vs. selonsertib 18 mg vs. cilofexor 30 mg vs. firsocostat 20 mg alone or in 2-drug combination	• No significance in improvement of ≥1 stage of fibrosis without worsening NASH • Combination of cilofexor/firsocostat ≥2-point ↓ in NAS score (steatosis, lobular inflammation, ballooning) ($p \leq 0.05$) • Improvement in AST, ALT, bile acids, eGFR, cytokeratin-18, insulin, ELF score, LS ($p \leq 0.05$)	• Pruritus in cilofexor group (20–29%) • Upper respiratory tract infection (10–16%)	No
Tropifexor	FLIGHT-FXR	2	• F2–F3 biopsy-proven NASH	• Tropifexor 200 µg vs. 140 µg vs. placebo	• ↓ in ALT, GGT, body weight, and dose-dependent ↓ ≥30% HFF in tropifexor vs. placebo • Dose-dependent ↓ in collagen with septa in tropifexor vs. placebo ($p = 0.006$)	• Pruritus (>60% in both tropifexor groups) • Dose-dependent ↑ in LDL	No
EDP-305	ARGON-1	2	• Noncirrhotic NASH	• EDP-305 2.5 mg vs. EDP-305 1 mg vs. placebo	• ↓ ALT in EDP-305 2.5 mg (−27.9 U/L in 2.5 mg EDP-305 vs. −15.4 U/L in 2.5 mg EDP-305, $p = 0.049$) • ↓ HFF with EDP-305 (−7.1% in 2.5 mg EDP-305, −3.3% in 1 mg EDP-305, vs. −2.4% in placebo, $p = 0.0009$)	• Pruritus (50.9% in 2.5 mg EDP 305, 9.1% in 1 mg EDP-305, 4.2% in placebo)	No

into two distinct categories: steroidal and nonsteroidal FXR agonists (see Table 13.1).

13.4.1.1 Steroidal FXR Agonists

13.4.1.1.1 Obeticholic Acid (OCA)

The first drug that showed potential promise for treatment of NASH was OCA, an FXR receptor agonist with approximately a 100-fold potency.[74] Initial clinical trials investigating the treatment of OCA in patients with type 2 diabetes and NAFLD showed patients had increased insulin sensitivity and decreased levels of γ-glutamyl transpeptidase (GGT) and alanine aminostransferase (ALT).[75] A subsequent phase II study was performed in 2015 investigating the role of OCA in NASH patients known as the FLINT (Farnesoid X Receptor Ligand Obeticholic Acid in NASH Treatment) trial.[76] In this multicenter, double-blind, randomized control trial, patients were either assigned 25 mg of OCA or placebo for a total of 72 weeks with the primary endpoint of improvement in the NAFLD activity score (NAS). Results showed a significant change in the NAS between the two groups. There was no significance in NASH resolution between the two groups, but there was significant improvement in fibrosis in the OCA-treated group. Liver chemistries revealed a significant decrease in ALT and aspartate aminotransferase (AST). Adverse effects noted in the OCA group revealed higher levels of LDL, decreased levels of HDL and the development of pruritus in over 33% of participants.[76]

In 2016, a phase III investigational study called the POISE (PBC OCA International Study of Efficacy) trial was performed with OCA investigating its role in the treatment of patients with primary biliary cholangitis (PBC).[77] Patients in this double-blind, randomized control study were assigned either OCA (5 mg up to 10 mg) or placebo with the primary endpoint of an ALP less than 1.67 times the upper limit of normal and a normal total bilirubin. Results showed the primary endpoint was achieved more in OCA patients than in the placebo group. Reports of increased LDL and decreased HDL were again noted in this trial, along with an increasing dose-dependent relationship on reports of pruritus.[77] This ultimately led to US FDA approval of OCA for treatment of PBC.[78] However, in 2021, it was revealed that use of OCA in patients with advanced cirrhosis could result in further hepatic decompensation. Thus, the FDA placed a restriction of OCA in cirrhotic patients with prior hepatic decompensation or portal hypertension.[79,80]

Given the findings of the FLINT trial and with US FDA approval of OCA for PBC, a phase III trial, called REGENERATE, is currently underway by Intercept Pharma investigating the role of OCA with NASH complicated by hepatic fibrosis.[81] In 2019, an 18-month interim analysis of the multicenter, double-blind, randomized control trial was released for patients with NASH and fibrosis stage F2–F3 receiving placebo, OCA 10 mg dose, or OCA 25 mg dose. The primary endpoint was improvement of fibrosis ≥1 stage or resolution of NASH. Results showed that treatment with OCA resulted in a statistically significant improvement in fibrosis. However, NASH resolution was not achieved. Elevations in LDL and pruritus were noted, consistent with adverse effects reported in prior studies.[81] In light of safety and efficacy concerns, REGENERATE is still ongoing and being monitored by drug regulatory agencies.

A phase 3 double-blind, randomized control trial, called REVERSE, was also performed to assess the safety and efficacy of OCA in patients with compensated NASH cirrhosis. Patients were randomized to receive either placebo, 10 mg OCA, or 10-to-25 mg OCA.[82] This study did not achieve its primary endpoint of ≥1-stage histological improvement in fibrosis without worsening of NASH after follow-up while on 18 months of therapy. However, despite not achieving its primary endpoint, it was reported that patients receiving 10 mg OCA and 10-to-25 mg OCA did have improvement in liver stiffness on transient elastography.

The safety profile of this trial revealed that treatment-emergent adverse events, treatment-emergent serious adverse events, and death were reportedly balanced among all arms. The most common reason for drug discontinuation was pruritus, reported in 37% of patients in the placebo arm, 41% in the 10 mg OCA arm, and 57% in the 10-to-25 mg OCA arm. Patients who received 10-to-25 mg of OCA also had a higher incidence of gallstones.[83]

Based upon the results of the interim analysis of the REGENERATE trial, a new drug application was submitted to the FDA in December 2022.[84] In May 2023, the FDA voted to defer approval of obeticholic acid for the treatment of NASH until further clinical outcome data became available.[85]

13.4.1.1.2 INT-767

Another agonist under current investigation is Intercept's INT-767, a dual FXR/TGR5 agonist. An in vitro study on NASH models has shown INT-767 to induce collagen reduction in a dose- and time-dependent manner.[86]

13.4.1.2 Nonsteroidal FXR Agonists

In light of current data on steroidal FXR agonists, there are concerns regarding their safety in long-term use. One limitation with the use of steroidal agents is its poor bioavailability. Additionally, steroid agonists exhibit partial agonism to GPBAR1 (also known as TGR5). While there has been a shown benefit with binding to FXR, the partial agonism to GPBAR1 may increase itching receptors on the skin, leading to pruritus.[87] As a result, the development of nonsteroidal FXR agonists is being investigated for the treatment of NASH. These nonsteroidal ligands are non-BA-type agonists and are unable to undergo enterohepatic circulation. They are therefore more gut-selective agonists of FXR as opposed to systemic agonists such as steroidal FXR ligands.[88,89] Nonsteroidal FXR agents currently in development include Cilofexor, Tropifexor and EDP-305.

13.4.1.2.1 Cilofexor

A phase 2 randomized controlled trial was undertaken in 2020 to assess the safety and efficacy of cilofexor in noncirrhotic NASH patients. Patients were randomized to receive either cilofexor 100 mg, cilofexor 30 mg or placebo for a total of 24 weeks. Results revealed that the hepatic fat content measured by the magnetic resonance imaging–proton density fat fraction (MRI-PDFF) was decreased in patients in the 100 mg cilofexor group. There was no significant difference between the 30 mg cilofexor group and placebo ($p = 0.87$). Additionally, patients in both cilofexor treatment groups had decreased GGT levels. There was no significant change in lipid levels while on cilofexor, but there was a dose-dependent increase in pruritus.[90]

In 2021, the ATLAS trial was completed, further assessing the role of cilofexor.[91] This was a phase 2b trial of NASH patients with F3–F4 fibrosis assessing the role of medication through three different pathways: FXR agonism, acetyl-CoA carboxylase (ACC) inhibition, and apoptosis signal-regulating kinase 1 (ASK1) inhibition. Cilofexor was assessed along with firsocostat (an inhibitor of ACC shown to improve hepatic steatosis, fibrosis and liver biochemistry) and selonsertib (an inhibitor of ASK1 believed to reduce inflammatory and apoptotic response that had been shown previously to have no efficacy in improvement of NASH fibrosis).[92,93] Patients were randomly assigned either monotherapy of each of these drugs or in combination. The primary endpoint of improvement of ≥1 stage of fibrosis without worsening NASH was not achieved in any of the monotherapy groups. However, while a combination of cilofexor/firsocostat over 48 weeks did not improve fibrosis by ≥1 stage, there was ≥2-point reduction in NAS scores with improvement in steatosis, lobular inflammation, ballooning, as well as improvement in AST, ALT, bile acids, estimated glomerular filtration rate (eGFR), cytokeratin-18, insulin, ELF score and liver stiffness (LS) ($p = \leq 0.05$).[91]

13.4.1.2.2 Tropifexor

Another nonsteroidal drug in phase II study is tropifexor, currently investigated in the FLIGHT-FXR trial.[94] In this randomized, double-blind trial, patients with NASH F2–F3 fibrosis were assigned to either tropifexor 140 μg, tropifexor 200 μg or placebo. At 48 weeks, there was a decrease in ALT, GGT and body weight and a dose-dependent decrease of ≥30% hepatic fat fraction (HFF) in patients on tropifexor compared to placebo. There was no significant difference in fibrosis improvement with no worsening NASH between tropifexor groups and placebo, but there was a dose-dependent reduction in collagen within septa in tropifexor groups compared to placebo ($p = 0.006$).[94] Pruritus was noted in >60% of the tropifexor groups along with an increase in LDL.

13.4.1.2.3 EDP-305

EDP-305 is a new investigational nonsteroidal FXR agonist drug currently in phase II study (ARGON-1). In this randomized controlled trial, patients with NASH were randomized to EDP-305 1 mg, EDP-305 2.5 mg or placebo over a period of 12 weeks. The primary endpoint of decreased ALT was achieved in patients on EDP-305 2.5 mg. A reduction in the HFF was also seen in patients receiving EDP-305. Additionally, pruritus was noted in over 50.9% of patients on 2.5 mg of EDP-305, compared to 9.1% and 4.2% in both 1 mg EDP-305 and placebo, respectively. There was no significant difference in LDL levels.[95] A follow-up phase 2b trial, called the ARGON-2 trial, by Enanta Pharmaceuticals is currently ongoing to assess the safety and efficacy of EDP-305 in biopsy-proven NASH.

13.4.2 FGF19 as a Drug Target - FGF19 Agonists

In addition to FXR agonists, FGF19 agonists are emerging as another potential target for the treatment of NASH. As previously mentioned, FGF19 is secreted in ileal enterocytes in response to BA activation of FXR, whereby it binds to the FGFR4/β-klotho complexes on hepatocytes.[29–31] As a product of the FXR activation pathway, FGF19 appears to have a similar role in the regulation of bile acids, glucose and energy.[96,97] Mice lacking FGF15 (a mouse ortholog of FGF19), FGFR4 and β-klotho have impaired bile acid homeostasis and impaired glucose levels.[98–101] Additionally, decreased levels of circulating FGF19 have been noted in patients with NASH.[102]

However, potential therapeutic use of FGF19 has been limited by its potential risk of malignancy.[103] This was noted when overexpression of FGF19 in skeletal muscle of transgenic mice led to liver dysplasia and ultimately hepatocellular carcinoma (HCC).[104] Future studies demonstrated that FGF19 and its interaction with FGFR4 may promote the proliferation of hepatocytes and induce the formation of HCC.[105,106]

The investigational drug in this class of medications is aldafermin.

13.5 ALDAFERMIN

Aldafermin (also known as NGM282 or M70) is a nontumorigenic analog of FGF19 that has shown therapeutic potential in NASH and has reached phase IIb clinical trials for NASH.[28,107,108] Aldafermin differs from wild-type FGF19 in amino acid composition in the amino terminus. With this change, aldafermin retains the ability to potently repress CYP7A1 expression but loses the ability to activate the signal transducer and activator of transcription 3 (STAT3), a signaling pathway essential for FGF19-mediated hepatocarcinogenesis.[107–109] In preclinical models, no liver tumors were observed in multiple animal models even after prolonged exposure to aldafermin.[108]

Preclinical studies in mice have demonstrated that treatment with aldafermin, via the FGFR4/KLB and FGFR1c/KLB receptor pathways, led to significant resolution of NASH and improvement in fibrosis.[107,110–113] Aldafermin caused a reduction in concentrations of ALT and AST, as well as a clear improvement in all histological features associated with NASH, including hepatic steatosis, inflammation, ballooning degeneration and fibrosis.[110] Aldafermin has since been studied in human clinical trials as well. Aldafermin was shown to be safe and well-tolerated in healthy volunteers and was associated with a reduction in serum concentrations of 7 α-hydroxy-4-cholesten-3-one (C4), a biomarker of hepatic CYP7A1 activity, indicating robust target engagement.[114] Of note, it has been established that aldafermin is also nonmitogenic in humans.[111] Subsequent phase 2 clinical trials evaluated treatment with aldafermin, in 4 cohorts of patients with biopsy-proven NASH and a recently completed study—the ALPINE 2/3 trial.[107,108,112,115–117]

Cohort 1 was a 12-week placebo-controlled, randomized, double-blind study that assessed the efficacy and safety of aldafermin.[107] This study represented the first-in-class controlled clinical investigation of an FGF19 analogue in the treatment of NASH.[107] The primary outcome was the absolute change in liver fat content from baseline to week 12, measured using MRI-PDFF. Overall, 23 (85%) of 27 and 24 (86%) of 28 patients receiving 3 mg or 6 mg aldafermin, respectively, achieved a "clinically meaningful" relative change in liver fat content (≥30% reduction), and the results were statistically significant.[118] In addition, NGM282 produced significant improvements in ALT, AST, and noninvasive serum fibrosis biomarkers (pro-C3 and ELF score). Cohort 2 was a dose-expansion study that evaluated aldafermin 0.3 mg, 1 mg and 3 mg for 12 weeks and also explored the use of concomitant statin therapies to support chronic administration of aldafermin.[115] Notably, albeit an expected consequence of CYP7A1 inhibition, treatment with aldafermin had ensuing increases in total cholesterol and LDL-C. This observed increase in total cholesterol and LDL-C were effectively managed with coadministration of aldafermin with rosuvastatin.[115] Cohort 3 was an open-label trial that assessed the histological efficacy of aldafermin in patients with biopsy-confirmed NASH.[112] In this 12-week study, 42% of the patients treated with aldafermin 3 mg had a decrease in fibrosis score from baseline of at least one stage.[112] Cohort 4 was a randomized, double-blind, placebo-controlled 24-week trial in patients with NASH and liver fibrosis.[108] The results of this trial extended the findings of the previous 12-week and open-label studies showing the benefits of aldafermin on liver fat and histology.[107,112,115] On post hoc analysis, aldafermin-treated patients achieved a statistically significant improvement in the combined endpoint of fibrosis improvement and resolution of NASH in just 24 weeks (22% vs. 0% placebo).[108] This significant improvement in fibrosis in patients with NASH being treated with aldafermin was, however, not shown in the most recently completed 24-week phase 2b study (the ALPINE 2/3 study) that evaluated aldafermin vs. placebo with a primary endpoint of histologic improvement in liver fibrosis with no worsening of NASH.[116,117] In line with the results of previous studies, however, results from the APLINE 2/3 trial showed that statistically significant improvement on multiple noninvasive measures of NASH were achieved in patients treated with aldafermin.[116,117] Unfortunately, the failure to meet the primary endpoint in the ALPINE 2/3 study has led to the decision to halt further pursuit of aldafermin as a potential drug in the treatment of NASH.[119]

13.6 SUMMARY

The beneficial effects of bile acid signaling on energy, glucose and lipid metabolism described in this chapter have motivated researchers to develop compounds that target these signaling pathways as a potential treatment for NASH. Activation of FXR in multiple tissues and cell types attenuates the severity of the major characteristics of NASH. There are several FXR agonists at various phases of clinical trials as reviewed. As with most drug targets, treatments working through the bile acid-FXR-FGF15/19 pathway have potential safety liabilities. In particular, safety concerns include the worsened serum lipid profile, side effects like pruritus, risk of hepatic decompensation and the potential carcinogenic risk of FGF19. Despite these challenges, the development of FXR and FGF 19 agonists provides hope for patients with NASH whose only treatment option currently is lifestyle modification. Taken as a whole, the data from clinical trials suggest that targeting bile acid signaling pathways and downstream mediators has significant potential to successfully treat patients with NASH.

REFERENCES

1. Williams CD, Stengel J, Asike MI, et al. Prevalence of nonalcoholic fatty liver disease and nonalcoholic steatohepatitis among a largely middle-aged population utilizing ultrasound and liver biopsy: a prospective study. *Gastroenterology*. 2011;140(1):124–131.
2. Byrne CD, Targher G. NAFLD: a multisystem disease. *Journal of Hepatology*. 2015;62(1):S47-S64.
3. Wong VW-S, Chitturi S, Wong GL-H, Yu J, Chan HL-Y, Farrell GC. Pathogenesis and novel treatment options for non-alcoholic steatohepatitis. *The Lancet Gastroenterology & Hepatology*. 2016;1(1):56–67.
4. Vilar-Gomez E, Martinez-Perez Y, Calzadilla-Bertot L, et al. Weight loss through lifestyle modification significantly reduces features of nonalcoholic steatohepatitis. *Gastroenterology*. 2015;149(2):367–378. e5.
5. Cusi K, Orsak B, Bril F, et al. Long-term pioglitazone treatment for patients with nonalcoholic steatohepatitis and prediabetes or type 2 diabetes mellitus: a randomized trial. *Annals of Internal Medicine*. 2016;165(5):305–315.
6. Armstrong MJ, Gaunt P, Aithal GP, et al. Liraglutide safety and efficacy in patients with non-alcoholic steatohepatitis (LEAN): a multicentre, double-blind, randomised, placebo-controlled phase 2 study. *The Lancet*. 2016;387(10019):679–690.
7. Arab JP, Karpen SJ, Dawson PA, Arrese M, Trauner M. Bile acids and nonalcoholic fatty liver disease: molecular insights and therapeutic perspectives. *Hepatology*. 2017;65(1):350–362.
8. Guo GL, Lambert G, Negishi M, et al. Complementary roles of farnesoid X receptor, pregnane X receptor, and constitutive androstane receptor in protection against bile acid toxicity. *Journal of Biological Chemistry*. 2003;278(46):45062–45071.
9. Yu Q, Jiang Z, Zhang L. Bile acid regulation: a novel therapeutic strategy in non-alcoholic fatty liver disease. *Pharmacology & Therapeutics*. 2018;190:81–90.
10. Bechmann LP, Kocabayoglu P, Sowa JP, et al. Free fatty acids repress small heterodimer partner (SHP) activation and adiponectin counteracts bile acid-induced liver injury in superobese patients with nonalcoholic steatohepatitis. *Hepatology*. 2013;57(4):1394–1406.
11. Kalhan SC, Guo L, Edmison J, et al. Plasma metabolomic profile in nonalcoholic fatty liver disease. *Metabolism*. 2011;60(3):404–413.
12. O'Brien KM, Allen KM, Rockwell CE, Towery K, Luyendyk JP, Copple BL. IL-17A synergistically enhances bile acid-induced inflammation during obstructive cholestasis. *The American Journal of Pathology*. 2013;183(5):1498–1507.
13. Chiang JY. Regulation of bile acid synthesis: pathways, nuclear receptors, and mechanisms. *Journal of Hepatology*. 2004;40(3):539–551.
14. Ferdinandusse S, Houten SM. Peroxisomes and bile acid biosynthesis. *Biochimica et Biophysica Acta (BBA)-Molecular Cell Research*. 2006;1763(12):1427–1440.
15. Russell DW. The enzymes, regulation, and genetics of bile acid synthesis. *Annual Review of Biochemistry*. 2003;72(1):137–174.
16. Zhu Y, Liu H, Zhang M, Guo GL. Fatty liver diseases, bile acids, and FXR. *Acta Pharmaceutica Sinica B*. 2016;6(5):409–412.
17. Pandak WM, Kakiyama G. The acidic pathway of bile acid synthesis: not just an alternative pathway. *Liver Research*. 2019;3(2):88–98.
18. Molinaro A, Wahlström A, Marschall H-U. Role of bile acids in metabolic control. *Trends in Endocrinology & Metabolism*. 2018;29(1):31–41.
19. Mertens KL, Kalsbeek A, Soeters MR, Eggink HM. Bile acid signaling pathways from the enterohepatic circulation to the central nervous system. *Frontiers in Neuroscience*. 2017;11:617.
20. Raufman J-P, Cheng K, Zimniak P. Activation of muscarinic receptor signaling by bile acids: physiological and medical implications. *Digestive Diseases and Sciences*. 2003;48(8):1431–1444.
21. Chiang JY. Bile acid metabolism and signaling. *Comprehensive Physiology*. 2013;3(3):1191.
22. Schaap FG, Trauner M, Jansen PL. Bile acid receptors as targets for drug development. *Nature Reviews Gastroenterology & Hepatology*. 2014;11(1):55–67.
23. Hundt M, Basit H, John S. *Physiology, Bile Secretion*. 2022. In: StatPearls [Internet]. Treasure Island (FL): StatPearls Publishing; 2023.

24. Wahlström A, Sayin SI, Marschall H-U, Bäckhed F. Intestinal crosstalk between bile acids and microbiota and its impact on host metabolism. *Cell Metabolism*. 2016;24(1):41–50.

25. Forman BM, Goode E, Chen J, et al. Identification of a nuclear receptor that is activated by farnesol metabolites. *Cell*. 1995;81(5):687–693.

26. Goldstein JL, Brown MS. Regulation of the mevalonate pathway. *Nature*. 1990;343(6257):425–430.

27. Makishima M, Okamoto A. Repa JJ, Tu H, Learned RM, Luk A, et al. Identification of a nuclear receptor for bile acids. *Science*. 1999;284:1362–1365.

28. Maliha S, Guo GL. FXR and FGF15/19 as pharmacological targets. *Liver Research*. 2021.

29. Inagaki T, Choi M, Moschetta A, et al. Fibroblast growth factor 15 functions as an enterohepatic signal to regulate bile acid homeostasis. *Cell Metabolism*. 2005;2(4):217–225.

30. Kong B, Wang L, Chiang JY, Zhang Y, Klaassen CD, Guo GL. Mechanism of tissue-specific farnesoid X receptor in suppressing the expression of genes in bile-acid synthesis in mice. *Hepatology*. 2012;56(3):1034–1043.

31. Maliha S, Guo GL. Farnesoid X receptor and fibroblast growth factor 15/19 as pharmacological targets. *Liver Research*. 2021;5(3):142–150. doi:10.1016/j.livres.2021.02.002

32. Kim I, Ahn S-H, Inagaki T, et al. Differential regulation of bile acid homeostasis by the farnesoid X receptor in liver and intestine. *Journal of Lipid Research*. 2007;48(12):2664–2672.

33. Plass JR, Mol O, Heegsma J, et al. Farnesoid X receptor and bile salts are involved in transcriptional regulation of the gene encoding the human bile salt export pump. *Hepatology*. 2002;35(3):589–596.

34. Landrier J-F, Eloranta JJ, Vavricka SR, Kullak-Ublick GA. The nuclear receptor for bile acids, FXR, transactivates human organic solute transporter-α and-β genes. *American Journal of Physiology-Gastrointestinal and Liver Physiology*. 2006;290(3):G476–G485.

35. Zollner G, Wagner M, Moustafa T, et al. Coordinated induction of bile acid detoxification and alternative elimination in mice: role of FXR-regulated organic solute transporter-α/β in the adaptive response to bile acids. *American Journal of Physiology-Gastrointestinal and Liver Physiology*. 2006;290(5):G923–G932.

36. Chen F, Ma L, Dawson PA, et al. Liver receptor homologue-1 mediates species-and cell line-specific bile acid-dependent negative feedback regulation of the apical sodium-dependent bile acid transporter. *Journal of Biological Chemistry*. 2003;278(22):19909–19916.

37. Denson LA, Sturm E, Echevarria W, et al. The orphan nuclear receptor, shp, mediates bile acid-induced inhibition of the rat bile acid transporter, NTCP. *Gastroenterology*. 2001;121(1):140–147.

38. Bell G, Lewis B, Petrie A, Dowling RH. Serum lipids in cholelithiasis: effect of chenodeoxycholic acid therapy. *British Medical Journal*. 1973;3(5879):520–523.

39. Miller N, Nestel P. Triglyceride-lowering effect of chenodeoxycholic acid in patients with endogenous hypertriglyceridaemia. *The Lancet*. 1974;304(7886):929–931.

40. Sinal CJ, Tohkin M, Miyata M, Ward JM, Lambert G, Gonzalez FJ. Targeted disruption of the nuclear receptor FXR/BAR impairs bile acid and lipid homeostasis. *Cell*. 2000;102(6):731–744.

41. Kast HR, Nguyen CM, Sinal CJ, et al. Farnesoid X-activated receptor induces apolipoprotein C-II transcription: a molecular mechanism linking plasma triglyceride levels to bile acids. *Molecular Endocrinology*. 2001;15(10):1720–1728.

42. Claudel T, Inoue Y, Barbier O, et al. Farnesoid X receptor agonists suppress hepatic apolipoprotein CIII expression. *Gastroenterology*. 2003;125(2):544–555.

43. Watanabe M, Houten SM, Wang L, et al. Bile acids lower triglyceride levels via a pathway involving FXR, SHP, and SREBP-1c. *The Journal of Clinical Investigation*. 2004;113(10):1408–1418.

44. Zhang Y, Castellani LW, Sinal CJ, Gonzalez FJ, Edwards PA. Peroxisome proliferator-activated receptor-γ coactivator 1α (PGC-1α) regulates triglyceride metabolism by activation of the nuclear receptor FXR. *Genes & Development*. 2004;18(2):157–169.

45. Hirokane H, Nakahara M, Tachibana S, Shimizu M, Sato R. Bile acid reduces the secretion of very low density lipoprotein by repressing microsomal triglyceride transfer protein gene expression mediated by hepatocyte nuclear factor-4. *Journal of Biological Chemistry*. 2004;279(44):45685–45692.

46. Schumacher JD, Guo GL. Pharmacologic modulation of bile acid-FXR-FGF15/FGF19 pathway for the treatment of nonalcoholic steatohepatitis. *Bile Acids and Their Receptors*. 2019:325–357.

47. Carr RM, Reid AE. FXR agonists as therapeutic agents for non-alcoholic fatty liver disease. *Current Atherosclerosis Reports*. 2015;17(4):1–14.

48. Ma K, Saha PK, Chan L, Moore DD. Farnesoid X receptor is essential for normal glucose homeostasis. *The Journal of Clinical Investigation*. 2006;116(4):1102–1109.

49. De Fabiani E, Mitro N, Gilardi F, Caruso D, Galli G, Crestani M. Coordinated control of cholesterol catabolism to bile acids and of gluconeogenesis via a novel mechanism of transcription regulation linked to the fasted-to-fed cycle. *Journal of Biological Chemistry*. 2003;278(40):39124–39132.

50. Yamagata K, Daitoku H, Shimamoto Y, et al. Bile acids regulate gluconeogenic gene expression via small heterodimer partner-mediated repression of hepatocyte nuclear factor 4 and Foxo1. *Journal of Biological Chemistry*. 2004;279(22):23158–23165.

51. Zhang Y, Lee FY, Barrera G, et al. Activation of the nuclear receptor FXR improves hyperglycemia and hyperlipidemia in diabetic mice. *Proceedings of the National Academy of Sciences*. 2006;103(4):1006–1011.

52. Li T, Owsley E, Matozel M, Hsu P, Novak CM, Chiang JY. Transgenic expression of cholesterol 7α-hydroxylase in the liver prevents high-fat diet-induced obesity and insulin resistance in mice. *Hepatology*. 2010;52(2):678–690.

53. Maruyama T, Miyamoto Y, Nakamura T, et al. Identification of membrane-type receptor for bile acids (M-BAR). *Biochemical and Biophysical Research Communications*. 2002;298(5):714–719.

54. Maruyama T, Tanaka K, Suzuki J, et al. Targeted disruption of G protein-coupled bile acid receptor 1 (Gpbar1/M-Bar) in mice. *Journal of Endocrinology*. 2006;191(1):197–205.

55. Keitel V, Cupisti K, Ullmer C, Knoefel WT, Kubitz R, Häussinger D. The membrane-bound

bile acid receptor TGR5 is localized in the epithelium of human gallbladders. *Hepatology*. 2009;50(3):861–870.

56. Reimann F, Habib AM, Tolhurst G, Parker HE, Rogers GJ, Gribble FM. Glucose sensing in L cells: a primary cell study. *Cell Metabolism*. 2008;8(6):532–539.

57. Thomas C, Gioiello A, Noriega L, et al. TGR5-mediated bile acid sensing controls glucose homeostasis. *Cell Metabolism*. 2009;10(3):167–177.

58. Cannon B, Nedergaard J. Brown adipose tissue: function and physiological significance. *Physiological Reviews*. 2004.

59. Zurlo F, Larson K, Bogardus C, Ravussin E. Skeletal muscle metabolism is a major determinant of resting energy expenditure. *The Journal of Clinical Investigation*. 1990;86(5):1423–1427.

60. Watanabe M, Houten SM, Mataki C, et al. Bile acids induce energy expenditure by promoting intracellular thyroid hormone activation. *Nature*. 2006;439(7075):484–489.

61. Ferrell JM, Pathak P, Boehme S, Gililand T, Chiang JY. Deficiency of both farnesoid X receptor and Takeda G protein-coupled receptor 5 exacerbated liver fibrosis in mice. *Hepatology*. 2019;70(3):955–970.

62. Zhang S, Wang J, Liu Q, Harnish DC. Farnesoid X receptor agonist WAY-362450 attenuates liver inflammation and fibrosis in murine model of non-alcoholic steatohepatitis. *Journal of Hepatology*. 2009;51(2):380–388.

63. Wang YD, Chen WD, Wang M, Yu D, Forman BM, Huang W. Farnesoid X receptor antagonizes nuclear factor κB in hepatic inflammatory response. *Hepatology*. 2008;48(5):1632–1643.

64. Liu T, Zhang L, Joo D, Sun S-C. NF-κB signaling in inflammation. *Signal Transduction and Targeted Therapy*. 2017;2(1):1–9.

65. Stofan M, Guo GL. Bile acids and FXR: novel targets for liver diseases. *Frontiers in Medicine*. 2020;7:544.

66. Friedman SL. Molecular regulation of hepatic fibrosis, an integrated cellular response to tissue injury. *Journal of Biological Chemistry*. 2000;275(4):2247–2250.

67. Koyama Y, Brenner DA. Liver inflammation and fibrosis. *The Journal of Clinical Investigation*. 2017;127(1):55–64.

68. Tsuchida T, Friedman SL. Mechanisms of hepatic stellate cell activation. *Nature Reviews Gastroenterology & Hepatology*. 2017;14(7):397–411.

69. Fickert P, Fuchsbichler A, Moustafa T, et al. Farnesoid X receptor critically determines the fibrotic response in mice but is expressed to a low extent in human hepatic stellate cells and periductal myofibroblasts. *The American Journal of Pathology*. 2009;175(6):2392–2405.

70. Fiorucci S, Rizzo G, Antonelli E, et al. Cross-talk between farnesoid-X-receptor (FXR) and peroxisome proliferator-activated receptor γ contributes to the antifibrotic activity of FXR ligands in rodent models of liver cirrhosis. *Journal of Pharmacology and Experimental Therapeutics*. 2005;315(1):58–68.

71. Renga B, Mencarelli A, Migliorati M, et al. SHP-dependent and -independent induction of peroxisome proliferator-activated receptor-γ by the bile acid sensor farnesoid X receptor counter-regulates the pro-inflammatory phenotype of liver myofibroblasts. *Inflammation Research*. 2011;60(6):577–587.

72. Kawamata Y, Fujii R, Hosoya M, et al. AG protein-coupled receptor responsive to bile acids. *Journal of Biological Chemistry*. 2003;278(11):9435–9440.

73. Keitel V, Donner M, Winandy S, Kubitz R, Häussinger D. Expression and function of the bile acid receptor TGR5 in Kupffer cells. *Biochemical and Biophysical Research Communications*. 2008;372(1):78–84.

74. Pellicciari R, Fiorucci S, Camaioni E, et al. 6α-ethyl-chenodeoxycholic acid (6-ECDCA), a potent and selective FXR agonist endowed with anticholestatic activity. *Journal of Medicinal Chemistry*. 2002;45(17):3569–3572.

75. Mudaliar S, Henry RR, Sanyal AJ, et al. Efficacy and safety of the farnesoid X receptor agonist obeticholic acid in patients with type 2 diabetes and nonalcoholic fatty liver disease. *Gastroenterology*. 2013;145(3):574–582. e1.

76. Neuschwander-Tetri BA, Loomba R, Sanyal AJ, et al. Farnesoid X nuclear receptor ligand obeticholic acid for non-cirrhotic, non-alcoholic steatohepatitis (FLINT): a multicentre, randomised, placebo-controlled trial. *The Lancet*. 2015;385(9972):956–965.

77. Nevens F, Andreone P, Mazzella G, et al. A placebo-controlled trial of obeticholic acid in primary biliary cholangitis. *New England Journal of Medicine*. 2016;375(7):631–643.

78. Administration USFaD. *FDA Approves Ocaliva for Rare, Chronic Liver Disease*, 2021. Updated 5/31/2016. Accessed 12/4/2021. www.fda.gov/news-events/press-announcements/fda-approves-ocaliva-rare-chronic-liver-disease

79. John BV, Schwartz K, Levy C, et al. Impact of obeticholic acid exposure on decompensation and mortality in primary biliary cholangitis and cirrhosis. *Hepatology Communications*. 2021.

80. Administration. USFaD. *Due to Risk of Serious Liver Injury, FDA Restricts Use of Ocaliva (Obeticholic Acid) in Primary Biliary Cholangitis (PBC) Patients with Advanced Cirrhosis*, 2021. Updated 06/03/2021. Accessed 11/26/2021. www.fda.gov/drugs/drug-safety-and-availability/due-risk-serious-liver-injury-fda-restricts-use-ocaliva-obeticholic-acid-primary-biliary-cholangitis

81. Younossi ZM, Ratziu V, Loomba R, et al. Obeticholic acid for the treatment of non-alcoholic steatohepatitis: interim analysis from a multicentre, randomised, placebo-controlled phase 3 trial. *The Lancet*. 2019;394(10215):2184–2196.

82. Pharmaceuticals I. *Study Evaluating the Efficacy and Safety of Obeticholic Acid in Subjects with Compensated Cirrhosis Due to Nonalcoholic Steatohepatitis (REVERSE)*, 2021. Updated 09/21/2021. Accessed 11/26/2021. https://clinicaltrials.gov/ct2/show/NCT03439254

83. Intercept Pharmaceuticals, Inc. (2022, September 30). Intercept Pharmaceuticals Announces REVERSE Phase 3 Study of Obeticholic Acid (OCA) in Compensated Cirrhosis due to NASH Did Not Meet its Primary Endpoint [Press release]. Retrieved from https://ir.interceptpharma.com/news-releases/news-release-details/intercept-pharmaceuticals-announces-reverse-phase-3-study

84. Intercept Pharmaceuticals, Inc. (2022, December 23). Intercept Resubmits New Drug Application to U.S. FDA for Obeticholic Acid [Press release]. Retrieved from https://ir.interceptpharma.com/news-releases/news-release-details/intercept-resubmits-new-drug-application-us-fda-obeticholic-acid

85. Intercept Pharmaceuticals, Inc. (2023, May 19). Intercept Announces Outcome of FDA Advisory Committee Meeting [Press release]. Retrieved from

https://ir.interceptpharma.com/news-releases/news-release-details/intercept-announces-outcome-fda-advisory-committee-meeting

86. Anfuso B, Tiribelli C, Adorini L, Rosso N. Obeticholic acid and INT-767 modulate collagen deposition in a NASH in vitro model. *Scientific Reports*. 2020;10(1):1–12.

87. Jiang L, Zhang H, Xiao D, Wei H, Chen Y. Farnesoid X receptor (FXR): structures and ligands. *Computational and Structural Biotechnology Journal*. 2021.

88. Trauner M, Fuchs CD, Halilbasic E, Paumgartner G. New therapeutic concepts in bile acid transport and signaling for management of cholestasis. *Hepatology*. 2017;65(4):1393–1404.

89. Sonne DP. Mechanisms in endocrinology: FXR signalling: a novel target in metabolic diseases. *European Journal of Endocrinology*. 2021;184(5):R193–R205.

90. Patel K, Harrison SA, Elkhashab M, et al. Cilofexor, a nonsteroidal FXR agonist, in patients with noncirrhotic NASH: a phase 2 randomized controlled trial. *Hepatology*. 2020;72(1):58–71.

91. Loomba R, Noureddin M, Kowdley KV, et al. Combination therapies including cilofexor and firsocostat for bridging fibrosis and cirrhosis attributable to NASH. *Hepatology*. 2021;73(2):625–643.

92. Loomba R, Kayali Z, Noureddin M, et al. GS-0976 reduces hepatic steatosis and fibrosis markers in patients with nonalcoholic fatty liver disease. *Gastroenterology*. 2018;155(5):1463–1473. e6.

93. Harrison SA, Wong VW-S, Okanoue T, et al. Selonsertib for patients with bridging fibrosis or compensated cirrhosis due to NASH: results from randomized phase III STELLAR trials. *Journal of Hepatology*. 2020;73(1):26–39.

94. Lucas K, Lopez P, Lawitz E, et al. Tropifexor, a highly potent FXR agonist, produces robust and dose-dependent reductions in hepatic fat and serum alanine aminotransferase in patients with fibrotic NASH after 12 weeks of therapy: FLIGHT-FXR Part C interim results. *Digestive and Liver Disease*. 2020;52:e38.

95. Ratziu V, Rinella ME, Neuschwander-Tetri BA, et al. EDP-305 in patients with NASH: a phase II double-blind placebo-controlled dose-ranging study. *Journal of Hepatology*. 2021.

96. Kliewer SA, Mangelsdorf DJ. Bile acids as hormones: the FXR-FGF15/19 pathway. *Digestive Diseases*. 2015;33(3):327–331.

97. Degirolamo C, Sabbà C, Moschetta A. Therapeutic potential of the endocrine fibroblast growth factors FGF19, FGF21 and FGF23. *Nature Reviews Drug Discovery*. 2016;15(1):51–69.

98. Yu C, Wang F, Kan M, et al. Elevated cholesterol metabolism and bile acid synthesis in mice lacking membrane tyrosine kinase receptor FGFR4. *Journal of Biological Chemistry*. 2000;275(20):15482–15489.

99. Ito S, Fujimori T, Furuya A, Satoh J, Nabeshima Y, Nabeshima Y-I. Impaired negative feedback suppression of bile acid synthesis in mice lacking βKlotho. *The Journal of Clinical Investigation*. 2005;115(8):2202–2208.

100. Tomiyama K-I, Maeda R, Urakawa I, et al. Relevant use of Klotho in FGF19 subfamily signaling system in vivo. *Proceedings of the National Academy of Sciences*. 2010;107(4):1666–1671.

101. Kir S, Beddow SA, Samuel VT, et al. FGF19 as a postprandial, insulin-independent activator of hepatic protein and glycogen synthesis. *Science*. 2011;331(6024):1621–1624.

102. Wojcik M, Janus D, Dolezal-Oltarzewska K, et al. A decrease in fasting FGF19 levels is associated with the development of non-alcoholic fatty liver disease in obese adolescents. *Journal of Pediatric Endocrinology and Metabolism*. 2012;25(11–12):1089–1093.

103. Zucman-Rossi J, Villanueva A, Nault J-C, Llovet JM. Genetic landscape and biomarkers of hepatocellular carcinoma. *Gastroenterology*. 2015;149(5):1226–1239. e4.

104. Nicholes K, Guillet S, Tomlinson E, et al. A mouse model of hepatocellular carcinoma: ectopic expression of fibroblast growth factor 19 in skeletal muscle of transgenic mice. *The American Journal of Pathology*. 2002;160(6):2295–2307.

105. Li Y, Zhang W, Doughtie A, et al. Up-regulation of fibroblast growth factor 19 and its receptor associates with progression from fatty liver to hepatocellular carcinoma. *Oncotarget*. 2016;7(32):52329.

106. Wu X, Ge H, Lemon B, et al. FGF19-induced hepatocyte proliferation is mediated through FGFR4 activation. *Journal of Biological Chemistry*. 2010;285(8):5165–5170.

107. Harrison SA, Rinella ME, Abdelmalek MF, et al. NGM282 for treatment of non-alcoholic steatohepatitis: a multicentre, randomised, double-blind, placebo-controlled, phase 2 trial. *The Lancet*. 2018;391(10126):1174–1185.

108. Harrison SA, Neff G, Guy CD, et al. Efficacy and safety of aldafermin, an engineered FGF19 analog, in a randomized, double-blind, placebo-controlled trial of patients with nonalcoholic steatohepatitis. *Gastroenterology*. 2021;160(1):219–231 e1. doi:10.1053/j.gastro.2020.08.004

109. Zhou M, Wang X, Phung V, et al. Separating tumorigenicity from bile acid regulatory activity for endocrine hormone FGF19. *Cancer Research*. 2014;74(12):3306–3316.

110. Zhou M, Learned RM, Rossi SJ, DePaoli AM, Tian H, Ling L. Engineered FGF19 eliminates bile acid toxicity and lipotoxicity leading to resolution of steatohepatitis and fibrosis in mice. *Hepatology Communications*. 2017;1(10):1024–1042.

111. Henriksson E, Andersen B. FGF19 and FGF21 for the treatment of NASH—Two sides of the same coin? Differential and overlapping effects of FGF19 and FGF21 from mice to human. *Frontiers in Endocrinology*. 2020;11

112. Harrison SA, Rossi SJ, Paredes AH, et al. NGM282 improves liver fibrosis and histology in 12 weeks in patients with nonalcoholic steatohepatitis. *Hepatology*. 2020;71(4):1198–1212.

113. Talukdar S, Kharitonenkov A. FGF19 and FGF21. In NASH we trust. *Molecular Metabolism*. 2020:101152.

114. Luo J, Ko B, Elliott M, et al. A nontumorigenic variant of FGF19 treats cholestatic liver diseases. *Science Translational Medicine*. 2014;6(247):247ra100–247ra100.

115. Rinella ME, Trotter JF, Abdelmalek MF, et al. Rosuvastatin improves the FGF19 analogue NGM282-associated lipid changes in patients with non-alcoholic steatohepatitis. *Journal of Hepatology*. 2019;70(4):735–744.

116. NGM Biopharmaceuticals I. *Evaluation of Efficacy, Safety and Tolerability of Aldafermin in a Phase 2b, Randomized, Double-blind, Placebo-controlled, Multi-center Study In Subjects With Nonalcoholic Steatohepatitis and Stage 2/3 Fibrosis (ALPINE 2/3)*, 2021. Updated 01/06/2022. Accessed 12/29/2021. https://clinicaltrials.gov/ct2/show/NCT03912532

117. NGM Biopharmaceuticals I. *Topline Results from the ALPINE 2/3 Study: A Randomized, Double-Blind, Placebo-Controlled, Multicenter, Phase 2b Trial Evaluating 3 Doses of the FGF19 Analogue Aldafermin on Liver Histology in Patients with Nonalcoholic Steatohepatitis and Stage 2 and 3 Fibrosis AASLD The Liver Meeting, Presidential Plenary Session, November 14, 2021.* NGM Biopharmaceuticals, Inc., 2021. Updated 11/14/2021. Accessed 12/30/2021. www.ngmbio.com/topline-results-from-the-alpine-2-3-study-a-randomized-double-blind-placebo-controlled-multicenter-phase-2b-trial-evaluating-3-doses-of-the-fgf19-analogue-aldafermin-on-liver-histology-in-patient/

118. Patel J, Bettencourt R, Cui J, et al. Association of noninvasive quantitative decline in liver fat content on MRI with histologic response in nonalcoholic steatohepatitis. *Therapeutic Advances in Gastroenterology.* 2016;9(5):692–701.

119. NGM Biopharmaceuticals I. *NGM Bio Reports Topline Results from 24-Week Phase 2b ALPINE 2/3 Study of Aldafermin in NASH.* NGM Biopharmaceuticals, Inc., 2021. Accessed 12/17/2021. https://ir.ngmbio.com/news-releases/news-release-details/ngm-bio-reports-topline-results-24-week-phase-2b-alpine-23-study

14 PPAR Agonists

Sven M. A. Francque

CONTENTS

14.1 INTRODUCTION

NonAlcoholic Fatty Liver Disease (NAFLD) and NonAlcoholic Steatohepatitis (NASH) are part of a multisystem disease with ramifications extending beyond the liver [1]. Morbidity and mortality are also related to the impact of the diseased liver on the cardiovascular (CV) system[2] and on organs involved in glycaemic control. People with NAFLD are two to five times more likely to develop type 2 diabetes mellitus (T2DM) [3,4], and NAFLD may add to coexisting metabolic risk factors [5]. Vice versa, patients with T2DM are at a high risk of having NAFLD. The global prevalence of NAFLD among patients with T2DM exceeds 55% [6].

The metabolic syndrome (MetS) or components of the MetS frequently occur with NAFLD [7], and the liver is involved in the pathogenesis of several components of the MetS. The liver is a key organ that is affected by nutritional overload (the so-called substrate-overload liver injury), adipose tissue dysfunction, insulin resistance (IR) and gut dysbiosis. The role of liver disease in the pathogenesis of T2DM and CV disease (CVD) shows that it is a driving force of a vicious circle [8,9]. For example, NAFLD increases the risk of T2DM [10] and CVD [11]. With the development of T2DM, there are a further increase in risk of CVD [12,13], a worsening of liver disease (fibrosis and cirrhosis) [14–16] and an increased risk of hepatocellular carcinoma [17]. Development of advanced liver fibrosis with NAFLD also increases the risk of CVD [18].

In light of the complex pathophysiology of NAFLD and the complex interorgan cross talk that drives both disease progression and outcomes, peroxisome proliferator-activated receptors (PPARs) are of particular interest because they are key regulators of lipid and glucose metabolism, as well as inflammation in different tissues. They are hence highly relevant to NAFLD when it is approached from the standpoint of a systemic disease involving metabolic changes in adipose tissue, skeletal muscle, liver and endothelium [19]. PPARs thus represent interesting therapeutic targets both in a liver-centered approach as well as in a systemic approach to NAFLD, in terms of improving liver function and liver-, CV- and diabetes-related outcomes. This chapter aims at comprehensively summarizing the current knowledge on the pleiotropic roles of PPARs in the pathophysiology of NASH viewed as an integrated part of metabolic and cardiovascular derangements, which must serve as a rationale for their use in the treatment of this condition.

14.2 NAFLD PATHOPHYSIOLOGY AND THE ROLE OF PPARS

NAFLD pathophysiology is extensively described in other chapters. In summary, the development of hepatic damage in persons with NASH requires both extra- and intrahepatic factors, which highlights the involvement of multiorgan systems. Chronic adipose dysfunction creates an imbalance between the release of anti-inflammatory insulin-sensitizing (e.g., adiponectin) and pro-inflammatory (e.g., interleukin-6, tumor necrosis factor-alpha) cytokines, which activate inflammatory pathways and IR in the liver [20]. Continuous oversupply of lipids to the liver also stimulates hepatic lipid oxidation, induces abnormal mitochondrial function and generates oxidative stress[21]. Finally, lipids may induce an unfolded protein response and endoplasmic reticulum (ER) stress [21]. All this results in tissue damage and inflammation, activating fibrogenesis. On the other hand, chronic liver damage will result via several mechanisms, including the altered release and clearance of lipoproteins and the release of several metabolic and inflammatory mediators, noy to mention the impact on distant organs and structures, including the cardiovascular system, muscle and adipose tissue [2,22,23].

PPARs were first described as members of the steroid hormone receptor superfamily of ligand-activated transcription factors causing proliferation of peroxisome [24,25]. As peroxisomes play an important role not only in fatty acid catabolism and in the pentose pathway and hence in energy metabolism but also in the reduction of reactive oxygen species [26], PPARs are critical regulators of fatty acid metabolism [24] and even so have an impact on glucose metabolism and inflammation. Although at first discovered to have an impact on peroxisomal proliferation, the actions of the PPAR target pathways involve several other cell organelles, most notably mitochondria, and numerous metabolic, inflammatory and fibrogenic pathways [24,27].

DOI: 10.1201/9781003386698-17

Three PPAR isotypes have been identified—α, β/δ and γ (with 2 subtypes: γ1 and γ2) [28,29]—the expression and actions of which differ according to isotype, organ and intraorgan cell type, resulting in a complex system of nuclear receptor-mediated interorgan cross talk [30] (Figure 14.1). Furthermore, substantial interspecies differences exist and need to be taken into account in translating findings in preclinical studies to patients[26]. This has been best documented for PPARα, the expression and activity of which have been shown to be lower in human livers compared to rodents. Also, differences between murine species and humans, but also guinea pigs, have been found at the level of PPARα expression, ligand activation and biological response. This is particularly of note when it comes to the role of peroxisome proliferation, which is relevant in rats and mice but not in humans [31–33]. PPARγ is more conserved across species, although some differences, for example in brown adipose tissue, have been documented [34,35]. Liver PPARγ expression, which is low in liver compared to adipose tissue, is induced by obesity in mice (the γ2 subtype [36]), but no increased expression has been noted in the human liver in relation to NASH [37].

14.2.1 PPARs and Steatosis

The main ligands for PPARs are fatty acids and their metabolites. Endogenous ligands can result from lipogenesis, lipolysis and fatty acid catabolism, explaining the mutual impact for example of PPARα pathways with acyl-CoA oxidase 1 (implicated in peroxisomal β-oxidation), fatty acid synthase (implicated in de novo lipogenesis) or hepatic adipose triglyceride lipase (implicated in triglyceride hydrolysis) [38–40].

PPARα, which is encoded by the *NR1C1* (Nuclear Receptor Subfamily 1 Group C Member 1) gene on the human chromosome 22, binds more saturated fatty acids than other PPAR isotypes and is predominantly expressed in tissues with a high rate of fatty acid oxidation, such as skeletal muscle, liver, heart, kidney and brown adipose tissue. Within the liver, it is expressed mainly in hepatocytes. In the vasculature, it is also expressed in various cell types within atherosclerotic plaques [41]. Notably, within the liver, expression has also been documented in endothelial cells and to some extent in hepatic stellate cells (HSC), where PPARα is implicated in maintaining these cells in the quiescent state [42].

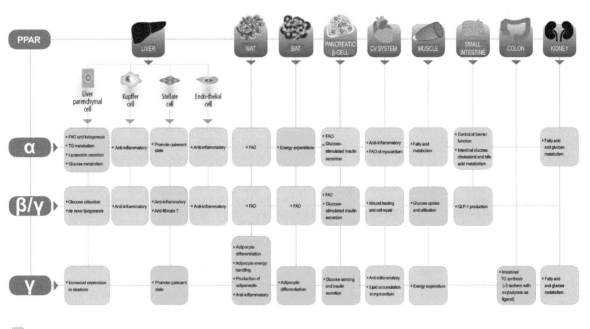

Figure 14.1 Complex role of PPARs

PPARs, composed of three different isotypes (α, β/δ, γ) are implicated in regulating lipids and carbohydrate metabolism, inflammation and fibrogenesis. The 3 isotypes are differentially expressed in the different tissues and cell types. The main sites of expression and the main functions are depicted. In NASH, PPARα could improve lipid metabolism by controlling lipid flux and regulating fatty acid transport as well as β-oxydation. It also reduces inflammation through its action on hepatocytes as well as reducing splanchnic inflammation and intestinal permeability. PPARα is also involved in decreasing portal pressure in the context of cirrhosis. PPARβ/δ is involved in glucose and lipoprotein metabolism and reduces insulin resistance in skeletal muscle. PPARβ/δ inhibits inflammatory macrophage phenotypes and favors the alternatively activated phenotype. PPARγ regulates insulin sensitivity within the adipose tissue and is a master regulator of HSC fate. PPARγ prevents HSC activation, which is a key event in fibrogenesis. Moreover, in the context of cirrhosis, PPARγ reduces portal pressure, splanchnic inflammation, angiogenesis and porto-systemic shunts. All together, the three PPAR isotypes, by acting within the different cells and organs, impact different pathways and mechanisms involved in NASH and fibrosis progression.

FAO: Fatty acid oxidation; GLP-1: Glucagon-like peptide 1; PPAR: Peroxisome proliferator-activated receptor; TG: Triglyceride.

As a key regulator of fatty acid metabolism and keto-genesis, PPARα regulates fatty acid transport, peroxisomal and mitochondrial β-oxidation and lipolysis and impacts the production of apolipoproteins. Overall, this leads to the reduction of triglyceride-rich lipoproteins and triglyceride accumulation in the liver, whereas plasma high-density lipoprotein (HDL) cholesterol (HDL-C) increases. In the fasting state, increased fatty acid oxidation produces acetyl-CoA, further converted into ketone bodies, involving the action of mitochondrial hydroxymethylglutaryl-CoA synthase, upregulated by PPARα. The mild phenotype of PPARα-deficient mice fed ad libitum indicate that PPARα is essentially involved in the fasting state since the phenotype becomes more pronounced during fasting, being character-ized by impaired fatty acid oxidation, lipid accumulation in the liver, as well as an inability to augment ketone body synthesis [43]. Transcriptomic studies in PPARα-deficient mice in fasting or fed condition have confirmed that major changes in the liver in gene expression occur in the fasting state [44]. Furthermore, PPARα seems to be implicated in the circadian clock [45–49]. It also regulates expression of a plethora of target genes by transactivation or transrepres-sion (the latter mainly of inflammatory genes), with about 50% conservation between rodents and humans in terms of gene ontology categories [50]. The latter is particularly relevant when it comes to drug development and transla-tion of preclinical data into patients.

All these aspects of PPARα physiology are relevant to NASH pathogenesis, and preclinical data point to an important role for alterations in PPARα, the deficiency of which leads to more severe NASH lesions [51], which PPARa agonists prevent or improve [52]. Mice with a PPARα mutant that only has transrepressive activity are protected against the development of NASH but not steato-sis, while mice with wild-type PPARα are protected from both NASH and steatosis [53]. Clinical data are in line with these experimental findings showing that liver PPARα expression inversely correlates with NASH severity and that improvement of liver histology accompanies increased hepatic PPARα expression [37].

PPARβ/δ also plays an important role in liver metabo-lism. Encoded by *NR1C2* on human chromosome 6, it is expressed in hepatocytes, sinusoidal endothelial cells, HSCs and Kupffer cells [30]. PPARβ/δ activates pathways of glucose utilisation and de novo lipogenesis in the liver. In PPARβ/δ-null mice, transcriptional profiling has revealed downregulation of genes associated with lipoprotein metabolism and glucose utilization pathways, indicating that these genes are positively regulated by PPARβ/δ [44]. In addition, it increases the production of monounsatu-rated fatty acids and protects against lipotoxicity and saturated fatty acid cytotoxicity [54]. Although PPARβ/δ and PPARα are both implicated in the fasting and fed states, PPARa seems to be predominantly important in the fasting state, whereas PPARβ/d is more equally involved in both [55]. PPARβ/δ ligands can mimic activation of PPARβ/δ pathways, although differential response may be seen between ligands [56], as it has been reported for other PPARs ligands, being attributed to the different capacities of these ligands to recruit various coactivators or corepres-sors [57].

14.2.2 PPARs and Inflammation

All 3 PPARs participate in the regulation of the inflam-matory process, a key component in the development of NASH. PPARγ, which is encoded by the *NR1C3* gene on human chromosome 3, binds to the p65 component of the NF-κB complex and induces inhibitory iκB, which attenu-ates NF-κB-driven inflammatory cytokine and chemokine production [58]. Upon ligand stimulation, PPARγ promotes the M2 macrophage phenotype by upregulating CD206 and CD163 [59]. In addition, PPARg improves endothelial cell function by lowering inflammation in diabetes and atherosclerosis [60], plays a significant role in controlling vascular homeostasis and decreases blood pressure in T2DM patients, thereby decreasing CV risk [61].

PPARα also has anti-inflammatory properties, mainly by transrepression of pro-inflammatory target genes [62]. This occurs not only in the liver but also in vascular endothelial cells, linking PPARα to systemic inflammation and athero-sclerosis [58].

PPARβ/δ is highly expressed in hepatocytes, liver sinusoidal endothelial cells and Kupffer cells [63]. It modulates expression of key genes involved in innate immunity and inflammation [44], although its role in inflammation is incompletely understood. Unligated PPARb/δ has pro-inflammatory effects in disease models, and its ligand engagement disrupts this complex and has anti-inflammatory effects, including suppression of pro-inflammatory adhesion molecules on vascular endothelial cells [64–66]. PPARβ/δ also activates Kupffer cells toward a more anti-inflammatory phenotype, which contributes to hepatic IR and NASH [67]. Conversely, increasing PPARβ/δ leads to alternatively activated Kupffer cells that have anti-inflammatory properties and result in less severe meta-bolic and hepatic derangements [68].

14.2.3 PPARs and Fibrosis

Fibrosis is the strongest predictor of adverse clinical out-comes in NASH, including liver-related death and overall mortality [69,70]. Fibrogenesis in HSCs is inhibited by PPARs [71]. PPARγ normally keeps HSCs quiescent, and its overexpression decreases its myofibroblastic charac-ter, resulting in reduced collagen production. Its reduced expression results in the progression of liver fibrosis and increased collagen production [42]. PPARγ and PPARβ/δ are expressed in a stimulus- and tissue-dependent manner in macrophages [72], which are a key factor for fibrosis, as inflammatory macrophages activate while restorative macrophages deactivate HSCs [73]. PPARβ/δ in fibroblasts and α-smooth muscle cells improve wound healing in skin diseases and myocardial infarction, through regulation of IL-1 signaling [74,75].

Human liver PPARα gene expression negatively cor-relates with NASH severity, visceral adiposity and IR [37]. Expression in the liver has also been documented in endothelial cells and to some extent in HSCs, where PPARα is implicated in maintaining these cells in the qui-escent state [42]. Interestingly, a liver biopsy transcriptomic analysis of NASH obese patients before and after bariatric surgery, combined with transcriptomic datasets from murine models of NASH and fibrosis, identified common clusters of genes with specific functions in inflammation and extracellular matrix homeostasis and in particular a role for PPARα-regulated dermatopontin in NASH-related fibrogenesis [76]. Dermatopontin is a protein involved in fibrinogenesis and collagen deposition, and its expression is lowered by PPARα activation [76,77].

14.2.4 PPARs in Nonhepatic Tissue

PPARs, in particular PPARg, play a key role in adipocyte biology and adaptation to nutrient supply [78,79]. PPARγ is highly expressed in adipose tissue where it plays an essential role in the regulation of adipocyte differentiation, adipogenesis and lipid metabolism [80]. As with the other PPARs, its distribution and actions are complex and differ also for its 2 subtypes. PPARγ1 is widely distributed in skeletal/cardiac muscle and the vascular bed, as well as in macrophages, colon epithelium and adipose tissue, whereas PPARγ2 is predominantly expressed in adipose tissue [29].

With central obesity, there is a switch in gene expression within adipocytes to a pattern that more closely resembles that of macrophages [81]. Thus, excess lipid storage associated with obesity, promotes adipose tissue inflammation. With obesity there is also an increased flux of free fatty acids from adipose tissue to the liver and to other organs, as well as altered secretion of adipokines [82]. The combination of altered adipokine secretion and increased flux of free fatty acids promotes development of ectopic triglyceride accumulation and an increase in the synthesis of toxic lipid mediators, in tissues other than adipose, such as liver, muscle and possibly pancreas [83].

Interventions that reduce fat mass/adipocyte hypertrophy (weight loss) or that pharmacologically restore adipose tissue insulin sensitivity (such as thiazolidinediones [TZD]) [84–87] restore adipose tissue biology and are beneficial in NAFLD given the dynamic cross talk between the liver and adipose tissue that adapts to day-to-day changes in energy needs. In humans, at least two-thirds of fatty acids reaching the liver are released from subcutaneous fat [81]. In NAFLD, there is a strong linear relationship between the severity of adipose tissue IR and that of hepatic steatosis [133], and patients with steatohepatitis tend to have worse IR than those with isolated steatosis [88]. However, hepatic and muscle IR, as well as atherogenic dyslipidaemia (elevated triglycerides, low HDL-C), and even hepatocyte necroinflammation, appear to be nearly fully established once patients develop steatosis [89].

14.3 PPAR-TARGETED TREATMENT FOR NASH

14.3.1 PPAR Agonistic Effects on the Severity of Liver Disease

Due to their key role in the transcriptional regulation of glucose and lipid metabolism, PPAR ligands hold promise as therapeutic agents for NAFLD [80]. Despite preclinical rationale [90], clinical data on PPARα single agonists are scarce. The PPARα agonist fenofibrate reduces lipid levels by activating PPARα, which is highly expressed in the liver, but has no effect on insulin sensitivity [91] or hepatic steatosis [92]. Rodents and humans differ substantially in terms of the differential expression and roles of the different PPAR isotypes [26,31–33,93], which may in part explain the fact that preclinical data on the efficacy of the isolated PPARα agonism [90] has not to date translated into histological improvement in NASH patients. As receptor binding and subsequent effects may substantially differ between molecules (the selective PPAR modulator concept [138]), studies are ongoing with other compounds. The PPARα agonist gemfibrozil improves lipid profiles in NAFLD patients [80]. Pemafibrate, which also showed benefits in preclinical NAFLD models and in patients with diabetes and dyslipidemia, has also been under clinical investigation for NAFLD treatment [94–96] (Table 14.1) but has failed to reduce liver fat content [97].

TZDs (PPARγ) improve IR by direct effects on adipose tissue, which appear to play an important role for the hepatic benefits of pioglitazone in patients with NASH

[98]. PPARγ activation in humans by TZDs is associated with a broad spectrum of metabolic effects in great part derived from restoring adipose tissue biology [81,99] and a decrease in chronic systemic inflammation [78,79], changes that are strongly associated with improvement in liver histology in patients with NASH [100]. In patients with biopsy-proven NASH, rosiglitazone improves hepatic steatosis and serum alanine aminotransferase (ALT), but not other histologic features of NASH, including fibrosis at 1 year [101] or with therapy for 2 years [102].

In rat models of fibrosis, pioglitazone prevented choline-deficient diet-induced fibrosis but was ineffective once hepatic fibrosis was established [103]. In patients with prediabetes or T2DM, pioglitazone 45 mg OD for 6 months improved NASH with a trend toward improvement in fibrosis compared to placebo [87]. This was followed by an 18-month randomized controlled trial (RCT) in 101 patients with biopsy-proven NASH [86]. Recently, in an RCT in 105 patients with T2DM, pioglitazone plus vitamin E improved steatosis, hepatocyte ballooning and inflammation [104]. In patients without T2DM, pioglitazone 30 mg daily for 12 months was reported to improve hepatic fibrosis [84], but this was not observed in the PIVENS study, where instead pioglitazone improved all other individual histological parameters and induced resolution of NASH in 47% of patients compared to 18% in the placebo arm [85]. A recent meta-analysis indicates that pioglitazone but not rosiglitazone significantly reduces fibrosis in NASH [105] in terms of the mean fibrosis stage but without reaching the endpoint of 1 stage improvement.

Why pioglitazone compared to rosiglitazone has drastically different efficacy in reversing steatohepatitis remains unclear, but it is often attributed to pioglitazone also being a weak agonist of the PPARα isotype [106]. However, the action of PPARα agonists alone seems unlikely to explain the broad effects of pioglitazone on liver histology in NASH. Pioglitazone improves mitochondrial function [107], but there are many other potential mechanisms by which it may have beneficial effects on the liver [78,79,108,109]. Evidently, each PPARγ agonist has a unique cardiometabolic signature and biology in the liver.

The PPARα/γ dual agonist saroglitazar has beneficial effects in experimental models of NASH [110] and in humans significantly decreases ALT levels and improves the cardiometabolic profile of subjects with biopsy-proven NASH [111]. A randomized, double-blind, phase 2 trial showed a significant effect on liver fat content after 16 weeks of treatment [112].

A study with histological endpoints is ongoing (NCT05011305).

The selective PPARδ agonist seladelpar (MBX-8025) improves insulin sensitivity and steatohepatitis in mouse models of NAFLD [113]. In humans, its effect is more on atherogenic dyslipidemia [114] and is rather modest on insulin sensitivity or steatosis compared to PPARδ agonists. A phase 2, double-blind RCT to evaluate the activity of seladelpar in NASH patients has been halted (NCT03551522) [115]. Preliminary results on 171 patients with NASH, with change in liver fat by MRI-PDFF as the primary endpoint, showed the 3 doses of seladelpar (10 mg, 20 mg and 50 mg) to be numerically worse vs. placebo (from 9.8 to 14.2% change vs. baseline compared to a 20.8% reduction with placebo). However, there was a significative dose–response reduction in ALT and GGT. The observation of some lesions on liver biopsy after treatment raised the suspicion on drug-induced liver injury. Careful

Table 14.1: Main Outcomes of PPAR Agonistic Drugs

	Action	Effect on Liver	Clinical Status	Safety Profile
Single PPAR agonists				
PPARα (fibrates)	Enhanced FFA metabolism; many antiatherogenic effects on lipoprotein metabolism: ↓plasma triglycerides ↑HDL-C	No effect on hepatic steatosis or NASH [91,92]	Pemafibrate [95,96] phase 2 (MRI-based endpoint) NCT03350165 finalized, failed to reduce liver fat content [97].	Toxic liver injury, impaired renal function (less with pemafibrate)
PPARγ (i.e., rosiglitazone)	Improved glucose and FFA metabolism; ↑LDL-C and HDL-C	Reduction of hepatic steatosis; no effect on resolution of NASH [101,102]	Phase 2 trials have been conducted	Weight gain, fluid retention and cardiac decompensation, bone fractures
PPARδ (i.e., seladelpar)	Improved FFA/lipid (LDL-C, TG, HDL-C) and glucose metabolism	No effect on hepatic steatosis [161]*	Phase 2 (MRI-based endpoint at 12 w, histological secondary endpoints at 52 w) (NCT03551522, halted)	Gastrointestinal side effects, headache, suspicion of drug-induced liver injury but not confirmed after careful data examination followed by FDA clearance
Dual PPAR agonists				
PPARα/γ (i.e., pioglitazone, saroglitazar)	Improved glucose and FFA metabolism; ↓plasma triglycerides ↑HDL-C Neutral effect on LDL-C	Pioglitazone may induce resolution of NASH [46]**, Saroglitazar improves ALT and steatosis [111,112,162]	Pioglitazone phase 2 trials have been conducted or are ongoing (NCT03646292, noninvasive endpoints and compared to empagliflozin or combination pioglitazone + empagliflozin), trials in patients with T2DM have also been labeled as phase 4; saroglitazar in phase 2 (NCT03061721, noninvasive endpoints) has reported results [112], and a study with histological endpoints is ongoing (NCT05011305).	Pioglitazone: weight gain, fluid retention and cardiac decompensation in patients with preexisting reduced cardiac function (pioglitazone improves overall cardiovascular outcomes), bone fractures; saroglitazar body weight neutral, gastritis and dyspepsia
PPARα/δ (i.e., elafibranor)	Improvement of atherogenic profile and FFA/glucose metabolism	May induce resolution of NASH [161], not confirmed in Phase 3 [121]	Phase 3 (with histological endpoint at interim analysis); NCT02704403 failed to achieve primary endpoint of NASH resolution; development in NASH halted	Body weight neutral; headache; increase in serum creatinine but no other markers of impaired renal function
Pan PPAR agonists				
PPAR a/d/g (i.e., lanifibranor)	Improved glucose and FFA metabolism; ↓plasma triglycerides ↑HDL-C Neutral effect on LDL-C	Resolution of NASH and regression of fibrosis and composite endpoint	Phase 2 (histological endpoint) NCT03459079 reported144, Phase 3 NCT04849728, EudraCT Number: 2020–004986–38).	Headache, dizziness, weight gain

* No detailed liver biopsy data available for seladelpar in NASH.
** Liver biopsy data only available for pioglitazone, not saroglitazar (ongoing studies).
FDA: Food and Drug Administration; FFA: Free fatty acids; HDL-C: High-density lipoprotein cholesterol; IR: Insulin resistance; LDL-C: Low-density lipoprotein cholesterol; MR: Magnetic resonance; NAFLD: Nonalcoholic fatty liver disease; NASH: Nonalcoholic steatohepatitis; PPAR: Peroxisome proliferator-activated receptors; T2DM: Type 2 diabetes mellitus.

examination of the data did not confirm this, and despite the Food and Drug Administration (FDA) clearance, the development of the drug in NASH was not resumed.

In rodent models of NASH and/or liver fibrosis, the dual PPARα/δ agonist elafibranor reduced liver fibrosis progression [116]. In the Phase 2b GOLDEN 505 study of 274 noncirrhotic patients with biopsy-proven NASH, elafibranor 120 mg daily was superior to placebo (20% vs. 11%; $p = 0.018$) in patients with a higher baseline NAFLD activity score (NAS ≥ 4) [117]. Further, a secondary post hoc analysis based on a revised definition for the resolution of NASH of disappearance of ballooning and disappearance of lobular inflammation or persistence of mild lobular inflammation (score of 0 or 1), without worsening in liver fibrosis (progression by ≥1 stage) was met in patients receiving elafibranor 120 mg daily (19% vs. 12%,

p = 0.045) [117]. Furthermore, in patients whose NASH improved, fibrosis also improved. Elafibranor has a positive effect on hepatic and muscle insulin sensitivity [118] and on steatohepatitis in NASH patients [119]. The phase 3 RESOLVE-IT trial (NCT02704403) [120] did not, however, confirm a significant benefit of elafibranor over placebo in inducing NASH resolution [121].

Activation of PPARβ/δ results in the modulation of lipid and glucose homeostasis, skeletal muscle function and brown adipose tissue activity, as well as PPARβ/δ agonists have been used to treat fibrosis in preclinical animal studies [122].

14.3.2 PPAR Agonist Treatment and Cardiovascular Effects

PPARα, -β/δ and -γ agonists improve endothelial dysfunction and regulate multiple pathways involved in subclinical inflammation and atherosclerosis [61,123]. PPARγ is also highly expressed in atherosclerotic lesions, and its activation reduces inflammatory pathways in cardiomyocytes and in the vascular bed [124–126].

The TZDs rosiglitazone and pioglitazone prevent the progression of prediabetes, which affects many NAFLD patients [127], to T2DM [128,129]. TZDs also exert longer-lasting glycaemic control than metformin or glibenclamide [130]. Rosiglitazone and pioglitazone increase HDL-C, and rosiglitazone (but not pioglitazone) increases low-density lipoprotein cholesterol (LDL-C) and is neutral on plasma triglycerides, which are reduced with pioglitazone treatment. This may account for the observed reduction of atherosclerosis progression [128,131,132] and reduction of CVD [133–135] observed with pioglitazone in T2DM patients. Moreover, in patients with prediabetes and good adherence to treatment (intake of ≥80% of prescribed dosage), pioglitazone reduces stroke by 36%, acute coronary syndromes by 53% and the combined endpoint of stroke/myocardial infarction/hospitalization for heart failure by 39% [136]. There still is a misperception that rosiglitazone increases the risk of death from CVD because of a controversial and significantly flawed meta-analysis [137]. A large RCT found no such increase [138], a conclusion shared in 2013 by the FDA that led to the removal of regulatory restrictions on rosiglitazone.

Use of a selective PPARβ/δ improves the lipid profile of patients with increased CV risk [139], but PPARα agonists (fibrates) have been more broadly tested in large RCTs and are often associated with reduction in CVD. Also, dual PPARα/γ agonism by saroglitazar improves the CV risk profile [111,140].

14.3.3 Pan-PPAR Agonism

Taken together, the concept of combining PPARα, -β/δ and -γ activation may represent a novel and potentially more efficacious therapeutic approach by targeting the large array of disturbances that contribute to the development and progression of NASH [141]. Lanifibranor (IVA337) is an indole sulfonamide PPAR agonist that activates all three subtypes (α, β/δ and γ), giving it the potential to address all the key features of NASH, namely inflammation, steatosis, ballooning and fibrosis [142]. In in vitro and in vivo preclinical studies, lanifibranor prevented and induced the regression of preexisting fibrotic damage in the liver and other organs without the classic effects on body weight, fluid retention and heart weight increase, reported with TZDs. Lanifibranor also improved metabolic features relevant to NASH [141] and was

investigated in the double-blind, randomized, placebo-controlled phase IIb NATIVE trial (NCT03008070) [143]. A 24-week treatment with 800 or 1,200 mg once daily showed dose-dependent significant effects on both the resolution of NASH without the worsening of fibrosis (45% for 1,200 mg vs. 19% on placebo, $p < 0.001$) and regression of fibrosis without worsening of NASH (42% vs. 24%, $p = 0.011$), as well as on the composite endpoint of NASH resolution and fibrosis stage improvement (31% vs. 7%, $p < 0.001$) with a good safety and tolerability profile [144] (see Table 14.1).

The drug improved glycaemic control and the lipid profile toward a less atherogenic type, including an increase in HDL cholesterol, a decrease in serum triglycerides and improvements in ApoB1 and the ApoB1/ApoA1 ratio. Lanifibranor did not change LDL-C. A significant decrease in diastolic blood pressure was also observed.

The compound is now being tested in a large phase 3 study (NCT04849728, EudraCT Number: 2020–004986–38).

14.3.4 Safety Profile of PPARs

In the phase 2 GOLDEN 505 study, elafibranor treatment was associated with a slight rise in creatinine [117], believed to be due to a rise in tubular reabsorption of creatinine. This is typical of all PPARa agonists and not deleterious to renal function as demonstrated with fenofibrate in the FIELD study, where it reduced the progression of CKD in patients with T2DM [145].

In practice, pioglitazone is the only TZD clinically in use today. There is increasing recognition of its cardiometabolic benefits [136,146,147], but it may alter bone metabolism and promote an increase in fractures with long-term use [135], although the risk remains relatively low and can be monitored and minimized with vitamin D and calcium supplementation [148]. Hematuria should be checked before and during treatment, although most studies have been negative in terms of the increased risk for bladder cancer [149].

Weight gain of 2–4% of body weight has been reported after 6–36 months of therapy in NASH trials [84–87] and in studies of longer duration in patients with T2DM [128,133,135]. These side effects may be treatment limiting but are reversible upon treatment discontinuation. Furthermore, this weight gain is associated with improved insulin sensitivity by shifting fat from ectopic tissues to subcutaneous and less metabolically deleterious depots [150], consistent with the observed reduction in CVD in RCTs [133–135]. In most patients, weight gain is exclusively from increased adiposity [151], but peripheral edema may occur in about 5% of patients and require treatment discontinuation.

Pioglitazone reduces the risk of CV events, but significant confusion remains about its effects on cardiac function. Heart failure was precipitated in more (~2%) patients on pioglitazone than on placebo in the PROACTIVE trial [133]. However, this was not observed in other placebo-controlled studies [85,86,128,131,132,135]. In a recent large RCT in 3,851 patients, the 5-year heart failure risk did not differ by treatment (4.1% pioglitazone, 4.2% placebo) [152]. While pioglitazone improves whole-body and myocardial insulin sensitivity, left ventricular diastolic and systolic function in healthy patients with T2DM [153,154], undiagnosed "diastolic dysfunction" (i.e., heart failure with preserved left ventricular function) may occur in ≥10% of patients with longstanding obesity, T2DM and/or NASH [155]. If fluid retention occurs during pioglitazone therapy in such patients, it may seem to be causing heart failure rather than unmasking established but subclinical heart disease. Therefore, in patients with established heart failure or with increased risk of heart failure, pioglitazone is contraindicated. In general, pioglitazone 15 mg/day is not associated with weight gain (~1%), edema or other side effects and may be the recommended dose for initiation in most patients. Up-titration to 30 mg/day may offer safe and maximal or near-maximal cardiometabolic [156] and liver histological [84,85] benefits for patients with NASH. Large RCTs with pioglitazone 15 mg/day are needed to assess its long-term CV and histological benefit in NASH.

The dual PPARα/γ agonist saroglitazar has not been associated with weight gain and edema, which have been reported with PPARγ agonists. No major serious adverse events have been reported. Long-term cardiovascular safety has not yet been established, but as mentioned, the overall CV risk factor profile improves [111,157]. The PPARβ/δ receptor agonist seladelpar, when investigated in a randomized phase 2 dose-finding study for patients with primary biliary cholangitis, was not associated with drug-induced transaminitis or pruritus [158].

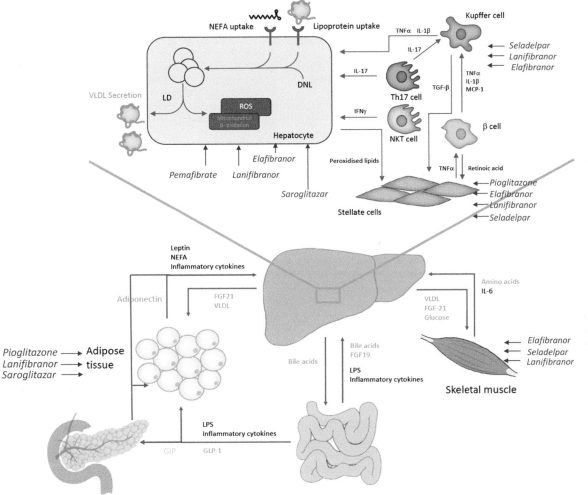

Figure 14.2 21PPAR therapeutic targets in the complex pathophysiology of NASH (Figure adapted from [22] [courtesy J. Haas] and [164].)

NASH is the result of a complex interplay of metabolic, inflammatory and fibrogenic processes. Within the liver, hepatocytes and several of its intracellular organels, most notably mitochondria, play an important role, alongside the stellate cells and several resident and infiltrating immune cells of different populations. NASH furthermore results from and impacts on an important cross talk between the liver, the adipose tissue, the gut (including the gut microbiome), the muscle and the pancreas. The cardiovascular system is even so implicated (not depicted, see reference [159]).

Numerous mediators are involved. PPAR drugs that have been tested in NASH or that are under development have differential targets inside and outside the liver to ultimately result in an improvement of the steatohepatitis and/or fibrosis.

ACC: Acetyl-CoA carboxylase; DNL: De novo lipogenesis; FAS: Fatty acid synthase; FGF19: Fibroblast growth factor 1; FGF21: Fibroblast growth factor 21; FXR: Farnesoid receptor X; GIP: Glucose-dependent insulinotropic polypeptide; GLP-1: Glucagon-like peptide 1; IFNg: Interferon gamma; IL1-b: Interleukin 1 beta; IL-6: Interleukin 6; IL-17: Interleukin 17; LD: Lipid droplets; LPS: Lipopolysaccharide; MCP-1: Monocyte chemoattractant protein 1; NEFA: Nonesterified fatty acids; NKT cell: Natural killer T cell; ROS: Reactive oxygen species; Th17: T helper 17 cell; TGFb: Tumor growth factor beta; TNFa: Tumor necrosis factor alpha; VLDL: Very-low-density lipoproteins.

The panPPAR agonist lanifibranor was generally well-tolerated with a low dropout rate (<5%) for adverse events (AEs). The vast majority of AEs were mild or moderate in intensity. The rate of severe treatment-emergent adverse events (TEAE) was low (<4%) and similar in the three groups. There were two drug-related serious TEAEs, both occurring in the placebo group (mild heart failure, urticaria). Compared to placebo, the most frequent TEAEs were diarrhea, nausea, weight increase and peripheral edema. One mild heart failure not requiring hospitalization was reported in the lanifibranor 1,200 mg arm. Peripheral edema was reported as a drug-related TEAE in 2.4% of patients in both lanifibranor arms, compared to none in placebo. One patient suffered from peripheral edema considered severe but recovered after stopping lanifibranor 1,200 mg for 12 days; treatment was resumed without edema reoccurrence. A mean weight increase from baseline on lanifibranor 1,200 mg and 800 mg (2.7 kg [3.1%] and 2.4 kg [2.6%], respectively) was also observed. Renal function was not impaired, nor were markers of bone turnover [144].

14.4 CONCLUSIONS

NAFLD is a multisystem disease with extrahepatic disease implications that include development of T2DM and CVD. Patients with NAFLD often present with many of the features of the MetS, and, with the progression of liver disease to NASH, there is development of hepatic inflammation and often fibrosis. PPARS are key regulators of many of the adversely affected mechanistic pathways that create this condition. This makes PPAR nuclear receptors attractive therapeutic targets in the treatment of NASH, not only to benefit the liver but also to ameliorate features of the MetS and to attenuate the risk of linked extrahepatic diseases such as T2DM and CVD. Although previous studies have shown limited efficacy of activation of individual PPARs (PPAR-α, PPAR-γ), ongoing clinical trials suggest that dual and pan-PPAR agonists may have broader and more efficacious therapeutic potential to affect the multisystem disease of NASH, by targeting different interrelated mechanisms in the pathophysiology of NASH.

14.5 ACKNOWLEDGMENT

This chapter was based on [23]. The author wishes to thank the PanNASH Initiative (https://pannash.org) for their assistance in drafting Figure 14.1.

List of Abbreviations

CVD: Cardiovascular disease; FDA: Food and Drug Administration; HDL-C: High-density lipoprotein cholesterol; HSC: Hepatic stellate cells; IR: Insulin resistance; LDL-C: Low-density lipoprotein cholesterol; MetS: Metabolic syndrome; NAFLD: Nonalcoholic fatty liver disease; NASH: Nonalcoholic steatohepatitis; PPAR: Proliferator-activated receptors; RCT: Randomized controlled trial; T2DM: Type 2 diabetes mellitus; TZD: Thiazolidinediones.

REFERENCE

[1] Byrne CD, Targher G. NAFLD: a multisystem disease. *Journal of Hepatology* 2015;62:S47–64. https://doi.org/10.1016/j.jhep.2014.12.012.

[2] Francque SM, van der Graaff D, Kwanten WJ. Non-alcoholic fatty liver disease and cardiovascular risk: pathophysiological mechanisms and implications. *Journal of Hepatology* 2016;65:425–443. https://doi.org/10.1016/j.jhep.2016.04.005.

[3] Tilg H, Moschen AR, Roden M. NAFLD and diabetes mellitus. *Nature Reviews Gastroenterology & Hepatology* 2017;14:32–42. https://doi.org/10.1038/nrgastro.2016.147.

[4] Lallukka S, Yki-Järvinen H. Non-alcoholic fatty liver disease and risk of type 2 diabetes. *Best Practice & Research Clinical Endocrinology & Metabolism* 2016;30:385–395. https://doi.org/10.1016/j.beem.2016.06.006.

[5] Adams LA, Anstee QM, Tilg H, Targher G. Non-alcoholic fatty liver disease and its relationship with cardiovascular disease and other extrahepatic diseases. *Gut* 2017;66:1138–1153. https://doi.org/10.1136/gutjnl-2017-313884.

[6] Younossi ZM, Golabi P, de Avila L, Paik JM, Srishord M, Fukui N, et al. The global epidemiology of NAFLD and NASH in patients with type 2 diabetes: a systematic review and meta-analysis. *Journal of Hepatology* 2019;71:793–801. https://doi.org/10.1016/j.jhep.2019.06.021.

[7] Targher G, Byrne CD. A perspective on metabolic syndrome and nonalcoholic fatty liver disease. *Metabolic Syndrome and Related Disorders* 2015;13:235–238. https://doi.org/10.1089/met.2015.1502.

[8] Yki-Järvinen H. Non-alcoholic fatty liver disease as a cause and a consequence of metabolic syndrome. *The Lancet Diabetes and Endocrinology* 2014;2:901–910. https://doi.org/10.1016/S2213-8587(14)70032-4.

[9] Wainwright P, Byrne C. Bidirectional relationships and disconnects between NAFLD and features of the metabolic syndrome. *International Journal of Molecular Sciences* 2016;17:367. https://doi.org/10.3390/ijms17030367.

[10] Mantovani A, Byrne CD, Bonora E, Targher G. Nonalcoholic fatty liver disease and risk of incident type 2 diabetes: a meta-analysis. *Diabetes Care* 2018;41:372–382. https://doi.org/10.2337/dc17-1902.

[11] Targher G, Byrne CD, Lonardo A, Zoppini G, Barbui C. Non-alcoholic fatty liver disease and risk of incident cardiovascular disease: a meta-analysis. *Journal of Hepatology* 2016;65:589–600. https://doi.org/10.1016/j.jhep.2016.05.013.

[12] Sattar N, Rawshani A, Franzén S, Rawshani A, Svensson A-M, Rosengren A, et al. Age at diagnosis of type 2 diabetes mellitus and associations with cardiovascular and mortality risks. *Circulation* 2019;139:2228–2237. https://doi.org/10.1161/CIRCULATIONAHA.118.037885.

[13] Millett ERC, Peters SAE, Woodward M. Sex differences in risk factors for myocardial infarction: cohort study of UK Biobank participants. *BMJ* 2018:k4247. https://doi.org/10.1136/bmj.k4247.

[14] Stepanova M, Rafiq N, Younossi ZM. Components of metabolic syndrome are independent predictors of mortality in patients with chronic liver disease: a population-based study. *Gut* 2010;59:1410–1415. https://doi.org/10.1136/gut.2010.213553.

[15] McPherson S, Hardy T, Henderson E, Burt AD, Day CP, Anstee QM. Evidence of NAFLD progression from steatosis to fibrosing-steatohepatitis using paired biopsies: implications for prognosis and clinical management. *Journal of Hepatology* 2015;62:1148–1155. https://doi.org/10.1016/j.jhep.2014.11.034.

[16] Tada T, Toyoda H, Sone Y, Yasuda S, Miyake N, Kumada T, et al. Type 2 diabetes mellitus: a risk factor for progression of liver fibrosis in middle-aged patients with non-alcoholic fatty liver disease. *Journal of Gastroenterology and Hepatology* 2019;34:2011–2018. https://doi.org/10.1111/jgh.14734.

[17] Yang JD, Ahmed F, Mara KC, Addissie BD, Allen AM, Gores GJ, et al. Diabetes is associated with increased risk of hepatocellular carcinoma in patients with cirrhosis from nonalcoholic fatty liver disease. *Hepatology* 2020;71:907–916. https://doi.org/10.1002/hep.30858.

[18] Angulo P, Kleiner DE, Dam-Larsen S, Adams LA, Bjornsson ES, Charatcharoenwitthaya P, et al. Liver fibrosis, but no other histologic features, is associated with long-term outcomes of patients with nonalcoholic fatty liver disease. *Gastroenterology* 2015;149:389–397.e10. https://doi.org/10.1053/j.gastro.2015.04.043.

[19] Derosa G, Sahebkar A, Maffioli P. The role of various peroxisome proliferator-activated receptors and their ligands in clinical practice. *Journal of Cellular Physiology* 2018;233:153–161. https://doi.org/10.1002/jcp.25804.

[20] Crewe C, An YA, Scherer PE. The ominous triad of adipose tissue dysfunction: inflammation, fibrosis, and impaired angiogenesis. *Journal of Clinical Investigation* 2017;127:74–82. https://doi.org/10.1172/JCI88883.

[21] Koliaki C, Szendroedi J, Kaul K, Jelenik T, Nowotny P, Jankowiak F, et al. Adaptation of hepatic mitochondrial function in humans with non-alcoholic fatty liver is lost in steatohepatitis. *Cell Metabolism* 2015;21:739–746. https://doi.org/10.1016/j.cmet.2015.04.004.

[22] Haas JT, Francque S, Staels B. Pathophysiology and mechanisms of nonalcoholic fatty liver disease. *Annual Review of Physiology* 2016;78:181–205. https://doi.org/10.1146/annurev-physiol-021115-105331.

[23] Francque S, Szabo G, Abdelmalek MF, Byrne CD, Cusi K, Dufour JF, et al. Nonalcoholic steatohepatitis: the role of peroxisome proliferator-activated receptors. *Nature Reviews Gastroenterology and Hepatology* 2021;18:24–39. https://doi.org/10.1038/S41575-020-00366-5.

[24] Dreyer C, Krey G, Keller H, Givel F, Helftenbein G, Wahli W. Control of the peroxisomal beta-oxidation pathway by a novel family of nuclear hormone receptors. *Cell* 1992;68:879–887. https://doi.org/10.1016/0092-8674(92)90031-7.

[25] Issemann I, Green S. Activation of a member of the steroid hormone receptor superfamily by peroxisome proliferators. *Nature* 1990;347:645–650. https://doi.org/10.1038/347645a0.

[26] Wanders RJA, Waterham HR. Biochemistry of mammalian peroxisomes revisited. *Annual Review of Biochemistry* 2006;75:295–332. https://doi.org/10.1146/annurev.biochem.74.082803.133329.

[27] Samuel VT, Shulman GI. Nonalcoholic fatty liver disease as a nexus of metabolic and hepatic diseases. *Cell Metabolism* 2018;27:22–41. https://doi.org/10.1016/j.cmet.2017.08.002.

[28] Michalik L, Auwerx J, Berger JP, Chatterjee VK, Glass CK, Gonzalez FJ, et al. International union of pharmacology. LXI. Peroxisome proliferator-activated receptors. *Pharmacological Reviews* 2006;58:726–741. https://doi.org/10.1124/pr.58.4.5.

[29] Fajas L, Auboeuf D, Raspé E, Schoonjans K, Lefebvre AM, Saladin R, et al. The organization, promoter analysis, and expression of the human PPARgamma gene. *The Journal of Biological Chemistry* 1997;272:18779–18789. https://doi.org/10.1074/jbc.272.30.18779.

[30] Tailleux A, Wouters K, Staels B. Roles of PPARs in NAFLD: potential therapeutic targets. *Biochimica et Biophysica Acta* 2012;1821:809–818. https://doi.org/10.1016/j.bbalip.2011.10.016.

[31] Cheung C, Akiyama TE, Ward JM, Nicol CJ, Feigenbaum L, Vinson C, et al. Diminished hepatocellular proliferation in mice humanized for the nuclear receptor peroxisome proliferator-activated receptor α. *Cancer Research* 2004;64:3849–3854. https://doi.org/10.1158/0008-5472.CAN-04-0322.

[32] Bell AR, Savory R, Horley NJ, Choudhury AI, Dickins M, Gray TJB, et al. Molecular basis of non-responsiveness to peroxisome proliferators: the guinea-pig PPARα is functional and mediates peroxisome proliferator-induced hypolipidaemia. *Biochemical Journal* 1998;332:689–693. https://doi.org/10.1042/bj3320689.

[33] Lawrence JW, Li Y, Chen S, DeLuca JG, Berger JP, Umbenhauer DR, et al. Differential gene regulation in human versus rodent hepatocytes by peroxisome proliferator-activated receptor (PPAR) α. *Journal of Biological Chemistry* 2001;276:31521–31527. https://doi.org/10.1074/jbc.M103306200.

[34] Pap A, Cuaranta-Monroy I, Peloquin M, Nagy L. Is the mouse a good model of human PPARγ-related metabolic diseases? *International Journal of Molecular Sciences* 2016;17:1236. https://doi.org/10.3390/ijms17081236.

[35] Su AI, Wiltshire T, Batalov S, Lapp H, Ching KA, Block D, et al. A gene atlas of the mouse and human protein-encoding transcriptomes. *Proceedings of the National Academy of Sciences* 2004;101:6062–6067. https://doi.org/10.1073/pnas.0400782101.

[36] Vidal-Puig A, Jimenez-Liñan M, Lowell BB, Hamann A, Hu E, Spiegelman B, et al. Regulation of PPAR gamma gene expression by nutrition and obesity in rodents. *Journal of Clinical Investigation* 1996;97:2553–2561. https://doi.org/10.1172/JCI118703.

[37] Francque S, Verrijken A, Caron S, Prawitt J, Paumelle R, Derudas B, et al. PPARα gene expression correlates with severity and histological treatment response in patients with non-alcoholic steatohepatitis. *Journal of Hepatology* 2015;63:164–173. https://doi.org/10.1016/j.jhep.2015.02.019.

[38] Kim SM, Lee B, An HJ, Kim DH, Park KC, Noh S-G, et al. Novel PPARα agonist MHY553 alleviates hepatic steatosis by increasing fatty acid oxidation and decreasing inflammation during aging. *Oncotarget* 2017;8:46273–46285. https://doi.org/10.18632/oncotarget.17695.

[39] Chakravarthy MV, Lodhi IJ, Yin L, Malapaka RRV, Xu HE, Turk J, et al. Identification of a physiologically relevant endogenous ligand for PPARα in liver. *Cell* 2009;138:476–488. https://doi.org/10.1016/j.cell.2009.05.036.

[40] Reid BN, Ables GP, Otlivanchik OA, Schoiswohl G, Zechner R, Blaner WS, et al. Hepatic overexpression of hormone-sensitive lipase and adipose triglyceride

lipase promotes fatty acid oxidation, stimulates direct release of free fatty acids, and ameliorates steatosis. *Journal of Biological Chemistry* 2008;283:13087–13099. https://doi.org/10.1074/jbc.M800533200.

[41] Lefebvre P. Sorting out the roles of PPAR in energy metabolism and vascular homeostasis. *Journal of Clinical Investigation* 2006;116:571–580. https://doi.org/10.1172/JCI27989.

[42] Zardi EM, Navarini L, Sambataro G, Piccinni P, Sambataro FM, Spina C, et al. Hepatic PPARs: their role in liver physiology, fibrosis and treatment. *Current Medicinal Chemistry* 2013;20:3370–3396. https://doi.org/10.2174/09298673113209990136.

[43] Kersten S, Seydoux J, Peters JM, Gonzalez FJ, Desvergne B, Wahli W. Peroxisome proliferator-activated receptor α mediates the adaptive response to fasting. *Journal of Clinical Investigation* 1999;103:1489–1498. https://doi.org/10.1172/JCI6223.

[44] Sanderson LM, Boekschoten MV, Desvergne B, Müller M, Kersten S. Transcriptional profiling reveals divergent roles of PPARα and PPARβ/δ in regulation of gene expression in mouse liver. *Physiological Genomics* 2010;41:42–52. https://doi.org/10.1152/physiolgenomics.00127.2009.

[45] Lemberger T, Saladin R, Vázquez M, Assimacopoulos F, Staels B, Desvergne B, et al. Expression of the peroxisome proliferator-activated receptor alpha gene is stimulated by stress and follows a diurnal rhythm. *The Journal of Biological Chemistry* 1996;271:1764–1769. https://doi.org/10.1074/jbc.271.3.1764.

[46] Canaple L, Rambaud J, Dkhissi-Benyahya O, Rayet B, Tan NS, Michalik L, et al. Reciprocal regulation of brain and muscle arnt-like protein 1 and peroxisome proliferator-activated receptor α defines a novel positive feedback loop in the rodent liver circadian clock. *Molecular Endocrinology* 2006;20:1715–1727. https://doi.org/10.1210/me.2006-0052.

[47] Guan D, Xiong Y, Borck PC, Jang C, Doulias P-T, Papazyan R, et al. Diet-induced circadian enhancer remodeling synchronizes opposing hepatic lipid metabolic processes. *Cell* 2018;174:831–842.e12. https://doi.org/10.1016/j.cell.2018.06.031.

[48] Tognini P, Murakami M, Liu Y, Eckel-Mahan KL, Newman JC, Verdin E, et al. Distinct circadian signatures in liver and gut clocks revealed by ketogenic diet. *Cell Metabolism* 2017;26:523–538.e5. https://doi.org/10.1016/j.cmet.2017.08.015.

[49] Gachon F, Leuenberger N, Claudel T, Gos P, Jouffe C, Fleury Olela F, et al. Proline- and acidic amino acid-rich basic leucine zipper proteins modulate peroxisome proliferator-activated receptor α (PPARα) activity. *Proceedings of the National Academy of Sciences* 2011;108:4794–4799. https://doi.org/10.1073/pnas.1002862108.

[50] Rakhshandehroo M, Hooiveld G, Müller M, Kersten S. Comparative analysis of gene regulation by the transcription factor PPARα between mouse and human. *PLoS ONE* 2009;4:e6796. https://doi.org/10.1371/journal.pone.0006796.

[51] Botta M, Audano M, Sahebkar A, Sirtori C, Mitro N, Ruscica M. PPAR agonists and metabolic syndrome: an established role? *International Journal of Molecular Sciences* 2018;19:1197. https://doi.org/10.3390/ijms19041197.

[52] Pawlak M, Lefebvre P, Staels B. Molecular mechanism of PPARα action and its impact on lipid

metabolism, inflammation and fibrosis in non-alcoholic fatty liver disease. *Journal of Hepatology* 2015;62:720–733. https://doi.org/10.1016/j.jhep.2014.10.039.

[53] Pawlak M, Baugé E, Bourguet W, de Bosscher K, Lalloyer F, Tailleux A, et al. The transrepressive activity of peroxisome proliferator-activated receptor alpha is necessary and sufficient to prevent liver fibrosis in mice. *Hepatology* 2014;60:1593–1606. https://doi.org/10.1002/hep.27297.

[54] Liu S, Hatano B, Zhao M, Yen C-C, Kang K, Reilly SM, et al. Role of peroxisome proliferator-activated receptor δ/β in hepatic metabolic regulation. *Journal of Biological Chemistry* 2011;286:1237–1247. https://doi.org/10.1074/jbc.M110.138115.

[55] Liu S, Brown JD, Stanya KJ, Homan E, Leidl M, Inouye K, et al. A diurnal serum lipid integrates hepatic lipogenesis and peripheral fatty acid use. *Nature* 2013;502:550–554. https://doi.org/10.1038/nature12710.

[56] Iwaisako K, Haimerl M, Paik Y-H, Taura K, Kodama Y, Sirlin C, et al. Protection from liver fibrosis by a peroxisome proliferator-activated receptor δ agonist. *Proceedings of the National Academy of Sciences* 2012;109. https://doi.org/10.1073/pnas.1202464109.

[57] Dietz M, Mohr P, Kuhn B, Maerki HP, Hartman P, Ruf A, et al. Comparative molecular profiling of the PPARα/γ activator aleglitazar: PPAR selectivity, activity and interaction with cofactors. *ChemMedChem* 2012;7:1101–1111. https://doi.org/10.1002/cmdc.201100598.

[58] Ricote M, Glass C. PPARs and molecular mechanisms of transrepression. *Biochimica et Biophysica Acta (BBA)—Molecular and Cell Biology of Lipids* 2007;1771:926–935. https://doi.org/10.1016/j.bbalip.2007.02.013.

[59] Zizzo G, Cohen PL. The PPAR-γ antagonist GW9662 elicits differentiation of M2c-like cells and upregulation of the MerTK/Gas6 axis: a key role for PPAR-γ in human macrophage polarization. *Journal of Inflammation* 2015;12:36. https://doi.org/10.1186/s12950-015-0081-4.

[60] Wilding JPH. PPAR agonists for the treatment of cardiovascular disease in patients with diabetes. *Diabetes, Obesity and Metabolism* 2012;14:973–982. https://doi.org/10.1111/j.1463-1326.2012.01601.x.

[61] Han L, Shen W-J, Bittner S, Kraemer FB, Azhar S. PPARs: regulators of metabolism and as therapeutic targets in cardiovascular disease. Part I: PPAR-α. *Future Cardiology* 2017;13:259–278. https://doi.org/10.2217/fca-2016-0059.

[62] Delerive P, de Bosscher K, Besnard S, vanden Berghe W, Peters JM, Gonzalez FJ, et al. Peroxisome proliferator-activated receptor alpha negatively regulates the vascular inflammatory gene response by negative cross-talk with transcription factors NF-kappaB and AP-1. *The Journal of Biological Chemistry* 1999;274:32048–32054. https://doi.org/10.1074/jbc.274.45.32048.

[63] Hoekstra M, Kruijt JK, van Eck M, van Berkel TJC. Specific gene expression of ATP-binding cassette transporters and nuclear hormone receptors in rat liver parenchymal, endothelial, and Kupffer cells. *Journal of Biological Chemistry* 2003;278:25448–25453. https://doi.org/10.1074/jbc.M301189200.

[64] Fan Y, Wang Y, Tang Z, Zhang H, Qin X, Zhu Y, et al. Suppression of Pro-inflammatory adhesion molecules by PPAR-δ in human vascular endothelial cells. *Arteriosclerosis, Thrombosis, and Vascular Biology* 2008;28:315–321. https://doi.org/10.1161/ATVBAHA.107.149815.

[65] Kilgore KS, Billin AN. PPARbeta/delta ligands as modulators of the inflammatory response. *Current Opinion in Investigational Drugs (London, England : 2000)* 2008;9:463–469.

[66] Liu Y, Colby J, Zuo X, Jaoude J, Wei D, Shureiqi I. The role of PPAR-δ in metabolism, inflammation, and cancer: many characters of a critical transcription factor. *International Journal of Molecular Sciences* 2018;19:3339. https://doi.org/10.3390/ijms19113339.

[67] Lanthier N, Molendi-Coste O, Horsmans Y, van Rooijen N, Cani PD, Leclercq IA. Kupffer cell activation is a causal factor for hepatic insulin resistance. *American Journal of Physiology-Gastrointestinal and Liver Physiology* 2010;298:G107–116. https://doi.org/10.1152/ajpgi.00391.2009.

[68] Odegaard JI, Ricardo-Gonzalez RR, Red Eagle A, Vats D, Morel CR, Goforth MH, et al. Alternative M2 activation of kupffer cells by PPARδ ameliorates obesity-induced insulin resistance. *Cell Metabolism* 2008;7:496–507. https://doi.org/10.1016/j.cmet.2008.04.003.

[69] Dulai PS, Singh S, Patel J, Soni M, Prokop LJ, Younossi Z, et al. Increased risk of mortality by fibrosis stage in nonalcoholic fatty liver disease: systematic review and meta-analysis. *Hepatology* 2017;65:1557–1565. https://doi.org/10.1002/hep.29085.

[70] Hagström H, Nasr P, Ekstedt M, Hammar U, Stål P, Hultcrantz R, et al. Fibrosis stage but not NASH predicts mortality and time to development of severe liver disease in biopsy-proven NAFLD. *Journal of Hepatology* 2017;67:1265–1273. https://doi.org/10.1016/j.jhep.2017.07.027.

[71] Weiskirchen R, Weiskirchen S, Tacke F. Organ and tissue fibrosis: molecular signals, cellular mechanisms and translational implications. *Molecular Aspects of Medicine* 2019;65:2–15. https://doi.org/10.1016/j.mam.2018.06.003.

[72] Lefere S, Tacke F. Macrophages in obesity and non-alcoholic fatty liver disease: crosstalk with metabolism. *JHEP Reports* 2019;1:30–43. https://doi.org/10.1016/j.jhepr.2019.02.004.

[73] Ritz T, Krenkel O, Tacke F. Dynamic plasticity of macrophage functions in diseased liver. *Cellular Immunology* 2018;330:175–182. https://doi.org/10.1016/j.cellimm.2017.12.007.

[74] Ham SA, Hwang JS, Yoo T, Lee WJ, Paek KS, Oh J-W, et al. Ligand-activated PPARδ upregulates α-smooth muscle actin expression in human dermal fibroblasts: a potential role for PPARδ in wound healing. *Journal of Dermatological Science* 2015;80:186–195. https://doi.org/10.1016/j.jdermsci.2015.10.005.

[75] Park JR, Ahn JH, Jung MH, Koh J-S, Park Y, Hwang S-J, et al. Effects of peroxisome proliferator-activated receptor-δ agonist on cardiac healing after myocardial infarction. *PLoS ONE* 2016;11:e0148510. https://doi.org/10.1371/journal.pone.0148510.

[76] Lefebvre P, Lalloyer F, Baugé E, Pawlak M, Gheeraert C, Dehondt H, et al. Interspecies NASH disease activity whole-genome profiling identifies a fibrogenic role of PPARα-regulated dermatopontin. *JCI Insight* 2017;2. https://doi.org/10.1172/jci.insight.92264.

[77] Kato A, Okamoto O, Wu W, Matsuo N, Kumai J, Yamada Y, et al. Identification of fibronectin binding sites in dermatopontin and their biological function. *Journal of Dermatological Science* 2014;76:51–59. https://doi.org/10.1016/j.jdermsci.2014.07.003.

[78] Soccio RE, Chen ER, Lazar MA. Thiazolidinediones and the promise of insulin sensitization in type 2 diabetes. *Cell Metabolism* 2014;20:573–591. https://doi.org/10.1016/j.cmet.2014.08.005.

[79] Ma X, Wang D, Zhao W, Xu L. Deciphering the roles of PPARγ in adipocytes via dynamic change of transcription complex. *Frontiers in Endocrinology* 2018;9:473. https://doi.org/10.3389/fendo.2018.00473.

[80] Liss KHH, Finck BN. PPARs and nonalcoholic fatty liver disease. *Biochimie* 2017;136:65–74. https://doi.org/10.1016/j.biochi.2016.11.009.

[81] Cusi K. Role of obesity and lipotoxicity in the development of nonalcoholic steatohepatitis: pathophysiology and clinical implications. *Gastroenterology* 2012;142:711–725.e6. https://doi.org/10.1053/j.gastro.2012.02.003.

[82] Lumeng CN, Saltiel AR. Inflammatory links between obesity and metabolic disease. *The Journal of Clinical Investigation* 2011;121:2111–2117. https://doi.org/10.1172/JCI57132.

[83] Byrne CD, Targher G. Ectopic fat, insulin resistance, and nonalcoholic fatty liver disease. *Arteriosclerosis, Thrombosis, and Vascular Biology* 2014;34:1155–1161. https://doi.org/10.1161/ATVBAHA.114.303034.

[84] Aithal GP, Thomas JA, Kaye P v., Lawson A, Ryder SD, Spendlove I, et al. Randomized, placebo-controlled trial of pioglitazone in nondiabetic subjects with nonalcoholic steatohepatitis. *Gastroenterology* 2008;135:1176–1184. https://doi.org/10.1053/j.gastro.2008.06.047.

[85] Sanyal AJ, Chalasani N, Kowdley KV, McCullough A, Diehl AM, Bass NM, et al. Pioglitazone, vitamin E, or placebo for nonalcoholic steatohepatitis. *New England Journal of Medicine* 2010;362:1675–1685. https://doi.org/10.1056/nejmoa0907929.

[86] Cusi K, Orsak B, Bril F, Lomonaco R, Hecht J, Ortiz-Lopez C, et al. Long-term pioglitazone treatment for patients with nonalcoholic steatohepatitis and prediabetes or type 2 diabetes mellitus a randomized trial. *Annals of Internal Medicine* 2016;165:305–315. https://doi.org/10.7326/M15-1774.

[87] Belfort R, Harrison SA, Brown K, Darland C, Finch J, Hardies J, et al. A placebo-controlled trial of pioglitazone in subjects with nonalcoholic steatohepatitis. *New England Journal of Medicine* 2006;355:2297–2307. https://doi.org/10.1056/NEJMoa060326.

[88] Lomonaco R, Bril F, Portillo-Sanchez P, Ortiz-Lopez C, Orsak B, Biernacki D, et al. Metabolic impact of nonalcoholic steatohepatitis in obese patients with type 2 diabetes. *Diabetes Care* 2016;39:632–638. https://doi.org/10.2337/dc15-1876.

[89] Bril F, Barb D, Portillo-Sanchez P, Biernacki D, Lomonaco R, Suman A, et al. Metabolic and histological implications of intrahepatic triglyceride content in nonalcoholic fatty liver disease. *Hepatology*

2017;65:1132–1144. https://doi.org/10.1002/hep.28985.

[90] Larter CZ, Yeh MM, van Rooyen DM, Brooling J, Ghatora K, Farrell GC. Peroxisome proliferator-activated receptor-α agonist, Wy 14,643, improves metabolic indices, steatosis and ballooning in diabetic mice with non-alcoholic steatohepatitis. *Journal of Gastroenterology and Hepatology* 2012;27:341–350. https://doi.org/10.1111/j.1440-1746.2011.06939.x.

[91] Belfort R, Berria R, Cornell J, Cusi K. Fenofibrate reduces systemic inflammation markers independent of its effects on lipid and glucose metabolism in patients with the metabolic syndrome. *The Journal of Clinical Endocrinology and Metabolism* 2010;95:829–836. https://doi.org/10.1210/jc.2009-1487.

[92] Fabbrini E, Mohammed BS, Korenblat KM, Magkos F, McCrea J, Patterson BW, et al. Effect of fenofibrate and niacin on intrahepatic triglyceride content, very low-density lipoprotein kinetics, and insulin action in obese subjects with nonalcoholic fatty liver disease. *The Journal of Clinical Endocrinology and Metabolism* 2010;95:2727–2735. https://doi.org/10.1210/jc.2009-2622.

[93] Palmer CN, Hsu MH, Griffin KJ, Raucy JL, Johnson EF. Peroxisome proliferator activated receptor-alpha expression in human liver. *Molecular Pharmacology* 1998;53:14–22.

[94] Honda Y, Kessoku T, Ogawa Y, Tomeno W, Imajo K, Fujita K, et al. Pemafibrate, a novel selective peroxisome proliferator-activated receptor alpha modulator, improves the pathogenesis in a rodent model of nonalcoholic steatohepatitis. *Scientific Reports* 2017;7:42477. https://doi.org/10.1038/srep42477.

[95] Araki E, Yamashita S, Arai H, Yokote K, Satoh J, Inoguchi T, et al. Efficacy and safety of pemafibrate in people with type 2 diabetes and elevated triglyceride levels: 52-week data from the PROVIDE study. *Diabetes, Obesity and Metabolism* 2019;21:1737–1744. https://doi.org/10.1111/dom.13686.

[96] Yokote K, Yamashita S, Arai H, Araki E, Suganami H, Ishibashi S. Long-term efficacy and safety of pemafibrate, a novel selective peroxisome proliferator-activated receptor-α modulator (SPPARMα), in dyslipidemic patients with renal impairment. *International Journal of Molecular Sciences* 2019;20:706. https://doi.org/10.3390/ijms20030706.

[97] Nakajima A, Eguchi Y, Yoneda M, Imajo K, Tamaki N, Suganami H, et al. Randomised clinical trial: pemafibrate, a novel selective peroxisome proliferator-activated receptor α modulator (SPPARMα), versus placebo in patients with non-alcoholic fatty liver disease. *Alimentary Pharmacology & Therapeutics* 2021;54:1263–1277. https://doi.org/10.1111/apt.16596.

[98] Gastaldelli A, Harrison SA, Belfort-Aguilar R, Hardies LJ, Balas B, Schenker S, et al. Importance of changes in adipose tissue insulin resistance to histological response during thiazolidinedione treatment of patients with nonalcoholic steatohepatitis. *Hepatology (Baltimore, Md)* 2009;50:1087–1093. https://doi.org/10.1002/hep.23116.

[99] Maeda N, Takahashi M, Funahashi T, Kihara S, Nishizawa H, Kishida K, et al. PPARgamma ligands increase expression and plasma concentrations of adiponectin, an adipose-derived protein. *Diabetes* 2001;50:2094–2099. https://doi.org/10.2337/diabetes.50.9.2094.

[100] Gastaldelli A, Harrison S, Belfort-Aguiar R, Hardies J, Balas B, Schenker S, et al. Pioglitazone in the treatment of NASH: the role of adiponectin. *Alimentary Pharmacology & Therapeutics* 2010;32:769–775. https://doi.org/10.1111/j.1365-2036.2010.04405.x.

[101] Ratziu V, Giral P, Jacqueminet S, Charlotte F, Hartemann-Heurtier A, Serfaty L, et al. Rosiglitazone for nonalcoholic steatohepatitis: one-year results of the randomized placebo-controlled fatty liver improvement with rosiglitazone therapy (FLIRT) trial. *Gastroenterology* 2008;135:100–110. https://doi.org/10.1053/j.gastro.2008.03.078.

[102] Ratziu V, Charlotte F, Bernhardt C, Giral P, Halbron M, LeNaour G, et al. Long-term efficacy of rosiglitazone in nonalcoholic steatohepatitis: results of the fatty liver improvement by rosiglitazone therapy (FLIRT 2) extension trial. *Hepatology* 2010;51:445–453. https://doi.org/10.1002/hep.23270.

[103] Leclercq IA. Limited therapeutic efficacy of pioglitazone on progression of hepatic fibrosis in rats. *Gut* 2006;55:1020–1029. https://doi.org/10.1136/gut.2005.079194.

[104] Bril F. Role of oral vitamin E for the treatment of nonalcoholic steatohepatitis (NASH) in patients with type 2 diabetes: a randomized controlled trial. *Diabetes Care* 2019.

[105] Musso G, Cassader M, Paschetta E, Gambino R. Thiazolidinediones and advanced liver fibrosis in nonalcoholic steatohepatitis: a meta-analysis. *JAMA Internal Medicine* 2017;177:633–640. https://doi.org/10.1001/jamainternmed.2016.9607.

[106] Sakamoto J, Kimura H, Moriyama S, Odaka H, Momose Y, Sugiyama Y, et al. Activation of human peroxisome proliferator-activated receptor (PPAR) subtypes by pioglitazone. *Biochemical and Biophysical Research Communications* 2000;278:704–711. https://doi.org/10.1006/bbrc.2000.3868.

[107] Kalavalapalli S, Bril F, Koelmel JP, Abdo K, Guingab J, Andrews P, et al. Pioglitazone improves hepatic mitochondrial function in a mouse model of nonalcoholic steatohepatitis. *American Journal of Physiology-Endocrinology and Metabolism* 2018;315:E163–173. https://doi.org/10.1152/ajpendo.00023.2018.

[108] Ahmadian M, Suh JM, Hah N, Liddle C, Atkins AR, Downes M, et al. PPARγ signaling and metabolism: the good, the bad and the future. *Nature Medicine* 2013;19:557–566. https://doi.org/10.1038/nm.3159.

[109] Devchand PR, Liu T, Altman RB, FitzGerald GA, Schadt EE. The pioglitazone trek via human PPAR Gamma: from discovery to a medicine at the FDA and beyond. *Frontiers in Pharmacology* 2018;9. https://doi.org/10.3389/fphar.2018.01093.

[110] Jain MR, Giri SR, Bhoi B, Trivedi C, Rath A, Rathod R, et al. Dual PPARα/γ agonist saroglitazar improves liver histopathology and biochemistry in experimental NASH models. *Liver International* 2018;38:1084–1094. https://doi.org/10.1111/liv.13634.

[111] Kaul U, Parmar D, Manjunath K, Shah M, Parmar K, Patil KP, et al. New dual peroxisome proliferator activated receptor agonist—Saroglitazar in diabetic dyslipidemia and non-alcoholic fatty liver disease: integrated analysis of the real world evidence. *Cardiovascular Diabetology* 2019;18:80. https://doi.org/10.1186/s12933-019-0884-3.

[112] Gawrieh S, Noureddin M, Loo N, Mohseni R, Awasty V, Cusi K, et al. Saroglitazar, a PPAR-α/γ agonist,

for treatment of NAFLD: a randomized controlled double-blind phase 2 trial. *Hepatology (Baltimore, Md)* 2021;74:1809–1824. https://doi.org/10.1002/hep.31843.

[113] Haczeyni F, Wang H, Barn V, Mridha AR, Yeh MM, Haigh WG, et al. The selective peroxisome proliferator-activated receptor-delta agonist seladelpar reverses nonalcoholic steatohepatitis pathology by abrogating lipotoxicity in diabetic obese mice. *Hepatology Communications* 2017;1:663–674. https://doi.org/10.1002/hep4.1072.

[114] Bays HE, Schwartz S, Littlejohn T, Kerzner B, Krauss RM, Karpf DB, et al. MBX-8025, a novel peroxisome proliferator receptor-δ agonist: lipid and other metabolic effects in dyslipidemic overweight patients treated with and without Atorvastatin. *The Journal of Clinical Endocrinology & Metabolism* 2011;96:2889–2897. https://doi.org/10.1210/jc.2011-1061.

[115] A study to evaluate seladelpar in subjects with nonalcoholic steatohepatitis (NASH) n.d.

[116] Staels B, Rubenstrunk A, Noel B, Rigou G, Delataille P, Millatt LJ, et al. Hepatoprotective effects of the dual peroxisome proliferator-activated receptor alpha/delta agonist, GFT505, in rodent models of nonalcoholic fatty liver disease/nonalcoholic steatohepatitis. *Hepatology* 2013;58:1941–1952. https://doi.org/10.1002/hep.26461.

[117] Ratziu V, Harrison SA, Francque S, Bedossa P, Lehert P, Serfaty L, et al. Elafibranor, an agonist of the peroxisome proliferator–Activated receptor–α and –δ, induces resolution of nonalcoholic steatohepatitis without fibrosis worsening. *Gastroenterology* 2016;150:1147–1159.e5. https://doi.org/10.1053/j.gastro.2016.01.038.

[118] Cariou B, Hanf R, Lambert-Porcheron S, Zaïr Y, Sauvinet V, Noël B, et al. Dual peroxisome proliferator-activated receptor α/δ agonist GFT505 improves hepatic and peripheral insulin sensitivity in abdominally obese subjects. *Diabetes Care* 2013;36:2923–2930. https://doi.org/10.2337/dc12-2012.

[119] Ratziu V, Harrison SA, Francque S, Bedossa P, Lehert P, Serfaty L, et al. Elafibranor, an agonist of the peroxisome proliferator-activated receptor-α and -δ, induces resolution of nonalcoholic steatohepatitis without fibrosis worsening. *Gastroenterology* 2016;150:1147–1159.e5. https://doi.org/10.1053/j.gastro.2016.01.038.

[120] Phase 3 study to evaluate the efficacy and safety of elafibranor versus placebo in patients with nonalcoholic steatohepatitis (NASH) n.d. https://ClinicalTrials.gov/show/NCT02704403 (accessed February 17, 2022).

[121] Stephen A. Harrison, Vlad Ratziu, Jean-François Dufour, Corné Kruger, Jörn Schattenberg, Sven Francque, et al. The dual PPARα/δ agonist elafibranor did not achieve resolution of NASH without worsening of fibrosis in adult patients with nonalcoholic steatohepatitis and significant fibrosis: 72 week surrogate endpoint analysis of the Phase 3 RESOLVE-IT trial 2020;72.

[122] McVicker BL, Bennett RG. Novel anti-fibrotic therapies. *Frontiers in Pharmacology* 2017;8. https://doi.org/10.3389/fphar.2017.00318.

[123] Han L, Shen W-J, Bittner S, Kraemer FB, Azhar S. PPARs: regulators of metabolism and as therapeutic targets in cardiovascular disease. Part II: PPAR-β/δ and PPAR-γ. *Future Cardiology* 2017;13:279–296. https://doi.org/10.2217/fca-2017-0019.

[124] Vallée A, Vallée J-N, Lecarpentier Y. Metabolic reprogramming in atherosclerosis: opposed interplay between the canonical WNT/β-catenin pathway and PPARγ. *Journal of Molecular and Cellular Cardiology* 2019;133:36–46. https://doi.org/10.1016/j.yjmcc.2019.05.024.

[125] Zhao N, Mi L, Zhang X, Xu M, Yu H, Liu Z, et al. Enhanced MiR-711 transcription by PPARγ induces endoplasmic reticulum stress-mediated apoptosis targeting calnexin in rat cardiomyocytes after myocardial infarction. *Journal of Molecular and Cellular Cardiology* 2018;118:36–45. https://doi.org/10.1016/j.yjmcc.2018.03.006.

[126] Peymani M, Ghaedi K, Irani S, Nasr-Esfahani MH. Peroxisome proliferator-activated receptor γ activity is required for appropriate cardiomyocyte differentiation. *Cell Journal* n.d.;18:221–228. https://doi.org/10.22074/cellj.2016.4317.

[127] Ortiz-Lopez C, Lomonaco R, Orsak B, Finch J, Chang Z, Kochunov VG, et al. Prevalence of prediabetes and diabetes and metabolic profile of patients with nonalcoholic fatty liver disease (NAFLD). *Diabetes Care* 2012;35:873–878. https://doi.org/10.2337/dc11-1849.

[128] DeFronzo RA, Tripathy D, Schwenke DC, Banerji M, Bray GA, Buchanan TA, et al. Pioglitazone for diabetes prevention in impaired glucose tolerance. *New England Journal of Medicine* 2011;364:1104–1115. https://doi.org/10.1056/NEJMoa1010949.

[129] Inzucchi SE, Viscoli CM, Young LH, Furie KL, Gorman M, Lovejoy AM, et al. Pioglitazone prevents diabetes in patients with insulin resistance and cerebrovascular disease. *Diabetes Care* 2016;39:1684–1692. https://doi.org/10.2337/dc16-0798.

[130] Kahn SE, Haffner SM, Heise MA, Herman WH, Holman RR, Jones NP, et al. Glycemic durability of rosiglitazone, metformin, or glyburide monotherapy. *New England Journal of Medicine* 2006;355:2427–2443. https://doi.org/10.1056/NEJMoa066224.

[131] Mazzone T, Meyer PM, Feinstein SB, Davidson MH, Kondos GT, D'Agostino RB, et al. Effect of pioglitazone compared with glimepiride on carotid intima-media thickness in type 2 diabetes. *JAMA* 2006;296:2572. https://doi.org/10.1001/jama.296.21.joc60158.

[132] Nissen SE, Nicholls SJ, Wolski K, Nesto R, Kupfer S, Perez A, et al. Comparison of pioglitazone vs glimepiride on progression of coronary atherosclerosis in patients with type 2 diabetes. *JAMA* 2008;299:1561. https://doi.org/10.1001/jama.299.13.1561.

[133] Dormandy JA, Charbonnel B, Eckland DJ, Erdmann E, Massi-Benedetti M, Moules IK, et al. Secondary prevention of macrovascular events in patients with type 2 diabetes in the PROactive study (PROspective pioglitAzone Clinical Trial In macroVascular Events): a randomised controlled trial. *The Lancet* 2005;366:1279–1289. https://doi.org/10.1016/S0140-6736(05)67528-9.

[134] Lincoff AM, Wolski K, Nicholls SJ, Nissen SE. Pioglitazone and risk of cardiovascular events in patients with type 2 diabetes mellitus. *JAMA* 2007;298:1180. https://doi.org/10.1001/jama.298.10.1180.

[135] Kernan WN, Viscoli CM, Furie KL, Young LH, Inzucchi SE, Gorman M, et al. Pioglitazone after ischemic stroke or transient ischemic attack. *New England*

Journal of Medicine 2016;374:1321–1331. https://doi.org/10.1056/NEJMoa1506930.

[136] Spence JD, Viscoli CM, Inzucchi SE, Dearborn-Tomazos J, Ford GA, Gorman M, et al. Pioglitazone therapy in patients with stroke and prediabetes: a post hoc analysis of the IRIS randomized clinical trial. *JAMA Neurology* 2019;76:526–535. https://doi.org/10.1001/jamaneurol.2019.0079.

[137] Nissen SE, Wolski K. Effect of rosiglitazone on the risk of myocardial infarction and death from cardiovascular causes. *New England Journal of Medicine* 2007;356:2457–2471. https://doi.org/10.1056/NEJMoa072761.

[138] Home PD, Pocock SJ, Beck-Nielsen H, Curtis PS, Gomis R, Hanefeld M, et al. Rosiglitazone evaluated for cardiovascular outcomes in oral agent combination therapy for type 2 diabetes (RECORD): a multicentre, randomised, open-label trial. *The Lancet* 2009;373:2125–2135. https://doi.org/10.1016/S0140-6736(09)60953-3.

[139] Choi Y-J, Roberts BK, Wang X, Geaney JC, Naim S, Wojnoonski K, et al. Effects of the PPAR-δ agonist MBX-8025 on atherogenic dyslipidemia. *Atherosclerosis* 2012;220:470–476. https://doi.org/10.1016/j.atherosclerosis.2011.10.029.

[140] Jani RH, Pai V, Jha P, Jariwala G, Mukhopadhyay S, Bhansali A, et al. A multicenter, prospective, randomized, double-blind study to evaluate the safety and efficacy of saroglitazar 2 and 4 mg compared with placebo in type 2 diabetes mellitus patients having hypertriglyceridemia not controlled with atorvastatin therapy (PRESS VI). *Diabetes Technology & Therapeutics* 2014;16:63–71. https://doi.org/10.1089/dia.2013.0253.

[141] Wettstein G, Luccarini J-M, Poekes L, Faye P, Kupkowski F, Adarbes V, et al. The new-generation pan-peroxisome proliferator-activated receptor agonist IVA337 protects the liver from metabolic disorders and fibrosis. *Hepatology Communications* 2017;1:524–537. https://doi.org/10.1002/hep4.1057.

[142] Boubia B, Poupardin O, Barth M, Binet J, Peralba P, Mounier L, et al. Design, synthesis, and evaluation of a novel series of indole sulfonamide peroxisome proliferator activated receptor (PPAR) α/γ/δ triple activators: discovery of lanifibranor, a new antifibrotic clinical candidate. *Journal of Medicinal Chemistry* 2018;61:2246–2265. https://doi.org/10.1021/acs.jmedchem.7b01285.

[143] Phase 2b study in NASH to assess IVA337, n.d.

[144] Francque SM, Bedossa P, Ratziu V, Anstee QM, Bugianesi E, Sanyal AJ, et al. A randomized, controlled trial of the pan-PPAR agonist lanifibranor in NASH. *The New England Journal of Medicine* 2021;385. https://doi.org/10.1056/NEJMoa2036205.

[145] Davis TME, Ting R, Best JD, Donoghoe MW, Drury PL, Sullivan DR, et al. Effects of fenofibrate on renal function in patients with type 2 diabetes mellitus: the Fenofibrate Intervention and Event Lowering in Diabetes (FIELD) study. *Diabetologia* 2011;54:280–290. https://doi.org/10.1007/s00125-010-1951-1.

[146] Lee M, Saver JL, Liao H-W, Lin C-H, Ovbiagele B. Pioglitazone for secondary stroke prevention. *Stroke* 2017;48:388–393. https://doi.org/10.1161/STROKEAHA.116.013977.

[147] DeFronzo RA, Inzucchi S, Abdul-Ghani M, Nissen SE. Pioglitazone: the forgotten, cost-effective cardioprotective drug for type 2 diabetes. *Diabetes and Vascular Disease Research* 2019;16:133–143. https://doi.org/10.1177/1479164118825376.

[148] Portillo-Sanchez P, Bril F, Lomonaco R, Barb D, Orsak B, Bruder JM, et al. Effect of pioglitazone on bone mineral density in patients with nonalcoholic steatohepatitis: a 36-month clinical trial. *Journal of Diabetes* 2019;11:223–231. https://doi.org/10.1111/1753-0407.12833.

[149] Filipova E, Uzunova K, Kalinov K, Vekov T. Pioglitazone and the risk of bladder cancer: a meta-analysis. *Diabetes Therapy* 2017;8:705–726. https://doi.org/10.1007/s13300-017-0273-4.

[150] Gastaldelli A, Sabatini S, Carli F, Gaggini M, Bril F, Belfort-DeAguiar R, et al. PPAR-γ-induced changes in visceral fat and adiponectin levels are associated with improvement of steatohepatitis in patients with NASH. *Liver International: Official Journal of the International Association for the Study of the Liver* 2021;41:2659–2670. https://doi.org/10.1111/liv.15005.

[151] Balas B, Belfort R, Harrison SA, Darland C, Finch J, Schenker S, et al. Pioglitazone treatment increases whole body fat but not total body water in patients with nonalcoholic steatohepatitis. *Journal of Hepatology* 2007;47:565–570. https://doi.org/10.1016/j.jhep.2007.04.013.

[152] Young LH, Viscoli CM, Schwartz GG, Inzucchi SE, Curtis JP, Gorman MJ, et al. Heart failure after ischemic stroke or transient ischemic attack in insulin-resistant patients without diabetes mellitus treated with pioglitazone. *Circulation* 2018;138:1210–1220. https://doi.org/10.1161/CIRCULATIONAHA.118.034763.

[153] van der Meer RW, Rijzewijk LJ, de Jong HWAM, Lamb HJ, Lubberink M, Romijn JA, et al. Pioglitazone improves cardiac function and alters myocardial substrate metabolism without affecting cardiac triglyceride accumulation and high-energy phosphate metabolism in patients with well-controlled type 2 diabetes mellitus. *Circulation* 2009;119:2069–2077. https://doi.org/10.1161/CIRCULATIONAHA.108.803916.

[154] Clarke GD, Solis-Herrera C, Molina-Wilkins M, Martinez S, Merovci A, Cersosimo E, et al. Pioglitazone improves left ventricular diastolic function in subjects with diabetes. *Diabetes Care* 2017;40:1530–1536. https://doi.org/10.2337/dc17-0078.

[155] Lehrke M, Marx N. Diabetes mellitus and heart failure. *The American Journal of Cardiology* 2017;120:S37–47. https://doi.org/10.1016/j.amjcard.2017.05.014.

[156] DeFronzo RA, Chilton R, Norton L, Clarke G, Ryder REJ, Abdul-Ghani M. Revitalization of pioglitazone: the optimum agent to be combined with a sodium-glucose co-transporter-2 inhibitor. *Diabetes, Obesity and Metabolism* 2016;18:454–462. https://doi.org/10.1111/dom.12652.

[157] Munigoti S, Harinarayan C. Role of Glitazars in atherogenic dyslipidemia and diabetes: two birds with one stone? *Indian Journal of Endocrinology and Metabolism* 2014;18:283. https://doi.org/10.4103/2230-8210.131134.

[158] Hirschfield G, Boudes P, Bowlus C, Gitlin N, Michael G, Harrison S, et al. Treatment efficacy and safety of seladelpar, a selective peroxisome proliferator-activated receptor delta agonist, in primary biliary cholangitis patients: 12- and 26-week analysis from an ongoing international, randomized, dose raging phase 2 study. *Journal of Hepatology* 2018;68:S105–106. https://doi.org/10.1016/S0168-8278(18)30429-X.

[159] Hampson SJ. Nursing interventions for the first three postpartum months. *Journal of Obstetric, Gynecologic, and Neonatal Nursing: JOGNN* n.d.;18:116–122. https://doi.org/10.1111/j.1552-6909.1989.tb00474.x.

[160] Francque S, Vonghia L. Pharmacological treatment for non-alcoholic fatty liver disease. *Advances in Therapy* 2019;36:1052–1074. https://doi.org/10.1007/s12325-019-00898-6.

[161] CymaBay Therapeutics reports topline 12-week data from an ongoing phase 2b study of seladelpar in patients with nonalcoholic steatohepatitis. n.d.

[162] Gawrieh S. *The Liver Meeting 2019—the 70th Annual Meeting of the AASLD*. Boston, MA, 2019.

15 Anti-Inflammatory Drugs

Metabolic Inflammation in NASH—A Drug Target?

Angelo Armandi and Jörn M. Schattenberg

CONTENTS

Key Points

- Nonalcoholic steatohepatitis (NASH) is a chronic inflammatory liver disease that can progress to end-stage liver disease.

- Preclinical models link the inflammatory component in NASH to stellate cell activation and progressive deposition of collagen that can build up to hepatic cirrhosis.

- In cross-sectional studies, NASH and in particular the disease activity defined by hepatic inflammation are linked to impaired quality of life and more advanced disease stages.

- Histologic endpoints are accepted as surrogate endpoints to reasonably likely predicted transplant-free survival by the Food and Drug Administration (FDA).

- Currently, no approved drug to treat NASH is available, but multiple mechanisms aiming to decrease hepatic inflammation are explored.

- Metabolic pathways act at multiple levels (the pathophysiological and insulin resistance levels), and lipid metabolism and energy metabolism are frequently disturbed in NASH.

- The use of anti-inflammatory drugs in NASH has a strong rationale, but currently the only compound that has shown a significant impact in phase 3 is an FXR agonist that exerts antifibrotic effects.

15.1 INTRODUCTION: WHY SHOULD INFLAMMATION BE TARGETED IN NAFLD?

Nonalcoholic fatty liver disease (NAFLD) is the most frequent liver disease globally, but, as of today, no effective therapy is approved. Based on multiple levels of preclinical evidence, hepatic inflammation is linked to both liver cell injury and activation of stellate cells, which are responsible for the deposition of collagen in the liver and progressive scaring. Currently, the US Food and Drug Administration (FDA) accepts two endpoints for conditional drug approval in precirrhotic nonalcoholic steatohepatitis (NASH). The first is the resolution of NASH without worsening of fibrosis, while the second is the improvement of fibrosis without worsening of NASH. In the context of the resolution of NASH, the absence of at least one of the two components of liver inflammation (lobular inflammation and ballooning) that comprise the histological NAFLD activity score (NAS), as described by Kleiner et al.,[1] is required. In contrast to the fibrosis stage, the presence of NASH on histology has not been linked with overall survival,[2,3] while lobular inflammation, which is a key feature of NASH, impacts the health-related quality of life.[4]

Fibrosing NASH represents a progressive liver injury that can lead to advanced liver disease, including cirrhosis, portal hypertension and hepatocellular carcinoma (HCC). A major obstacle in assessing NASH—both as an endpoint in trials or as a disease—is related to its definition, which involves the overall impression of a pathologist assessing the specific piece of liver tissue obtained for the assessment. This is refined in the regulatory context, when a 3- to 5-tier scoring system semiquantitatively grades lobular inflammation, hepatocellular ballooning, steatosis, in addition to fibrosis to define NASH disease activity. In addition, the inter- and intrapathologist agreement for grading of ballooning and inflammation is low and represents one major challenge.[5] This has diagnostic implications, because ballooning is the key feature of NASH, and its absence supports the efficacy of experimental drugs.

These challenges need to be considered when discussing the natural history of NASH and the potential to address hepatic inflammation as a drug target. There is little controversy around hepatic inflammation as the driver of hepatic fibrogenesis. However, in the absence of studies performing repeated liver biopsies over time, all estimations beyond hard outcomes are vague. A meta-analysis has proposed that a patient with NASH progresses one histological fibrosis stage every 7 years on average.[6] After reaching the precirrhotic stage (histological stage F3) or even cirrhosis (F4), about 20% of patients develop the endpoint of either liver cirrhosis (for the precirrhotic population) or decompensation (for the cirrhotic population) within 48 weeks.[7] Importantly, hepatic inflammation in NASH can be affected by the type of diet, weight changes and cofactors of liver disease. This contrasts with fibrosis, which builds up and regresses at a significant

DOI: 10.1201/9781003386698-18

slower rate, making it a good measure of inflammation that has occurred over time. The traditional risk factors of NASH, including increased waist circumference, insulin resistance, dyslipidemia, as well as defined genetic risk profiles, impact on the severity of hepatic inflammation in NASH.[8] Patients go through phases of progression, plateaus and regressions of hepatic inflammation during the disease evaluation. and this variable slowly and progressively accounts for difficulties in studying NASH in validated animal models. In fact, most preclinical models that are used to generate evidence to support anti-inflammatory and antifibrotic drugs do not recapitulate the complexity of the human disease with multiple environmental and intrinsic factors.[9]

The strongest evidence that anti-inflammatory drugs will be successful comes from lifestyle interventions aiming at weight loss that have shown resolution of steatohepatitis with a weight loss of 7% and more. Importantly, this can only be achieved by approximately 10% of patients over a 1-year time span.[10] This highlights the great and currently unmet need to develop effective and safe pharmacotherapy for NASH. Additionally, patients developing NASH in the absence of obesity or additional metabolic risk factors, including lean individuals,[11] could be of special interest for anti-inflammatory compounds. One challenge for the field has been to identify and define the right study population for a specific mechanism of action (MoA) in a trial exploring anti-inflammatory drugs. While the obvious answer is that all patients with NASH should benefit, it can be assumed that the underlying triggers of inflammation can differ among individual patients and that, as such, the responses to the drug could differ. It can be expected that the development of prognostic and predictive biomarkers that are currently explored in large, multicenter prospective registry studies will help in this regard.[12] In the end, there is overwhelming evidence that a drug aimed at decreasing hepatocellular inflammation will help to stabilize or even reverse fibrotic NASH, and, based on this, many clinical trials explore investigational products for the resolution of steatohepatitis in individuals with biopsy-proven NASH. The following section summarize these compounds (see Tables 15.1 and 15.2).

15.2 NUCLEAR RECEPTOR AGONISTS: SELECTIVE MODULATION AND TAILORED APPROACHES

Nuclear receptors regulate the expression of key drivers of inflammation and fibrosis in the hepatic compartment. Additionally, they are critically involved in energy metabolism acting as ligands and activate transcription factors for a variety of genes involved in energy homeostasis. Investigational products targeting key regulators of metabolic inflammation, like peroxisome proliferator-activated receptors (PPARs)[13] or farnesoid-X receptor (FXR)[14] in individuals with major metabolic diseases have shown positive effects on surrogate markers of hepatic inflammation.

15.2.1 Class of PPARs

PPARs are well-known to modulate lipid and glucose metabolism but are also acting on immune-cell populations making them an attractive target for drug development in NASH. In 2010, strong evidence on the benefit of PPARs in NASH was generated within the PIVENS trial, a placebo-controlled, 3-arm study that compared pioglitazone (30 mg daily), vitamin E (800 IU daily) and placebo in nondiabetic fibrosing NASH for 96 weeks.[15] The

composite outcome was the improvement in inflammation and fibrosis, with a predefined significance level at $p < 0.025$ in this multicomparator setup. The most striking finding was that the antioxidant vitamin E resulted in a significant improvement in NASH when compared to placebo (43% vs. 19%, $p = 0.001$) in this nondiabetic population. Pioglitazone, a thiazolidinedione that improves insulin sensitivity and has an established role in the treatment of type 2 diabetes, showed no superiority vs. placebo (34% vs. 19%, $p = 0.04$). This came as a surprise, as pioglitazone is an agonist of PPAR gamma, which has proven effects on lipid metabolism and insulin sensitivity. Aligned with this MoA, pioglitazone led to improvement of steatosis but not fibrosis stage. This response was different in patients with prediabetes or type 2 diabetes, where pioglitazone led to both resolution of NASH (treatment difference of 32%, $p < 0.001$) and improvement in fibrosis score (treatment difference of 0.5, $p = 0.039$).[16]

In subsequent clinical trials, several different PPAR agonists—addressing the three receptor subclasses alpha, delta and gamma differentially—were subsequently investigated. Elafibranor is a dual PPAR alpha-delta agonist that has shown promising results on dyslipidemia, insulin resistance and surrogate markers of liver inflammation (transaminases, gamma-glutamyl transferase) in patients with NASH in a phase 2 clinical trial. A significantly higher proportion of patients receiving elafibranor in a phase 2b study showed NASH resolution when compared to placebo (19% vs. 12%, $p = 0.045$). This effect was pronounced in the subgroup with a higher NAS (equal or above 4) and more advanced fibrosis compared to mild disease (NAS 3) on post hoc analysis.[17] However, the subsequent phase 3 study failed to demonstrate the same efficacy. Here, the effect was only 4% over placebo, leading to a high, comparable response rate in the placebo arm (15% as compared to 19% of treated patients). Importantly, there was an overall improvement in the cardiometabolic profile of all patients in the study, which was deemed to be related to lifestyle changes. Since improvement of the metabolism has deep implications upon the liver metabolic pathways, this could also explain placebo response rates. Overall, standardization of lifestyle recommendations in phase 2 and phase 3 clinical trials appear to be crucial when exploring anti-inflammatory drugs in NASH.[18]

Despite these limitations, the role of other PPARs was subsequently explored. In a phase 2b study, the pan-PPAR agonist lanifibranor demonstrated a 2-point improvement in NASH using the SAF (steatosis, activity, fibrosis) scoring system[19] without worsening of fibrosis, which was significantly higher than placebo (55% vs. 33%, $p = 0.007$). Improvements in the fibrosis stage of at least 1 without worsening of NASH and a resolution of NASH with additional improvement in the fibrosis stage were observed.[20] These findings supported the further assessment of lanifibranor in a phase 3 trial, which is currently in progress. Finally, the dual PPAR alpha-gamma agonist saroglitazar has been shown to improve NASH in animal models[21] and has been evaluated in a phase 2 trial on nonbiopsied NAFLD and elevated transaminases, with the primary endpoint of percentage in changes of alanine aminotransferase from baseline to week 16.[22] The treated arm achieved the endpoint with a significantly higher proportion when compared to placebo (−44% vs. 4.1%, $p < 0.001$). In addition, saroglitazar led to an improvement in liver fat content measured by proton density fat

Table 15.1: Investigational Products Exploring Anti-Inflammatory Mechanisms in Nonalcoholic Steatohepatitis (NASH) with Fibrosis

Investigational Drug	Mechanism of Action (MoA)	Clinical Trial Phase (Name)	Primary Endpoint	Efficacy	Reference
Vitamin E	Antioxidant effect	Phase 3 (PIVENS)	Improvement in the NAS score and fibrosis*	Improvement in NASH, ALT, AST, steatosis, lobular inflammation	Sanyal et al. 2010
Pioglitazone	PPAR-gamma agonist	Phase 3 (PIVENS)	Improvement in the NAS score and fibrosis*	Improvement in ALT, AST, steatosis, lobular inflammation	Sanyal et al. 2010
Liraglutide	GLP-1 receptor agonist	Phase 2 (LEAN)	Resolution of NASH without worsening of fibrosis	Resolution of NASH without worsening of fibrosis	Armstrong et al. 2016
Cenicriviroc	Chemokine receptor 2/5 antagonist	Phase 2b	Improvement of $\geq$ 2 points in NAS without worsening in fibrosis	Fibrosis improvement of at least 1 stage without worsening of NASH	Friedman et al. 2018
Obethicholic acid	FXR agonist	Phase 3, month 18—planed interim analysis (REGENERATE)	Fibrosis improvement of at least 1 stage without worsening of NASH or NASH resolution without worsening of fibrosis	Fibrosis improvement of at least 1 stage without worsening of NASH	Younossi et al. 2019
Resmetirom	TH-receptor beta agonist	Phase 2 (MAESTRO)	Absolute liver fat content at PDFF-MR after 12 weeks	Reduction in absolute liver fat content	Harrison et al. 2019
Tropifexor/cenicriviroc	Combined FXR agonist/chemokine receptor 2/5 antagonist	Phase 2b (TANDEM study)	Fibrosis improvement of at least 1 stage or NASH resolution	Completed—data pending	Pedrosa et al. 2020
Lanifibranor	Pan-PPAR agonist	Phase 2b (NATIVE)	Decrease of at least 2 points of SAF score	Decrease of at least 2 points of SAF score, resolution of NASH without worsening of fibrosis, improvement of at least 1 fibrosis stage without worsening of NASH, resolution of NASH and improvement of at least 1 fibrosis stage, improvement in ALT, AST, lipid profile, inflammatory and fibrosis biomarkers	Francque et al. 2021
Saroglitazar	PPAR alpha-gamma agonist	Phase 2a	Percentage change of ALT at 16 weeks	Improvement in ALT levels, liver fat content by PDFF-MR, adiponectin, triglycerides, HOMA-IR	Gawrieh et al. 2021
Semglutide	GLP-1 receptor agonist	Phase 2	Resolution of NASH without worsening of fibrosis	Resolution of NASH without worsening of fibrosis	Newsome et al. 2021
Aldafermin	FGF19 analogue	Phase 2	Absolute liver fat content at PDFF-MR after 24 weeks	Reduction in absolute liver fat content, ALT, AST, PRO-C3	Harrison et al. 2021
BIO89–100	FGF21 analogue	Phase 1b/2a	Absolute liver fat content at PDFF-MR after 12 weeks	Reduction in absolute liver fat content, liver fat volume, ALT, triglycerides, LDL cholesterol; increase in adiponectin	Frias et al. 2021
Aramchol	SCD1 partial inhibitor	Phase 2b	Absolute liver fat content at PDFF-MR after 52 weeks	NASH resolution without worsening in fibrosis, fibrosis improvement of at least 1 stage without worsening of NASH, ALT improvement	Ratziu et al. 2021
Tropifexor	FXR agonist	Phase 2 (FLIGHT-FXR)	Absolute liver fat content at PDFF-MR after 12 weeks, percentage change of ALT and AST levels after 12 weeks	Completed—data pending.	ClinicalTrials.gov: NCT02855164
Tirzepatide	GLP-1/GIP agonist	Phase 2b	Resolution of NASH without worsening of fibrosis	Ongoing	ClicalTrials.gov: NCT0416773
JKB-122	TLR4 antagonist	Phase 2	Fibrosis improvement of at least 1 stage or NASH resolution	Ongoing	ClicalTrials.gov: NCT0455069

* With an improvement by 1 or more in ballooning; no increase in fibrosis score; and either a decrease in the NAS < 3 or NAS decrease by 2 points, with at least a 1-point decrease in either the lobular inflammation or steatosis score

ALT: Alanine aminotransferase; AST: Aspartate aminotransferase; FGF: Fibroblast growth factor; FXR: Farnesoid-X receptor; GIP: Gastric inhibitory peptide; GLP-1: Glucagon-like peptide-1; HOMA-IR: Homeostatic model assessment—insulin resistance; LDL: Low-density lipoprotein; NAS: Nonalcoholic fatty liver disease (NAFLD) activity score; PDFF-MR: Proton density fat fraction-magnetic resonance; PPAR: Peroxisome proliferator-activated receptors; PRO-C3: N-terminal propeptide of type III collagen; SAF: Steatosis activity fibrosis (score); SCD1: Stearoyl-CoA desaturase 1; TLR4: Toll-like receptor 4; TH: Thyroid hormone.

Table 15.2: Overview of Randomized Clinical Trials of Investigational Products That Have Been Withdrawn from Treatment of Nonalcoholic Steatohepatitis (NASH) with Fibrosis

Name of the Compound	Authors	Drug Target	Phase of the Study	Primary Endpoints	Reasons for Failure
Elafibranor	Ratziu et al. 2016	PPAR alfa-delta agonist	Phase 2	Resolution of NASH without worsening in fibrosis	High placebo response rate in the phase 3
Simtuzumab	Harrison et al. 2018	LOXL-2 inhibitor	Phase 2b	Changes in hepatic collagen content for bridging fibrosis; changes in HVPG for cirrhosis	Ineffective in reducing fibrosis stage, preventing progression to cirrhosis and preventing liver decompensation
Cilofexor	Patel et al. 2020	FXR agonist	Phase 2	Changes in liver fat content by PDFF-MR and liver stiffness by MRE	No significant differences in liver fat content changes between the treated and placebo arms; no changes in liver stiffness
MSDC-0602K	Harrison et al. 2020	mTOT agonist	Phase 2b	Improvement of ≥ 2 points in NAS with a ≥ 1 point reduction in either ballooning or lobular inflammation and no worsening in fibrosis	No significant differences in the histology endpoints
Selorsentib	Harrison et al. 2020	ASK1 inhibitor	Phase 3	Fibrosis improvement of at least 1 stage without NASH worsening	No antifibrotic effect in both bridging fibrosis and compensated cirrhosis
Emricasan	Harrison et al. 2020	Pan-caspase inhibitor	Phase 2	Fibrosis improvement of at least 1 stage without NASH worsening	High placebo response rate

ASK1: Apoptosis signal-regulating kinase 1; FXR: Farnesoid-X receptor; HVPG: Hepatic venous portal gradient; LOXL2: Lysyl oxidase homolog 2; mTOT: Mitochondrial target of thiazolidinediones; MRE: Magnetic resonance elastography; NAS: Nonalcoholic fatty liver disease (NAFLD) activity score; PDFF-MR: Proton density fat fraction-magnetic resonance; PPAR: Peroxisome proliferator-activated receptors.

fraction magnetic resonance (MRI-PDFF), in insulin resistance as measured by the surrogate homeostatic model for insulin resistance (HOMA-IR) index, and in atherogenic lipids.

15.2.2 Farnesoid X-Receptor (FXR)

FXRs are regulators of hepatic cholesterol metabolism and bile acid synthesis, and through these actions they affect hepatic inflammation and fibrogenesis. This involves prominent inflammatory signaling systems including tumor necrosis factor alpha, nuclear factor kappa B in hepatocytes and transforming growth factor beta in stellate cells.[23] Additionally, FXR agonism in the intestine leads to the liberation of fibroblast growth factor 19 (FGF19) that, in turn, acts on the liver compartment and augments its anti-inflammatory and antifibrotic effects. The selective, steroidal FXR agonist obeticholic acid (OCA) is the only drug so far that has demonstrated histological benefit in patients with NASH in both a phase 2b and a phase 3 clinical trial.[24] In the phase 3 REGENERATE study, OCA used at 25 mg achieved a significant reduction of fibrosis at month 18 vs. placebo (23% vs. 12%) but, not disappointingly, did not show superiority in NASH resolution.[25] Nonetheless, when exploring key features of steatohepatitis including lobular inflammation and hepatocyte ballooning or when abandoning the overall scoring system and exploring resolution of NASH based on the pathologist assessment, a significant effect with OCA was observed. Also, noninvasive including liver enzymes (transaminases) and noninvasive fibrosis tests (FIB-4; FibroTest) showed a sustained reduction

along with the fibrosis improvement.[26] The challenging question in this regard is how the pleiotropic effects of OCA translate into a predominantly antifibrotic effect without showing a robust anti-inflammatory signal. One possible explanation has to do with the vulnerability of the currently used endpoints including the semiquantitative assessment of a small piece of liver tissue. On the other hand, the paradigm of a tailored, individualized therapy may represent a way forward, with the combination of antifibrotic and specific anti-inflammatory medications.

The concept of FXR agonism is being explored in several other studies. Cilofexor is a selective, nonsteroidal FXR agonist, leading to a strong intestinal activation of FXR and FGF19 release and, through this, partly circumventing some of the unwanted direct FXR effects including dyslipidemia and pruritus. Based on encouraging data from a proof-of concept study,[27] a phase 2 trial was developed on a larger cohort of patients with NASH diagnosed noninvasively by MRI-PDFF and magnetic resonance elastography (MRE) or liver biopsy. Albeit showing reductions in liver fat and liver enzymes (a 24-week median decrease in liver fat of −22.7% in the treated arm, compared to the increase of 1.9% of the placebo arm, $p = 0.003$), in the absence of a histological endpoint, the changes in NASH are difficult to determine. In addition, pruritus was observed in a major proportion of treated patients than placebo.[28] Another FXR agonist, tropifexor, has shown to be effective in preclinical models of NASH[29] and has been recently evaluated in a phase 2 study.[30] In addition, a combination strategy with tropifexor and cenicriviroc has been designed into a current phase 2 trial on fibrosing NASH, with the primary endpoint of resolution of NASH or improvement in fibrosis.[31] Results of the FLIGHT-FXR study will be presented in the fall of 2022.

15.3 ADDRESSING METABOLIC DERANGEMENTS TO IMPROVE LIVER INFLAMMATION

The initial trigger of hepatic inflammation is thought to arise in the context of metabolic disturbances including insulin resistance and dyslipidemia. Therefore, addressing the key regulators of metabolic pathways has been explored as a treatment strategy for NASH individuals. NAFLD is inserted into a complex picture of systemic inflammation driven by multiple metabolic dysregulations.[32,33] In addition, intrahepatic lipid incomplete oxidation is a major source of injury leading to oxidative stress and lipoapoptosis.

15.3.1 Insulin Sensitivity: Incretins

Given the central role of insulin resistance in NASH, numerous clinical trials have addressed specific targets involved in glucose metabolism. Of great interest is the glucagon metabolism, which controls lipid oxidation and mitochondrial function. Glucagon-like peptide-1 (GLP-1) is a gut-derived hormone that improves insulin secretion, reduces appetite and delays gastric emptying. Based on their robust weight loss effects, GLP-1 are a promising class of drugs for the treatment of NASH.

The first trials with GLP-1 agonists conducted on diabetic individuals had shown marked improvement in transaminases as a surrogate of liver inflammation.[34] Accordingly, in a phase 2 trial conducted on NASH (LEAN trial), the GLP-1 agonist liraglutide led to NASH resolution in a significant proportion of treated patients when compared to placebo ($p = 0.019$). Interestingly, this study did not show fibrosis regression by at least one stage,[35] albeit weight loss occurred in the range of expectance. In a larger phase 2b study enrolling 320 patients, the long-acting GLP-1 agonist semaglutide was studied and showed a significant improvement in NASH resolution, with 59% in the treated arm vs. 17% in the placebo group ($p < 0.001$) in the placebo group at 72 weeks but again without improving fibrosis. These results suggest that the two endpoints that are being studied for conditional drug approval—resolution of NASH and regression of fibrosis—can appealingly be disassociated. A large phase 3 trial on the effects of semaglutide in noncirrhotic NASH are underway to explore its efficacy in this population.[36]

Dual agonists of the GLP-1 receptor and the Glucagon receptor or the glucose-dependent insulinotropic polypeptide (GIP) are under development to exploit the agnostic activities of these incretin signals. Tirzepatide, which is a GLP-1/GIP coagonist, is currently being explored in a phase 2 study[37] after showing improvements in liver inflammatory and fibrosis biomarkers in diabetic patients[38] and strong effects on body weight. The increased efficacy of this drug class is offset by side effects, including nausea, that need consideration.

15.3.2 Glucose Metabolism: FGF19 and FGF21

FGF19 has been identified as a key regulator of metabolic processes including hepatic glycogen synthesis and suppression of gluconeogenesis in the liver through altered bile acid and cholesterol metabolism.[39] The short half-life of FGF19 prohibits its use as a drug; however, the engineered

FGF-19 analog aldafermin exhibits acceptable pharmacokinetic and pharmacodynamic profiles and has been explored in patients with NASH. Based on its mechanism of action, the anti-inflammatory effects achieved through metabolic benefits were anticipated. In a phase 2 study, at 24 weeks, the absolute liver fat reduction exceeded 5% measured on MRI-PDFF: a median reduction of 7.7% in the treated arm vs. 2.7% in the placebo group ($p = 0.002$) were observed. Parallel improvements of the histological features steatosis, inflammation, and fibrosis were observed, despite lacking statistical significance.[40] These data informed the phase 2b ALPINE 2/3 studies using aldafermin for 24 weeks in noncirrhotic NASH. While the full study report has not been published, the development program was halted because the predefined dose-dependent effect on fibrosis regression was not seen. Nonetheless, aldafermin demonstrated a numerically higher rate of NASH resolution in all three doses over placebo and reached significance in the highest dose group (3 mg) at week 24.[41]

Similarly, FGF21 is a hormone involved in the glucose, lipid end energy metabolism.[42] The engineered long-acting glyco-pegylated FGF21 analogue BIO89-100 has been tested in a population of either biopsy-proven NASH or "phenotypic" NASH (central obesity with either diabetes mellitus or alterations in liver stiffness or transaminases). BIO89-100 has led to significant improvements in liver fat content and liver fat volume by PDFF-MR[43], and a phase 2b study is currently enrolling.

Based on these available data, overall there is a rationale to support the use of FGF in NASH. The challenge to this type of drug—and one reason for the discontinuation of the development of aldafermin in the noncirrhotic population—could be the limitations associated with the subcutaneous application. On the other hand, the option to have a combination partner with other subcutaneous drugs that is capable of reducing hepatic inflammation could be one option for these drugs in the near future.

15.3.3 Thyroid Hormones and Lipid Metabolism

An interesting approach to modulate hepatic inflammation are thyromimetics that are affecting liver lipid metabolism. Thyroid hormones act directly on thyroid hormone receptors (THR), and the beta subtype (THR beta) is a key player of hepatic lipid metabolism. The unwanted THR alpha effects—that are mediating bone turnover and promoting cardiovascular side effects—can be avoided by drugs that are specifically designed to activate the beta receptor or thyromimetics that are specifically targeted to the hepatic compartment.[44] The link of "hepatic hypothyroidism"—being in part responsible for increased low-density lipoprotein (LDL) cholesterol secretion and liver steatosis—to hepatic inflammation has been addressed in a number or clinical trials. Resmetirom, a selective THR beta agonist, was firstly developed in dyslipidemia but subsequently also showed improvement of hepatic steatosis and oxidative stress in animal models.[45] A 36-week phase 2 study in NASH demonstrated a robust effect with improvement in liver fat assessed by MRI-PDFF after 12 weeks (−39% in the treated arm vs. −10.4% in the placebo arm, $p < 0.05$), as well as after 36 weeks −37.7% in the treated arm vs. −10.4% of placebo ($p < 0.05$). In parallel, surrogates of hepatic inflammation including liver enzymes, atherogenic lipids and noninvasive markers of inflammation (including an enhanced liver fibrosis [ELF] test and cytokeratin-18) improved. With regard to histology, the proportion of patients with 2-point NAS improvement at week 36 was significantly higher in the treated arm when compared to placebo: 46% vs. 19% ($p = 0.017$).[46] A phase 3 study of resmetirom in patients with noncirrhotic but also cirrhotic NASH patients is currently underway and will report interim data in the fall of 2022.

15.3.4 Linking Metabolism and Inflammation

Other metabolic active compounds have been explored in the context of NASH. Aramchol is a cholic-arachidic acid conjugate that inhibits de novo lipogenesis by targeting stearoyl-CoA desaturase 1 (SCD1). In a trial with HIV-associated NAFLD, Aramchol did not lead to a significant change in liver fat content by MRI-PDFF.[47] However, in a follow-up phase 2b trial in NASH patients, histological improvement of steatosis, inflammation and ballooning, along with a slight, nonsignificant improvement in fibrosis, was observed at 52 weeks.[48] Aramchol is currently under evaluation in a large phase 3 clinical trial. Another interesting approach is the regulation of insulin sensitivity using a molecule targeting the mitochondrial target of thiazolidinediones (mTOT). The investigational product, named MSDC-0602K, is a second-generation insulin sensitizer that has been shown to improve lipid oxidation and to reduce de novo lipogenesis and gluconeogenesis.[49] In a phase 2b study conducted on NASH patients, the drug did not meet the histological endpoints but showed a positive impact on insulin sensitivity and surrogates of liver inflammation and fibrosis.[50]

15.4 WHY IT IS CRUCIAL TO RESOLVE HEPATIC INFLAMMATION WHEN TARGETING FIBROTIC NASH

These summarized data from completed and ongoing clinical trials have painted a picture in which NASH resolution and fibrosis regression are two interchangeable and separately achievable endpoints. From a regulatory perspective—which aims at quantifying benefit to determine whether a drug should receive accelerated approval in the regulator landscape—this seems like a valid approach. However, from the patient's perspective and the pathophysiology of the disease, NASH and hepatic fibrosis cannot be separated from one another (Figure 15.1). There is ample evidence that hepatic inflammation driven by metabolic disturbance is the key driver of hepatic fibrogenesis in NASH. Inflammation and fibrosis are parts of a disease continuum that continuously shapes this liver disease.[51] All attempts to develop an antifibrotic treatment that will not decrease hepatic necroinflammation or is given in parallel to significant weight loss will fail to achieve clinically meaningful endpoints. The data that are generated within clinical trials have many facets, and the limitations that arise from the semiquantitative scoring system of the histological endpoint is one of them. Another important aspect to consider is the different dynamics of hepatic inflammation and hepatic fibrogenesis. While hepatic inflammation is much more volatile and susceptible to lifestyle decisions changing potentially within hours, hepatic fibrolysis or fibrogenesis is changing at a much slower pace taking weeks or months.

A number of unsuccessful drug development programs can inform the field on its path forward (see reference 12 for details on the "graveyard" of NASH development). Cenicriviroc is a dual antagonist of chemokine receptors 2 and 5, leading to the inhibition of hepatic stellate cells and macrophages, which are linked to inflammation and fibrogenesis.[52] Hence, there was a strong rational to explore its efficacy in NASH. However, the phase 2b

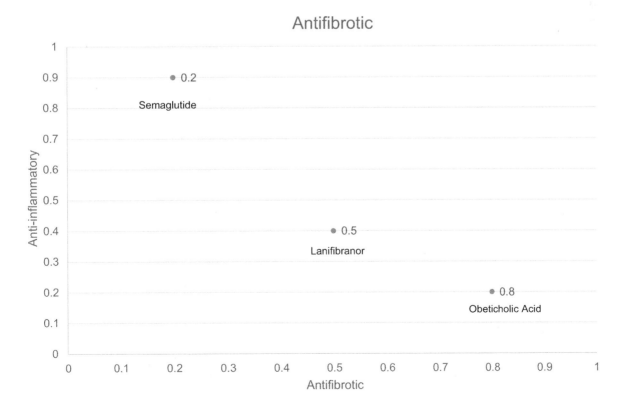

Figure 15.1 Relative potency of different NASH drugs on the inflammation and fibrosis axes

study did not meet the inflammatory endpoint (improvement of 2 points of NAS).[53] Likewise, the apoptosis signal-regulating kinase 1 (ASK1) inhibitor selonsertib was supported by excellent preclinical data and had suggested a benefit on fibrosis in an open-label phase 2 trial on NASH.[54] However, the subsequent trials conducted in fibrosing NASH and compensated cirrhosis failed to reach the fibrosis endpoint at 48 weeks.[55] The pan-caspase inhibitor emricasan that was coined at the prevention of apoptosis and inflammation, failed in both the phase 2b trial conducted in fibrosing NASH and also the cirrhotic trial that was design to explore reduction of portal hypertension measured by hepatic venous portal gradient (HVPG).[56,57] Likewise, toll-like receptor 4 (TLR4) signaling, which is involved in the activation of the immune system, insulin resistance and metabolic inflammation driven by visceral adipose tissue,[58,59] was a strong target for pharmacotherapy. Even though preclinical studies in TLR4-knockout mice showed an improvement in obesity, insulin resistance, liver fat content, and inflammation,[60] JKB-121—an antagonist of TLR4—failed to show a meaningful effect.[61]

15.5 CONCLUSIONS: Current Pitfalls and Future Perspectives

The available evidence supports the concept that hepatic necroinflammation is a druggable target. The challenges on the path forward have become obvious from failed development programs. At this stage, the high placebo response rates that account for a great proportion of trial failures highlights the great need to validate a robust and noninvasive endpoint for conditional regulatory approval. The limitations of liver histology that capture a static picture from a "snapshot" biopsy at one point in time during the evolution of a complex disease is the major hurdle that has made NASH resolution look like a seemingly unachievable endpoint. Augmentation of liver histology by introducing artificial intelligence algorithm can partly account for some but, by far, not all the challenges.[62] Also, the improvement that can be seen on surrogate markers of liver inflammation or in parallel metabolic parameters (lipid profile, weight loss) are not robust enough to predict outcomes. The seemingly high discrepancies between phase 2a trials—achieving a positive endpoint on liver inflammation—and later stage clinical trials failing to demonstrate histology improvement highlight tall these aspects. To overcome these challenges, large academia-driven research consortia (LITMUS, NIMBLE, GOLDMINE, NAIL-NIT) have undertaken an enormous scientific effort to define and approve novel biomarkers that will close this gap and allow for an easier path forward.

In conclusion, despite the difficulties surrounding drug development in NASH, the current landscape of pharmacological therapy is very promising. The constant efforts to better understand the challenges in this field will help to improve the individual patient's perspectives and the understanding of the pathophysiology of NAFLD and will guide clinicians toward a better approach for its management—in the end leading to the approval of an urgently required pharmacotherapy for fibrosing NASH.

REFERENCES

1. Kleiner DE, Brunt EM, Van Natta M, Behling C, Contos MJ, Cummings OW, et al. Design and validation of a histological scoring system for nonalcoholic fatty liver disease. *Hepatology.* 2005;41(6):1313–1321.

2. Sanyal AJ, Van Natta ML, Clark J, Neuschwander-Tetri BA, Diehl A, Dasarathy S, et al. Prospective study of outcomes in adults with nonalcoholic fatty liver disease. *N Engl J Med.* 2021;385(17):1559–1569.

3. Hagström H, Nasr P, Ekstedt M, Hammar U, Stål P, Hultcrantz R, et al. Fibrosis stage but not NASH predicts mortality and time to development of severe liver disease in biopsy-proven NAFLD. *J Hepatol.* 2017;67(6):1265–1273.

4. Huber Y, Boyle M, Hallsworth K, Tiniakos D, Straub BK, Labenz C, et al. Health-related quality of life in nonalcoholic fatty liver disease associates with hepatic inflammation. *Clin Gastroenterol Hepatol.* 2019;17(10):2085–2092.e1.

5. Brunt EM, Clouston AD, Goodman Z, Guy C, Kleiner DE, Lackner C, et al. Complexity of ballooned hepatocyte feature recognition: defining a training atlas for artificial intelligence-based imaging in NAFLD. *J Hepatol.* 2022;76(5):1030–1041.

6. Dulai PS, Singh S, Patel J, Soni M, Prokop LJ, Younossi Z, et al. Increased risk of mortality by fibrosis stage in nonalcoholic fatty liver disease: systematic review and meta-analysis. *Hepatology.* 2017;65(5):1557–1565.

7. Loomba R, Adams LA. The 20% rule of NASH progression: the natural history of advanced fibrosis and cirrhosis caused by NASH. *Hepatology.* 2019;70(6):1885–1888.

8. Armandi A, Rosso C, Caviglia GP, Bugianesi E. Insulin resistance across the spectrum of nonalcoholic fatty liver disease. *Metabolites.* 2021;11(3):155.

9. Farrell G, Schattenberg JM, Leclercq I, Yeh MM, Goldin R, Teoh N, et al. Mouse models of nonalcoholic steatohepatitis: toward optimization of their relevance to human nonalcoholic steatohepatitis. *Hepatology.* 2019;69(5):2241–2257.

10. Vilar-Gomez E, Martinez-Perez Y, Calzadilla-Bertot L, Torres-Gonzalez A, Gra-Oramas B, Gonzalez-Fabian L, et al. Weight loss through lifestyle modification significantly reduces features of nonalcoholic steatohepatitis. *Gastroenterology.* 2015;149(2):367–378.e5; quiz e14–15.

11. Younes R, Govaere O, Petta S, Miele L, Tiniakos D, Burt A, et al. Caucasian lean subjects with non-alcoholic fatty liver disease share long-term prognosis of non-lean: time for reappraisal of BMI-driven approach? *Gut.* 2022;71(2):382–390.

12. Drenth JPH, Schattenberg JM. The nonalcoholic steatohepatitis (NASH) drug development graveyard: established hurdles and planning for future success. *Expert Opin Investig Drugs.* 2020;29(12):1365–1375.

13. Pawlak M, Lefebvre P, Staels B. Molecular mechanism of PPARα action and its impact on lipid metabolism, inflammation and fibrosis in non-alcoholic fatty liver disease. *J Hepatol.* 2015;62(3):720–733.

14. Radun R, Trauner M. Role of FXR in bile acid and metabolic homeostasis in NASH: pathogenetic concepts and therapeutic opportunities. *Semin Liver Dis.* 2021;41(4):461–475.

15. Sanyal AJ, Chalasani N, Kowdley KV, McCullough A, Diehl AM, Bass NM, et al. Pioglitazone, vitamin E, or placebo for nonalcoholic steatohepatitis. *N Engl J Med.* 2010;362(18):1675–1685.

16. Cusi K, Orsak B, Bril F, Lomonaco R, Hecht J, Ortiz-Lopez C, Tio F, Hardies J, Darland C, Musi N, Webb A, Portillo-Sanchez P. Long-term pioglitazone treatment for patients with nonalcoholic steatohepatitis and

prediabetes or type 2 diabetes mellitus: a randomized trial. *Ann Intern Med.* 2016;165(5):305–315.

17. Ratziu V, Harrison SA, Francque S, Bedossa P, Lehert P, Serfaty L, et al. Elafibranor, an agonist of the peroxisome proliferator-activated receptor-alpha and -delta, induces resolution of nonalcoholic steatohepatitis without fibrosis worsening. *Gastroenterology.* 2016;150(5):1147–1159.e5.

18. Glass O, Filozof C, Noureddin M, Berner-Hansen M, Schabel E, Omokaro SO, et al. Standardisation of diet and exercise in clinical trials of NAFLD-NASH: recommendations from the liver forum. *J Hepatol.* 2020;73(3):680–693.

19. Bedossa P. FLIP Pathology Consortium. Utility and appropriateness of the fatty liver inhibition of progression (FLIP) algorithm and steatosis, activity, and fibrosis (SAF) score in the evaluation of biopsies of nonalcoholic fatty liver disease. *Hepatology.* 2014;60(2):565–575.

20. Francque SM, Bedossa P, Ratziu V, Anstee QM, Bugianesi E, Sanyal AJ, et al. A randomized, controlled trial of the pan-PPAR agonist lanifibranor in NASH. *N Engl J Med.* 2021;385(17):1547–1558.

21. Akbari R, Behdarvand T, Afarin R, Yaghooti H, Jalali MT, Mohammadtaghvaei N. Saroglitazar improved hepatic steatosis and fibrosis by modulating inflammatory cytokines and adiponectin in an animal model of non-alcoholic steatohepatitis. *BMC Pharmacol Toxicol.* 2021;22(1):53.

22. Gawrieh S, Noureddin M, Loo N, Mohseni R, Awasty V, Cusi K, et al. Saroglitazar, a PPAR-α/γ agonist, for treatment of NAFLD: a randomized controlled double-blind phase 2 trial. *Hepatology.* 2021;74(4):1809–1824.

23. Chávez-Talavera O, Tailleux A, Lefebvre P, Staels B. Bile acid control of metabolism and inflammation in obesity, type 2 diabetes, dyslipidemia, and nonalcoholic fatty liver disease. *Gastroenterology.* 2017;152(7):1679–1694.e3.

24. Neuschwander-Tetri BA, Loomba R, Sanyal AJ, Lavine JE, Van Natta ML, Abdelmalek MF, Chalasani N, Dasarathy S, Diehl AM, Hameed B, Kowdley KV, McCullough A, Terrault N, Clark JM, Tonascia J, Brunt EM, Kleiner DE, Doo E. NASH Clinical Research Network. Farnesoid X nuclear receptor ligand obeticholic acid for non-cirrhotic, non-alcoholic steatohepatitis (FLINT): a multicentre, randomised, placebo-controlled trial. *Lancet.* 2015;385(9972):956–965.

25. Younossi ZM, Ratziu V, Loomba R, Rinella M, Anstee QM, Goodman Z, et al. Obeticholic acid for the treatment of non-alcoholic steatohepatitis: interim analysis from a multicentre, randomised, placebo-controlled phase 3 trial. *Lancet.* 2019;394(10215):2184–2196.

26. Rinella ME, Dufour JF, Anstee QM, Goodman Z, Younossi Z, Harrison SA, et al. Non-invasive evaluation of response to obeticholic acid in patients with NASH: results from the REGENERATE study. *J Hepatol.* 2022;76(3):536–548.

27. Lawitz E, Herring R Jr, Younes ZH, Gane E, Ruane P, Schall RA, et al. PS-105 – Proof of concept study of an apoptosis-signal regulating kinase (ASK1) inhibitor (selonsertib) in combination with an acetyl-CoA carboxylase inhibitor (GS-0976) or a farnesoid X receptor agonist (GS-9674) in NASH. *J Hepatol.* 2018;68:S57.

28. Patel K, Harrison SA, Elkhashab M, Trotter JF, Herring R, Rojter SE, et al. Cilofexor, a nonsteroidal FXR agonist, in patients with noncirrhotic NASH: a phase 2 randomized controlled trial. *Hepatology.* 2020;72(1):58–71.

29. Hernandez ED, Zheng L, Kim Y, Fang B, Liu B, Valdez RA, et al. Tropifexor-mediated abrogation of steatohepatitis and fibrosis is associated with the antioxidative gene expression profile in rodents. *Hepatol Commun.* 2019;3(8):1085–1097.

30. https://clinicaltrials.gov/ct2/show/NCT02855164

31. Pedrosa M, Seyedkazemi S, Francque S, Sanyal A, Rinella M, Charlton M, et al. A randomized, double-blind, multicenter, phase 2b study to evaluate the safety and efficacy of a combination of tropifexor and cenicriviroc in patients with nonalcoholic steatohepatitis and liver fibrosis: study design of the TANDEM trial. *Contemp Clin Trials.* 2020;88:105889.

32. Gehrke N, Schattenberg JM. Metabolic inflammation-a role for hepatic inflammatory pathways as drivers of comorbidities in nonalcoholic fatty liver disease? *Gastroenterology.* 2020;158(7):1929–1947.e6.

33. Rosso C, Kazankov K, Younes R, Esmaili S, Marietti M, Sacco M, et al. Crosstalk between adipose tissue insulin resistance and liver macrophages in non-alcoholic fatty liver disease. *J Hepatol.* 2019;71(5):1012–1021.

34. Buse JB, Klonoff DC, Nielsen LL, Guan X, Bowlus CL, Holcombe JH, et al. Metabolic effects of two years of exenatide treatment on diabetes, obesity, and hepatic biomarkers in patients with type 2 diabetes: an interim analysis of data from the open-label, uncontrolled extension of three double-blind, placebo-controlled trials. *Clin Ther.* 2007;29(1):139–153.

35. Armstrong MJ, Gaunt P, Aithal GP, Barton D, Hull D, Parker R, et al. Liraglutide safety and efficacy in patients with non-alcoholic steatohepatitis (LEAN): a multicentre, double-blind, randomised, placebo-controlled phase 2 study. *Lancet.* 2016;387(10019):679–690.

36. Newsome PN, Buchholtz K, Cusi K, Linder M, Okanoue T, Ratziu V, et al. A placebo-controlled trial of subcutaneous semaglutide in nonalcoholic steatohepatitis. *N Engl J Med.* 2021;384(12):1113–1124.

37. https://clinicaltrials.gov/ct2/show/NCT04166773

38. Hartman ML, Sanyal AJ, Loomba R, Wilson JM, Nikooienejad A, Bray R, et al. Effects of novel dual GIP and GLP-1 receptor agonist tirzepatide on biomarkers of nonalcoholic steatohepatitis in patients with type 2 diabetes. *Diabetes Care.* 2020;43(6):1352–1355.

39. Sanyal AJ, Ling L, Beuers U, DePaoli AM, Lieu HD, Harrison SA, et al. Potent suppression of hydrophobic bile acids by aldafermin, an FGF19 analogue, across metabolic and cholestatic liver diseases. *JHEP Rep.* 2021;3(3):100255.

40. Harrison SA, Neff G, Guy CD, Bashir MR, Paredes AH, Frias JP, et al. Efficacy and safety of aldafermin, an engineered FGF19 analog, in a randomized, double-blind, placebo-controlled trial of patients with nonalcoholic steatohepatitis. *Gastroenterology.* 2021;160(1):219–231.e1.

41. www.globenewswire.com/news-release/2021/05/24/2234585/35057/en/NGM-Bio-Reports-Topline-Results-from-24-Week-Phase-2b-ALPINE-2-3-Study-of-Aldafermin-in-NASH.html

42. BonDurant LD, Ameka M, Naber MC, Markan KR, Idiga SO, Acevedo MR, et al. FGF21 regulates metabolism through adipose-dependent and -independent mechanisms. *Cell Metab.* 2017;25(4):935–944.e4.

43. Frias JP, Lawitz EJ, Ortiz-LaSanta G, Franey B, Morrow L, Chen CY, et al. BIO89–100 demonstrated robust reductions in liver fat and liver fat volume (LFV) by

MRI-PDFF, favorable tolerability and potential for weekly (QW) or every 2 weeks (Q2W) dosing in a phase 1b/2a placebo-controlled, double-blind, multiple ascending dose study in NASH. *J Endocr Soc.* 2021;5(Suppl 1):A5–6. doi:10.1210/jendso/bvab048.010.

44. Johansson L, Rudling M, Scanlan TS, Lundåsen T, Webb P, Baxter J, et al. Elective thyroid receptor modulation by GC-1 reduces serum lipids and stimulates steps of reverse cholesterol transport in euthyroid mice. *Proc Natl Acad Sci USA.* 2005;102(29):10297–10302.

45. Sinha RA, Bruinstroop E, Singh BK, Yen PM. Nonalcoholic fatty liver disease and hypercholesterolemia: roles of thyroid hormones, metabolites, and agonists. *Thyroid.* 2019;29(9):1173–1191.

46. Harrison SA, Bashir MR, Guy CD, Zhou R, Moylan CA, Frias JP, et al. Resmetirom (MGL-3196) for the treatment of non-alcoholic steatohepatitis: a multicentre, randomised, double-blind, placebo-controlled, phase 2 trial. *Lancet.* 2019;394(10213):2012–2024.

47. Ajmera VH, Cachay E, Ramers C, Vodkin I, Bassirian S, Singh S, et al. MRI assessment of treatment response in HIV-associated NAFLD: a randomized trial of a stearoyl-coenzyme-a-desaturase-1 inhibitor (ARRIVE trial). *Hepatology.* 2019;70(5):1531–1545.

48. Ratziu V, de Guevara L, Safadi R, Poordad F, Fuster F, Flores-Figueroa J, et al. Aramchol in patients with nonalcoholic steatohepatitis: a randomized, double-blind, placebo-controlled phase 2b trial. *Nat Med.* 2021;27(10):1825–1835.

49. Colca JR, McDonald WG, Adams WJ. MSDC-0602K, a metabolic modulator directed at the core pathology of non-alcoholic steatohepatitis. *Expert Opin Investig Drugs.* 2018;27(7):631–636.

50. Harrison SA, Alkhouri N, Davison BA, Sanyal A, Edwards C, Colca JR, et al. Insulin sensitizer MSDC-0602K in non-alcoholic steatohepatitis: a randomized, double-blind, placebo-controlled phase IIb study. *J Hepatol.* 2020;72(4):613–626.

51. Schuppan D, Surabattula R, Wang XY. Determinants of fibrosis progression and regression in NASH. *J Hepatol.* 2018;68(2):238–250.

52. Tacke F. Cenicriviroc for the treatment of non-alcoholic steatohepatitis and liver fibrosis. *Expert Opin Investig Drugs.* 2018;27(3):301–311.

53. Friedman SL, Ratziu V, Harrison SA, Abdelmalek MF, Aithal GP, Caballeria J, et al. A randomized, placebo-controlled trial of cenicriviroc for treatment of nonalcoholic steatohepatitis with fibrosis. *Hepatology.* 2018;67(5):1754–1767.

54. Loomba R, Lawitz E, Mantry PS, Jayakumar S, Caldwell SH, Arnold H, et al. The ASK1 inhibitor selonsertib in patients with nonalcoholic steatohepatitis: a randomized, phase 2 trial. *Hepatology.* 2018;67(2):549–559.

55. Harrison SA, Wong VW, Okanoue T, Bzowej N, Vuppalanchi R, Younes Z, et al. Selonsertib for patients with bridging fibrosis or compensated cirrhosis due to NASH: results from randomized phase III STELLAR trials. *J Hepatol.* 2020;73(1):26–39.

56. Harrison SA, Goodman Z, Jabbar A, Vemulapalli R, Younes ZH, Freilich B, et al. A randomized, placebo-controlled trial of emricasan in patients with NASH and F1-F3 fibrosis. *J Hepatol.* 2020;72(5):816–827.

57. Frenette C, Kayali Z, Mena E, Mantry PS, Lucas KJ, Neff G, et al. Emricasan to prevent new decompensation in patients with NASH-related decompensated cirrhosis. *J Hepatol.* 2021;74(2):274–282.

58. Cengiz M, Ozenirler S, Elbeg S. Role of serum toll-like receptors 2 and 4 in non-alcoholic steatohepatitis and liver fibrosis. *J Gastroenterol Hepatol.* 2015;30(7):1190–1196.

59. Shi H, Kokoeva MV, Inouye K, Tzameli I, Yin H, Flier JS. TLR4 links innate immunity and fatty acid-induced insulin resistance. *J Clin Invest.* 2006;116(11):3015–3025.

60. Yu J, Zhu C, Wang X, Kim K, Bartolome A, Dongiovanni P, Yates KP, Valenti L, Carrer M, Sadowski T, Qiang L, Tabas I, Lavine JE, Pajvani UB. Hepatocyte TLR4 triggers inter-hepatocyte Jagged1/Notch signaling to determine NASH-induced fibrosis. *Sci Transl Med.* 2021;13(599): eabe1692.

61. Diehl AM, Harrison S, Caldwell S, Rinella M, Paredes A, Moylan C, et al. JKB-121 in patients with nonalcoholic steatohepatitis: a phase 2 double blind randomized placebo control study. *J Hepatol.* 2018;68(1):S103.

62. Taylor-Weiner A, Pokkalla H, Han L, Jia C, Huss R, Chung C, et al. A machine learning approach enables quantitative measurement of liver histology and disease monitoring in NASH. *Hepatology.* 2021;74(1):133–147.

16 Practical Aspects of Pharmacologic Management

Naim Alkhouri and Stephen A. Harrison

CONTENTS

16.1 INTRODUCTION

Currently, there are no FDA-approved medications for the treatment of NASH-associated fibrosis or cirrhosis. A recent study that we conducted in Texas to evaluate the prevalence of NASH in asymptomatic middle-aged Americans revealed that 14% of participants had evidence of NASH on liver biopsy with even higher prevalence in Hispanics at 25% and those with type 2 diabetes at 36% (1). Moreover, 6% had evidence of significant fibrosis (stage 2 fibrosis or higher i.e., ≥F2) suggesting that NASH will likely become a significant public health crisis in the coming years.

In previous chapters, detailed discussions of the main mechanisms of action for NASH therapeutic agents and their development programs have been provided by experts in the field.

In this chapter, we articulate our vision on how the therapeutic field will shape up over the next few years in terms of identifying the appropriate patients for pharmacotherapy and best practices for selecting the appropriate drug and monitoring patient response.

16.2 SELECTING THE APPROPRIATE PATIENTS FOR PHARMACOLOGIC TREATMENT

Given the fact that patients with fibrotic NASH, defined as the presence of NAS ≥4 and ≥F2, are considered at high risk for progression to cirrhosis and developing major adverse liver event (MALO), most pharmacologic agents in development are targeting this specific subset of the NAFLD population (2). Several longitudinal studies have demonstrated that among the histologic parameters of NASH, the fibrosis stage has the highest prognostic values in predicting the risk of clinical outcomes and that patients with cirrhosis (F4) have the highest risk of developing MALO (3–5). Therefore, patients with NASH cirrhosis have the highest unmet need for pharmacologic agents that can potentially reverse cirrhosis (improvement from F4 to F3 or less).

Identifying patients with fibrotic NASH and NASH cirrhosis that may benefit from pharmacologic treatment based on liver biopsy is problematic for several reasons including but not limited to the invasive nature of the biopsy and intra- and interpathologist variability in interpreting NASH histology (6).

In the previous chapters, several noninvasive tests (NITs) that can identify high-risk NASH patients including serologic and radiologic tests were discussed. Some of these tests rely on readily available clinical characteristics and blood tests to calculate a score such as the FIB4 index to rule out the presence of advanced fibrosis (7). Other serologic tests measure more specific fibrosis biomarkers such as the enhanced liver fibrosis (ELF) panel that consists of three extracellular matrix (ECM) turnover proteins: hyaluronic acid (HA), tissue inhibitor of metalloproteinase 1 (TIMP-1) and N-terminal procollagen III-peptide (PIIINP) (8). Imaging tests can determine the severity of steatosis, inflammation and fibrosis such as MRI-proton density fat fraction (MRI-PDFF), corrected T1 by Liver MultiScan™, liver stiffness measurement by vibration controlled transient elastography (VCTE) and MR elastography (MRE) (9).

16.3 MONITORING RESPONSE TO TREATMENT

In order for pharmaceutical companies to obtain the Food and Drug Administration (FDA) conditional approval for a specific therapeutic agent for fibrotic (noncirrhotic) NASH (NASH with F2–F3), there is a need to demonstrate efficacy in a phase 3 trial on one of these two primary endpoints: (1) NASH resolution without worsening of fibrosis or (2) fibrosis improvement of at least 1 fibrosis stage without worsening of steatohepatitis. Both histologic endpoints require a repeat liver biopsy at the end of treatment (10, 11).

Importantly, major issues are related to the accuracy and reproducibility of pathologists' interpretation of liver biopsy samples (intra- and interreader reliability) that have been highlighted in the literature (12, 13). These issues with histologic interpretation are likely to cause major problems for identifying appropriate patients for pharmacologic treatment and their response to therapy, especially when relying on the local community pathologists. Recently, artificial intelligence (AI) and machine learning (ML) algorithms were developed to address pathologists' variability when interpreting NASH biopsies. These algorithms are trained on the derivation set of slides based on the annotation by the pathologist of NASH main histologic features (steatosis, ballooning, inflammation and fibrosis) and then applied to external slide sets for validation (14). Unfortunately, these AI algorithms will not resolve the issues related to the invasive nature of a biopsy and the heterogeneity of the disease that is not captured by the small size of the biopsy.

Therefore, the development and validation of noninvasive tests (NITs) that accurately predict the presence of NASH and significant fibrosis, as well as the treatment

DOI: 10.1201/9781003386698-19

histological response, is an essential need for the practical management of NASH once the drugs are FDA approved (15, 16). Reliable and accurate NITs that can predict treatment response early on may help improve the efficiency of delivering effective therapy and allow personalization of treatment based on response by reducing unnecessary drug exposure in patients unlikely to respond and switching to other therapeutic agents if changes in the NIT suggest an unlikely response.

16.3.1 ALT Response Criteria

Although ALT is not sensitive for detecting NASH or staging fibrosis (17, 18), reduction in ALT levels during treatment for NASH has been shown to predict improvement in histology. In fact, an ALT decrease of more than 17 U/L at week 24 was an independent predictor of histological improvement in the FLINT trial, which studied the effects of the drug obeticholic acid (OCA) on NASH (19). Similar significance in treatment response was noted in trials achieving the primary histological endpoint of NASH resolution with the drugs pioglitazone and vitamin E (PIVENS trial) and demaglutide (20, 21).

16.3.2 MRI-PDFF Response Criteria

A relative decline in liver fat content (LFC) as assessed by MRI-PDFF by ≥30% has been established and validated in several large multicenter randomized controlled trials (RCTs) (22–24) as a predictor of achieving ≥2 point improvements in NAS with at least 1-point improvement in lobular inflammation or ballooning as well as NASH resolution (25). In fact, a systematic review that included 346 subjects from seven trials showed that reaching the 30% threshold of relative decline in LFC from baseline is associated with an odds ratio (OR) of 5.45 (95% CI 1.53–19.46, $P = 0.009$) for achieving histologic NASH resolution and OR of 6.98 (95% CI 2.38–20.43, $P < 0.001$) for achieving histologic response defined as a 2-point improvement in NAS with at least a 1-point improvement in ballooning or lobular inflammation (26).

16.3.3 Corrected T1 (cT1) Response Criteria

By eliminating the confounding effects of iron, cT1 mapping by multiparametric MRI accurately calculates the T1 relaxation time and provides a good marker of liver inflammation and fibrosis (27). cT1 technique has been utilized for predicting clinical outcomes in patients with chronic liver disease including those with NAFLD (28). In a subset of patients from the phase 3 REGENERATE trial, treatment with OCA resulted in dose-dependent improvements in cT1 on multiparametric MRI (29).

In a retrospective longitudinal analysis pooled together from 4 independent interventional NASH clinical trials, a cT1 change of 80 ms corresponded to a 2-point change in NAS, and the median reduction in cT1 was significantly different for responders and nonresponders (30).

Instead of relying on just one biomarker, the combination of serologic and imaging biomarkers in one score is an attractive strategy to improve the accuracy of identifying fibrotic NASH and its response to therapy. For example, the FAST (FibroScan® + AST) score combines two FibroScan® biomarkers (CAP for steatosis and VCTE for fibrosis) with AST as a biomarker of inflammation in a score that ranges from 0 to 1 with values >0.67 providing a high positive predictive value for fibrotic NASH (31). More recently, the MAST (MRI + AST) score combined MRI-PDFF for steatosis, MRE for fibrosis, and AST to identify patients with fibrotic NASH with high accuracy in the derivation and validation cohorts (32).

We would like to emphasize that several of these biomarkers, such as VCTE, MRE, and cT1, have their own prognostic value in predicting MALO (28,33–35) and that therefore we foresee a future where the inclusion of patients in registration trials will be solely based on NITs with known prognostic values.

16.4 SELECTING THE APPROPRIATE THERAPEUTIC AGENT

Although significant progress in the field of drug development for NASH has taken place over the past decade, there are currently no FDA-approved drugs for NASH, and the quest to develop safe and effective treatments has been daunting. Several drugs with promising results in early phase trials have subsequently failed to replicate significant efficacy in late-stage trials. Luckily, several drugs are successfully advancing through the different phases of trials with few agents already in phase 3 trials such as resmetirom, obeticholic acid, semaglutide and lanifibranor (36,37). Selected data from noncirrhotic NASH trials that demonstrate the rates of NASH resolution and fibrosis regression are shown in Figures 16.1 and 16.2.

The mechanism of action for agents in development ranges from drugs that target obesity and insulin resistance, to inhibiting de novo lipogenesis in the liver, to modulating the response to lipotoxic lipid species, and finally to targeting liver inflammation and fibrosis (38).

It is very clear that the main driving pathogenic mechanism in NASH varies among different individuals based on their genetic background, epigenetics, microbiome, ethnicity, comorbidities and other factors that need further characterization. Despite the fact that some drugs have pleiotropic effects on the liver, their efficacy in clinical trials remains suboptimal, indicating that one drug is unlikely to be the answer for all patients with NASH and highlighting the need for more personalized medicine.

When evaluating a new therapeutic agent for fibrotic NASH, multiple aspects should be considered in addition to the efficacy in terms of liver endpoints and outcomes. It is of utmost importance to evaluate the effects of any novel NASH drug on cardiovascular risk factors such as type 2 diabetes, weight and hypercholesterolemia due to the fact that cardiovascular disease (CVD) is the major cause of mortality in patients with NASH. Therefore, a drug that increases LDL cholesterol or the TG/HDL ratio may not be ideal for NASH patients with extensive CV history that are on several medications to manage their dyslipidemia. Based on patient-reported outcomes, their quality of life can determine their compliance with a specific drug and ability to remain on the drug for a prolonged period of time. For example, gastrointestinal adverse events such as nausea and vomiting may limit the ability to use GLP1 agonists and FGF21 analogues in certain patients. Similarly, pruritus has emerged as the major adverse event of FXR agonists, limiting patients' tolerability at higher doses. As a way to help clinicians evaluate the safety and efficacy of NASH drugs and to facilitate comparisons among different classes of medications, we have developed the NASH Drug Score Card (36).

16.5 COMBINATION THERAPY

The development of NASH and liver fibrosis are mediated by biologically heterogenous mechanisms providing a rationale for combination therapy with agents that have complementary effects (39).

Drug Development Landscape: NASH Resolution

Proportion of Subjects with Resolution of NASH and No Worsening of Fibrosis

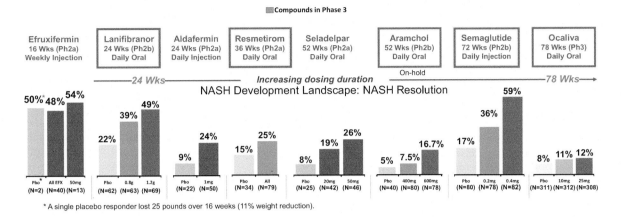

Figure 16.1 Data from selected trials demonstrating the different response rates in terms of NASH resolution with several therapeutic agents (not a head-to-head comparison; these trials have variable durations)

Drug Development Landscape: Fibrosis Improvement

Proportion of Subjects With ≥1 Stage Improvement in Fibrosis and No Worsening of NAS[1]

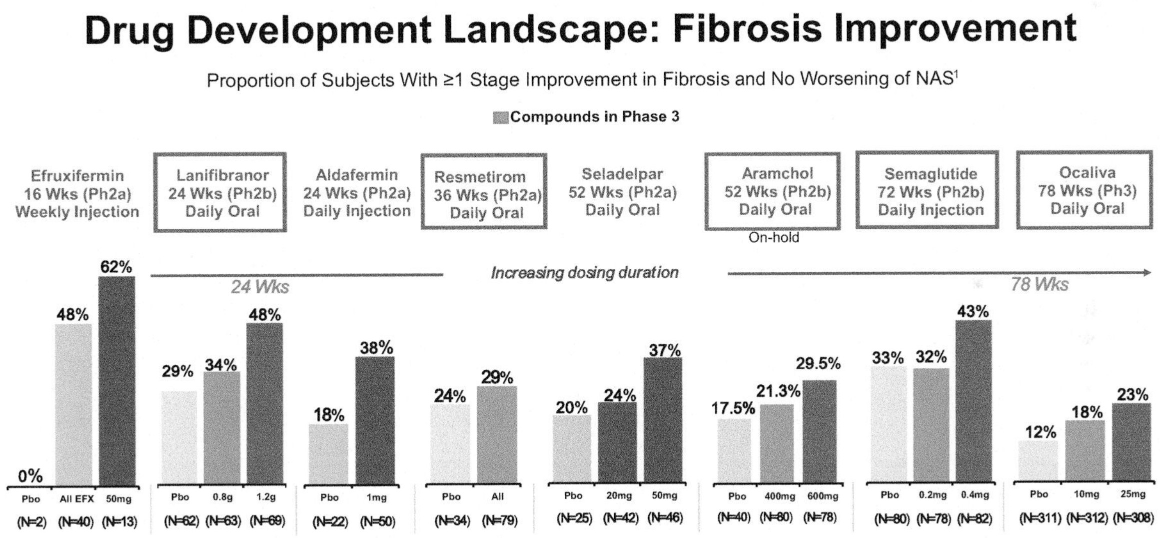

Figure 16.2 Data from selected trials demonstrating the different response rates in terms of fibrosis regression by one stage with several therapeutic agents (not a head-to-head comparison; these trials have variable durations)

In the ATLAS trial, 392 patients with bridging fibrosis or NASH cirrhosis were randomized to several arms that compared the efficacy of firsocostat (acetyl-Co A carboxylase [ACC] inhibitor that inhibits de novo lipogenesis) and cilofexor (FXR agonist) as monotherapies or in combination compared to placebo. Patients who received combination therapy were more likely to have improvement in fibrosis by 1 stage or more without worsening of NASH compared to those on placebo, although the difference did not reach statistical significance (21% vs. 11%, $p = 0.17$) (40).

A subsequent proof-of-concept trial assessed the effects of the GLP-1 agonist semaglutide alone or in combination with firsocostat and cilofexor in 108 patients with fibrotic NASH. The triple combination regimen was associated with greater reduction in liver fat on MRI-PDFF, in liver stiffness on transient elastography, and in ALT levels compared to semaglutide monotherapy, supporting the concept that combination therapy may provide additional benefits. Importantly, tolerability and the rates of adverse events leading to discontinuation of drugs were similar in all arms (41).

At this time, the ideal duration of NASH treatment is not clearly understood. Most advanced trials (phases 3 and 4) plan to follow patients longitudinally for 5–8 years to assess treatment efficacy on relevant clinical endpoints such as MALO and overall mortality. However, evidence suggests that most patients with NASH progress slowly (42) and that the development of cirrhosis and its complications can take several decades, making the duration of these trials potentially inadequate. Similarly to type 2 diabetes, it is possible that most patients with NASH will need lifelong therapy (43).

16.6 MANAGEMENT OF NASH CIRRHOSIS

There are several factors to take into consideration in the management of cirrhotic NASH.

First is the need for surveillance for hepatocellular carcinoma with ultrasonography/cross-sectional imaging + alpha fetoprotein every 6 months (44). Second, with the ability to identify the presence of clinically significant portal hypertension (CSPH) in these patients noninvasively with liver stiffness measurement by transient elastography and the presence of thrombocytopenia, the prevention of hepatic decompensation in patients with CSPH is potentially feasible with nonselective beta-blockers regardless of the presence of varices on endoscopic evaluation (45). Third, a relatively small retrospective study demonstrated that vitamin E at 800 units/day was associated with improvement in transplant-free survival and less hepatic decompensation (46). Fourth, a recent analysis of data from the simtuzumab and selonsertib NASH cirrhosis trials showed that cirrhosis regression on the end-of-treatment biopsy was associated with an 84% reduction in the risk for MALO vs. nonregression (HR, 0.16; 95% CI, 0.04, 0.65 [$p = 0.0104$]) (47). Therefore, designing trials based on the endpoint of fibrosis regression by 1 stage in those with NASH cirrhosis is a reasonable choice.

It is important to note that the FDA has provided a list of prespecified clinical events that constitute acceptable efficacy endpoints for NASH cirrhosis trials with a suggestion to perform a time-to-event analysis compared with placebo. These clinical events include (1) ascites needing treatment or complication of ascites such as spontaneous bacterial peritonitis; (2) variceal bleeding; (3) hepatic encephalopathy requiring hospitalization; (4) worsening of the MELD score ≥15; (5) liver transplantation; (6) death from any cause [33].

16.7 CONCLUSIONS

In the near future, we anticipate that the identification of high-risk patients with fibrotic NASH will be done completely with accurate NITs that will eliminate the need for costly liver biopsies. High-risk patients will be managed with pharmacologic agents and monitored for response using the same NITs. Determining the optimal first-line drug for a specific patient will rely on several factors including (1) the severity of NASH and stage of fibrosis with patients with F3–F4 requiring the most aggressive management strategies with drugs that have antifibrotic activities; (2) the safety and adverse events of the drug, keeping in mind its effects on CV risk factors (weight, insulin resistance, dyslipidemia) and the patient's quality of life (pruritus); (3) NAFLD phenotype, for example, patients with lean NAFLD may not be good candidates for medications such as GLP1 agonists where the mechanism of improvement is believed to be mediated through weight loss; (4) route of administration and patient comfort level with drugs that require SQ injection or IV infusions as opposed to oral agents (36).

The recent discovery of several genetic polymorphisms that play a role in NAFLD such as PNPLA3 and HSD17b13, coupled with the ability to alter gene expression with RNA interference and oligonucleotide-based therapeutics, has provided a rationale for several clinical studies that are currently evaluating the effectiveness of oligonucleotide therapies targeting the relevant NAFLD genetic variants (48). This opens the door for high-level personalized medicine based on the knowledge of specific genetic polymorphisms and using drugs that can alter their expression (49).

When patients are started on first-line therapy, NITs will be used to determine response after 6- to 12-month period with several possible scenarios that depend on efficacy and tolerability.

If the drug shows adequate response with good tolerability, then it will be continued, and the response should be assessed with the same NITs on a yearly basis. If the drug shows no efficacy after a period of 6–12 months, then this will define futility, necessitating the cessation of this drug and starting a new agent. Some patients may

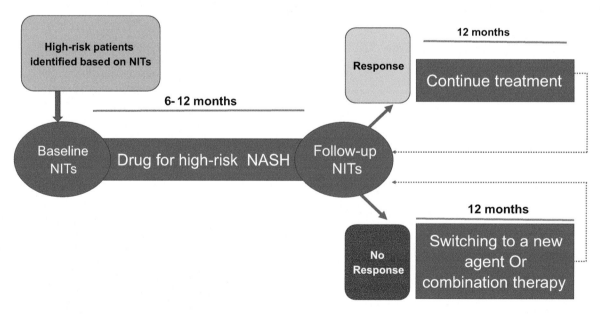

Figure 16.3 Future management of high-risk NASH patients

Patients will be identified using accurate noninvasive tests (NITs), then started on treatment and monitored for response/futility by NITs.

have partial response or may improve in certain aspects of NAFLD while worsening other aspects. In that case, a decision to switch therapy or add another agent will be up to the treating physician (Figure 16.3).

In conclusion, the management of NAFLD/NASH will witness a complete transformation in the next 5 years where high-risk patients will be identified by NITs and triaged to the best treatment modalities, including personalized and effective therapeutic agents.

REFERENCES

1. Harrison SA, Gawrieh S, Roberts K, Lisanti CJ, Schwope RB, Cebe KM, Paradis V, et al. Prospective evaluation of the prevalence of non-alcoholic fatty liver disease and steatohepatitis in a large middle-aged US cohort. *J Hepatol* 2021;75:284–291.
2. Kleiner DE, Brunt EM, Wilson LA, Behling C, Guy C, Contos M, Cummings O, et al. Association of histologic disease activity with progression of nonalcoholic fatty liver disease. *JAMA Netw Open* 2019;2:e1912565.
3. Angulo P, Kleiner DE, Dam-Larsen S, Adams LA, Bjornsson ES, Charatcharoenwitthaya P, Mills PR, et al. Liver fibrosis, but no other histologic features, is associated with long-term outcomes of patients with nonalcoholic fatty liver disease. *Gastroenterology* 2015;149:389–397 e310.
4. Ekstedt M, Hagstrom H, Nasr P, Fredrikson M, Stal P, Kechagias S, Hultcrantz R. Fibrosis stage is the strongest predictor for disease-specific mortality in NAFLD after up to 33 years of follow-up. *Hepatology* 2015;61:1547–1554.
5. Younossi ZM, Stepanova M, Rafiq N, Makhlouf H, Younoszai Z, Agrawal R, Goodman Z. Pathologic criteria for nonalcoholic steatohepatitis: interprotocol agreement and ability to predict liver-related mortality. *Hepatology* 2011;53:1874–1882.
6. Thomaides-Brears HB, Alkhouri N, Allende D, Harisinghani M, Noureddin M, Reau NS, French M, et al. Incidence of complications from percutaneous biopsy in chronic liver disease: a systematic review and meta-analysis. *Dig Dis Sci* 2021.
7. Chalasani N, Younossi Z, Lavine JE, Charlton M, Cusi K, Rinella M, Harrison SA, et al. The diagnosis and management of nonalcoholic fatty liver disease: practice guidance from the American association for the study of liver diseases. *Hepatology* 2018;67:328–357.
8. Sanyal AJ, Harrison SA, Ratziu V, Abdelmalek MF, Diehl AM, Caldwell S, Shiffman ML, et al. The natural history of advanced fibrosis due to nonalcoholic steatohepatitis: data from the simtuzumab trials. *Hepatology* 2019;70:1913–1927.
9. Ajmera V, Loomba R. Imaging biomarkers of NAFLD, NASH, and fibrosis. *Mol Metab* 2021:101167.
10. Sanyal AJ, Brunt EM, Kleiner DE, Kowdley KV, Chalasani N, Lavine JE, Ratziu V, et al. Endpoints and clinical trial design for nonalcoholic steatohepatitis. *Hepatology (Baltimore, Md.)* 2011;54:344–353.
11. Noncirrhotic Nonalcoholic Steatohepatitis with Liver Fibrosis: Developing Drugs for Treatment. Guidance for Industry. *U.S. Department of Health and Human Services Food and Drug Administration Center for Drug Evaluation and Research (CDER)*, 2018. www.fda.gov/media/119044/download.
12. Brunt EM, Clouston AD, Goodman Z, Guy C, Kleiner DE, Lackner C, Tiniakos DG, et al. Complexity of ballooned hepatocyte feature recognition: defining a training atlas for artificial intelligence-based imaging in NAFLD. *J Hepatol* 2022.
13. Davison BA, Harrison SA, Cotter G, Alkhouri N, Sanyal A, Edwards C, Colca JR, et al. Suboptimal reliability of liver biopsy evaluation has implications for randomized clinical trials. *J Hepatol* 2020;73:1322–1332.
14. Pokkalla H, Pethia K, Glass B, Kerner JK, Gindin Y, Han L, Huss R, et al. Machine learning models accurately interpret liver histology in patients with nonalcoholic steatohepatitis (NASH). *Hepatology*. 2019;70(suppl.1):121A–2A.
15. Filozof C, Chow SC, Dimick-Santos L, Chen YF, Williams RN, Goldstein BJ, Sanyal A. Clinical endpoints and adaptive clinical trials in precirrhotic nonalcoholic steatohepatitis: facilitating development approaches for an emerging epidemic. *Hepatol Commun* 2017;1:577–585.
16. Younossi ZM, Ratziu V, Loomba R, Rinella M, Anstee QM, Goodman Z, Bedossa P, et al. Obeticholic acid for the treatment of non-alcoholic steatohepatitis: interim analysis from a multicentre, randomised, placebo-controlled phase 3 trial. *Lancet* 2019;394:2184–2196.
17. Fracanzani AL, Valenti L, Bugianesi E, Andreoletti M, Colli A, Vanni E, Bertelli C, et al. Risk of severe liver disease in nonalcoholic fatty liver disease with normal aminotransferase levels: a role for insulin resistance and diabetes. *Hepatology* 2008;48:792–798.
18. Gawrieh S, Wilson LA, Cummings OW, Clark JM, Loomba R, Hameed B, Abdelmalek MF, et al. Histologic findings of advanced fibrosis and cirrhosis in patients with nonalcoholic fatty liver disease who have normal aminotransferase levels. *Am J Gastroenterol* 2019;114:1626–1635.
19. Loomba R, Sanyal AJ, Kowdley KV, Terrault N, Chalasani NP, Abdelmalek MF, McCullough AJ, et al. Factors associated with histologic response in adult patients with nonalcoholic steatohepatitis. *Gastroenterology* 2019;156:88–95 e85.
20. Sanyal AJ, Chalasani N, Kowdley KV, McCullough A, Diehl AM, Bass NM, Neuschwander-Tetri BA, et al. Pioglitazone, vitamin E, or placebo for nonalcoholic steatohepatitis. *N Engl J Med* 2010;362:1675–1685.
21. Newsome PN, Buchholtz K, Cusi K, Linder M, Okanoue T, Ratziu V, Sanyal AJ, et al. A placebo-controlled trial of subcutaneous semaglutide in nonalcoholic steatohepatitis. *N Engl J Med* 2021;384:1113–1124.
22. Loomba R. MRI-PDFF treatment response criteria in nonalcoholic steatohepatitis. *Hepatology* 2020.
23. Loomba R, Neuschwander-Tetri BA, Sanyal A, Chalasani N, Diehl AM, Terrault N, Kowdley K, et al. Multicenter validation of association between decline in MRI-PDFF and histologic response in NASH. *Hepatology* 2020;72:1219–1229.
24. Loomba R, Bedossa, P, Guy, C, Taub, R, Bashir, M, Harrison, SA. Magnetic resonance imaging-proton density fat fraction (MRI-PDFF) to predict treatment response on NASH liver biopsy: a secondary analysis of the resmetirom randomized placebo controlled Phase 2 clinical trial. *J Hepatol* 2020;73:S56.
25. Stine JG, Munaganuru N, Barnard A, Wang JL, Kaulback K, Argo CK, Singh S, et al. Change in MRI-PDFF and histologic response in patients with nonalcoholic steatohepatitis: a systematic review and meta-analysis. *Clin Gastroenterol Hepatol* 2020.
26. Stine JG, Munaganuru N, Barnard A, Wang JL, Kaulback K, Argo CK, Singh S, et al. Change in MRI-PDFF and histologic response in patients with

nonalcoholic steatohepatitis: a systematic review and meta-analysis. *Clin Gastroenterol Hepatol* 2021;19:2274–2283 e2275.

27. Dennis A, Mouchti S, Kelly M, Fallowfield JA, Hirschfield G, Pavlides M, Banerjee R. A composite biomarker using multiparametric magnetic resonance imaging and blood analytes accurately identifies patients with non-alcoholic steatohepatitis and significant fibrosis. *Sci Rep* 2020;10:15308.

28. Pavlides M, Banerjee R, Sellwood J, Kelly CJ, Robson MD, Booth JC, Collier J, et al. Multiparametric magnetic resonance imaging predicts clinical outcomes in patients with chronic liver disease. *J Hepatol* 2016;64:308–315.

29. Anstee Q, Digpal K. P21 Obeticholic acid improves hepatic fibroinflammation as assessed by multiparametric MRI: interim results of the REGENERATE trial. *Gut* 2020;69:A17.

30. Noureddin M, Alkhouri N, Denis A, Kelly M, Harrison SA. Decreases in liver cT1 accurately reflect histological improvement induced by therapies in NASH with enhanced sensitivity to fibrosis change: a multi-centre pooled cohort analysis. *J Hepatol* 2022; ILC.

31. Aggarwal P, Harrington A, Singh T, Cummings-John O, Kohli A, Noureddin M, Alkhouri N. Identifying patients who require pharmacotherapy for nonalcoholic steatohepatitis (NASH) using the fast score. *Hepatology* 2020;72:922A–923A.

32. Noureddin M, Truong E, Gornbein JA, Saouaf R, Guindi M, Todo T, Noureddin N, et al. MRI-based (MAST) score accurately identifies patients with NASH and significant fibrosis. *J Hepatol* 2021.

33. Are VS, Vuppalanchi R, Vilar-Gomez E, Chalasani N. Enhanced liver fibrosis score can be used to predict liver-related events in patients with nonalcoholic steatohepatitis and compensated cirrhosis. *Clin Gastroenterol Hepatol* 2021;19:1292–1293 e1293.

34. Boursier J, Vergniol J, Guillet A, Hiriart JB, Lannes A, Le Bail B, Michalak S, et al. Diagnostic accuracy and prognostic significance of blood fibrosis tests and liver stiffness measurement by FibroScan in non-alcoholic fatty liver disease. *J Hepatol* 2016;65:570–578.

35. Gidener T, Ahmed OT, Larson JJ, Mara KC, Therneau TM, Venkatesh SK, Ehman RL, et al. Liver stiffness by magnetic resonance elastography predicts future cirrhosis, decompensation, and death in NAFLD. *Clin Gastroenterol Hepatol* 2020.

36. Alkhouri N, Tincopa M, Loomba R, Harrison SA. What does the future hold for patients with nonalcoholic steatohepatitis: diagnostic strategies and treatment options in 2021 and beyond? *Hepatol Commun* 2021.

37. Vuppalanchi R, Noureddin M, Alkhouri N, Sanyal AJ. Therapeutic pipeline in nonalcoholic steatohepatitis. *Nat Rev Gastroenterol Hepatol* 2021;18:373–392.

38. Neuschwander-Tetri BA. Hepatic lipotoxicity and the pathogenesis of nonalcoholic steatohepatitis: the central role of nontriglyceride fatty acid metabolites. *Hepatology* 2010;52:774–788.

39. Dufour JF, Caussy C, Loomba R. Combination therapy for non-alcoholic steatohepatitis: rationale, opportunities and challenges. *Gut* 2020.

40. Loomba R, Noureddin M, Kowdley KV, Kohli A, Sheikh A, Neff G, Bhandari BR, et al. Combination therapies including cilofexor and firsocostat for bridging fibrosis and cirrhosis due to NASH. *Hepatology* 2020.

41. Alkhouri N, Herring R, Kabler H, Kayali Z, Hassanein T, Kohli A, Huss R, et al. Safety and efficacy of combination therapies including semaglutide, cilofexor, and firsocostat in patients with NASH. *Hepatology* 2020;72:Abstract LO2.

42. Singh S, Allen AM, Wang Z, Prokop LJ, Murad MH, Loomba R. Fibrosis progression in nonalcoholic fatty liver vs nonalcoholic steatohepatitis: a systematic review and meta-analysis of paired-biopsy studies. *Clin Gastroenterol Hepatol* 2015;13:643–654 e641–649; quiz e639–640.

43. Alkhouri N, Poordad F, Lawitz E. Management of non-alcoholic fatty liver disease: lessons learned from type 2 diabetes. *Hepatol Commun* 2018;2:778–785.

44. Marrero JA, Kulik LM, Sirlin CB, Zhu AX, Finn RS, Abecassis MM, Roberts LR, et al. Diagnosis, staging, and management of hepatocellular carcinoma: 2018 practice guidance by the american association for the study of liver diseases. *Hepatology* 2018;68:723–750.

45. Garcia-Tsao G, Abraldes JG. Nonselective beta-blockers in compensated cirrhosis: preventing variceal hemorrhage or preventing decompensation? *Gastroenterology* 2021;161:770–773.

46. Vilar-Gomez E, Vuppalanchi R, Gawrieh S, Ghabril M, Saxena R, Cummings OW, Chalasani N. Vitamin E improves transplant-free survival and hepatic decompensation among patients with nonalcoholic steatohepatitis and advanced fibrosis. *Hepatology* 2018.

47. Sanyal AJ, Anstee QM, Trauner M, Lawitz EJ, Abdelmalek MF, Ding D, Han L, et al. Cirrhosis regression is associated with improved clinical outcomes in patients with nonalcoholic steatohepatitis. *Hepatology* 2021.

48. Alkhouri N, Reddy GK, Lawitz E. Oligonucleotide-based therapeutics: an emerging strategy for the treatment of chronic liver diseases. *Hepatology* 2021;73:1581–1593.

49. Alkhouri N, Gawrieh S. A perspective on RNA interference-based therapeutics for metabolic liver diseases. *Expert Opin Investig Drugs* 2021;30:237–244.

SECTION IV

EXTRAHEPATIC MANIFESTATIONS

17 Endocrinology

Diabetes and other Endocrinopathies

Scott Isaacs and Julio Leey

CONTENTS

Key Points

- NAFLD is the hepatic complication of T2D.

- NAFLD and T2D have a bidirectional deleterious association stemming from common pathophysiology allowing one condition to exacerbate the other.

- T2D is the most important risk enhancer for severe steatosis, progression of fibrosis, cirrhosis and hepatocellular carcinoma among patients with NAFLD.

- Clinicians should be proactive in the early diagnosis and treatment of T2D patients with NAFLD, which provides an opportunity to prevent or slow disease progression and earlier detection of HCC.

- Management of NAFLD and T2D should be focused on simultaneously improving both conditions and their comorbidities.

- All persons with T2D and NAFLD should be considered at high risk for cardiometabolic outcomes and aggressively managed for hyperglycemia, hypertension and atherogenic dyslipidemia.

- Although there are currently no FDA-approved medications to treat NAFLD or NASH, optimal management includes improved dietary patterns and exercise to promote weight loss, consideration for antiobesity medications and/or bariatric surgery for enhanced weight loss, cardiovascular disease screening and prevention and optimal diabetes management using medications with proven efficacy in NAFLD (i.e., GLP-1 RA, pioglitazone and SGLT2i).

- Screening for NAFLD in T1D is only necessary in persons with other risk factors such as obesity, metabolic syndrome, elevated plasma aminotransferases or incidentally found hepatic steatosis on imaging.

- Patients with endocrinopathies do not need to be routinely evaluated for NAFLD, beyond the risk associated with the presence of T2D, metabolic syndrome or obesity.

17.1 INTRODUCTION

The increasing prevalence of NAFLD has paralleled global increases in obesity and T2D, making it the leading cause of chronic liver disease. NAFLD and T2D have a complex, bidirectional and mutually detrimental relationship mediated through insulin resistance, visceral adiposity and lipotoxicity. Although disease awareness is low among patients and providers, there is a growing understanding that NAFLD is a complication of T2D with broad cardiometabolic, hepatic and neoplastic repercussions. There are associations between NAFLD and other endocrinopathies including type 1 diabetes, growth hormone deficiency, hypogonadism, hypothyroidism and polycystic ovary syndrome; however, the associations appear to be largely due to increased insulin resistance and visceral adiposity, in some cases, a consequence of the underlying endocrinopathy.

17.2 PATHOPHYSIOLOGY OF T2D AND NAFLD

Although exact pathophysiological mechanisms for the development of NAFLD and progression are still being fully elucidated, it is understood that hepatic and systemic insulin resistance interfere with lipid metabolism, leading to visceral adiposity and hepatic steatosis. Insulin resistance is fueled by systemic inflammation, oxidative stress, mitochondrial dysfunction, and endothelial dysfunction, leading to impaired glucose tolerance, glucotoxicity and lipotoxicity. Hyperglycemia stimulates de novo lipogenesis, increasing free fatty acid exposure to the hepatocyte and atherogenic dyslipidemia. The common pathophysiology allows one condition to exacerbate the other, leading to more severe diabetes, diabetes comorbidities, as well as increased prevalence and severity of liver disease. T2D is the most important risk enhancer for severe steatosis, progression of fibrosis, cirrhosis and hepatocellular carcinoma (HCC). By promoting hepatic insulin resistance and increasing gluconeogenesis, NAFLD, especially NASH, magnifies T2D risk and, if disease is already present, exacerbates its severity, making it more difficult to manage. In the presence of T2D, the risk of cardiovascular disease increases in conjunction with increasing severity of NAFLD and fibrosis. NAFLD enhances cardiovascular risk in T2D by promoting atherogenic dyslipidemia, inducing hypertension and increasing proinflammatory, procoagulant and proatherogenic mediators.

DOI: 10.1201/9781003386698-21

17.3 EPIDEMIOLOGY

The global prevalence of NAFLD in T2D ranges from 20 to 80% depending on the diagnostic tool used for evaluation. Many studies have underestimated the prevalence of hepatic steatosis because they use liver ultrasound or liver enzymes for screening, which are considered less sensitive than controlled attenuation parameter (CAP) or magnetic resonance-based imaging techniques. Plasma liver aminotransferase levels are normal in 50–90% of patients with NAFLD and T2D. CAP is one of the most sensitive methods of detecting steatosis, with studies showing prevalence rates in persons with T2D approaching 80%. However, the accuracy of CAP is hindered by the presence of T2D as well as the extent of obesity and steatosis present.

NAFLD is associated with a 2.2 times greater risk for developing T2D. Persons with NASH are even more likely to develop T2D, and the risk is further increased among those with advanced fibrosis. The presence of NAFLD results in hyperglycemia that is more difficult to control. Reciprocally, the presence of T2D doubles the risk for NAFLD, and it occurs at younger ages. Although the prevalence of NAFLD is very high in persons with T2D, the main burden of disease is from NASH and advanced liver fibrosis. T2D is the most important predictor of liver-related outcomes. T2D increases the risk for NASH with more severe fibrosis and accelerates disease progression. The prevalence of NASH in persons with T2D is 30 to 40%, 2- to 3-fold the rate in the general population. Persons with diabetes tend to have more advanced NASH. Although the rate of disease progression is slow in most people, it may be faster in individuals with poorly controlled diabetes or with additional metabolic risk factors.

The prevalence of advanced liver fibrosis (stage >F2) is 12–21% in persons with T2D. Overall, T2D is associated with a 2-fold higher risk of cirrhosis. Additional factors that increase fibrosis, cirrhosis and mortality risk in persons with T2D include age (>50 years), insulin resistance and more features of the metabolic syndrome (dyslipidemia, hypertension, visceral adiposity). Approximately 15% of persons with NASH develop cirrhosis, which increases the risk of complications of end-stage liver disease and HCC.

Among patients with T2D and NAFLD, the risk for HCC is increased by 2-fold, and the risk of death is increased by 1.5-fold with even higher risk in persons with more advanced fibrosis. Having more features of the metabolic syndrome along with T2D increases the risk of HCC by 5-fold and having a BMI > 35 kg/m^2 increases the risk of HCC by 4-fold. It is interesting to note that visceral obesity in both nonobese and obese groups increases the risk for HCC, demonstrating the importance of assessing waist circumference as a metabolic risk factor for HCC. Early detection of NAFLD in this high-risk population can lead to enhanced screening for HCC, potentially diagnosing and treating smaller tumors at less advanced stages.

There is a lack of patient awareness of NAFLD with less than 5% of persons being aware of having liver disease compared to liver disease awareness in 38% of persons with viral hepatitis. Referrals to hepatology for high-risk patients remains low. Most persons with T2D or prediabetes, who have underlying NAFLD, are seen in primary care or endocrinology settings, but many remain undiagnosed and untreated. Clinicians tend to underestimate the risk for NAFLD with advanced fibrosis in high-risk groups such as those with T2D. In fact, most patient with NAFLD are diagnosed incidentally with ultrasound, CT or MRI when screening for another medical condition. Most patients with T2D and NAFLD have normal liver enzymes and symptoms, if present, are vague and mainly consist of fatigue and right upper abdominal pain. In an outpatient clinic setting, 70% of persons with T2D and an A1c of ≥7.5% had hepatic steatosis, and 9% had previously undiagnosed precirrhosis or cirrhosis (F3 or F4). In this setting, fewer than 30% of patients with T2D and moderate-to-advanced fibrosis (>F2) had elevated liver enzyme levels. NAFLD and T2D prevalence, with a disproportionate increase in advanced disease, is expected to rise in the future corresponding to predicted increases in obesity rates. Interventions that improve NAFLD and hepatic insulin resistance will likely decrease the risk of developing T2D, although not definitively established. It has been estimated that there are approximately 18 million people in the United States who have both T2D and NAFLD, of which 6.4 million have NASH. Health care costs to account for transplants, cardiovascular-related deaths and liver-related deaths in this group are estimated to be $50 to $100 billion over the next 20 years.

17.4 NAFLD AND MICROVASCULAR COMPLICATIONS

The association of NAFLD and diabetes complications is not well-known. NAFLD has also been associated with an increase in the rate of microvascular diabetic complications, especially chronic kidney disease. One meta-analysis found that NAFLD resulted in a 2-fold increased prevalence of CKD in persons with diabetes. Another meta-analysis found that NAFLD was associated with an 80% increase in CKD and that advanced fibrosis was associated with an even greater risk for CKD. The relationship between diabetic retinopathy and NAFLD remains controversial. Some studies have found an association between NAFLD and diabetic retinopathy. However, a recent meta-analysis did not find an association. In a meta-analysis of 9,000 patients, it was found that diabetic peripheral neuropathy is more frequent in persons who had both T2D and NAFLD.

17.5 NAFLD DIAGNOSIS AND FIBROSIS RISK STRATIFICATION IN T2D

Clinicians should be proactive in the early diagnosis and treatment of patients with NAFLD and T2D. Early detection provides an opportunity to prevent or slow disease progression as well as earlier detection of HCC. Plasma aminotransferases are elevated in a minority of persons with NAFLD and T2D. A liver ultrasound is not recommended for routine clinical diagnosis, although many cases are discovered incidentally on imaging studies (US, CT or MRI). The FIB-4 is the most validated noninvasive test (NIT) for diagnosis and risk stratification in patients with T2D among the many NITs assessed to this end. The NAFLD fibrosis score (NFS), on the other hand, may overestimate the prevalence of advanced liver fibrosis in T2D and should be avoided in patients with T2D. The FIB-4 has good ability to predict changes in hepatic fibrosis over time and allows risk stratification for future liver-related morbidity and mortality. FIB-4 can be used as a first-line test, followed by a liver stiffness measurement (e.g., Fibroscan®) or biomarker (e.g., ELF) to stratify persons with indeterminate scores. Shear wave elastography (SWE) is a newer technique for assessing liver stiffness that seems to have accuracy similar to elastography but less than magnetic resonance-based imaging;

however, it has been less well-validated. Magnetic resonance-based imaging is considered the most accurate over time but, due to the high cost and limited availability, has limited use.

17.6 MANAGEMENT OF PATIENTS WITH NAFLD AND T2D

There are limitations of the literature regarding the management of NAFLD. Although multiple lifestyle studies have been published, they have small sample sizes, and none has been longer than 12 months. Randomized controlled trials to assess the effectiveness of pioglitazone have a duration of 2–3 years and GLP-1 RAs of 1.5 years. Trials with SGLT2 inhibitors have had an open-label design, and there are no studies with paired biopsies to assess the effect on liver histology.

Because T2D is known to accelerate progression to cirrhosis in NASH, aggressive and individualized management is critical. Available treatments should be focused on simultaneously improving both diabetes and NASH and their comorbidities in addition to timely referral to specialists when indicated. All persons with T2D should be considered at high risk for cardiometabolic outcomes and routinely evaluated for hypertension, atherogenic dyslipidemia and cardiovascular disease. Clinicians should manage persons with NAFLD and T2D for cardiometabolic risk enhancers including obesity, dyslipidemia and hypertension and should screen for cardiovascular disease based on current standards of care. Although no FDA-approved medications are currently available to treat NAFLD or NASH, treatment should focus on weight loss, cardiovascular disease prevention and optimal diabetes management. In addition to hepatic and diabetes benefits, there is a cardiometabolic benefit from a minimum of 5% weight loss and even greater cardiometabolic and liver histologic benefit with at least 10% weight loss. There is a dose–response relationship between the magnitude of weight loss and the degree of steatosis improvement, as well as resolution of NASH, but not for fibrosis.

First and foremost, clinicians must emphasize lifestyle changes including a low-calorie meal plan, restriction of saturated fat, starch and sugar, and improved eating patterns (e.g., Mediterranean diet, minimally processed whole foods) and exercise. Even without weight loss, a better-quality dietary composition has been shown to improve liver histology. A structured weight loss program is preferred and, when possible, tailored to the individual's lifestyle and personal preferences. Although exercise has a limited effect on weight loss, exercise helps weight loss maintenance, improves cardiometabolic health and has benefits with respect to visceral fat and liver fat that are independent of weight loss. Liver histology benefits from increasing exercise are associated with adherence and intensity rather than a specific type of exercise.

Diabetes medications, such as glucagon-like peptide 1 receptor agonists, pioglitazone and sodium glucose cotransporter 2 inhibitors are all considered preferred agents in NAFLD because they reduce liver fat and have been shown to reduce cardiovascular risk, the most common cause of mortality. GLP-1 RA and pioglitazone are preferred agents for those with T2D and biopsy-proven NASH because of demonstrated benefits for liver histology.

Pioglitazone improves insulin resistance, reduces adipose tissue dysfunction, improves lipid storage/redistribution and glucose utilization and provides histologic improvement in patients with NASH with and without diabetes. Pioglitazone has also been shown to be effective in preventing diabetes and cardiovascular disease. Side effects of pioglitazone include weight gain, increased fracture risk, edema, heart failure and bladder cancer.

GLP-1 RAs are effective pharmacotherapy for obesity and T2D with strong clinical benefits including weight loss, glycemic control, reduction in CKD and cardiometabolic improvements. GLP-1 RAs normalize plasma aminotransferases, reduce liver fat, and improve liver histology, such as resolution of NASH but not fibrosis stage. The side effects of GLP-1 RAs include gastrointestinal symptoms, mainly nausea, and risk for pancreatitis and medullary thyroid carcinoma.

SGLT2 inhibitors reduce liver fat by decreasing the lipid burden on the liver from glycosuria, creating energy deficit and weight loss; however, there is no evidence of benefit for steatohepatitis. This class of drugs also offers cardiovascular and heart failure benefits as well as renal protective benefits The most common side effects of SGLT2 inhibitors are genital yeast infections, increased urination, as well as a risk for euglycemic diabetic ketoacidosis.

Metformin, acarbose, DPP-IV inhibitors and insulin are not recommended to treat steatohepatitis due to a lack of evidence of efficacy on hepatocyte necrosis or inflammation but should be continued as needed for appropriate diabetes management. There is not enough evidence to recommend the use of vitamin E in patients with T2D. Management of patients with NAFLD and T2D should also promote cardiometabolic health and reduce the increased cardiovascular risk with aggressive management of blood pressure and lipids.

As an adjunct to lifestyle, weight loss treatment includes consideration of weight loss medications, particularly glucagon-like peptide 1 receptor agonists and bariatric surgery. Weight loss assisted by any of the available FDA-approved medications for the treatment of obesity can improve NAFLD and NASH by reducing adipose tissue mass. Medications for the chronic treatment of obesity include phentermine/topiramate ER and naltrexone/bupropion ER, orlistat, liraglutide and semaglutide and are approved for individuals with T2D and BMI 27–29.9 kg/m^2. When combined with lifestyle modification, weight loss with a medication is 7–18% of baseline weight at 1 year.

Table 17.1: Diabetes Medications and Effect on NAFLD

Medication	Hepatic Steatosis	Steatohepatitis	Fibrosis
Pioglitazone	Decreased	Decreased	Decreased
GLP-1 RA	Decreased	Decreased	Unknown
SGLT2 inhibitors	Decreased	Unknown	Unknown
DPP-IV inhibitors	Unchanged	Unknown	Unknown
Metformin	Unchanged	Neutral	Unknown
Insulin	Decreased	Neutral	Unknown

Greater initial weight loss predicts better long-term success. Of the medications currently approved for chronic obesity, semaglutide, has the best efficacy in achieving 10, 15 and even ≥20% weight loss in some patients.

Bariatric surgery is the most effective treatment to achieve sustained weight loss and has been demonstrated to produce resolution or improvement of diabetes, steatosis, fibrosis and reduction in risk for HCC. In addition, bariatric surgery improves other comorbidities in NAFLD such as hypertension, sleep apnea, atherogenic dyslipidemia, and it reduces the risk of cardiovascular disease. In a recent study, bariatric surgery, compared with nonsurgical management, was associated with an 88% lower risk of major adverse liver outcomes as well as a 70% reduction in adverse cardiovascular events.

17.7 NAFLD AND TYPE 1 DIABETES

Because approximately one-third of persons with type 1 diabetes (T1D) have obesity, more attention has been directed to the risk for NAFLD in this population. A large meta-analysis published in 2020 found that the prevalence of NAFLD in adults with T1D was 22%. However, rates differed significantly due to different imaging modalities and heterogeneous populations. In a study using magnetic resonance-based imaging, the prevalence of NAFLD was approximately 9% in T1D, which was much lower than the 68% rate seen in persons with T2D. Because NAFLD is most closely linked to insulin resistance and obesity, it is understandable that some studies have not found persons with T1D to have a higher risk of NAFLD. Through increased hepatic insulin resistance, NAFLD is associated with the need for higher insulin doses for comparable glycemic control in T1D. Persons with NAFLD and T1D have a greater risk of atherogenic dyslipidemia, cardiovascular disease, arrhythmias and other cardiac complications. It is difficult to fully assess the influence of T1D and the risk for NAFLD due to significant discrepancies among studies; however, obesity and insulin resistance appear to be the most important driving factors. Screening for NAFLD in T1D is only necessary in persons with risk factors such as obesity, metabolic syndrome, elevated plasma aminotransferases or incidentally found hepatic steatosis on imaging.

17.8 NAFLD AND GROWTH HORMONE

Patients with hypopituitarism and/or hypothalamic disease frequently develop central obesity, diabetes and NAFLD. Although the pathophysiology of this phenomenon is not well-understood, it appears to be related to growth hormone (GH) deficiency. In the liver, GH is known to cause gluconeogenesis and glycogenolysis antagonizing insulin signaling. GH promotes an anabolic effect in most tissues except in adipose tissue where the catabolic effect causes lipolysis. GH excess as seen in acromegaly causes glucose intolerance.

Clinical studies have shown that both serum IGF-1 and GH levels are lower in patients with NAFLD and adult patients with GH deficiency have a higher prevalence of NAFLD compared to controls adjusted by age, gender and BMI. Interestingly, lower levels of GH correlate to worse histological severity of NAFLD. Patients with congenital defects of GH deficiency, either isolated or as part of multiple hormone deficiencies, also have more central obesity and NAFLD.

In animal models, GH and IGF-1 deficiency replicate NAFL/NASH features with abnormal mitochondrial morphology and the restoration of GH and/or IGF-1 levels prevented the onset of NAFL/NASH features in rodents. Clinically, the treatment of GH deficiency in adults led to biochemical improvement of liver enzymes and better histology, and in an observational study of adults with childhood/onset GH deficiency, a high percentage of them developed NALFD after GH therapy cessation.

A few small clinical studies have assessed the effect of GH on NAFLD. In a small double-blind, placebo-controlled, randomized study of 40 post-menopausal women with abdominal obesity, treatment with GH for 12 months resulted in decreased hepatic fat, visceral fat and improved insulin sensitivity. Similar results were found in premenopausal females and in males. At this point, larger and longer studies are needed to assess the efficacy and long-term effects of GH therapy in NAFLD.

17.9 NAFLD AND HYPOGONADISM

Characterized by reduced testosterone secretion and/or spermatogenesis, hypogonadism can be caused by a disease of the testes (primary hypogonadism) or hypothalamic-pituitary axis (secondary hypogonadism). Several studies show the association between low testosterone and increased visceral fat, insulin resistance and dyslipidemia, though this association has the confounder effect of obesity. More recently, in an observational study using liver biopsy and MRI, low testosterone level was more common in NAFLD patients; however, this association disappeared when adjusted for insulin resistance and obesity. The evidence in hypogonadal females is even more limited; one retrospective study found that estrogen was a protective factor against worsening fibrosis, but this effect dissipated after age 50.

17.10 NAFLD AND THYROID

Thyroid hormones are involved in many metabolic processes including fat distribution, lipid utilization, energy expenditure and glucose homeostasis. Abnormal levels of both thyroid hormones and thyroid-stimulating hormone (TSH) can affect hepatic steatosis and levels of free fatty acids. T3 and T4 are activators of several enzymes that lead to the hepatic fatty acid synthesis. TSH also acts on hepatic TSH receptors that stimulate PPARα pathway and SREBP-1c and increases hepatic gluconeogenesis.

Although the prevalence of hypothyroidism ranges is higher (15 and 36%) among patients with NAFLD, a causal relationship is not clear as the severity of hypothyroidism does not correlate consistently with the severity of NAFLD. This lack of association could be explained by obesity, which is common in both conditions. In a cross-sectional study using ^{1}H-MRS, a modest relationship was observed between steatosis and low free T4 but not with the insulin resistance or histological features of NASH. Treatment with low-dose levothyroxine for 16 weeks in euthyroid patients with NAFLD resulted in significant improvement of liver fat; however, this study only had a "before-and-after" design, lacking a control group.

17.11 NAFLD AND PCOS

PCOS is associated with cardiovascular risk factors such as obesity, NAFLD and insulin resistance. Between 35 and 70% of women with PCOS have NAFLD. A meta-analysis of 17 observational studies showed that PCOS per se is not a risk factor for the development of NAFLD and that hyperandrogenism could be a contributing factor to the high prevalence of NAFLD in females with PCOS. One factor to consider is that the diagnosis of PCOS relies in different criteria that lead to different phenotypes.

17.12 CONCLUSIONS

NAFLD is the hepatic complication of T2D with a 70–80% prevalence. Insulin resistance and lipotoxicity mediate a common pathophysiological pathway. NAFLD and T2D have a bidirectional deleterious relationship where one condition exacerbates the other. Patients with NAFLD and T2D are at high risk for cardiovascular events and should be aggressively managed for hyperglycemia, hypertension and atherogenic dyslipidemia. Despite various associations between NAFLD and several endocrinopathies, more studies are needed to elucidate the role of hormonal therapy for NAFLD. Patients with T1D or other endocrinopathies do not need to be routinely evaluated for NAFLD, unless there are risk factors such as T2D, obesity, metabolic syndrome, elevated plasma aminotransferases or incidentally found hepatic steatosis on imaging. Currently, it is recommended to use GH, testosterone and thyroid hormone replacement following current medical guidelines for their respective hormone-deficient states and to avoid use for the specific purpose of NAFLD treatment.

REFERENCES

1. Adams LA, Feldstein A, Lindor KD, Angulo P. Nonalcoholic fatty liver disease among patients with hypothalamic and pituitary dysfunction. *Hepatology*. 2004;39(4):909–914.
2. Bredella MA, Gerweck AV, Lin E, et al. Effects of GH on body composition and cardiovascular risk markers in young men with abdominal obesity. *J Clin Endocrinol Metab*. 2013;98(9):3864–3872. doi:10.1210/jc.2013-2063
3. Bredella MA, Lin E, Brick DJ, et al. Effects of GH in women with abdominal adiposity: a 6-month randomized, double-blind, placebo-controlled trial. *Eur J Endocrinol*. 2012;166(4):601–611. doi:10.1530/EJE-11-1068
4. Bril F, Cusi K. Management of nonalcoholic fatty liver disease in patients with type 2 diabetes: a call to action. *Diabetes Care*. 2017;40(3):419–430.
5. Bril F, Cusi K. Nonalcoholic fatty liver disease: the new complication of type 2 diabetes mellitus. *Endocrinol Metab Clin N Am*. 2016;45(4):765–781.
6. Bril F, Kadiyala S, Portillo Sanchez P, Sunny NE, Biernacki D, Maximos M, Kalavalapalli S, Lomonaco R, Suman A, Cusi K. Plasma thyroid hormone concentration is associated with hepatic triglyceride content in patients with type 2 diabetes. *J Investig Med*. 2016;64(1):63–68. doi:10.1136/jim-2015-000019. Epub 2015 Dec 16. PMID: 26755815.
7. Bruinstroop E, Dalan R, Cao Y, et al. Low-dose levothyroxine reduces intrahepatic lipid content in patients with type 2 diabetes mellitus and NAFLD. *J Clin Endocrinol Metab*. 2018;103(7):2698–2706. doi:10.1210/jc.2018-00475
8. Budd J, Cusi K. Role of agents for the treatment of diabetes in the management of nonalcoholic fatty liver disease. *Curr Diabetes Rep*. 2020;20(11):59.
9. Chavez C, Cusi K, Kadiyala S. The emerging role of glucagon-like peptide-1 receptor agonists for the management of NAFLD. *J Clin Endocrinol Metab*. 2022;107(1):29–38.
10. Cusi K, Isaacs S, et al. American association of clinical endocrinology (AACE) clinical practice guideline for the diagnosis and management of non-alcoholic fatty liver disease in primary care and endocrinology settings. *Endocr Pract*. 2022 (in press).
11. Cusi K, Sayyal A, et al. Non-alcoholic fatty liver disease (NAFLD) prevalence and its metabolic associations in patients with type 1 diabetes and type 2 diabetes. *Diabetes Obes Metab*. 2017;19(11):1630–1634.
12. Cusi K. A diabetologist's perspective of non-alcoholic steatohepatitis (NASH): knowledge gaps and future directions. *Liver Int*. 2020;40(Suppl 1):82–88.
13. Cusi K. Time to include nonalcoholic steatohepatitis in the management of patients with type 2 diabetes. *Diabetes Care*. 2020;43(2):275–279.
14. Dayton KA, Bril F, Barb D, Lai J, Kalavalapalli S, Cusi K. Severity of non-alcoholic steatohepatitis is not linked to testosterone concentration in patients with type 2 diabetes. *PLoS ONE*. 2021;16(6):e0251449. Published 2021 Jun 2. doi:10.1371/journal.pone.0251449
15. Donaghy A, Ross R, Wicks C, et al. Growth hormone therapy in patients with cirrhosis: a pilot study of efficacy and safety. *Gastroenterology*. 1997;113(5):1617–1622. doi:10.1053/gast.1997.v113.pm9352864
16. Franco C, Brandberg J, Lönn L, Andersson B, Bengtsson BA, Johannsson G. Growth hormone treatment reduces abdominal visceral fat in postmenopausal women with abdominal obesity: a 12-month placebo-controlled trial. *J Clin Endocrinol Metab*. 2005;90(3):1466–1474. doi:10.1210/jc.2004-1657
17. Fukuda I, Hizuka N, Yasumoto K, Morita J, Kurimoto M, Takano K. Metabolic co-morbidities revealed in patients with childhood-onset adult GH deficiency after cessation of GH replacement therapy for short stature. *Endocr J*. 2008;55(6):977–984.
18. Gastaldelli A, Cusi K. From NASH to diabetes and from diabetes to NASH: mechanisms and treatment options. *JHEP Rep*. 2019;1(4):312–328.
19. Greco C, et al. Association of nonalcoholic fatty liver disease (NAFLD) with peripheral diabetic polyneuropathy: a systematic review and meta-analysis. *J Clin Med*. 2021;10(19):4466.
20. He W, An X, Li L, et al. Relationship between hypothyroidism and non-alcoholic fatty liver disease: a systematic review and meta-analysis. *Front Endocrinol (Lausanne)*. 2017;8:335. Published 2017 Nov 29. doi:10.3389/fendo.2017.00335
21. Johannsson G, Mårin P, Lönn L, et al. Growth hormone treatment of abdominally obese men reduces abdominal fat mass, improves glucose and lipoprotein metabolism, and reduces diastolic blood pressure. *J Clin Endocrinol Metab*. 1997;82(3):727–734. doi:10.1210/jcem.82.3.3809
22. Kanwal F, Shubrock J, et al. Clinical care pathway for the risk stratification and management of patients with nonalcoholic fatty liver disease. *Gastroenterology*. 2021;161(5):1657–1669.
23. Khan R, Bril F. et al. Modulation of insulin resistance in nonalcoholic fatty liver disease. *Hepatology*. 2019;70(2):711–724.
24. Kopchick JJ, Berryman DE, Puri V, Lee KY, Jorgensen JOL. The effects of growth hormone on adipose tissue: old observations, new mechanisms. *Nat Rev Endocrinol*. 2020;16(3):135–146. doi:10.1038/s41574-019-0280-9

25. Li Y, Wang L, Zhou L, et al. Thyroid stimulating hormone increases hepatic gluconeogenesis via CRTC2. *Mol Cell Endocrinol*. 2017;446:70–80. doi:10.1016/j.mce.2017.02.015

26. Lomonaco R, Levia E, et al. Advanced liver fibrosis is common in patients with type 2 diabetes followed in the outpatient setting: the need for systematic screening. *Diabetes Care*. 2021;44(2):399–406.

27. Mantovani A, Nascimbeni F, Lonardo A, et al. Association between primary hypothyroidism and nonalcoholic fatty liver disease: a systematic review and meta-analysis. *Thyroid*. 2018;28(10):1270–1284. doi:10.1089/thy.2018.0257

28. Mavromati M, Jornayvaz FR. Hypothyroidism-associated dyslipidemia: potential molecular mechanisms leading to NAFLD. *Int J Mol Sci*. 2021;22(23):12797. Published 2021 Nov 26. doi:10.3390/ijms222312797

29. Mody A, White D, Kanwal F, Garcia JM. Relevance of low testosterone to non-alcoholic fatty liver disease. *Cardiovasc Endocrinol*. 2015;4(3):83–89.

30. Møller N, Schmitz O, Jøorgensen JO, et al. Basal- and insulin-stimulated substrate metabolism in patients with active acromegaly before and after adenomectomy. *J Clin Endocrinol Metab*. 1992;74(5):1012–1019. doi:10.1210/jcem.74.5.1569148

31. Nishizawa H, Iguchi G, Murawaki A, et al. Nonalcoholic fatty liver disease in adult hypopituitary patients with GH deficiency and the impact of GH replacement therapy. *Eur J Endocrinol*. 2012;167(1):67–74.

32. Nishizawa H, Takahashi M, Fukuoka H, Iguchi G, Kitazawa R, Takahashi Y. GH-independent IGF-I action is essential to prevent the development of nonalcoholic steatohepatitis in a GH-deficient rat model. *Biochem Biophys Res Commun*. 2012;423(2):295–300.

33. Sharma R, Kopchick JJ, Puri V, Sharma VM. Effect of growth hormone on insulin signaling. *Mol Cell Endocrinol*. 2020;518:111038. doi:10.1016/j.mce.2020.111038

34. Singeap AM, Stanciu C, Huiban L, et al. Association between nonalcoholic fatty liver disease and endocrinopathies: clinical implications. *Can J Gastroenterol Hepatol*. 2021;2021:6678142. Published 2021 Jan 11. doi:10.1155/2021/6678142

35. Sumida Y, Yonei Y, Tanaka S, et al. Lower levels of insulin-like growth factor-1 standard deviation score are associated with histological severity of non-alcoholic fatty liver disease. *Hepatol Res*. 2015;45(7):771–781.

36. Wu J, Yao XY, Shi RX, Liu SF, Wang XY. A potential link between polycystic ovary syndrome and non-alcoholic fatty liver disease: an update meta-analysis. *Reprod Health*. 2018;15(1):77. Published 2018 May 10. doi:10.1186/s12978-018-0519-2

37. Wu ZY, Li YL, Chang B. Pituitary stalk interruption syndrome and liver changes: from clinical features to mechanisms. *World J Gastroenterol*. 2020;26(44):6909–6922. doi:10.3748/wjg.v26.i44.6909

38. Xu L, Xu C, Yu C, et al. Association between serum growth hormone levels and nonalcoholic fatty liver disease: a cross-sectional study. *PLoS ONE*. 2012;7(8):e44136.

39. Yang JD, Abdelmalek MF, Pang H, et al. Gender and menopause impact severity of fibrosis among patients with nonalcoholic steatohepatitis. *Hepatology*. 2014;59(4):1406–1414. doi:10.1002/hep.26761

40. Younossi A, Henry L. Fatty liver through the ages: nonalcoholic steatohepatitis. *Endocr Pract*. 2022;28(2):204–213.

41. Younossi Z, Corey K, et al. Clinical assessment for high-risk patients with non-alcoholic fatty liver disease in primary care and diabetology practices. *Aliment Pharmacol Ther*. 2020;52(3):513–526.

42. Younossi Z, Golabi P, et al. The global epidemiology of NAFLD and NASH in patients with type 2 diabetes: a systematic review and meta-analysis. *J Hepatol*. 2019;71(4):793–801.

18 Obstructive Sleep Apnea and Nonalcoholic Fatty Liver Disease

Dania Brigham and Shikha S. Sundaram

CONTENTS

INTRODUCTION

Obstructive sleep apnea (OSA) occurs when there is partial or complete obstruction of the upper airways while an individual is sleeping. It has been broadly associated with insulin resistance, obesity and the metabolic syndrome and is a risk factor for both Type 2 diabetes mellitus and cardiovascular disease. Emerging evidence has increasingly linked OSA to the development of NAFLD as well. OSA affects 4–5% of the general population and 35–45% of the obese population.[1-3] Men are more commonly affected (4–24%) by OSA than women (2–9%). The prevalence of OSA in pediatrics varies widely based on the criteria used and has been reported in up to 13% of children.[4] Most studies, however, report a prevalence of 1–4%. Symptomatically, patients may experience snoring, increased respiratory efforts, restless sleep, excessive daytime sleepiness, morning headaches, difficulty concentrating, anxiety, depression and poor quality of life. Sleep fragmentation may be experienced as recurrent arousals from sleep and contribute to excessive daytime sleepiness. Physiologically, repetitive episodes of shallow or paused breathing translate to reduced blood oxygen saturations and hypercapnia.[5] Hypoxia is sensed by the carotid body receptors, with resultant sympathetic activation, arousal from sleep and reoxygenation.[6]

Sleep-disordered breathing may be accompanied by chronic intermittent hypoxia (CIH), with important physiologic consequences. CIH in animal models has been shown to cause a cyclic reduction in oxygen tension in liver, fat and muscle tissue and the circulation.[7] This results in further disruption at the molecular and cellular level, including the generation of increased reactive oxygen species and oxidative stress. Chronic intermittent hypoxia may also increase sympathetic nervous system output due to increased catecholamine release.[8-10] Furthermore, CIH may cause changes in respiratory patterns, which then impact the frequency of presympathetic neuron discharge and sympathetic outflow.[11]

The gold standard for OSA diagnosis is multichannel polysomnography to assess multiple physiologic parameters simultaneously. These include an electroencephalogram, electrooculogram, electromyogram, and nasal and oral airflow measurements.[12] Apnea is defined as the cessation of airflow for ≥10 seconds despite inspiratory effort. Hypopnea is defined as isolated significant (≥50%) reduction in airflow or moderate (<50%) airflow reduction, coupled with either desaturations or awakening noted on electroencephalography.[12] Using data from the polysomnography, an apnea hypopnea index (AHI) can be calculated by dividing the number of events by hours of sleep. OSA is classified as severe with an AHI >30, moderate with an AHI of 15–30 or mild if the AHI is 5–15.

PATHOPHYSIOLOGY

Hypoxic stress associated with OSA and CIH may elicit a broad range of pathologic events that include sympathetic activation, systemic inflammation, impaired glucose and lipid metabolism and endothelial dysfunction. OSA and CIH contribute several interrelated mechanistic links to the development and progression of NAFLD. OSA/CIH may exacerbate dyslipidemia by driving de novo lipogenesis. Liver fat may be generated by dietary intake of lipids and carbohydrates, de novo lipogenesis and peripheral lipolysis with flux of free fatty acids. These can then be stored as triglycerides, the FFA can be oxidized, or the triglycerides can be exported to very-low-density lipoproteins.[13] The transcription factor sterol receptor element binding protein (SREBP) is crucial in hepatic de novo lipogenesis, mediating the expression of genes such as fatty acid synthase and acyl-coA carboxylase to promote de novo free fatty acid and triglyceride synthesis.[14] It also increases the activity of stearoylcoenzyme-A desaturase (SCD)-1, which converts polyunsaturated fatty acids into monounsaturated fatty acids, which are further converted to cholesterol esters and triglycerides and then secreted. Moreover, CIH increases hepatic lipid content by activating influx from adipose tissue through both lipid biosynthetic pathways via SREBP-1c and the SREBP-1 regulated enzyme stearoyl coA desaturase.[15,16] Animal studies have shown that CIH enhances the expression of these lipogenic genes with resultant increased hepatic triglyceride content. Experimentally, interrupting SREBP and SCD-1 signaling prevents hyperlipidemia in the presence of CIH.[16-18] OSA/CIH may further exacerbate dyslipidemia by enhancing peripheral lipolysis. CIH also increases sympathetic activity, which induces insulin resistance, thereby promoting adipose tissue lipolysis and FFA flux into the liver. Normally, free fatty acids (FFA) are metabolized by oxygen-dependent beta-oxidation. However, excess flux of FFA, compounded by an inability to metabolize all of the FFA, results in more FFA availability for triglyceride and cholesterol synthesis and worsening hepatic steatosis.[13] CIH also exacerbates dyslipidemia by reducing lipoprotein clearance, selectively inactivating adipose tissue lipoprotein lipase and reducing VLDL clearance from the circulation.[11].

Insulin resistance plays a crucial role in NAFLD pathogenesis. In mice with diet and genetic-induced obesity, the presence of CIH- induced insulin resistance and severe glucose intolerance, mediated by sympathetic nervous system CIH, stimulates the carotid bodes, which then activate central sympathetic outflow and catecholamine efflux by the adrenal medulla, with resulting suppression of insulin secretion and stimulation of hepatic gluconeogenesis and glucose output.[19-21] The presence of OSA/CIH may further

DOI: 10.1201/9781003386698-22

exacerbate insulin resistance in affected individuals independent of body mass index.[22] Following two nights of auditory and mechanical sleep fragmentation, healthy volunteers developed reduced insulin sensitivity, elevated morning cortisol levels and increased sympathetic tone.[23] Increased cortisol levels and sympathetic tone promote insulin resistance by reducing pancreatic insulin secretion, inhibiting insulin-mediated glucose uptake and increasing hepatic gluconeogenesis.[13] Animal models of OSA also suggest roles for pancreatic beta cell apoptosis and ROS generation in the development of insulin resistance.[24]

Obese patients with OSA have increased visceral fat and visceral-to-total-fat ratios as compared to obese patients without OSA.[25] OSA/CIH contribute to adipose tissue dysfunction, which may exacerbate NAFLD in affected individuals. Adipose tissue stores triglycerides and energy but also functions as an endocrine organ, secreting cytokines and inflammatory factors that regulate glucose and lipid metabolism. Animal models have demonstrated that local adipose tissue hypoxia is partially responsible for the dysregulated production of adipokines.[26] Adiponectin secretion, protective in its regulation of FA oxidation and insulin sensitivity, is decreased in patients with OSA and correlates inversely with OSA severity based on the AHI.[27] Upregulation of leptin mRNA levels also occurs in adipocytes exposed to hypoxia.[25] Furthermore, serum leptin levels correlate strongly with OSA severity as measured by AHI and prolonged hypoxemia.[25] Intermittent hypoxia also induces adipose tissue inflammation, with changes in inflammatory gene expression, inflammatory cytokine release and an increased presence of pro-inflammatory macrophages.[13] CIH also induces nuclear factor kappa B (NF-KB), a master regulator of the inflammatory response, and NFKB-regulated proinflammatory cytokines, TNF-1α, IL1-βa and IL-16.[28]

In addition to the indirect contribution of hypoxia on dyslipidemia, insulin resistance and visceral fat changes in NAFLD pathogenesis, the hypoxia signaling system has a direct impact on NAFLD pathogenesis. The liver has an inherent oxygen gradient, with higher oxygen partial pressures in periportal regions and lower oxygen pressures in perivenular regions. OSA and CIH may inherently worsen this oxygen gradient. Dysregulation of this oxygen gradient may occur due to increase hepatocyte size from steatosis or alternately from increased oxygen consumption due to fat oxidation.[29] Hypoxia-inducible factors (HIFs) are central to the hepatic response to hypoxia. Cellular adaptations to hypoxia rely on the transcription of HIF, which is inactive during normoxia but is activated in hypoxic condition. HIF is a heterodimer, consisting of alpha and beta subunits. Oxygen=dependent hydroxylation of the HIF alpha subunit occurs by prolyl hydroxylases under normoxia, creating a binding site for the von Hippel Lindau gene product, which combines with a component of the E3 ubiquitin ligase complex. This complex is subsequently destroyed in the proteosome. Under hypoxic conditions, however, this degradation is inhibited, allowing the alpha and beta subunits to heterodimerize. The heterodimer can then translocate to the nucleus, bind to hypoxia response elements of hypoxia-responsive genes and regulate gene transcription.[30,31] Beyond hypoxia, HIF stabilization also occurs in response to increased ROS generation, which is known to occur in human NAFLD.[32]

HIF activation may contribute to the progression of NAFLD in numerous ways. Chronic HIF activation, particularly HIF-2α, may inhibit fatty acid oxygenation and thereby worsen hepatic lipid accumulation.[33] Metabolically, HIFs may also worsen diet-induced steatosis by activating lipogenic gene expression. HIF signaling also contributes to fibrosis in NAFLD by upregulating fibrogenic mediator expression in Kupffer and hepatic stellate cells.[34] Mouse hepatocytes exposed to hypoxia demonstrate increased plasminogen activator-inhibitor-1 (PAI-1), which contributes to fibrosis by inhibiting matrix metalloproteinase activity, thereby allowing for increased collagen and extracellular matrix accumulation.[34,35] Hepatocyte-specific knockouts of the oxygen-sensing HIF-1 alpha subunit were protected from liver fibrosis development as their presence is necessary for collagen cross-linking.[36] HIF signaling may also increase the production of hepatic stellate cell activators, such as platelet-derived growth factor 1 (PDGF-1) and increased Type 1 collagen expression in activated hepatic stellate cells. Hepatic stellate cells and fibroblasts make fibrillar collagen and lysyl oxidase (LOX). Hypoxia potentiates LOX activity, which contributes to cross-linking collagen and elastin and increasing liver stiffness. The mechanical tension caused by this stiffness further stems hepatic stellate cell differentiation and portal fibroblasts into myofibroblasts, which lay down more extracellular collagen and thereby fibrosis. Hypoxia may induce HIF-1α, which may induce LOX enzyme expression and thereby worsen fibrosis.[36] HIF-1α mediated expression of VEGF may also contribute to fibrosis by means of aberrant angiogenesis. VEGF expression in hypoxic hepatocytes is increased in an HIF-1α dependent manner. In bile duct ligation models of liver fibrosis, blocking VEGF can prevent fibrosis.[37,38] CIH also activates the hedgehog signaling pathway, which may further allow for functional activation of HIF-1α and induce genes important in the epithelial to mesenchymal transition, such as sonic hedgehog.[39]

CLINICAL IMPLICATIONS

With mounting experimental evidence linking OSA/CIH with NAFLD, it is important to understand the clinical implications for patients with both obesity-related conditions. Two meta-analyses have attempted to synthesize the evidence regarding the risk of NAFLD in patients with and without OSA to determine the impact of OSA on NAFLD disease severity. Musso et al. reviewed observational studies in which OSA was diagnosed by polysomnogram, cardiorespiratory polygraphy or nocturnal oximetry, and the diagnosis of NAFLD was made by liver histology, radiologic imaging (ultrasound, CT scan or MRI) and/or biochemistry.[40] Fifteen cross-sectional studies were included, 8 of which enrolled bariatric patients, with a total of 2,183 participants. Ten studies assessed histology (80% of which enrolled morbidly obese bariatric surgery candidates), 6 assessed radiologic steatosis and 2 assessed only liver enzymes in their NAFLD diagnosis. The pooled odds ratio of NAFLD based on histology, radiology or elevated aminotransferases in the presence of OSA was 2.10.[40] In subjects with OSA, the OR was 2.37 for the presence of NASH on biopsy and remained similar (OR = 2.81) when restricted to studies enrolling nonmorbidly obese patients. Additionally, the pooled OR in participants with OSA for the presence of any stage fibrosis was 2.16 and 2.3 for the presence of advanced (stage F3–F4) fibrososis.[40] Finally, the pooled OR of severe vs. mild to moderate OSA and the presence of histologic NASH was 1.89, and the OR for advanced fibrosis was 2.68.[40] Similarly, a slightly older meta-analysis that included 9 studies with 2,272 participants with and without OSA showed a significant association between OSA and histologic lobular inflammation (OR 2.84), ballooning (OR 2.31), steatosis (OR 3.22) and fibrosis (OR 2.77).[41] Using a slightly different approach, a recent meta-analysis sought to evaluate liver steatosis using the Hepatic Steatosis Index and fibrosis using Fibrotest or Fibrometer in an individual participant meta-analysis.[42] They found that 75% of the 2,120 patients enrolled had steatosis, with an AHI >5 being a risk factor. The prevalence of steatosis increased with OSA severity with an OR of 2.33 for an AHI between 5 and 30 and an OR of 2.80 for AHI >30 events per hour.[42] However, there was no association between AHI and fibrosis in 185 subjects.[42] In contrast, a prospective observational study of 51 nonbariatric patients with biopsy-proven NAFLD, those with moderate to severe OSA had a slightly increased risk of hepatic fibrosis (OR 1.22).[43] Therefore, while some conflicting data exist, most studies in adults show a strong relationship between OSA and NAFLD disease severity. However, little is known about the impact of chronic intermittent hypoxia on NAFLD disease severity.

Small pediatric studies have provided some insight into the role of OSA/CIH on NAFLD disease severity in children. Early-onset NAFLD is associated with an increased risk of complications later in life, including cirrhosis and hepatocellular carcinoma.[44] Sundaram et al. first demonstrated in obese children with biopsy-proven NAFLD that OSA/CIH was common, occurring in 60% of the studied subjects. They focused on the impact of CIH, noting that children with OSA/CIH had significantly more severe histologic hepatic fibrosis, which was related to a worsening oxygen nadir. In addition, increasing time with oxygen saturations below 90% was related to NAFLD histologic inflammation, steatosis and NAS score, as well as aminotransferase elevation.[45] They went on to further show that nocturnal hypoxia was a trigger for localized oxidative stress, an important factor associated with NASH progression and hepatic fibrosis in children.[32] They also demonstrated that mechanistically, the hedgehog pathway was activated in pediatric patients with NAFLD and nocturnal hypoxia, which again related to disease severity.[39] Nobili et al. also studied children with biopsy-proven NAFLD, noting that the duration of oxygen desaturations correlated with increased intrahepatic leukocytes and activated macrophages (Kupffer cells), circulating markers of hepatocyte apoptosis (CK-18) and hepatic fibrogenesis (hyaluronic acid).[46] A recent meta-analysis by Chen et al. aimed to evaluate the relationship between OSA and NAFLD in children and adolescents based on 9 pediatric studies. Both AST and ALT were significantly higher in children with OSA than control groups. Subgroup analyses revealed that both mild and severe OSA were significantly correlated to elevated liver enzymes. Focusing on the 2 studies that evaluated NAFLD histologically, they found NAFLD inflammation tended to be higher in OSA patients and that OSA was significantly associated with worse hepatic fibrosis.[47]

TREATMENT

Continuous positive airway pressure (CPAP) is the gold standard treatment for OSA. It precludes upper airway collapse, thereby improving sleep fragmentation, symptoms such as daytime sleepiness, and overall quality of life.[48,49] Importantly, in patients with OSA, CPAP treatment decreases mortality risk.[50] Given the emerging relationship between OSA and NAFLD, CPAP treatment for NAFLD

is an intriguing concept. To date, published studies have yielded conflicting results for several reasons. First, NAFLD and NASH have been variably defined in the published studies. Histologic confirmation and determination of NAFLD severity by the gold standard of liver biopsy is a rarity in this segment of the published literature. Most commonly, abnormal aminotransferases have been used to define patients as having NAFLD. Additional criteria used to define NAFLD in these studies include the presence of steatosis on radiologic imaging (ultrasound, CT scan or MRI), as well abnormal controlled attenuation parameter (CAP) on FibroScan® testing. Post-CPAP outcomes measures have also been variable, including the markers used to determine outcomes. Moreover, individual studies have had relatively small sample sizes. The length of CPAP treatment has also been quite variable, with few studies extending beyond 12 months, as would be common in pharmacologic trials. Finally, details regarding adherence to CPAP therapy are scarce and likely further impact the interpretation of studies' results. As such, each study must be interpreted in the context of these potential shortcomings.

CPAP therapy has most extensively been studied to determine its effects on aminotransferases in NAFLD. An observational study utilized nasal CPAP, demonstrating decreased AST after 1 month, with sustained improvements over 6 months of CPAP therapy.[51] A very small prospective cohort study of 6 subjects treated with CPAP for 3 years demonstrated significant reduction in liver enzymes as compared to 5 controls, without changes in BMI confounding these results.[52] A study of 28 patients with ultrasound-defined NAFLD had significant improvements in both AST and ALT, without any change in BMI, after 3 months of CPAP (mean usage: 6 hours per day).[53] More recently, an observational study utilizing an institutional database of 351 subjects receiving CPAP for at least 3 months found significant improvement in liver enzymes.[54] This study suggested that those with better adherence had greater decreases in their aminotransferases.[54] Sundaram et al. studied adolescents with biopsy-proven NAFLD, severe OSA/CIH and evidence of significant oxidative stress. Despite an increase in body mass index, 3 months of home CPAP therapy reduced ALT, metabolic syndrome markers and oxidative stress, as measured by F(2)-isoprostanes.[55] Kohler et al. conducted a 4-week randomized control trial of patients with NAFLD based on elevated liver enzymes. In this study, no beneficial effect on aminotransferases in the 47 subjects receiving CPAP was found as compared to 47 controls who received subtherapeutic CPAP.[56] Using a slightly different approach, Sivam et al. studied 27 subjects in a randomized control crossover trial. They all received CPAP for 8 weeks, with no changes in aminotransferase levels detected.[57] A recent meta-analysis examined the clinical utility of CPAP treatment for NAFLD, which included 5 articles with 7 patient cohorts and 192 adult subjects. This meta-analysis showed that CPAP use was associated with significant decreases in both AST and ALT in patients with OSA, without concurrent changes in BMI. Importantly, subgroup analyses indicated that 3 or more months of CPAP treatment were required to garner this clinical benefit.[53] As such, while non-RCTs and a meta-analysis suggest CPAP therapy may be beneficial in improving aminotransferases in NAFLD, small RCTs do not support this treatment. The relatively short duration of therapy in these RCTs may have these negative results.

CPAP has also been evaluated for its utility in treating the hepatic steatosis central to NAFLD physiology. In their small cohort study, Shpirer et al. found that 2–3 years of CPAP partially reversed moderate to severe steatosis assessed by CT scan, with no accompanying changes in the BMI or triglyceride levels of participants.[52,58] In an observational cohort study, 6–12 months of CPAP improved severe steatosis without changes in BMI.[59] Toyama et al. conducted an observational study of 61 subjects. In those with hepatic steatosis at baseline, there was decreased accumulation of liver fat after 31 months of CPAP therapy, despite stable BMI and worsening visceral and subcutaneous fat accumulations, suggesting longer therapy may be needed to alter hepatic steatosis.[60] In 50 subjects with OSA, hepatic steatosis was assessed by CAP score using FibroScan®. After 6 months of CPAP, CAP scores for steatosis did not improve. Furthermore, a subgroup analysis of 17 subjects with stable BMI and good CPAP adherence also did not show improved CAP measurements.[61] In contrast, the previously mentioned RCT with crossover design of 8 weeks of CPAP therapy did not improve hepatic fat as measured by magnetic resonance imaging and spectroscopy. Kritikou et al. also found no improvement in hepatic steatosis by CT scan in an RCT of 38 subjects receiving either CPAP or sham CPAP for 2 months.[62] Similarly, an RCT of 65 subjects found no significant change in liver fat after 24 weeks of either CPAP or sham CPAP.[63] Most recently, an RCT of 106 subjects with clinical NAFLD (criteria not defined) and OSA (based on a home sleep test, not polysomnography) received 6 months of either autoadjusting or subtherapeutic CPAP. Again, no differences in hepatic fat measured by MR spectroscopy and controlled attenuation parameter (CAP) scores by transient elastography were found, even when only looking at subjects with at least 4 hours of CPAP usage per night.[64] CPAP treatment for hepatic steatosis thereby yields results similar to outcomes with liver enzymes; observational studies suggest the potential benefit of CPAP while RCTs do not.

Limited data are available on the impact of CPAP for NAFLD hepatic fibrosis treatment, although fibrosis may be the most important indicator of long-term prognosis. Kim et al. used an institutional database of 221 subjects with OSA and clinically suspected NAFLD based on elevated ALT. In subjects treated with CPAP for at least 3 months, a potential reduction in advanced fibrosis as assessed by APRI (AST-to-platelet ratio index) score, a surrogate for fibrosis, was seen.[54,65] Liver fibrosis based on serum lysyl oxidase, which cross-links collagen and may be a biomarker of fibrosis, was also significantly reduced in 35 subjects after 3 months of CPAP therapy.[66] However, 50 subjects with OSA and NAFLD, demonstrated no changes in liver stiffness measurements indicating fibrosis by FibroScan®.[61] Similarly, Buttacavoli studied 15 patients before and after 6–12 months of CPAP and found no improvement in fibrosis by transient elastography.[59] An RCT to assesses liver fibrosis improvement using CPAP vs. sham treated 103 patients for 6–12 weeks without improvements in Fibromax scores.[67] FibroMax is a proprietary noninvasive test that uses an algorithm that includes gender, age, weight and height with 10 serum biomarkers. FibroMax includes three tests, SteatoTest, NashTest and FibroTest, in order to evaluate steatosis, NASH and liver fibrosis, respectively.[67] Most recently, an RCT of 106 subjects with clinical NAFLD received 6 months of either autoadjusting or subtherapeutic CPAP with no improvements in liver stiffness as measured by transient elastography, even when focusing only on the subgroup with at least 4 hours of CPAP usage per night.[64]

The clinical benefit of screening every patient with NAFLD for OSA and vice versa is unclear. However, simple clinical screening tools in clinic and liver function tests could help determine who needs further assessment or evaluation. As the availability of noninvasive point of

Table 18.1: Studies Examining the Therapeutic Benefit of CPAP on NAFLD

Author	Study Design	Sample Size	CPAP Duration	Outcome of interest	Therapeutic Benefit
Chin[51]	Observational	40	6 months	Aminotransferases	Yes
Shpirer[52]	Prospective Cohort	11 (6 CPAP, 5 control)	3 years	Aminotransferases and steatosis	Yes and yes
Chen[68]	Prospective Cohort	160	3 months	Aminotransferases	Yes
Kim[54]	Observational	351	3 months	Aminotransferases and fibrosis	Yes and yes
Sundaram[55]	Prospective Cohort	12	3 months	Aminotransferases and oxidative stress	Yes and yes
Kohler[56]	RCT*	94 (47 CPAP, 47 Sham)	1 month	Aminotransferases	No
Sivam[57]	RCT*, cross over	27	8 weeks	Aminotransferases	No
Chen[53]	Meta-analysis	192	≥ 3months	Aminotransferases	Yes
Buttacavoli[59]	Observational	15	6–12 months	Steatosis and Fibrosis	Yes and no
Toyama[60]	Observational	61	32 months	Steatosis	Yes
Hirono[61]	Prospective cohort	123	6 months	Aminotransferases and Steatosis	Yes and No
Kritikou[62]	RCT*	38	2 months	Steatosis	No
Hoyos[63]	Prospective cohort	65	3–6 months	Steatosis	No
Ng[64]	RCT*	106 (53 CPAP, 53 subtherapeutic CPAP)	6	Steatosis and fibrosis	No and no
Mesarwi[66]	Prospective cohort	35	3 months	Fibrosis	Yes
Jullian-Desayes[67]	RCT*	103 (51 CPAP, 52 sham)	1.5–3 months	Steatosis and fibrosis	No and No

RCT: Randomized control trial.

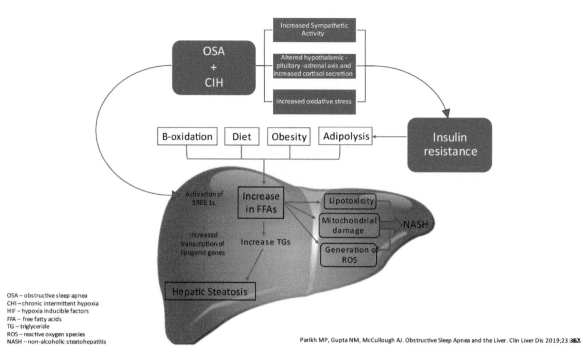

Parikh MP, Gupta NM, McCullough AJ. Obstructive Sleep Apnea and the Liver. Clin Liver Dis 2019;23:363.

Figure 18.1 Impact of obstructive sleep apnea and chronic intermittent hypoxia on NAFLD pathogenesis[13]

care testing and biomarkers improves, it may be easier and more cost-effective to both screen and diagnose NAFLD in children and adults with OSA and vice versa. Furthermore, in the future, as pharmacologic therapies begin to play a bigger role in the care of NAFLD patients, early identification of risk factors for advanced disease will become increasingly important.

REFERENCES

1. Heinzer R, Vat S, Marques-Vidal P, et al. Prevalence of sleep-disordered breathing in the general population: the HypnoLaus study. *Lancet Respir Med* 2015;3:310–318.
2. Young T, Palta M, Dempsey J, Skatrud J, Weber S, Badr S. The occurrence of sleep-disordered breathing among middle-aged adults. *N Engl J Med* 1993;328:1230–1235.
3. Lindberg E, Gislason T. Epidemiology of sleep-related obstructive breathing. *Sleep Med Rev* 2000;4:411–433.
4. Lumeng JC, Chervin RD. Epidemiology of pediatric obstructive sleep apnea. *Proc Am Thorac Soc* 2008;5:242–252.
5. Mannarino MR, Di Filippo F, Pirro M. Obstructive sleep apnea syndrome. *Eur J Intern Med* 2012;23:586–593.
6. Prabhakar NR, Kumar GK. Mechanisms of sympathetic activation and blood pressure elevation by intermittent hypoxia. *Respir Physiol Neurobiol* 2010;174:156–161.
7. Reinke C, Bevans-Fonti S, Drager LF, Shin MK, Polotsky VY. Effects of different acute hypoxic regimens on tissue oxygen profiles and metabolic outcomes. *J Appl Physiol (1985)* 2011;111:881–890.
8. Sundar KM, Prchal JT. The cornerstone of the aberrant pathophysiology of obstructive sleep apnea: tissue responses to chronic sustained versus intermittent hypoxia. *Am J Respir Cell Mol Biol* 2017;56:419–420.
9. Skelly JR, Rowan SC, Jones JF, O'Halloran KD. Upper airway dilator muscle weakness following intermittent and sustained hypoxia in the rat: effects of a superoxide scavenger. *Physiol Res* 2013;62:187–196.
10. Ramirez TA, Jourdan-Le Saux C, Joy A, et al. Chronic and intermittent hypoxia differentially regulate left ventricular inflammatory and extracellular matrix responses. *Hypertens Res* 2012;35:811–818.
11. Drager LF, Li J, Shin MK, et al. Intermittent hypoxia inhibits clearance of triglyceride-rich lipoproteins and inactivates adipose lipoprotein lipase in a mouse model of sleep apnoea. *Eur Heart J* 2012;33:783–790.
12. Sleep-related breathing disorders in adults: recommendations for syndrome definition and measurement techniques in clinical research. The Report of an American Academy of Sleep Medicine Task Force. *Sleep* 1999;22:667–689.
13. Parikh MP, Gupta NM, McCullough AJ. Obstructive sleep apnea and the liver. *Clin Liver Dis* 2019;23:363–382.
14. Hazlehurst JM, Lim TR, Charlton C, et al. Acute intermittent hypoxia drives hepatic de novo lipogenesis in humans and rodents. *Metabol Open* 2022;14:100177.
15. Li J, Grigoryev DN, Ye SQ, et al. Chronic intermittent hypoxia upregulates genes of lipid biosynthesis in obese mice. *J Appl Physiol (1985)* 2005;99:1643–1648.
16. Li J, Thorne LN, Punjabi NM, et al. Intermittent hypoxia induces hyperlipidemia in lean mice. *Circ Res* 2005;97:698–706.
17. Li J, Nanayakkara A, Jun J, Savransky V, Polotsky VY. Effect of deficiency in SREBP cleavage-activating protein on lipid metabolism during intermittent hypoxia. *Physiol Genomics* 2007;31:273–280.
18. Savransky V, Jun J, Li J, et al. Dyslipidemia and atherosclerosis induced by chronic intermittent hypoxia are attenuated by deficiency of stearoyl coenzyme a desaturase. *Circ Res* 2008;103:1173–1180.
19. Polotsky M, Elsayed-Ahmed AS, Pichard L, et al. Effects of leptin and obesity on the upper airway function. *J Appl Physiol (1985)* 2012;112:1637–1643.
20. Drager LF, Li J, Reinke C, Bevans-Fonti S, Jun JC, Polotsky VY. Intermittent hypoxia exacerbates

metabolic effects of diet-induced obesity. *Obesity (Silver Spring)* 2011;19:2167–2174.

21. Shin MK, Yao Q, Jun JC, et al. Carotid body denervation prevents fasting hyperglycemia during chronic intermittent hypoxia. *J Appl Physiol (1985)* 2014;117:765–776.

22. Ip MS, Lam B, Ng MM, Lam WK, Tsang KW, Lam KS. Obstructive sleep apnea is independently associated with insulin resistance. *Am J Respir Crit Care Med* 2002;165:670–676.

23. Stamatakis KA, Punjabi NM. Effects of sleep fragmentation on glucose metabolism in normal subjects. *Chest* 2010;137:95–101.

24. Xu J, Long YS, Gozal D, Epstein PN. Beta-cell death and proliferation after intermittent hypoxia: role of oxidative stress. *Free Radic Biol Med* 2009;46:783–790.

25. Li M, Li X, Lu Y. Obstructive sleep apnea syndrome and metabolic diseases. *Endocrinology* 2018;159:2670–2675.

26. Hosogai N, Fukuhara A, Oshima K, et al. Adipose tissue hypoxia in obesity and its impact on adipocytokine dysregulation. *Diabetes* 2007;56:901–911.

27. Chen DD, Huang JF, Lin QC, Chen GP, Zhao JM. Relationship between serum adiponectin and bone mineral density in male patients with obstructive sleep apnea syndrome. *Sleep Breath* 2017;21:557–564.

28. Savransky V, Bevans S, Nanayakkara A, et al. Chronic intermittent hypoxia causes hepatitis in a mouse model of diet-induced fatty liver. *Am J Physiol Gastrointest Liver Physiol* 2007;293:G871–877.

29. Holzner LMW, Murray AJ. Hypoxia-inducible factors as key players in the pathogenesis of non-alcoholic fatty liver disease and non-alcoholic steatohepatitis. *Front Med (Lausanne)* 2021;8:753268.

30. Jaakkola P, Mole DR, Tian YM, et al. Targeting of HIF-alpha to the von Hippel-Lindau ubiquitylation complex by O2-regulated prolyl hydroxylation. *Science* 2001;292:468–472.

31. Benita Y, Kikuchi H, Smith AD, Zhang MQ, Chung DC, Xavier RJ. An integrative genomics approach identifies Hypoxia Inducible Factor-1 (HIF-1)-target genes that form the core response to hypoxia. *Nucleic Acids Res* 2009;37:4587–4602.

32. Sundaram SS, Halbower A, Pan Z, et al. Nocturnal hypoxia-induced oxidative stress promotes progression of pediatric non-alcoholic fatty liver disease. *J Hepatol* 2016;65:560–569.

33. Morello E, Sutti S, Foglia B, et al. Hypoxia-inducible factor 2alpha drives nonalcoholic fatty liver progression by triggering hepatocyte release of histidine-rich glycoprotein. *Hepatology* 2018;67:2196–2214.

34. Copple BL, Bustamante JJ, Welch TP, Kim ND, Moon JO. Hypoxia-inducible factor-dependent production of profibrotic mediators by hypoxic hepatocytes. *Liver Int* 2009;29:1010–1021.

35. Mesarwi OA, Moya EA, Zhen X, et al. Hepatocyte HIF-1 and intermittent hypoxia independently impact liver fibrosis in murine nonalcoholic fatty liver disease. *Am J Respir Cell Mol Biol* 2021;65:390–402.

36. Mesarwi OA, Shin MK, Bevans-Fonti S, Schlesinger C, Shaw J, Polotsky VY. Hepatocyte hypoxia inducible factor-1 mediates the development of liver fibrosis in a mouse model of nonalcoholic fatty liver disease. *PLoS ONE* 2016;11:e0168572.

37. Mejias M, Garcia-Pras E, Tiani C, Miquel R, Bosch J, Fernandez M. Beneficial effects of sorafenib on splanchnic, intrahepatic, and portocollateral circulations in portal hypertensive and cirrhotic rats. *Hepatology* 2009;49:1245–1256.

38. Yang L, Kwon J, Popov Y, et al. Vascular endothelial growth factor promotes fibrosis resolution and repair in mice. *Gastroenterology* 2014;146:1339–1350 e1.

39. Sundaram SS, Swiderska-Syn M, Sokol RJ, et al. Nocturnal hypoxia activation of the hedgehog signaling pathway affects pediatric nonalcoholic fatty liver disease severity. *Hepatol Commun* 2019;3:883–893.

40. Musso G, Cassader M, Olivetti C, Rosina F, Carbone G, Gambino R. Association of obstructive sleep apnoea with the presence and severity of non-alcoholic fatty liver disease. A systematic review and meta-analysis. *Obes Rev* 2013;14:417–431.

41. Jin S, Jiang S, Hu A. Association between obstructive sleep apnea and non-alcoholic fatty liver disease: a systematic review and meta-analysis. *Sleep Breath* 2018;22:841–851.

42. Jullian-Desayes I, Trzepizur W, Boursier J, et al. Obstructive sleep apnea, chronic obstructive pulmonary disease and NAFLD: an individual participant data meta-analysis. *Sleep Med* 2021;77:357–364.

43. Krolow GK, Garcia E, Schoor F, Araujo FBS, Coral GP. Obstructive sleep apnea and severity of nonalcoholic fatty liver disease. *Eur J Gastroenterol Hepatol* 2021;33:1104–1109.

44. Chalasani N, Younossi Z, Lavine JE, et al. The diagnosis and management of non-alcoholic fatty liver disease: practice Guideline by the American Association for the Study of Liver Diseases, American College of Gastroenterology, and the American Gastroenterological Association. *Hepatology* 2012;55:2005–2023.

45. Sundaram SS, Sokol RJ, Capocelli KE, et al. Obstructive sleep apnea and hypoxemia are associated with advanced liver histology in pediatric nonalcoholic fatty liver disease. *J Pediatr* 2014;164:699–706 e1.

46. Nobili V, Cutrera R, Liccardo D, et al. Obstructive sleep apnea syndrome affects liver histology and inflammatory cell activation in pediatric nonalcoholic fatty liver disease, regardless of obesity/insulin resistance. *Am J Respir Crit Care Med* 2014;189:66–76.

47. Chen LD, Chen MX, Chen GP, et al. Association between obstructive sleep apnea and non-alcoholic fatty liver disease in pediatric patients: a meta-analysis. *Pediatr Obes* 2021;16:e12718.

48. Patel SR, White DP, Malhotra A, Stanchina ML, Ayas NT. Continuous positive airway pressure therapy for treating sleepiness in a diverse population with obstructive sleep apnea: results of a meta-analysis. *Arch Intern Med* 2003;163:565–571.

49. D'Ambrosio C, Bowman T, Mohsenin V. Quality of life in patients with obstructive sleep apnea: effect of nasal continuous positive airway pressure-a prospective study. *Chest* 1999;115:123–129.

50. Marin JM, Carrizo SJ, Vicente E, Agusti AG. Long-term cardiovascular outcomes in men with obstructive sleep apnoea-hypopnoea with or without treatment with continuous positive airway pressure: an observational study. *Lancet* 2005;365:1046–1053.

51. Chin K, Nakamura T, Takahashi K, et al. Effects of obstructive sleep apnea syndrome on serum aminotransferase levels in obese patients. *Am J Med* 2003;114:370–376.

52. Shpirer I, Copel L, Broide E, Elizur A. Continuous positive airway pressure improves sleep apnea associated fatty liver. *Lung* 2010;188:301–307.

53. Chen LD, Lin L, Zhang LJ, et al. Effect of continuous positive airway pressure on liver enzymes in obstructive sleep apnea: a meta-analysis. *Clin Respir J* 2018;12:373–381.

54. Kim D, Ahmed A, Kushida C. Continuous positive airway pressure therapy on nonalcoholic fatty liver disease in patients with obstructive sleep apnea. *J Clin Sleep Med* 2018;14:1315–1322.

55. Sundaram SS, Halbower AC, Klawitter J, et al. Treating obstructive sleep apnea and chronic intermittent hypoxia improves the severity of nonalcoholic fatty liver disease in children. J Pediatr 2018;198:67–75 e1.

56. Kohler M, Pepperell JC, Davies RJ, Stradling JR. Continuous positive airway pressure and liver enzymes in obstructive sleep apnoea: data from a randomized controlled trial. *Respiration* 2009;78:141–146.

57. Sivam S, Phillips CL, Trenell MI, et al. Effects of 8 weeks of continuous positive airway pressure on abdominal adiposity in obstructive sleep apnoea. *Eur Respir J* 2012;40:913–918.

58. OPTN-RHSA final rule with comment period. *Fed Regist* 1998:16296–16338.

59. Buttacavoli M, Gruttad'Auria CI, Olivo M, et al. Liver steatosis and fibrosis in OSA patients after long-term CPAP treatment: a preliminary ultrasound study. *Ultrasound Med Biol* 2016;42:104–109.

60. Toyama YMK, Azume M, Hamada S, et al. Chin K. Impacts of long-term CPAP therapy on fatty liver in male OSA patients with abdominal obesity. *Eur Respir J* 2014;44.

61. Hirono H, Watanabe K, Hasegawa K, Kohno M, Terai S, Ohkoshi S. Impact of continuous positive airway

pressure therapy for nonalcoholic fatty liver disease in patients with obstructive sleep apnea. *World J Clin Cases* 2021;9:5112–5125.

62. Kritikou I, Basta M, Tappouni R, et al. Sleep apnoea and visceral adiposity in middle-aged male and female subjects. *Eur Respir J* 2013;41:601–609.

63. Hoyos CM, Killick R, Yee BJ, Phillips CL, Grunstein RR, Liu PY. Cardiometabolic changes after continuous positive airway pressure for obstructive sleep apnoea: a randomised sham-controlled study. *Thorax* 2012;67:1081–1089.

64. Ng SSS, Wong VWS, Wong GLH, et al. Continuous positive airway pressure does not improve nonalcoholic fatty liver disease in patients with obstructive sleep apnea. A randomized clinical trial. *Am J Respir Crit Care Med* 2021;203:493–501.

65. Wai CT, Greenson JK, Fontana RJ, et al. A simple noninvasive index can predict both significant fibrosis and cirrhosis in patients with chronic hepatitis C. *Hepatology* 2003;38:518–526.

66. Mesarwi OA, Shin MK, Drager LF, et al. Lysyl oxidase as a serum biomarker of liver fibrosis in patients with severe obesity and obstructive sleep apnea. *Sleep* 2015;38:1583–1591.

67. Jullian-Desayes I, Tamisier R, Zarski JP, et al. Impact of effective versus sham continuous positive airway pressure on liver injury in obstructive sleep apnoea: data from randomized trials. *Respirology* 2016;21:378–385.

68. Chen LD, Zhang LJ, Lin XJ, et al. Association between continuous positive airway pressure and serum aminotransferases in patients with obstructive sleep apnea. *Eur Arch Otorhinolaryngol* 2018;275:587–594.

19 Extrahepatic Gastrointestinal Manifestations of Nonalcoholic Fatty Liver Disease

Rinjal Brahmbhatt and Mousab Tabbaa

CONTENTS

Key Points

- Nonalcoholic fatty liver disease (NAFLD) is a manifestation of metabolic disturbances and pathophysiologic pathways that impact all organ systems, and the gastrointestinal tract is no exception.

- Esophageal, gastric, small bowel, colonic and pancreaticobiliary diseases are prevalent in this population. This has important implications in the management of NAFLD as a multisystem disease.

- Of note, NAFLD is associated with several GI malignancies, and with earlier recognition and diagnosis, this may alter their disease course.

- In this chapter, we will review the impact of NAFLD on the gastrointestinal tract outside the parenchymal liver.

19.1 INTRODUCTION

NAFLD is a multisystem disease associated with a myriad of extrahepatic gastrointestinal manifestations. Visceral adiposity and hepatic steatosis promote a state of systemic inflammation, predisposing individuals with NAFLD to a variety of gastrointestinal diseases and extrahepatic neoplasias. Different mechanisms for this association have been proposed, including activation of the inflammatory pathway by lipotoxicity that results in extrahepatic tissue damage. Herein, we describe the extrahepatic gastrointestinal manifestations of NAFLD and highlight studies that provide mechanistic explanations for these manifestations, as well as identify potentially modifiable or clinically detectable relationships between NAFLD and these associated conditions.

19.2 NAFLD AND THE ESOPHAGUS

19.2.1 Gastroesophageal Reflux Disease

Multiple studies have shown that NAFLD is independently associated with an increased risk of gastroesophageal reflux disease (GERD) symptoms as well as erosive esophagitis (EE). The detrimental effect of NAFLD on EE might be greater than those of generalized and visceral obesity (1–3). Specifically, Mikolasevic et al. demonstrated a positive association between controlled attenuation parameter (CAP) on transient elastography and a higher prevalence of GERD. In particular, they found a higher prevalence of LA grades B and C erosive esophagitis in this cohort of NAFLD patients (4).

Interestingly, GERD may not only be associated with NAFLD but also may worsen it, representing a viscous cycle. Taketani et al. reported that nearly 30% of Japanese patients with biopsy-proven NAFLD had insomnia, which was independently associated with GERD symptoms (5). They also demonstrated that treatment with a proton pump inhibitor could relieve both insomnia and GERD symptoms. Correspondingly, Spiegel et al. demonstrated that a shorter sleep duration may increase the risk of obesity and diabetes due to changes in the secretion of hormones such as cortisol, leptin and ghrelin and to increased insulin resistance (6).

Several plausible mechanisms to explain the relationship between NAFLD and GERD have been proposed. Increased serum levels of interleukin-1 and interleukin-6 in patients with NAFLD have been found to contribute to the development of GERD. Interleukin-6 could decrease esophageal contraction, impair acid clearance and thus increase reflux episodes. Furthermore, increased systemic oxidative stress and impaired antioxidant capacity in

DOI: 10.1201/9781003386698-23

patients with NAFLD may contribute to esophageal mucosal injuries, suggesting the critical role of oxidative stress in the pathogenesis of GERD. Finally, obesity, especially visceral adiposity in NAFLD patients, might increase intra-abdominal pressure leading to increased lower esophageal sphincter relaxation and therefore acid reflux. Similarly, gastroparesis in NAFLD patients with diabetes may also increase the propensity for GERD.

19.2.2 Barrett's Esophagus

Obesity has been a well-established risk factor for Barrett's esophagus (BE). Multiple studies have demonstrated an association between increased visceral adiposity and an increase in the risk of BE. In one study of a Japanese population with NAFLD, obesity tended to be associated with the risk of BE, and this risk appeared to be mediated for the most part by visceral adiposity (7–10).

Apfel et al. reported an increased risk of progression of BE with low-grade dysplasia in one population of patients with cirrhosis, the majority of which had NASH as the etiologic cause of their liver disease. Furthermore, due to this association, the authors recommended increased surveillance of BE in such patients and, in particular, those with higher Child–Pugh scores (11).

19.2.3 Esophageal Cancer

Esophageal cancer is the eighth most common form of cancer worldwide, and obesity has been identified as a major risk factor. The risk of esophageal cancer has been found to be up to 4-fold higher in patients with obesity compared to lean populations and is even more pronounced in those with visceral fat distribution as compared to those with an increased BMI (12). Interestingly, the association between visceral obesity and esophageal adenocarcinoma is independent of GERD and possibly mediated by adipose tissue insulin resistance and chronic inflammation (13–15).

Purported mechanisms include upregulation of GGT, which is increased after oxidative stress. Previous studies have reported on the associations of serum GGT level with the risk of cancer. As essential parts of the cellular defense apparatus, GGT and GSH combat oxidative stress (16). Increased GGT has been regarded as a marker of exposure to certain carcinogens and its levels can be affected by environmental and lifestyle factors such as diet, tobacco use and alcohol use.

Importantly, compared to patients without NAFLD, patients with NAFLD with incidental esophageal, stomach or colorectal cancer showed significantly increased all-cause mortality during the observation period in one study. Given the increased mortality in cancer patients with NAFLD, adipocytokines might link obesity-related disorders with neoplasm development both intra- and extrahepatically. The steatotic and inflamed liver may secrete growth factors, such as NAFLD-derived plasminogen activator inhibitor 1, vascular endothelial growth factor (VEGF), or angiopoietin, into the systemic circulation and may therefore be involved in metastasis and cancer progression (17).

19.3 NAFLD AND THE STOMACH

19.3.1 Helicobacter pylori

The possible association between Helicobacter pylori infection and NAFLD initially stemmed from the isolation of Helicobacter pylori (HP) in the livers of patients with NAFLD. Although there have been conflicting results, several subsequent clinical trials have demonstrated a higher rate of fatty liver and NASH in HP-positive patients compared to HP-negative patients. In one meta-analysis, the pooled overall odds ratio of H. pylori infection in NAFLD patients compared with controls was 1.36 (95% CI: 1.22–1.53, $I = 89.6\%$, $P=0.000$), and there was a 36% increased risk of NAFLD in patients with HP infection (18). Additionally, small trials examining the effect of HP eradication have shown improvement in markers of NAFLD activity, further supporting a link between these two conditions (19). Specifically, treatment of HP resulted in an improved metabolic profile as defined by insulin resistance, the fatty liver index and imaging characteristics after HP was eradicated (20). Mechanisms include metabolic insults from inflammatory cytokines such as CRP, TNF-α and IL-6, which trigger insulin resistance (21). Furthermore, HP may influence leptin and adiponectin production, thereby influencing fat metabolism and transporting relevant enzymes or by insulin signal transduction. Previous studies have also shown that the existence of HP itself was associated with increased intestinal permeability and may affect the normal gut microbiota, which is associated with metabolism and gut inflammation. Some speculate that HP may invade the intestinal mucosa, increasing gut permeability and gut dysbiosis, thus facilitating the passage of bacterial endotoxin, mainly lipopolysaccharide, via the portal vein to the liver where it promotes the inflammatory response leading to NAFLD (22) (Figure 19.1).

19.3.2 Gastric Cancer

A possible direct link between NAFLD and gastric cancer has been suggested in a few studies (23). In one Turkish study, 1,840 patients underwent upper endoscopies over a 6-month period, and the prevalence of NAFLD in subjects with gastric cancer was higher than average (24).

19.4 NAFLD AND THE SMALL INTESTINES

19.4.1 Celiac Disease

NAFLD patients have a higher incidence of celiac disease compared to the general population, despite celiac patients having a lower risk for metabolic syndrome before the start of a gluten-free diet. In turn, patients with celiac disease have a higher risk of developing NAFLD compared to the general population. In about 3.5% of patients with NAFLD, celiac disease represents the only extrahepatic manifestation of the disease. The incidence is highest in the first year after diagnosis and was found to be persistently higher than in the general population over the ensuing 15 years (25). The pathophysiologic mechanism of this is unclear but may be related to cellular stress and apoptosis caused by celiac disease (26). Intestinal permeability is increased in both celiac disease and NAFLD, perhaps mediated by intestinal dysbiosis which has been shown to serve as a trigger for the development of NASH in patients with hepatic steatosis (27).

19.4.1.1 Small Intestinal Bacterial Overgrowth

As the gut microbiome is altered in NAFLD (as previously discussed in Chapter 5), small intestinal bacterial overgrowth (SIBO) may also contribute to the pathogenesis of NAFLD. SIBO has been shown to be up to 65% more prevalent in the NAFLD than the non-NAFLD population (28). In one study evaluating liver biopsies of patients with NAFLD and SIBO, histological characteristics that were associated with SIBO included higher steatosis and fibrosis grade, lobular and portal inflammation, and ballooning grade (29). In comparison with those without SIBO,

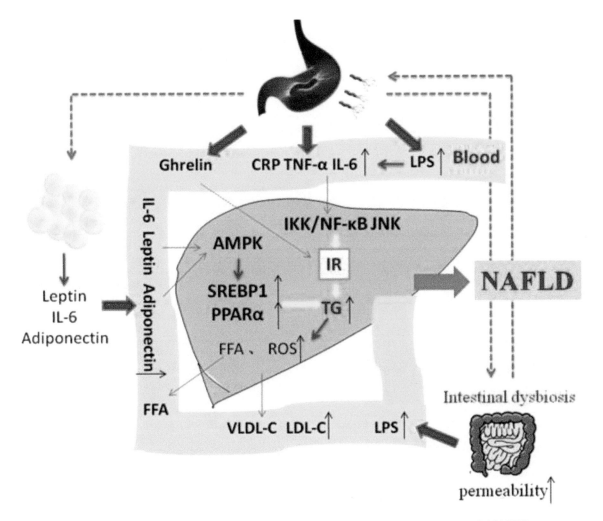

Figure 19.1 Possible mechanism explaining the increased prevalence of HP in patients with NAFLD

HP is purported to cause chronic low-grade systemic inflammation, resulting in increased levels of inflammatory cytokines such as IL-6 and TNF-α, which may affect insulin action and its level and thus promote insulin resistance. Additionally HP infection may also stimulate the release of leptin and adiponectin from adipose tissue, activating AMPK and upregulating SREBP1c and PPARα (22).

patients with SIBO had significantly higher endotoxin levels and higher CD14 mRNA, nuclear factor kappa beta mRNA, and toll-like receptor 4 (TLR4) protein expression. Patients with NASH had significantly higher endotoxin levels and higher intensity of TLR4 protein expression in comparison with patients without NASH (30). TLR expression in innate immune cells, such as dendritic cells and natural killer T cells, can trigger a pro-inflammatory cascade leading to hepatocyte damage and the development of NASH. NASH subjects have elevated plasma levels of lipopolysaccharide associated with a rise in tumor necrosis factor (TNF)-α gene expression in the hepatic tissue. Additionally, SIBO is associated with increased gut permeability characterized by disruption of the intercellular tight junctions leading to bacterial translocation (31). Further studies are needed to determine whether therapy of SIBO reduces the risk of NAFLD, fibrosis and cirrhosis.

19.4.2 Inflammatory Bowel Disease

Various hepatic manifestations of IBD are well-described and beyond the scope of this chapter. However, in IBD patients with abnormal liver enzymes, NAFLD remains

the most common cause, affecting more than 30% of IBD patients (up to 55% of patients with UC and up to 40% of patients with Crohn's disease) (32). NAFLD is more commonly seen in Crohn's patients with a longer duration of IBD, older age, higher BMI and diabetes (33). A recent systematic review found prevalence rates up to 39.5% and from 1.5 to 55% in CD and UC patients, respectively (34). IBD behavior, extension, activity and drug response do not appear to be affected by the presence of NAFLD (35). IBD patients develop NAFLD with fewer metabolic risk factors than non-IBD NAFLD patients. The IBD-related intestinal inflammatory state could be invoked to explain the higher prevalence of NAFLD in this population. In IBD, inflammation causes breakdown of the gut barrier, leading to the translocation of bacteria and the release of cytokines (such as TNF alpha). These mediators may contribute to the pathophysiology behind NAFLD in such patients. Furthermore, alteration of the gut microbiome, well-described in IBD, may play a role in NAFLD progression in these patients (36,37). In one study, among 223 NAFLD patients, 78 patients with IBD were younger, were less likely to have altered liver enzymes, had lower mean body weight, smaller waist circumference and lower BMI and a lower prevalence of metabolic syndrome. Within the IBD population, patients with severe IBD and also those with a lower BMI had a higher prevalence of S3 on transient elastography (see discussion of lean NAFLD in Chapter 35). Independent risk factors for S3 in IBD patients were more than one IBD relapse per year during disease history, surgery for IBD and more extensive intestinal involvement. Anti-TNF therapy was the only independent factor found to be protective against abnormal liver enzymes. In another study, higher CDAI scores were seen among patients with NAFLD. Therefore, NAFLD in IBD patients appears to be different from that in non-IBD patients (38,39). IBD patients appear to develop NAFLD as a result of an increased inflammatory load and not because of metabolic risk factors.

19.5 NAFLD AND THE COLON
19.5.1 Irritable Bowel Syndrome
There is increasing interest in the possibility of an association between NAFLD and irritable bowel syndrome (IBS) due to similar etiologic factors for both diseases. The prevalence in the literature of both NAFLD and IBS occurring concomitantly is variable and ranges from 12 to 74%. One similar risk factor for both NAFLD and IBS is obesity. There is evidence that IBS is more prevalent in patients who are obese. It has been noted that increased

visceral adiposity enhances perception of luminal stimuli, dysmotility and abdominal pain. Higher body mass index has been associated with accelerated colonic and rectosigmoid transit and increased stool frequency. Additionally, dysregulation of the microbiome has been shown to be a component for the development of both NAFLD, as previously discussed, and IBS (40). As in NAFLD, altered intestinal motility and sensitivity, reduced microbial diversity, and the presence of a pro-inflammatory state are also implicated in IBS (Figure 19.2). As depression and anxiety are both more prevalent in IBS and bowel symptoms significantly impact quality of life, a multidisciplinary approach may be needed for NAFLD patients who have coexistent IBS.

19.5.2 Diverticular Disease
Both NAFLD and diverticular disease are associated with metabolic syndrome. In one study, an increased severity of diverticulitis was associated with the presence of hepatic steatosis. In a retrospective study investigating accompanying diseases in patients with NAFLD, Kempiński et al. found that colonic diverticulosis is the second most frequent concomitant gastrointestinal disease, second only to GERD. Colonic diverticulosis was significantly more prevalent in the study group than in the controls (23.7 vs. 15.8%). In addition to shared factors such as obesity, diets low in fiber and high in fats and red meat, and altered gut

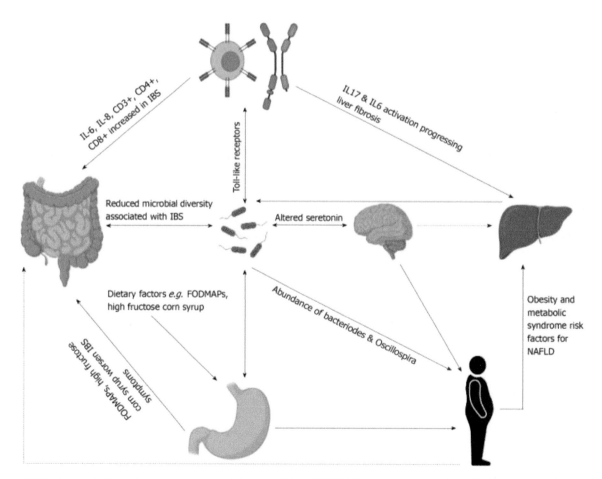

Figure 19.2 Several etiologic factors overlap between IBS and NAFLD: obesity, alterations in the gut microbiome, dietary factors and immune-mediated causes (41)

microbiome, arterial hypertension has importantly also been implicated in the development of both NAFLD and diverticulosis. Arterial hypertension can over time lead to structural changes in the bowel wall by damaging blood vessels and further reducing blood supply in vulnerable anatomical areas (42).

19.5.3 *Clostridioides difficile*

NAFLD has been shown to be associated not only with *Clostridioides difficile* infection (CDI) but also recurrent CDI. Hospitalized CDI patients with NAFLD in one study had more intestinal complications with either perforation or obstruction compared to CDI patients with liver disease of another etiology such as viral hepatitis or alcoholic liver disease. On the other hand, NAFLD was found to be an independent predictor of CDI in another study (43). Gut dysbiosis may contribute to the pathogenesis of CDI as in NAFLD. *Bacteroides* and *Bifidobacterium* play an important role in preventing colonization by *C. difficile*, and patients with NAFLD were shown to have a relative decrease in the proportion of *Bacteroides* to *Firmicutes*. The chronic low-level inflammation associated with NAFLD and the resultant impaired immune response might predispose patients to CDI as well as other infections.

19.5.4 Colonic Adenomas and Colorectal Cancer

NAFLD is associated with an increased risk of developing colorectal adenomatous polyps. This is true even after adjusting for diabetes, obesity and hyperlipidemia. Furthermore, adenomatous polyps are more common in those NAFLD patients with advanced fibrosis compared to no fibrosis and in those with NASH compared to simple steatosis (44). In a retrospective cohort study, Hwang et al. evaluated 2,917 patients who had undergone colonoscopy and found an ultrasound-diagnosed NAFLD prevalence of 41.5% in the patients with adenomas compared to 30.2% among patients without adenomas, and this was independent of the presence of metabolic syndrome (45).

A population-based study in Korea and prospective study in China have shown an increased prevalence of not only colonic adenomas but also of advanced neoplasia such as colonic cancer, high-grade dysplasia and villous histology in patients with NAFLD (46,47).

In one large cohort study, sigmoid colon adenocarcinoma and highly differentiated colorectal adenocarcinoma were more common among NAFLD patients (48). Lifestyle factors, such as a high-fat/low-fiber diet, increased consumption of red processed meat and a sedentary lifestyle, can cause insulin resistance and alter the gut microbiome. These, in turn, can cause mitochondrial dysfunction, increased oxidative stress, intestinal barrier destruction and increased production and absorption of gut-derived toxic and pro-inflammatory metabolites, such as advanced glycation end products (AGEs), IL-6, IL-8 and plasminogen activator inhibitor-1 (PAI-1). These proinflammatory metabolites have been implicated in the pathogenesis of NAFLD and also disrupt intestinal cell repair and apoptosis, thus potentiating tumorigenesis (49). Furthermore, NAFLD patients have disordered adipocytokine metabolism. Typically, adiponectin has anticarcinogenic effects as it suppresses cell growth of carcinoma through the AMPc-activated protein kinase. Decreased adiponectin and increased leptin serum levels have been demonstrated in NAFLD patients. These hormones, secreted by adipocytes, have been proposed to play an important role in the development of colorectal cancer (50).

19.6 NAFLD AND THE PANCREATICOBILIARY TRACT

19.6.1 Biliary Disease and Cancer

NAFLD and gallbladder disease share similar risk factors, such as obesity, insulin resistance, dyslipidemia, and high dietary cholesterol intake. In particular, female sex, increased age, higher BMI, and the presence of NASH and fibrosis are associated with the development of cholelithiasis in NAFLD patients. In one meta-analysis, the pooled prevalence of gallbladder disease in NAFLD patients was 17%, which is higher than in the general population (51). In other studies, the prevalence of cholelithiasis in NAFLD patients was found to be as high as 47% (52). It is well-known that in obesity, diabetes and hypertriglyceridemia, secretion of biliary cholesterol as well as gallbladder motility are disrupted and that biliary composition and gallbladder emptying are affected. At the cellular level, NAFLD patients were found to have a decreased level of farnesoid X receptor and its mRNA in liver tissue. This nuclear receptor plays an important role in regulating the transcription of ATP-binding cassette transporters on the hepatocyte canalicular membrane, resulting in decreased activity of bile salt export pumps. Consequently, there is a decrease in biliary concentration of bile acids and phospholipids, leading to reduced solubility of cholesterol and thus increased risk of gallstone formation.

Biliary tract cancers, including cholangiocarcinoma (CCA) and gallbladder cancer, are the second most common type of hepatobiliary cancer worldwide. NAFLD is associated with an increased risk of CCA, particularly intrahepatic CCA, and the risk is further increased in NASH patients (53,54). This is primarily thought to occur via the induction of hepatic inflammation. As with colorectal cancer, it is mediated through NAFLD-associated gut dysbiosis, which can promote carcinogenesis via the gut-liver axis. The hypothesized mechanism consists of increased intestinal permeability and hepatic production and systemic release of numerous pro-inflammatory cytokines that promote carcinogenesis through proliferation, antiapoptosis and angiogenesis. This effect appears to be independent of other factors such as obesity (55).

19.6.2 Pancreatitis

NAFLD has been associated with acute pancreatitis (AP), independent of obesity. In hospitalized patients, the presence of NAFLD was shown to increase the risk of death, more severe AP, necrotizing pancreatitis, SIRS and length of hospital stay. Furthermore, in one study, NAFLD was found to be a risk factor for postendoscopic retrograde cholangiopancreatography pancreatitis. Such patients may benefit from prophylactic pancreatic stenting and/or rectal NSAID therapy (56).

19.6.3 Pancreatic Cancer

NAFLD may be an important risk factor for pancreatic cancer, presumably related to high BMI and visceral adiposity. In one study, NAFLD was also found to be an independent risk factor for pancreatic cancer and was associated with decreased survival following diagnosis. The role of NAFLD in pancreatic cancer may be driven by dysregulated cytokine activity, promoting the progression of pancreatic cancer. Insulin resistance results in the release of pro-inflammatory cytokines from excess. Cytokines, such as adiponectin, IGF-1, TNF-α, IL-6 and

VEGF, contribute to the development of cancer through angiogenesis, cell migration and mitogenesis (57).

19.7 SUMMARY

Nonalcoholic fatty liver disease (NAFLD) is associated with a variety of extrahepatic gastrointestinal manifestations. The prevalence of esophageal, gastric, small bowel, colonic and pancreaticobiliary diseases in this patient population has important implications in the management of NAFLD as a multisystem disease. Alterations in the gut microbiome, insulin resistance and the release of pro-inflammatory cytokines may account for these associated conditions. Further studies are needed to determine the optimal methods by which to manage NAFLD patients as they pertain to extrahepatic manifestations of the disease, including the potential impact on surveillance for malignancy among patients with NAFLD.

REFERENCES

1. Miele L, Cammarota G, Vero V, Racco S, Cefalo C, Marrone G, Pompili M, Rapaccini G, Bianco A, Landolfi R, Gasbarrini A, Grieco A. Non-alcoholic fatty liver disease is associated with high prevalence of gastro-oesophageal reflux symptoms. *Dig Liver Dis.* 2012;44(12):1032–1036. doi:10.1016/j.dld.2012.08.005. Epub 2012 Sep 7. PMID: 22963909

2. Hung WC, Wu JS, Yang YC, Sun ZJ, Lu FH, Chang CJ. Nonalcoholic fatty liver disease vs. obesity on the risk of erosive oesophagitis. *Eur J Clin Invest.* 2014;44(12):1143–1149. doi:10.1111/eci.12348. Epub 2014 Nov 3. PMID: 25293867

3. Yang HJ, Chang Y, Park SK, Jung YS, Park JH, Park DI, Cho YK, Ryu S, Sohn CI. Nonalcoholic fatty liver disease is associated with increased risk of reflux esophagitis. *Dig Dis Sci.* 2017;62(12):3605–3613. doi:10.1007/s10620-017-4805-6. Epub 2017 Oct 23. PMID: 29063416

4. Mikolasevic I, Poropat G, Filipec Kanizaj T, Skenderevic N, Zelic M, Matasin M, Vranic L, Kresovic A, Hauser G. Association between gastroesophageal reflux disease and elastographic parameters of liver steatosis and fibrosis: controlled attenuation parameter and liver stiffness measurements. *Can J Gastroenterol Hepatol.* 2021;2021:6670065. doi:10.1155/2021/6670065. PMID: 33688490; PMCID: PMC7925017

5. Taketani H, Sumida Y, Tanaka S, Imajo K, Yoneda M, Hyogo H, Ono M, Fujii H, Eguchi Y, Kanemasa K, Chayama K, Itoh Y, Yoshikawa T, Saibara T, Fujimoto K, Nakajima A, Japan Study Group of NAFLD. The association of insomnia with gastroesophageal reflux symptoms in biopsy-proven nonalcoholic fatty liver disease. *J Gastroenterol.* 2014;49(7):1163–1174. doi:10.1007/s00535-013-0871-5. Epub 2013 Aug 22. PMID: 23975270

6. Spiegel K, Leproult R, L'Hermite-Balériaux M, Copinschi G, Penev PD, Van Cauter E. Leptin levels are dependent on sleep duration: relationships with sympathovagal balance, carbohydrate regulation, cortisol, and thyrotropin. *J Clin Endocrinol Metab.* 2004;89:5762–5771. doi:10.1210/jc.2004-1003

7. Akiyama T, Yoneda M, Inamori M, Iida H, Endo H, Hosono K, Yoneda K, Fujita K, Koide T, Tokoro C, Takahashi H, Goto A, Abe Y, Kirikoshi H, Kobayashi N, Kubota K, Saito S, Nakajima A. Visceral obesity and the risk of Barrett's esophagus in Japanese patients with non-alcoholic fatty liver disease. *BMC Gastroenterol.* 2009;9:56. doi:10.1186/1471-230X-9-56. PMID: 19622165; PMCID: PMC2718904

8. Kubo A, Cook M, Shaheen N, Vaughan T, Whiteman D, Murray L, Corley DA. Sex specific associations between body mass index, waist circumference and the risk of Barrett's oesophagus: a pooled analysis from the international BEACON consortium. *Gut* 2013;62:1684–1691.

9. El-Serag H, Hashmi A, Garcia J, Richardson P, Alsarraj A, Fitzgerald S, Vela M, Shaib Y, Abraham NS, Velez M, et al. Visceral abdominal obesity measured by CT scan is associated with an increased risk of Barrett's oesophagus: a case-control study. *Gut* 2014;63:220–229.

10. Garcia J, Splenser A, Kramer J, Alsarraj A, Fitzgerald S, Ramsey D, El-Serag HB. Circulating inflammatory cytokines and adipokines are associated with increased risk of Barrett's esophagus: a case-control study. *Clin Gastroenterol Hepatol.* 2014;12:229–238.

11. Apfel T, Lopez R, Sanaka MR, Thota PN. Risk of progression of Barrett's esophagus in patients with cirrhosis. *World J Gastroenterol.* 2017;23(18):3287–3294. doi:10.3748/wjg.v23.i18.3287. PMID: 28566888; PMCID: PMC5434434

12. Singh S, Sharma AN, Murad MH, Buttar NS, El-Serag HB, Katzka DA, Iyer PG. Central adiposity is associated with increased risk of esophageal inflammation, metaplasia, and adenocarcinoma: a systematic review and meta-analysis. *Clin Gastroenterol Hepatol.* 2013;11:1399–1412.

13. Beddy P, Howard J, McMahon C, Knox M, de Blacam C, Ravi N, Reynolds JV, Keogan MT. Association of visceral adiposity with oesophageal and junctional adenocarcinomas. *Br J Surg.* 2010;97:1028–1034.

14. Merry A, Schouten L, Goldbohm R, van Den Brandt P. Body mass index, height and risk of adenocarcinoma of the oesophagus and gastric cardias: a prospective cohort study. *Gut.* 2007;56:1503–1511.

15. El-Serag H, Ergun G, Pandolfino J, Fitzgerald S, Tran T, Kramer J. Obesity increases oesophageal acid exposure. *Gut.* 2007;56:749–755.

16. Choi YJ, Lee DH, Han KD, Yoon H, Shin CM, Park YS, et al. Elevated serum gamma-glutamyltransferase is associated with an increased risk of oesophageal carcinoma in a cohort of 8,388,256 Korean subjects. *PLoS ONE.* 2017;12(5):e0177053. Epub 2017/05/06. doi:10.1371/journal.pone.0177053

17. Wong VW, Hui AY, Tsang SW, Chan JL, Tse AM, Chan KF, et al. Metabolic and adipokine profile of Chinese patients with nonalcoholic fatty liver disease. *Clin Gastroenterol Hepatol.* 2006;4(9):1154–1161. Epub 2006/08/15. doi:10.1016/j.cgh.2006.06.011

18. Ning L, Liu R, Lou X, Du H, Chen W, Zhang F, Li S, Chen X, Xu G. Association between Helicobacter pylori infection and nonalcoholic fatty liver disease: a systemic review and meta-analysis. *Eur J Gastroenterol Hepatol.* 2019;31(7):735–742. doi:10.1097/MEG.0000000000001398. PMID: 30950907

19. Hossain IA, Akter S, Bhuiyan FR, Shah MR, Rahman MK, Ali L. Subclinical inflammation in relation to insulin resistance in prediabetic subjects with nonalcoholic fatty liver disease. *BMC Res Notes.* 2016;9:266. doi:10.1186/s13104-016-2071-x

20. Abenavoli L, Milic N, Masarone M, Persico M. Association between non-alcoholic fatty liver disease, insulin resistance and *Helicobacter pylori*. *Med Hypotheses.* 2013;81:913–915. doi:10.1016/j.mehy.2013.08.011

21. Tsai CC, Kuo TY, Hong ZW, Yeh YC, Shih KS, Du SY, et al. *Helicobacter pylori* neutrophil-activating protein

induces release of histamine and interleukin-6 through G protein-mediated MAPKs and PI3K/Akt pathways in HMC-1 cells. *Virulence*. 2015;6:755–765. doi:10.1080/21505594.2015.1043505

22. Cheng DD, He C, Ai HH, Huang Y, Lu NH. The possible role of *Helicobacter pylori* infection in non-alcoholic fatty liver disease. *Front Microbiol*. 2017;8:743. Published 2017 May 10. doi:10.3389/fmicb.2017.00743

23. Hamaguchi M, Hashimoto Y, Obora A, Kojima T, Fukui M. Non-alcoholic fatty liver disease with obesity as an independent predictor for incident gastric and colorectal cancer: a population-based longitudinal study. *BMJ Open Gastroenterol*. 2019;6(1):e000295. doi:10.1136/bmjgast-2019-000295. PMID: 31275587; PMCID: PMC6577367

24. Uzel M, Sahiner Z, Filik L. Non-alcoholic fatty liver disease, metabolic syndrome and gastric cancer: single center experience. *J Buon*. 2015;20(2):662. PMID: 26011365

25. Reilly NR, Lebwohl B, Hultcrantz R, Green PHR, Ludvigsson JF. Increased risk of non-alcoholic fatty liver disease after diagnosis of celiac disease. *J Hepatol*. 2015;62:1405–1411. doi:10.1016/j.jhep.2015.01.013

26. Kälsch J, Bechmann LP, Manka P, Kahraman A, Schlattjan M, Marth T, Rehbehn K, Baba HA, Canbay A. Non-alcoholic steatohepatitis occurs in celiac disease and is associated with cellular stress. *Z Gastroenterol*. 2013;51(1):26–31. doi:10.1055/s-0032-1330421. Epub 2013 Jan 11. PMID: 23315648

27. Miele L, Valenza V, La Torre G, Montalto M, Cammarota G, Ricci R, et al. Increased intestinal permeability and tight junction alterations in nonalcoholic fatty liver disease. *Hepatology*. 2009;49:1877–1887.

28. Fitriakusumah Y, Lesmana CRA, Bastian WP, Jasirwan COM, Hasan I, Simadibrata M, Kurniawan J, Sulaiman AS, Gani RA. The role of Small Intestinal Bacterial Overgrowth (SIBO) in Non-alcoholic Fatty Liver Disease (NAFLD) patients evaluated using Controlled Attenuation Parameter (CAP) Transient Elastography (TE): a tertiary referral center experience. *BMC Gastroenterol*. 2019;19(1):43. doi:10.1186/s12876-019-0960-x. PMID: 30894137; PMCID: PMC6427876

29. Mikolasevic I, Delija B, Mijic A, Stevanovic T, Skenderevic N, Sosa I, Krznaric-Zrnic I, Abram M, Krznaric Z, Domislovic V, Filipec Kanizaj T, Radic-Kristo D, Cubranic A, Grubesic A, Nakov R, Skrobonja I, Stimac D, Hauser G. Small intestinal bacterial overgrowth and non-alcoholic fatty liver disease diagnosed by transient elastography and liver biopsy. *Int J Clin Pract*. 2021;75(4):e13947. doi:10.1111/ijcp.13947. Epub 2021 Feb 16. PMID: 33406286

30. Kapil S, Duseja A, Sharma BK, Singla B, Chakraborti A, Das A, Ray P, Dhiman RK, Chawla Y. Small intestinal bacterial overgrowth and toll-like receptor signaling in patients with non-alcoholic fatty liver disease. *J Gastroenterol Hepatol*. 2016;31(1):213–221. doi:10.1111/jgh.13058. PMID: 26212089

31. Ferolla SM, Armiliato GN, Couto CA, Ferrari TC. The role of intestinal bacteria overgrowth in obesity-related nonalcoholic fatty liver disease. *Nutrients*. 2014;6(12):5583–5599. Published 2014 Dec 3. doi:10.3390/nu6125583

32. Cappello M, Randazzo C, Bravata I, et al. Liver function test abnormalities in patients with inflammatory bowel diseases: a hospital-based survey. *Clin Med Insights Gastroenterol*. 2014;7:25–31.

33. Glassner K, Malaty HM, Abraham BP. Epidemiology and risk factors of nonalcoholic fatty liver disease among patients with inflammatory bowel disease. *Inflamm Bowel Dis*. 2017;23:998–1003.

34. Gizard E, Ford AC, Bronowicki JP, Peyrin-Biroulet L. Systematic review: the epidemiology of the hepatobiliary manifestations in patients with inflammatory bowel disease. *Aliment Pharmacol Ther*. 2014;40:3–15.

35. Principi M, Iannone A, Losurdo G, Mangia M, Shahini E, Albano F, Rizzi SF, La Fortezza RF, Lovero R, Contaldo A, Barone M, Leandro G, Ierardi E, Di Leo A. Nonalcoholic fatty liver disease in inflammatory bowel disease: prevalence and risk factors. *Inflamm Bowel Dis*. 2018;24(7):1589–1596. doi:10.1093/ibd/izy051. PMID: 29688336

36. Bessissow T, Le NH, Rollet K, et al. Incidence and predictors of nonalcoholic fatty liver disease by serum biomarkers in patients with inflammatory bowel disease. *Inflamm Bowel Dis*. 2016;22:1937–1944.

37. Wiest R, Albillos A, Trauner M, et al. Targeting the gut-liver axis in liver disease. *J Hepatol*. 2017;67:1084–1103.

38. Sartini A, Gitto S, Bianchini M, et al. Non-alcoholic fatty liver disease phenotypes in patients with inflammatory bowel disease. *Cell Death Dis*. 2018;9(2):87. Published 2018 Jan 24. doi:10.1038/s41419-017-0124-2

39. Likhitsup A, Dundulis J, Ansari S, et al. High prevalence of non-alcoholic fatty liver disease in patients with inflammatory bowel disease receiving anti-tumor necrosis factor therapy. *Ann Gastroenterol*. 2019;32(5):463–468. doi:10.20524/aog.2019.0405

40. Scalera A, Di Minno MN, Tarantino G. What does irritable bowel syndrome share with non-alcoholic fatty liver disease?. *World J Gastroenterol*. 2013;19(33):5402–5420. doi:10.3748/wjg.v19.i33.5402

41. Purssell H, Whorwell PJ, Athwal VS, Vasant DH. Non-alcoholic fatty liver disease in irritable bowel syndrome: more than a coincidence? *World J Hepatol*. 2021;13(12):1816–1827. doi:10.4254/wjh.v13.i12.1816. PMID: 35069992; PMCID: PMC8727221

42. Milovanovic T, Pantic I, Dragasevic S, Lugonja S, Dumic I, Rajilic-Stojanovic M. The interrelationship among non-alcoholic fatty liver disease, colonic diverticulosis and metabolic syndrome. *J Gastrointestin Liver Dis*. 2021;30(2):274–282. doi:10.15403/jgld-3308. PMID: 33951119

43. Papić N, Jelovčić F, Karlović M, Marić LS, Vince A. Nonalcoholic fatty liver disease as a risk factor for Clostridioides difficile infection. *Eur J Clin Microbiol Infect Dis*. 2020;39(3):569–574. doi:10.1007/s10096-019-03759-w. Epub 2019 Nov 28. PMID: 31782025

44. Blackett JW, Verna EC, Lebwohl B. Increased prevalence of colorectal adenomas in patients with nonalcoholic fatty liver disease: a cross-sectional study. *Dig Dis*. 2020;38(3):222–230. doi:10.1159/000502684. Epub 2019 Aug 30. PMID: 31473746

45. Hwang ST, Cho YK, Park JH, Kim HJ, Park DI, Sohn CI, et al. Relationship of non-alcoholic fatty liver disease to colorectal adenomatous polyps. *J Gastroenterol Hepatol*. 2010;25(3):562–567

46. Seo JY, Bae JH, Kwak MS, Yang JI, Chung SJ, Yim JY, Lim SH, Chung GE. The risk of colorectal adenoma in nonalcoholic or metabolic-associated fatty liver disease. *Biomedicines*. 2021;9(10):1401. doi:10.3390/biomedicines9101401. PMID: 34680518; PMCID: PMC8533199

47. Li Y, Liu S, Gao Y, Ma H, Zhan S, Yang Y, Xin Y, Xuan S. Association between NAFLD and risk of

colorectal adenoma in Chinese Han population. *J Clin Transl Hepatol.* 2019;7(2):99–105. doi:10.14218/JCTH.2019.00010. Epub 2019 May 4. PMID: 31293908; PMCID: PMC6609839

48. Lin XF, Shi KQ, You J, Liu WY, Luo YW, Wu FL, Chen YP, Wong DK, Yuen MF, Zheng MH. Increased risk of colorectal malignant neoplasm in patients with nonalcoholic fatty liver disease: a large study. *Mol Biol Rep.* 2014;41(5):2989–2997. doi:10.1007/s11033-014-3157-y. Epub 2014 Jan 22. PMID: 24449368

49. Chen J, Bian D, Zang S, Yang Z, Tian G, Luo Y, Yang J, Xu B, Shi J. The association between non-alcoholic fatty liver disease and risk of colorectal adenoma and cancer incident and recurrence: a meta-analysis of observational studies. *Expert Rev Gastroenterol Hepatol.* 2019;13(4):385–395. doi:10.1080/17474124.2019.1580143. Epub 2019 Feb 19. PMID: 30791768

50. An W, Bai Y, Deng SX, Gao J, Ben QW, Cai QC, Zhang HG, Li ZS. Adiponectin levels in patients with colorectal cancer and adenoma: a meta-analysis. *Eur J Cancer Prev.* 2012;21:126–133.

51. Shen SS, Gong JJ, Wang XW, Chen L, Qin S, Huang LF, Chen YQ, Ren H, Yang QB, Hu HD. Promotional effect of nonalcoholic fatty liver disease on Gallstone disease: a systematic review and meta-analysis. *Turk J Gastroenterol.* 2017;28(1):31–39. doi:10.5152/tjg.2016.0357. Epub 2016 Dec 19. PMID: 27991855

52. Koller T, Kollerova J, Hlavaty T, Huorka M, Payer J. Cholelithiasis and markers of nonalcoholic fatty liver disease in patients with metabolic risk factors. *Scand J Gastroenterol.* 2012;47(2):197–203. doi:10.3109/00365521.2011.643481. Epub 2011 Dec 19. PMID: 22182015

53. Ghidini M, Ramai D, Facciorusso A, Singh J, Tai W, Rijavec E, Galassi B, Grossi F, Indini A. Metabolic disorders and the risk of cholangiocarcinoma. *Expert Rev Gastroenterol Hepatol.* 2021;15(9):999–1007. doi:10.1080/17474124.2021.1946393. Epub 2021 Aug 21. PMID: 34423721

54. Wongjarupong N, Assavapongpaiboon B, Susantitaphong P, Cheungpasitporn W, Treeprasertsuk S, Rerknimitr R, Chaiteerakij R. Nonalcoholic fatty liver disease as a risk factor for cholangiocarcinoma: a systematic review and meta-analysis. *BMC Gastroenterol.* 2017;17(1):149. doi:10.1186/s12876-017-0696-4. PMID: 29216833; PMCID: PMC5721586

55. Park JH, Hong JY, Kwon M, Lee J, Han K, Han IW, Kang W, Park JK. Association between non-alcoholic fatty liver disease and the risk of biliary tract cancers: a South Korean nationwide cohort study. *Eur J Cancer.* 2021;150:73–82. doi:10.1016/j.ejca.2021.03.024. Epub 2021 Apr 20. PMID: 33892409

56. Hou S, Tang X, Cui H, Liu C, Bai X, Shi L, Shi Y. Fatty liver disease is associated with the severity of acute pancreatitis:A systematic review and meta-analysis. *Int J Surg.* 2019;65:147–153. doi:10.1016/j.ijsu.2019.04.003. Epub 2019 Apr 12. PMID: 30986497

57. Chang CF, Tseng YC, Huang HH, Shih YL, Hsieh TY, Lin HH. Exploring the relationship between nonalcoholic fatty liver disease and pancreatic cancer by computed tomographic survey. *Intern Emerg Med.* 2018;13(2):191–197. doi:10.1007/s11739-017-1774-x. Epub 2017 Dec 12. PMID: 29235054

20 Extrahepatic and Hepatic Cancers

Maryam Ibrahim and Tracey G. Simon

CONTENTS

Key Points

- NAFLD is a multisystem disease associated with extrahepatic complications and cancers.

- Carcinogenesis is mediated through changes in lipid metabolism, growth and proliferation pathways, oxidative stress, immune signaling, genetics and microbiome.

- Robust evidence is available for the increased incidence of HCC (hepatocellular carcinoma) in NAFLD.

- NAFLD has been linked to increased cholangiocarcinoma risk, with a stronger association for intrahepatic cholangiocarcinoma.

- There appears to be a higher prevalence of colorectal lesions in NAFLD.

- More evidence is still needed for associations between NAFLD and esophageal, gastric, pancreatic, renal, prostate, breast, uterine, lung and hematologic cancers.

20.1 INTRODUCTION

NAFLD is now viewed as a multisystem disease that is associated with extrahepatic complications [1]. Increasing evidence now links NAFLD with various diseases, including diabetes, kidney disease, cardiovascular disease and cancer. Recently, there has been increased attention to the possible association between NAFLD and cancer development. Malignancies, whether within or outside the GI tract, represent significant contributors to death in patients with NAFLD [1]. While the precise mechanisms linking NAFLD to carcinogenesis are largely undefined, NAFLD is viewed as the hepatic manifestation of metabolic syndrome, and a body of evidence indicates an increased

risk of cancer—particularly gastrointestinal and hepatic cancers—in patients with metabolic syndrome [2]. In this setting, NAFLD can either share common risk factors (such as obesity or type 2 diabetes), or it may actively mediate various pathogenic mechanisms, leading to cancer [2]. In this chapter, we review the current evidence and potential mechanisms underpinning observed associations between NAFLD and both hepatic and extrahepatic cancers (with a focus on cholangiocarcinoma, colorectal, esophageal, gastric, pancreatic, genitourinary, breast, uterine, lung and hematologic cancers).

20.2 CARCINOGENESIS IN NAFLD: Potential Mechanisms

20.2.1 Hepatic Cancers

It has been hypothesized that the pathogenesis of cancer in patients with NAFLD is related to a complex range of environmental factors (lifestyle, diet, microbiome) acting upon a susceptible genetic or epigenetic background in order to modify responses to caloric excess [3]. Obesity, diabetes and the metabolic syndrome are essential elements of the association between NAFLD and HCC [4,5]. Dyslipidemia and hypertension, two additional components of metabolic syndrome, have also been shown to contribute to HCC risk in a recent analysis of US patients from the Veterans Healthcare Administration [4]. As such, NASH-HCC pathogenesis is influenced by derangements that occur in the setting of obesity and the metabolic syndrome, which include oxidative stress and aberrant lipid metabolism [4]. In particular, the excess accumulation of intrahepatic lipids promotes mitochondrial dysfunction and oxidative stress, which in turn ignites a cascade of carcinogenic and pro-inflammatory processes including changes in

DOI: 10.1201/9781003386698-24

lipid metabolism, activation of growth and proliferation pathways, as well as changes in the immune response [4] (see Figure 20.1).

While the precise mechanism linking obesity and the metabolic syndrome to the pathogenesis of NAFLD-HCC is still undefined, several have been proposed. One proposed mechanism is through changes in lipid metabolism. In order for hepatocytes to escape lipotoxicity, they downregulate carnitine palmitoyltransferase 2 (CPT2), which drives malignant transformation through the accumulation of acylcarnitine [6]. Moreover, sterol regulatory element-binding proteins transcription factors (SREBPs), which are known to interact with p53, are modified in the setting of oxidative stress, and this may contribute to hepatocarcinogenesis [7] (see Figure 20.1).

NAFLD-related HCC may also arise through changes in growth and proliferation pathways, which are directly affected by the metabolic syndrome. Fatty acid accumulation induces junctional protein associated with coronary artery disease (JCAD), a protein which promotes the progression of NASH to HCC by inhibiting LATS2 kinase activity [8]. The Hedgehog (Hh) pathway is consistently activated in NASH, with a level of activity that correlates with liver disease severity, and increased Hh pathway activity has also been observed in hepatic carcinogenesis

[9]. Insulin resistance and insulin-like growth factor (IGF) signaling have also been implicated in NASH-HCC. Insulin resistance and subsequent hyperinsulinemia increase the activity of IGF-1, which stimulates hepatocyte growth via Akt and mTOR, potentially driving liver carcinogenesis [10]. IGF-1 demonstrates antiapoptotic effects in NASH animal models, but the paradoxical upregulation of IGF-1R in HCC tissue suggests that the antiapoptotic effect might be driving abnormal growth [11]. Oxidative stress induces caspase-2, which drives apoptosis and the subsequent compensatory proliferation of hepatocytes [12,13]. Finally, it has been proposed that oxidative stress could promote hepatocarcinogenesis by impacting immune signaling pathways [4]. Specifically, CD4+T cells which play a pivotal role in antitumor surveillance are selectively lost due to susceptibility to oxidative stress [14]. Obesity-related chronic inflammation activates Kupffer cells through TREM1 receptor, which drives the secretion of inflammatory cytokines such as IL-6 and TNF-a. This causes alterations in NF-kB signaling, hepatocyte proliferation and subsequent HCC development [15,16] (see Figure 20.1).

Other mechanisms implicated in NASH-HCC development include genetic variants and gut microbiota [4]. Genetic variants associated with HCC include patatin-like

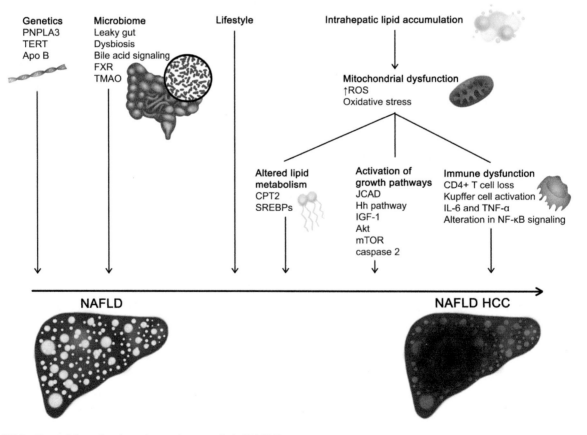

Figure 20.1 Potential mechanisms for carcinogenesis in NAFLD

PNPLA3: Patatin-like phospholipase domain-containing protein 3; TERT: Telomerase reverse transcriptase; Apo B: Apolipoprotein B; FXR: Farnesoid X receptor; TMAO: Trimethylamine N-oxide; ROS: Reactive oxygen species; CPT2: Carnitine palmitoyltransferase 2; SREBP: Sterol regulatory element-binding proteins; JCAD: Junctional protein associated with coronary artery disease; Hh: Hedgehog; IGF-1: Insulin-like growth factor-1; Akt: Protein kinase B; mTOR: Mammalian target of rapamycin; IL-6: Interleukin-6; NF-kB: Nuclear factor kappa light chain enhancer of activated B cells.

phospholipase domain-containing protein 3 (*PNPLA3*) polymorphisms, telomerase reverse transcriptase (*TERT*) promoter mutations and apolipoprotein B mutations, among others [17–19]. Moreover, increasing evidence suggests the role of gut dysbiosis in cirrhosis and subsequent HCC development. In a study of patients with NASH cirrhosis, patients with HCC had increased levels of *Bacteroides* and *Ruminococcaceae*, whereas *Akkermansia* and *Bifidobacterium* were reduced in comparison to NASH-cirrhosis without HCC [20]. NASH-HCC has also been linked to dysbiosis through bile acid signaling to liver cells, which triggers upregulation in growth pathways such as mTOR [21,22]. The gut microbiome regulates bile acids and consequently the farnesoid X receptor (FXR), a bile acid sensor [23]. FXR helps to prevent hepatocarcinogenesis by protecting against bile acid-related liver injury and modulating fibrosis in mouse models [23]. Further studies are needed to investigate the role of FXR signaling in metabolic syndrome, NASH, and NASH to HCC transition [24]. Other metabolites through which the gut microbiome could contribute to HCC development include trimethylamine (TMA) and its metabolite trimethylamine *N*-oxide (TMAO) as well as ethanol, which are generated by gut bacteria [22]. High TMAO levels are associated with insulin resistance, suggesting that it could contribute to NAFLD progression and possibly NASH-HCC [22]. Ethanol, a known hepatotoxin and carcinogen, is produced by gut microbiota and is increased in patients with NASH [22]. Whether this contributes to NAFLD progression and HCC development is currently unknown (see Figure 20.1).

20.2.2 Extrahepatic Cancers

Several mechanisms have been suggested to link NAFLD to extrahepatic cancers, mainly through obesity-related chronic inflammation, dysbiosis, insulin resistance and changes in adiponectin and leptin levels [4,25]. However, the exact mechanism by which NAFLD might promote extrahepatic tumorigenesis remains unclear. It was suggested that visceral adipose tissue accumulation in NAFLD may affect other organs by releasing cytokines such as growth factors, adipocytokines and proinflammatory factors [26]. Emerging data support the fact that local ectopic fat may affect the paracrine pathway to induce cancer development in the pancreas and breast [27,28]. However, these findings remain preliminary, and future research is needed to precisely define the mechanisms and pathways that might link NAFLD to the development of extrahepatic cancers.

20.3 NAFLD AND GI MALIGNANCIES: Clinical and Epidemiological Data
20.3.1 Hepatocellular Carcinoma

HCC is one of very few cancers with growing incidence and mortality in the US and worldwide [29], and it now represents the fourth leading cause of cancer death in the world [30,31]. In parallel with the growing epidemics of obesity and type 2 diabetes, NAFLD is a growing cause of HCC in the US [4]. Studies from South Korea, Europe and southeast Asia have shown a similar rapid increase in NAFLD-HCC over the last two decades [23]. In the US, it is now the fastest growing cause of HCC among listed liver transplant candidates as well as transplant recipients [32].

In cohorts of patients with NASH in Europe and the US, the annual incidence of HCC ranges from 0.7 to 2.6% [33,34]. The incidence of HCC in patients with NASH is higher in men, older patients, Hispanics and patients with

higher alcohol intake and diabetes [5,33,35]. A prospective cohort of biopsy-proven NASH cirrhosis from Japan had an 11.3% 5-year incidence of HCC [36]. This cohort was older and had a higher prevalence of diabetes, which could account for the higher observed HCC incidence [23]. In a population-based cohort study conducted by Simon et al. including 8,892 adults with histologically defined NAFLD in Sweden, NAFLD patients had significantly increased overall cancer incidence (10.9 vs. 13.8/1,000 person-years [PYs]; aHR, 1.27 [95%CI, 1.18–1.36]), driven primarily by HCC (aHR, 17.08 [95%CI, 11.56–25.25]) [37].

The mean age of NAFLD-related HCC is 73 years, which is higher than the mean age of patients with viral hepatitis-related HCC [38]. NASH-HCC is diagnosed at a later stage, and the mortality appears to be higher than HCC from other liver conditions [38,39]. The lack of public awareness surrounding NAFLD and its progression, as well as the lack of HCC screening guidelines in high-risk patients with NAFLD without cirrhosis contributes to the late diagnosis and treatment [23].

It is estimated that 3–5% of the current adult US population have NASH, with a projected increase in the prevalence rate by 2030 [40]. It has also been reported that HCC may arise in patients with NASH even in the absence of cirrhosis; thus the rising NASH prevalence is quite alarming [4]. In two large studies in the Veterans Healthcare Administration, 20 to 36% of NASH-HCC cases did not have underlying cirrhosis, and NAFLD was the leading etiology of HCC in patients without cirrhosis [35,41]. An Italian multicenter cohort of patients with NAFLD-HCC found that 50% of the patients were without cirrhosis but rather had advanced fibrosis [39]. This suggests that the fibrosis stage might be relevant in future efforts to risk-stratify NAFLD patients according to their future HCC risk [23]. Similarly, in a Japanese multicenter cohort, 72% of the patients with biopsy-proven NAFLD-HCC had advanced fibrosis (F3 and F4) [42], further underscoring that HCC may develop in NASH with advanced fibrosis [23].

The proportions of patients with HCC attributable to NAFLD varies widely across different counties/regions, with percentages ranging between 1 and 38% [23], due in large part to discrepancies in definitions of NAFLD and its ascertainment [23]. Several US studies have used either primary diagnoses reported in national transplantation databases or ICD-9 codes from large national registries [23]. Many studies have expanded their study definitions to include patients with cryptogenic cirrhosis and components of the metabolic syndrome, as NAFLD is often underreported [43,44]. Some studies also include patients with cryptogenic cirrhosis even without the metabolic syndrome [45]. However, a notable prior study by Thuluvath et al., looking at the United Network for Organ Sharing database, found that patients with cryptogenic cirrhosis have a different risk factor profile than patients with NASH cirrhosis and concluded that NASH cirrhosis and cryptogenic cirrhosis are not equivalent [46]. Further adjustment in the definitions of suspected cryptogenic cirrhosis and NASH cirrhosis would be important for a more precise estimate of the proportion of patients with NAFLD-HCC without cirrhosis, as well as the risk of HCC in patients with cirrhosis of either etiology [23].

Several studies around the world have specifically investigated the relationship between diabetes and HCC risk among patients with NAFLD. In a Mayo Clinic study, the presence of diabetes was associated with a 4-fold increase in the risk of HCC in patients with NASH cirrhosis. This was validated using liver transplant registrants identified within the United Network for Organ Sharing, whereby diabetes was an independent risk factor for HCC development in patients with NASH cirrhosis [5]. Diabetes was also the strongest independent risk factor for HCC development in patients with NAFLD in a large European population-based study [47]. Moreover, Kanwal et al. found that among patients with NAFLD, the presence of additional, comorbid metabolic traits led to a stepwise increase in HCC risk and that diabetes was associated with the highest risk of development of HCC [48]. Collectively, these findings underscored the importance of regular screening for diabetes and rigorous attention to blood sugar control, among patients with NAFLD [23].

20.3.2 HCC Surveillance/Screening

NASH-HCC has a unique natural history and pathogenesis that makes HCC surveillance in patients with NASH quite challenging [4]. There is no current high-level, NAFLD-specific evidence to support or refute the clinical impact and cost-effectiveness of established HCC surveillance protocols in the setting of NAFLD or NASH cirrhosis [23]. Accordingly, it is recommended that all patients with NAFLD cirrhosis—as in all etiologies of cirrhosis—undergo regular semiannual HCC screening [49]. However, there is increasing attention paid to the need for more personalized HCC surveillance protocols. Importantly, as NAFLD patients without cirrhosis can develop HCC, HCC surveillance might be considered in selected, high-risk patients with advanced fibrosis on a case-by-case basis [23].

The American Gastroenterology Association (AGA) Clinical Practice Update recommends considering HCC screening in patients with noninvasive markers that indicate the presence of advanced fibrosis (F3) or cirrhosis [50]. The AGA recommends combining 2 or more noninvasive fibrosis tests of separate categories (imaging based and blood based) in order to minimize the likelihood of misclassification [23]. If the test results are concordant for either advanced fibrosis or cirrhosis, the AGA recommends consideration of HCC surveillance [23]. The European Association for the Study of the Liver (EASL) guidelines recommend individual risk assessment for HCC surveillance in patients with liver disease of any etiology with advanced fibrosis (F3) [51]. No specific recommendations for HCC surveillance in NAFLD patients without cirrhosis are provided by the Asian Pacific Association for the Study of Liver disease (APASL) clinical practice guidelines [52,53].

Patients without advanced fibrosis have too low an HCC risk, and as such routine screening is not currently recommended [35]. The recommended modality for HCC surveillance in the AASLD, APASL and EASL practice guidelines is ultrasonography with or without concomitant alpha-fetoprotein level [51,52,54]. In a study of 941 patients with cirrhosis undergoing ultrasonography, the quality was inadequate to exclude liver lesions in 20% of the scans [55]. Elevated BMI and NASH cirrhosis were independent factors associated with inadequate quality of scans [55]. Thus it is imperative for future clinical and implementation research to focus on improving both the methods of assessment and the reporting of the quality of HCC surveillance ultrasonography in order to improve early detection of NAFLD-HCC tumors.

20.3.3 Challenges and Future Prospects

There continues to be a debate over the cost-effectiveness and potential harm from overinvestigating false positive tests for HCC screening [24]. The debate is especially pertinent for NAFLD patients, as they are more likely to have unrecognized liver disease and are at high risk of having low-quality imaging studies for HCC screening. Even in known NAFLD-associated cirrhosis, surveillance is less likely to detect early NAFLD-associated HCC than HCC arising from other etiologies [24]. This is also relevant when considering initiation of HCC surveillance in patients with advanced NAFLD, who do not have cirrhosis. This represents an enormous and growing population, which is exposed to a relatively small—albeit devastating—risk, and in that setting it has thus far been felt that the cost of ultrasound surveillance is prohibitive [24]. Currently, the hope is that further research will identify combinations of factors that can better risk-stratify patients with NAFLD, in order to create more targeted, cost-effective surveillance strategies [24]. To that end, the combination GALAD serum score has shown promising diagnostic performance, and its prospective evaluation as an HCC surveillance biomarker is eagerly awaited [24]. Other candidates awaiting validation include the serum glycoproteins osteopontin and dickkopf (24), panels of nucleic acids and extracellular vesicles (EVs), as well as circulating tumor DNA (ctDNA) [24] or proteomic signatures in serum EVs [24].

Another challenge arises in the management of patients with NAFLD-associated HCC. The Barcelona Clinic for Liver Cancer (BCLC) is the algorithm employed in the AASLD and EASL guidelines, which guide staging and treatment selection [24]. Unfortunately, it is rare to detect NAFLD-HCC at the BCLC-0 or BCLA-A stage [24]. Even when the tumor is small, advanced age and metabolic syndrome-associated comorbidity make curative procedures more challenging. Rather, the vast majority of NAFLD-HCC are classified as BCLC-C or BCLC-D, owing largely to the performance status test (PST) [24]. PST has a major effect on survival; however, it is a subjective measure that can be more difficult to assess in patients with metabolic syndrome [24]. Thus improved strategies for early detection and preventive strategies remain an urgent necessity to avoid the alarming projected increases in NAFLD-HCC incidence and mortality. The ongoing challenge for all patients with HCC, including those with NAFLD-HCC, will be to identify robust biomarkers that will improve risk stratification and guide both treatment selection and monitoring

20.3.4 Intra- and Extrahepatic Cholangiocarcinoma (CCA)

NAFLD has been linked to increased CCA risk, with some studies indicating a stronger association with intrahepatic CCA, suggesting underlying common mechanisms to HCC [56]. In a systematic review and meta-analysis by Liu et al., which included studies from USA, Europe and Asia, NAFLD was associated with a significantly higher risk of developing both intrahepatic and extrahepatic CCA [1]. Another meta-analysis by Wongjarupong et al. included seven case-control studies with a total of 9,102 CCA patients and observed similarly increased intrahepatic and extrahepatic CCA risk in patients with NAFLD [56].

Despite the preceding meta-analyses, the association between NAFLD and extrahepatic CCA is still controversial. Recently, Corrao et al. performed a meta-analysis as well as trial sequential analyses to study the association between NAFLD and CCA [57]. They found that NAFLD determines an increased risk of total as well as intrahepatic CCA incidence, but they observed no association for extrahepatic CCA [57]. The subsequent trial sequential analyses proved that the associations were conclusive, and the authors thereby concluded that there is no association between NAFLD and extrahepatic CCA [57]. As such, further studies are still needed to study the existence or magnitude of this association.

20.3.5 Colorectal Cancer (CRC) and Adenomas

To date, the majority of prior studies has found a higher prevalence of colorectal lesions in patients with NAFLD [2]. Hwang et al. provided the first evidence for the association between colorectal adenomatous polyps and NAFLD [58]. In their study of 2,917 patients, NAFLD was more prevalent in the adenomatous polyp group as compared to controls, and it was associated with 3-fold increased odds of colorectal adenomas [58]. These findings were confirmed in a large Korean retrospective cohort study, whereby NAFLD patients had a 3-fold increase in the risk of CRC and a 2-fold increase in the occurrence of polyps [59]. In a cross-sectional study by Wong et al., the presence of NASH was associated with the highest CRC risk, among NAFLD patients [60]. Although they further reported a high prevalence of right-sided CRC [60], it remains unclear whether NAFLD or its histological features are linked to specific CRC subtypes, and larger, prospective studies are still needed to clarify this question.

Longitudinal studies have largely replicated these findings [2]. For example, the incidence of de novo adenoma was increased by 45% in patients with NAFLD in a prospective study where patients had paired colonoscopies, with negative index colonoscopies [61]. In a Danish cohort study of hospitalized patients, an increased risk of CRC was seen with fatty liver as compared to the general population [62]. A recent meta-analysis of 10 studies showed that NAFLD patients have a significantly higher risk of developing colorectal adenomas and CRC [1]. In another meta-analysis, the presence and severity of NAFLD were again associated with an increased risk of incident CRC or adenomas [63]. Finally, in asymptomatic adults undergoing a screening colonoscopy, a meta-analysis by Mantovani et al. found similar positive associations for colorectal adenoma and cancer [64]. In contrast, only two studies failed to demonstrate a statistically significant increase in the incidence of colorectal adenomas in patients with NAFLD [2].

20.3.6 CRC Screening in Patients with NAFLD

Given the observed associations between NAFLD, NASH and the formation of adenomatous colon polyps, including right-sided polyps, polyps with high-grade dysplasia and CRC [2,60], some authors have suggested enhanced CRC screening and surveillance in this population [60]. However, to date the available body of evidence is still limited, and it is unclear whether patients with NAFLD would derive benefit from early or increased CRC screening and surveillance strategies. Thus, at present, it is important for clinicians to continue recommending that patients with NAFLD undergo appropriate CRC screening as per published guidelines [65].

20.3.7 Liver Metastasis from CRC

The "seed-soil" hypothesis suggests that metastatic cancer cells will migrate to an area where the local microenvironment is favorable. The "soil" has unique biological characteristics and microenvironment with special molecular components and cells that promote metastasis formation [66]. Several studies have addressed the role of the liver with NAFLD as "soil" in the metastasis of CRC cells as "seeds" [66]. Yan et al. found that in patients with CRC, the presence of NAFLD was associated with an increased incidence of synchronous liver metastasis, detected on or prior to the primary CRC tumor [66]. These findings are supported by preclinical data demonstrating that hepatic steatosis increases colon tumor metastasis to the liver [67,68]. However, other studies have found that liver metastases of CRC arise less frequently in the setting of NAFLD [69,70]; thus prospective research is still needed in populations with well-phenotyped NAFLD, which also carefully distinguishes between synchronous and metachronous CRC metastasis [66,69,70].

20.3.8 Other GI Malignancies

20.3.8.1 Esophageal, Gastric and Pancreatic CA

While central adiposity may represent an important, shared risk factor for NAFLD and for esophageal adenocarcinoma [71], a link between NAFLD and esophageal or gastric cancer is less clear. Although very few clinical studies have studied these links, it has been reported that NAFLD is associated with the risk of developing esophageal cancer [1], and a meta-analysis of 3 high-quality studies suggested that NAFLD patients have an elevated risk of developing gastric cancer [1]. However, most prior studies to date have been limited by small sample sizes with few cancer outcomes or by a limited ability to accurately phenotype NAFLD and its severity [71]. More recently, in a large retrospective analysis of patients with biopsy-confirmed NAFLD, Simon et al. found no significant association between NAFLD and incident gastric or esophageal cancer [37].

Pancreatic cancer has been shown to be highly associated with NAFLD [71]. A meta-analysis of 3 high-quality studies suggested that NAFLD patients have an elevated risk of developing pancreatic cancer [1,72,73], while a more recent retrospective study showed significant higher crude incidence but nonsignificant adjusted risk [74]. Emerging epidemiologic and translational data support the role of local ectopic fat as a paracrine mechanism for the development of pancreatic cancer, where the local adipose tissue microenvironment impacts tumor progression. As such, it would be biologically plausible for NAFLD to contribute to the development of pancreatic cancer, and further research is needed to better characterize these potential associations [73] (see Table 20.1).

20.4 NAFLD AND NON-GI MALIGNANCIES

20.4.1 Renal Cell Carcinoma (RCC)

To date, NAFLD has been linked to increased RCC incidence in 3 large retrospective cohort studies [62,72,74], but only one study showed a statistically significant risk [62,71]. Watanabe et al. found that in Japanese populations, NAFLD might be associated with more severe RCC and shorter overall survival [75]. In their large retrospective study, Simon et al. found that NAFLD patients had significantly higher rates of developing kidney/bladder cancer [37]. Further research in large populations is still needed to better clarify this potential relationship (see Table 20.1).

Table 20.1: Summary of Studies That Investigated the Association between NAFLD and Extrahepatic Cancers

Extrahepatic Cancer	Study	Type of Study	Country	Findings
Colorectal	Hwang S. T. et al., (2009) [58]	Cross-sectional	South Korea	NAFLD was associated with increased risk of colorectal adenomas (OR 1.28,95% CI: 1.03–1.6). Higher prevalence of NAFLD among adenoma group vs. nonadenoma group (41.5 vs. 30.2%).
Colorectal	Stadlmayr A. et al., (2011) [79]	Cross-sectional	Austria	Independent association between NAFLD and increased risk of colorectal adenomas (aOR 1.47, 95% CI 1.08–2).
Colorectal	Wong V. W. et al., (2011) [60]	Cross-sectional	China	Higher prevalence of colorectal adenomas (34.7 vs. 21.5%), as well as advanced neoplasms (18.6 vs. 5.5%) in NAFLD group as compared to healthy controls. Among the biopsy group, there was higher prevalence of adenomas (51 vs. 25.6%) and advanced neoplasms (34.7 vs. 14%) in patients with NASH as compared to those with simple steatosis. NASH was associated with adenomas (aOR 4.89, 95% CI 2.04–11.7) and advanced neoplasms (OR 5.34, 95% CI 1.92–14.84).
Colorectal	Lee Y. I. et al. (2012) [59]	Retrospective cohort	South Korea	NAFLD was associated with adenomatous polyps (aRR 1.94, 95% CI 1.11–3.4) and colorectal cancer (aRR 3.08, 95% CI 1.02–9.34).
Colorectal	Huang K. W. et al. (2013) [61]	Retrospective Cohort	Taiwan	Higher prevalence of NAFLD in the adenoma group as compared to the nonadenoma group (55.6 vs. 38.8%). After adjusting, NAFLD was an independent risk factor for development of colorectal adenoma (OR 1.45; 95% CI: 1.07–1.98).
Colorectal	Lin X. F. et al. (2014) [80]	Cross-sectional	China	Higher prevalence of colorectal cancer in NAFLD group (29.3 vs. 18%). NAFLD was independently associated with increased colorectal cancer risk (aOR 1.87, 95% CI 1.36–2.57).
Colorectal	Sun L. M. et al. (2015) [74]	Retrospective cohort	Taiwan	Higher incidence of colorectal cancer in NAFLD with cirrhosis group (aHR 2.58, 95% CI 1.59–4.18).
Colorectal	Bhatt B. D. et al.,(2015) [81]	Retrospective cohort	USA	Higher prevalence of polyps (59 vs. 40%) and adenomas (32 vs. 21%) in NAFLD group. NAFLD was predictive of finding a polyp on colonoscopy (OR 2.42, $P = 0.001$) and associated with adenoma (OR 1.95, $P = 0.02$).
Colorectal	Lee T. et al. (2016) [82]	Cross-sectional	South Korea	aOR for colorectal cancer with varying severity of NAFLD was 1.13 for mild, 1.12 for moderate, and 1.56 for severe ($P = 0.007$).
Colorectal	Yang Y. J. et al. (2017) [83]	Retrospective cohort	South Korea	Cumulative incidence rates of colorectal neoplasm at 3 and 5 years in the NAFLD group were 9.1 and 35.2% vs. 5.0 and 25.3% in non-NAFLD group. NAFLD was associated with increased risk of overall colorectal tumors (aHR 1.31, 95% CI 1.01–1.71), and the development of ≥3 adenomas at the time of surveillance colonoscopy (aHR: 2.49, 95% CI: 1.20–5.20).
Colorectal	Ahn J. S. et al., (2017) [84]	Cross-sectional	South Korea	Higher prevalence of any colorectal neoplasia (38% vs. 28.9%) and advanced colorectal neoplasia (2.8% vs. 1.9%) in NAFLD patients. The aOR in NAFLD patients was 1.1 (95% CI:1.03–1.17) for any colorectal neoplasia and 1.21 (95% CI: 0.99–1.47) for advanced colorectal neoplasia.
Colorectal	Kim G. A. et al., (2017) [72]	Retrospective cohort	South Korea	Higher incidence of colorectal cancer in NAFLD patients (69.4 vs. 34.1 per 100,000 person-years; IRR 2.04; 95% CI 1.3–3.19).
Colorectal	Kim M. C. et al. (2019) [85]	Cross-Sectional	South Korea	NAFLD is an independent risk factor for colorectal adenoma (aOR 1.15; 95%CI 1.02–1.3), advanced adenoma (aOR 1.5; 95% CI 1.12–2.01), and multiple adenomas (aOR 1.32; 95%CI 1.01–1.73).
Colorectal	Cho Y. et al. (2019) [86]	Cross-sectional	South Korea	NASH was an independent risk factor for colorectal polyps (OR 2.08; 95% CI 1.12–3.86) and advanced colorectal neoplasm (OR 2.81; 95% CI 1.01–7.87).
Colorectal	Allen A. M., et al. (2019) [73]	Retrospective cohort	USA	Higher incidence of colon cancer in NAFLD patients IRR 1.76 (95% CI 1.08–2.8).
Colorectal	Simon TG, et al. (2021) [37]	Retrospective cohort	Sweden	No significant associations between NAFLD and colon cancer (aHR 1.05, 95% CI [0.85–1.28]).
Esophageal	Sorensen HT et al. (2003) [62]	Retrospective cohort	Denmark	The standardized incidence ratio of esophageal cancer was SIR 2.9, 95% CI 0.4–10.3 in the NAFLD group.
Gastric	Uzel M et al. (2015) [87]	Retrospective cohort	Turkey	The prevalence of NAFLD was higher in gastric cancer as compared to the Turkish general population.

Extrahepatic Cancer	Study	Type of Study	Country	Findings
Esophageal and gastric	Sun L. M. et al., (2015) [74]	Retrospective cohort	Taiwan	Significantly higher incidence of esophageal cancer in the NAFLD with cirrhosis group (aHR 7.25; 95% CI 2.44–21.6) and gastric cancer (aHR 5.5; 95% CI 2.78–10.9).
Gastric	Allen A. M. et al. (2019) [73]	Retrospective cohort	USA	Higher incidence of gastric cancer in NAFLD patients (IRR 2.3, 95% CI 1.3–4.1).
Esophageal and gastric	Simon TG, et al. (2021) [37]	Retrospective cohort	Sweden	No significant associations between NAFLD and cancer of the esophagus or stomach (aHR 1.15, 95% CI 0.77–1.71).
Pancreas	Sorensen H. T. et al. (2003) [62]	Retrospective cohort	Denmark	The standardized incidence ratio of pancreatic cancer was SIR 3, 95% CI 1.3–5.8 in the NAFLD group.
Pancreas	Sun L. M. et al. (2015) [74]	Retrospective cohort	Taiwan	Higher crude and adjusted incidence risk of pancreatic cancer in NAFLD with cirrhosis group (HR 4.18; 95% CI 1.67–10.4 and aHR 2.72; 95% CI 0.93–7.95), but the adjusted incidence risk was statistically insignificant.
Pancreas	Kim G. A. et al. (2017) [72]	Retrospective cohort	South Korea	Higher incidence of pancreatic cancer in NAFLD patients (16 vs. 13.8 per 100,000 person-years) but was statistically insignificant (IRR 1.16; 95% CI 0.51–2.65).
Pancreas	Chang C. F. et al. (2017) [88]	Case control	Taiwan	NAFLD was an independent risk factor for pancreatic cancer (OR 2.63, 95% CI 1.24–5.58).
Pancreas	Allen A. M. et al. (2019) [73]	Retrospective cohort	USA	Higher incidence of pancreatic cancer in NAFLD patients (IRR 2.1, 95% CI 1.2–3.3)
Pancreas	Simon T. G. et al. (2021) [37]	Retrospective cohort	Sweden	NAFLD patients had significantly higher rates of developing pancreatic cancer (aHR, 2.15 [95% CI 1.40–3.30)
Kidney	Sorensen H. T. et al. (2003) [62]	Retrospective cohort	Denmark	Standardized incidence ratio of renal cancer in the NAFLD group: SIR 2.7, 95% CI 1.1–5.6.
Kidney	Sun L.M. et al. (2015) [74]	Retrospective cohort	Taiwan	Higher crude and adjusted hazard ratios of urinary system cancer (HR 1.19; 95% CI 0.53–2.66; aHR 1.60; 95% CI 0.69–3.72) in NAFLD with cirrhosis group; however, both were statistically insignificant.
Kidney	Kim G. A. et al. (2017) [72]	Retrospective cohort	South Korea	Higher incidence of renal cancer in NAFLD patients (35.6 vs. 20.3 per 100,000 person-years) but was statistically insignificant (IRR 1.76; 95% CI 0.96–3.22).
Kidney/bladder	Simon T.G., et al. (2021) [37]	Retrospective cohort	Sweden	NAFLD patients had significantly higher rates of developing kidney/bladder cancer (aHR, 1.41, 95% CI, 1.07–1.86).
Prostate	Sorensen H.T. et al. (2003) [62]	Retrospective cohort	Denmark	The standardized incidence ratio of prostate cancer in the NAFLD group: SIR 1.3, 95% CI 0.5–2.8.
Prostate	Kim G.A. et al. (2017) [72]	Retrospective cohort	South Korea	Lower incidence of prostate cancer in NAFLD patients (126 vs. 138.9 per 100,000 person-years) but statistically insignificant (IRR 0.91; 95% CI 0.63–1.31).
Prostate	Simon TG, et al. (2021) [37]	Retrospective cohort	Sweden	No significant associations between NAFLD and prostate cancer (aHR 0.91, 95% CI 0.77–1.09)
Breast	Sorensen H.T. et al. (2003) [62]	Retrospective cohort	Denmark	Standardized incidence ratio of breast cancer in the NAFLD group: SIR 0.9, 95% CI 0.4–1.7.
Breast	Sun L. M. et al. (2015) [74]	Retrospective cohort	Taiwan	Higher adjusted incidence risk in the NAFLD with cirrhosis group (aHR 1.23; 95% CI 0.28–5.38) compared to the control group but not statistically significant.
Breast	Chu C. H. et al. (2003) [77]	Case control	China	45.2% of breast cancer patients vs. 20.3% of the controls had NAFLD (OR 3.23; 95% CI 2.1–5.1, P < 0.0001).
Breast	Kim G. A. et al. (2017) [72]	Retrospective cohort	South Korea	Higher incidence of breast cancer in the NAFLD group (181.6 vs. 102.5 per 100,000 person-years) than non-NAFLD group, with IRR 1.77, 95% CI 1.15–2.74.
Breast	Kwak M.-S., et al. (2018) [89]	Case control	South Korea	NAFLD was independently associated with breast cancer (OR 1.63, 95% CI 1.01–2.62; P = 0.046).
Breast	Allen AM, et al. (2019) [73]	Retrospective cohort	USA	Higher incidence of breast cancer in NAFLD vs. controls, SIR 1.68 (95% CI 1.05–2.76)
Breast	Simon TG, et al. (2021) [37]	Retrospective cohort	Sweden	No significant associations between NAFLD and breast cancer (aHR 0.99, 95% CI [0.79–1.24])
Uterine	Sun L. M. et al. (2015) [74]	Retrospective cohort	Taiwan	Higher crude and adjusted hazard ratio of uterine cancer in the NAFLD with cirrhosis group (HR 2.11; 95% CI 0.67–6.63; and aHR 2.03; 95% CI 0.6–6.8), but both statistically insignificant.

(Continued)

Table 20.1 (Continued)

Extrahepatic Cancer	Study	Type of Study	Country	Findings
Uterine	Kim G. A. et al. (2017) [72]	Retrospective cohort	South Korea	Higher incidence of uterine/cervical/ovarian cancers in NAFLD patients (48.4 vs. 23.5 per 100,000 person-years) but statistically insignificant (IRR 2.06; 95% CI 0.86–4.91).
Uterine	Allen A. M. et al. (2019) [73]	Retrospective cohort	USA	Higher incidence of uterine cancer in NAFLD patients (IRR 2.3, 95% CI 1.4–4.1).
Uterine/cervical/ovarian	Simon T. G. et al. (2021) [37]	Retrospective cohort	Sweden	No significant associations between NAFLD and uterine cancer (aHR 0.82, 95% CI 0.61–1.09).
Lung	Allen A.M. et al. (2019) [73]	Retrospective cohort	USA	No significant increase in the incidence rates of lung cancer in NAFLD patients (IRR 1.34, 95% CI 0.87–2.07).
Lung	Simon TG, et al. (2021) [37]	Retrospective cohort	Sweden	No significant associations between NAFLD and lung cancer (aHR 1.06, 95%CI 0.82–1.39).
Hematologic	Sun L. M. et al. (2015) [74]	Retrospective cohort	Taiwan	Significantly higher adjusted incidence of hematologic cancer in the NAFLD with cirrhosis group (aHR 3.12; 95% CI 1.34–7.25).
Hematologic	Allen A.M. et al. (2019) [73]	Retrospective cohort	USA	No significant increase in the incidence rates of non-Hodgkin lymphoma in NAFLD patients (IRR 0.94, 95% CI 0.52–1.7).
Hematologic	Simon T. G. et al. (2021) [37]	Retrospective cohort	Sweden	NAFLD patients had modest yet significantly higher rates of developing hematologic cancers (0.7 vs. 1.0/1,000 PYs; aHR, 1.46, 95% CI, 1.12–1.90).

OR: Odds ratio; CI: Confidence interval; aOR: Adjusted odds ratio; aRR: Adjusted relative risk; aHR: Adjusted hazard ratio; IRR: Incidence rate ratio; SIR: Standardized incidence ratio; HR: Hazard ratio; PY: Person-year.

20.4.2 Prostate CA

Large-scale studies have examined the incidence of prostate cancer in patients with NAFLD; however, the results have been inconsistent [71]. A large study from South Korea that included over 10 million males from a national database registry showed a significant higher incidence of prostate cancer in patients with NAFLD, defined using surrogate measures (i.e., a hepatic steatosis index ³ 36 or fatty liver index ³ 60) [71,76]. In a subsequent meta-analysis of 3 large studies (including the aforementioned Korean study), NAFLD was associated with a significantly elevated risk of developing prostate cancer [1,72,73,76]. In contrast, other studies failed to show a statistically significant association [37], and so whether prostate cancer constitutes a significant threat in men with NAFLD remains unclear [71] (see Table 20.1).

20.4.3 Breast CA

The association between breast cancer and obesity is well-described [71], and with each 5 kg of weight gain, the risk of breast cancer development increases by 11% [71]. Accordingly, several retrospective studies have shown a similar positive association between NAFLD and breast cancer [71–73,77], the largest of which estimated a 3-fold higher prevalence [77] and a 60–70% increase in incidence [72,73]. In a meta-analysis by Liu et al. that included 4 of these high-quality studies, it was concluded that NAFLD patients are more susceptible to the development of breast cancer [1]. However, other, smaller studies have failed to show a significant relationship between NAFLD and the incidence or prevalence of breast cancer [62,71,74], and further research is needed to disentangle the risk associated with obesity from any related specifically to NAFLD (see Table 20.1).

20.4.4 Uterine CA

Very few studies have provided evidence for or against an association between NAFLD and uterine cancer, to date [37,71–74] (see Table 20.1).

20.4.5 Lung CA

Large retrospective cohort studies showed no increased rates of lung cancer in NAFLD patients [37,73] (see Table 20.1).

20.4.6 Hematologic CA

A statistically significant higher incidence of hematologic cancer was found in a single retrospective cohort study investigating the incidence of cancers in over 2000 NAFLD patients [74]. Similarly, Simon et al. showed that NAFLD patients had modest yet significantly higher rates of developing hematologic cancers [37]. The mechanisms that might underpin an association between NAFLD and hematologic cancer development remains undefined, and further research is needed to better characterize these relationships (see Table 20.1).

20.4.7 Is It Time to Change Our Extrahepatic Cancer Screening Strategies for Patients with NAFLD?

Given emerging data supporting an increased risk of some extrahepatic cancers in patients with NAFLD, increased clinical awareness is warranted. However, as previously outlined, these data remain preliminary, and further research from large-scale cohorts with well-phenotyped NAFLD and carefully adjudicated clinical outcomes are urgently needed, so that these risks can be confirmed and quantified at the population level. In the interim, it is important that clinicians ensure that their patients with NAFLD are up-to-date with their recommended cancer surveillance, based on current guidelines. Patients should also be counseled regarding behaviors that may be associated with increased cancer risk [78].

20.5 CONCLUSION

Substantial evidence is accumulating for a role of NAFLD as an independent risk factor for several cancers, particularly hepatic cancers. Data are also accumulating regarding the molecular mechanisms that drive HCC in NAFLD, which hold promise for future biomarker development and prevention strategies [24]. In contrast, evidence linking NAFLD to extrahepatic cancer incidence is still scarce, and well-designed cohort studies with long-term follow-up are still needed. Such work is crucial to define precise, population-level risk estimates for various cancer types in patients with NAFLD, which in turn will help improve personalized strategies for risk counselling, screening and surveillance, in high-risk patients with NAFLD.

REFERENCES

1. Liu, S.-S., Ma, X.F., Zhao, J., Du, S.X., Zhang, J., Dong, M.Z., Xin, Y.N. Association between nonalcoholic fatty liver disease and extrahepatic cancers: a systematic review and meta-analysis. *Lipids in Health and Disease*. 2020; **19**(1): 1–10.

2. Sanna, C., Rosso, C., Marietti, M., Bugianesi, E. Non-alcoholic fatty liver disease and extra-hepatic cancers. *International Journal of Molecular Sciences*. 2016; **17**(5): 717.

3. Buzzetti, E., Pinzani, M., Tsochatzis, E.A. The multiple-hit pathogenesis of non-alcoholic fatty liver disease (NAFLD). *Metabolism*. 2016; **65**(8): 1038–1048.

4. Wegermann, K., Hyun, J., Diehl, A.M. Molecular mechanisms linking nonalcoholic steatohepatitis to cancer. *Clinical Liver Disease*. 2021; **17**(1): 6.

5. Yang, J.D., Ahmed, F., Mara, K.C., Addissie, B.D., Allen, A.M., Gores, G.J., Roberts, L.R. Diabetes is associated with increased risk of hepatocellular carcinoma in patients with cirrhosis from nonalcoholic fatty liver disease. *Hepatology*. 2020; **71**(3): 907–916.

6. Fujiwara, N., Nakagawa, H., Enooku, K., Kudo, Y., Hayata, Y., Nakatsuka, T., Tanaka, Y., Tateishi, R., Hikiba, Y., Misumi, K. CPT2 downregulation adapts HCC to lipid-rich environment and promotes carcinogenesis via acylcarnitine accumulation in obesity. *Gut*. 2018; **67**(8): 1493–1504.

7. Wu, H., Ng, R., Chen, X., Steer, C.J., Song, G. MicroRNA-21 is a potential link between non-alcoholic fatty liver disease and hepatocellular carcinoma via modulation of the HBP1-p53-Srebp1c pathway. *Gut*. 2016; **65**(11): 1850–1860.

8. Ye, J., Li, T.-S., Xu, G., Zhao, Y.-M., Zhang, N.-P., Fan, J., Wu, J. JCAD promotes progression of nonalcoholic steatohepatitis to liver cancer by inhibiting LATS2 kinase activity. *Cancer Research*. 2017; **77**(19): 5287–5300.

9. Verdelho Machado, M., Diehl, A.M., The hedgehog pathway in nonalcoholic fatty liver disease. *Critical Reviews in Biochemistry and Molecular Biology*. 2018; **53**(3): 264–278.

10. Farrell, G. Insulin resistance, obesity, and liver cancer. *Clinical Gastroenterology and Hepatology*. 2014; **12**(1): 117–119.

11. Adamek, A., Kasprzak, A. Insulin-like growth factor (IGF) system in liver diseases. *International Journal of Molecular Sciences*. 2018; **19**(5): 1308.

12. Hirsova, P., Bohm, F., Dohnalkova, E., Nozickova, B., Heikenwalder, M., Gores, G.J., Weber, A. Hepatocyte apoptosis is tumor promoting in murine nonalcoholic steatohepatitis. *Cell Death & Disease*. 2020; **11**(2): 1–12.

13. Kanda, T., Matsuoka, S., Yamazaki, M., Shibata, T., Nirei, K., Takahashi, H., Kaneko, T., Fujisawa, M., Higuchi, T., Nakamura, H. Apoptosis and non-alcoholic fatty liver diseases. *World Journal of Gastroenterology*. 2018; **24**(25): 2661.

14. Ma, C., Kesarwala, A.H., Eggert, T., Medina-Echeverz, J., Kleiner, D.E., Jin, P., Stroncek, D.F., Terabe, M., Kapoor, V., ElGindi, M. NAFLD causes selective CD4+ T lymphocyte loss and promotes hepatocarcinogenesis. *Nature*. 2016; **531**(7593): 253–257.

15. Ritz, T., Krenkel, O., Tacke, F. Dynamic plasticity of macrophage functions in diseased liver. *Cellular Immunology*. 2018; **330**: 175–182.

16. Ma, C., Zhang, Q., Greten, T.F. Nonalcoholic fatty liver disease promotes hepatocellular carcinoma through direct and indirect effects on hepatocytes. *The FEBS Journal*. 2018; **285**(4): 752–762.

17. Liu, Y.-L., Patman, G.L., Leathart, J.B.S., Piguet, A.C., Burt, A.D., Dufour, J.-F., Day, C.P., Daly, A.K., Reeves, H.L., Anstee, Q.M. Carriage of the PNPLA3 rs738409 C> G polymorphism confers an increased risk of non-alcoholic fatty liver disease associated hepato-cellular carcinoma. *Journal of Hepatology*. 2014; **61**(1): 75–81.

18. Llovet, J.M., Chen, Y., Wurmbach, E., Roayaie, S., Fiel, M.I., Schwartz, M., Thung, S.N., Khitrov, G., Zhang, W., Villanueva, A. A molecular signature to discriminate dysplastic nodules from early hepatocellular carci-noma in HCV cirrhosis. *Gastroenterology*. 2006; **131**(6): 1758–1767.

19. Ally, A., Balasundaram, M., Carlsen, R., Chuah, E., Clarke, A., Dhalla, N., Holt, R.A., Jones, S.J.M., Lee, D., Ma, Y. Comprehensive and integrative genomic characterization of hepatocellular carcinoma. *Cell*. 2017; **169**(7): 1327–1341.

20. Ponziani, F.R., Bhoori, S., Castelli, C., Putignani, L., Rivoltini, L., Del Chierico, F., Sanguinetti, M., Morelli, D., Paroni Sterbini, F., Petito, V. Hepatocellular car-cinoma is associated with gut microbiota profile and inflammation in nonalcoholic fatty liver disease. *Hepatology*. 2019; **69**(1): 107–120.

21. Boursier, J., Diehl, A.M. Nonalcoholic fatty liver disease and the gut microbiome. *Clinics in Liver Disease*. 2016; **20**(2): 263–275.

22. Schwabe, R.F., Greten, T.F. Gut microbiome in HCC—Mechanisms, diagnosis and therapy. *Journal of Hepatology*. 2020; **72**(2): 230–238.

23. Huang, D.Q., El-Serag, H.B., Loomba, R. Global epidemiology of NAFLD-related HCC: trends, pre-dictions, risk factors and prevention. *Nature Reviews Gastroenterology & Hepatology*. 2021; **18**(4): 223–238.

24. Anstee, Q.M., Reeves, H.L., Kotsiliti, E., Govaere, O., Heikenwalder, M. From NASH to HCC: cur-rent concepts and future challenges. *Nature Reviews Gastroenterology & Hepatology*. 2019; **16**(7): 411–428.

25. Tilg, H., Diehl, A.M. NAFLD and extrahepatic cancers: have a look at the colon. *Gut*. 2011; **60**(6): 745–746.

26. Després, J.-P., Lemieux, I. Abdominal obesity and meta-bolic syndrome. *Nature*. 2006; **444**(7121): 881–887.

27. Hori, M., Takahashi, M., Hiraoka, N., Yamaji, T., Mutoh, M., Ishigamori, R., Furuta, K., Okusaka, T., Shimada, K., Kosuge, T. Association of pancreatic fatty infiltration with pancreatic ductal adenocarcinoma. *Clinical and Translational Gastroenterology*. 2014; **5**(3): e53.

28. Lashinger, L.M., Malone, L.M., McArthur, M.J., Goldberg, J.A., Daniels, E.A., Pavone, A., Colby, J.K., Smith, N.C., Perkins, S.N., Fischer, S.M. Genetic reduction of insulin-like growth factor-1 mimics the anticancer effects of calorie restriction on cyclooxygenase-2—driven pancreatic neoplasia. *Cancer Prevention Research*. 2011; **4**(7): 1030–1040.

29. Beste, L.A., Leipertz, S.L., Green, P.K., Dominitz, J.A., Ross, D., Ioannou, G.N. Trends in burden of cirrhosis and hepatocellular carcinoma by underlying liver disease in US veterans, 2001–2013. *Gastroenterology*. 2015; **149**(6): 1471–1482.

30. Akinyemiju, T., Abera, S., Ahmed, M., Alam, N., Alemayohu, M.A., Allen, C., Al-Raddadi, R., Alvis-Guzman, N., Amoako, Y., Artaman, A. The burden of primary liver cancer and underlying etiologies from 1990 to 2015 at the global, regional, and national level: results from the global burden of disease study 2015. *JAMA Oncology*. 2017; **3**(12): 1683–1691.

31. Yang, J.D., Hainaut, P., Gores, G.J., Amadou, A., Plymoth, A., Roberts, L.R. A global view of hepatocellular carcinoma: trends, risk, prevention and management. *Nature Reviews Gastroenterology & Hepatology*. 2019; **16**(10): 589–604.

32. Younossi, Z., Stepanova, M., Ong, J.P. Jacobson, I.M., Bugianesi, E., Duseja, A., Eguchi, Y., Wong, V.W., Negro, F., Yilmaz, Y. Nonalcoholic steatohepatitis is the fastest growing cause of hepatocellular carcinoma in liver transplant candidates. *Clinical Gastroenterology and Hepatology*. 2019; **17**(4): 748–755.

33. Ascha, M.S., Hanouneh, I.A., Lopez, R., Tamimi, T.A., Feldstein, A., Zein, N.N. The incidence and risk factors of hepatocellular carcinoma in patients with nonalcoholic steatohepatitis. *Hepatology*. 2010; **51**(6): 1972–1978.

34. Sanyal, A.J., Banas, C., Sargeant, C., Luketic, V.A., Sterling, R.K., Stravitz, R.T., Shiffman, M.L., Heuman, D., Coterrell, A., Fisher, R.A. Similarities and differences in outcomes of cirrhosis due to nonalcoholic steatohepatitis and hepatitis C. *Hepatology*. 2006; **43**(4): 682–689.

35. Kanwal, F., Kramer, J.R., Mapakshi, S., Natarajan, Y., Chayanupatkul, M., Richardson, P.A., Li, L., Desiderio, R., Thrift, A.P., Asch, S.M. Risk of hepatocellular cancer in patients with non-alcoholic fatty liver disease. *Gastroenterology*. 2018; **155**(6): 1828–1837.

36. Yatsuji, S., Hashimoto, E., Tobari, M., Taniai, M., Tokushige, K., Shiratori, K. Clinical features and outcomes of cirrhosis due to non-alcoholic steatohepatitis compared with cirrhosis caused by chronic hepatitis C. *Journal of Gastroenterology and Hepatology*. 2009; **24**(2): 248–254.

37. Simon, T.G., Roelstraete, B., Sharma, R., Khalili, H., Hagström, H., Ludvigsson, J.F. Cancer risk in patients with biopsy-confirmed nonalcoholic fatty liver disease: a population-based cohort study. *Hepatology*. 2021; **74**(5): 2410–2423.

38. Younossi, Z.M., Otgonsuren, M., Henry, L., Venkatesan, C., Mishra, A., Erario, M., Hunt, S. Association of non-alcoholic fatty liver disease (NAFLD) with hepatocellular carcinoma (HCC) in the United States from 2004 to 2009. *Hepatology*. 2015. **62**(6): 1723–1730.

39. Piscaglia, F., Svegliati-Baroni, G., Barchetti, A., Pecorelli, A., Marinelli, S., Tiribelli, C., Bellentani, S. Clinical patterns of hepatocellular carcinoma in nonalcoholic fatty liver disease: a multicenter prospective study. *Hepatology*. 2016; **63**(3): 827–838.

40. Estes, C., Razavi, H., Loomba, R., Younossi, Z., Sanyal, A.J. Modeling the epidemic of nonalcoholic fatty liver disease demonstrates an exponential increase in burden of disease. *Hepatology*. 2018; **67**(1): 123–133.

41. Mittal, S., El-Serag, H.B., Sada, Y.H., Kanwal, F., Duan, Z., Temple, S., May, S.B., Kramer, J.R., Richardson, P.A., Davila, J.A. Hepatocellular carcinoma in the absence of cirrhosis in United States veterans is associated with nonalcoholic fatty liver disease. *Clinical Gastroenterology and Hepatology*. 2016; **14**(1): 124–131.

42. Yasui, K., Hashimoto, E., Komorizono, Y., Koike, K., Arii, S., Imai, Y., Shima, T., Kanbara, Y., Saibara, T., Mori, T. Characteristics of patients with nonalcoholic steatohepatitis who develop hepatocellular carcinoma. *Clinical Gastroenterology and Hepatology*. 2011; **9**(5): 428–433.

43. Alexander, M., Loomis, A.K., Fairburn-Beech, J., Van der Lei, J., Duarte-Salles, T., Prieto-Alhambra, D., Ansell, D., Pasqua, A., Lapi, F., Rijnbeek, P. Real-world data reveal a diagnostic gap in non-alcoholic fatty liver disease. *BMC Medicine*. 2018; **16**(1): 1–11.

44. Mercado-Irizarry, A., Torres, E.A. Cryptogenic cirrhosis: current knowledge and future directions. *Clinical Liver Disease*. 2016; **7**(4): 69.

45. Caldwell, S., Marchesini, G. Cryptogenic vs. NASH-cirrhosis: the rose exists well before its name. *Journal of Hepatology*. 2018; **68**(3): 391–392.

46. Thuluvath, P.J., Kantsevoy, S., Thuluvath, A.J., Savva, Y. Is cryptogenic cirrhosis different from NASH cirrhosis? *Journal of Hepatology*. 2018; **68**(3): 519–525.

47. Alexander, M., Loomis, A.K., Van Der Lei, J., Duarte-Salles, T., Prieto-Alhambra, D., Ansell, D., Pasqua, A., Lapi, F., Rijnbeek, P., Mosseveld, M. Risks and clinical predictors of cirrhosis and hepatocellular carcinoma diagnoses in adults with diagnosed NAFLD: real-world study of 18 million patients in four European cohorts. *BMC Medicine*. 2019; **17**(1): 1–9.

48. Kanwal, F., Kramer, J.R., Li, L., Dai, J., Natarajan, Y., Yu, X., Asch, S.M., El-Serag, H.B. Effect of metabolic traits on the risk of cirrhosis and hepatocellular cancer in nonalcoholic fatty liver disease. *Hepatology*. 2020; **71**(3): 808–819.

49. Chalasani, N., Younossi, Z., Lavine, J.E., Charlton, M., Cusi, K., Rinella, M., Harrison, S.A., Brunt, E.M., Sanyal, A.J. The diagnosis and management of nonalcoholic fatty liver disease: practice guidance from the American Association for the Study of Liver Diseases. *Hepatology*. 2018; **67**(1): 328–357.

50. Loomba, R., Lim, J.K., Patton, H., El-Serag, H.B. AGA clinical practice update on screening and surveillance for hepatocellular carcinoma in patients with nonalcoholic fatty liver disease: expert review. *Gastroenterology*. 2020; **158**(6): 1822–1830.

51. EASL. EASL clinical practice guidelines: management of hepatocellular carcinoma. *J Hepatol*. 2018; **69**(1): 182–236.

52. Omata, M., Cheng, A. L., Kokudo, N., Kudo, M., Lee, J. M., Jia, J., Tateishi, R., Han, K. H., Chawla, Y. K., Shiina, S., Jafri, W., Payawal, D. A., Ohki, T., Ogasawara, S., Chen, P. J., Lesmana, C. R. A., Lesmana, L. A., Gani, R. A., Obi, S., Dokmeci, A. K., Sarin, S. K. Asia-Pacific clinical practice guidelines on the management of hepatocellular carcinoma: a 2017 update. *Hepatology International*. 2017; **11**(4): 317–370.

53. Eslam, M., Sarin, S.K., Wong, V.W., Fan, J.G., Kawaguchi, T., Ahn, S.H., Zheng, M.-H., Shiha, G., Yilmaz, Y., Gani, R. The Asian pacific association for the study of the liver clinical practice guidelines for the diagnosis and management of metabolic associated fatty liver disease. *Hepatology International*. 2020; **14**(6): 889–919.

54. Marrero, J.A., Kulik, L.M., Sirlin, C.B., Zhu, A.X., Finn, R.S., Abecassis, M.M., Roberts, L.R., Heimbach, J.K.

Diagnosis, staging, and management of hepatocellular carcinoma: 2018 practice guidance by the American association for the study of liver diseases. *Hepatology*. 2018; **68**(2): 723–750.

55. Simmons, O., Fetzer, D.T., Yokoo, T., Marrero, J.A., Yopp, A., Kono, Y., Parikh, N.D., Browning, T., Singal, A.G. Predictors of adequate ultrasound quality for hepatocellular carcinoma surveillance in patients with cirrhosis. *Alimentary Pharmacology & Therapeutics*. 2017; **45**(1): 169–177.

56. Wongjarupong, N., Assavapongpaiboon, B., Susantitaphong, P., Cheungpasitporn, W., Treeprasertsuk, S., Rerknimitr, R., Chaiteerakij, R. Non-alcoholic fatty liver disease as a risk factor for cholangiocarcinoma: a systematic review and meta-analysis. *BMC Gastroenterology*. 2017; **17**(1): 1–8.

57. Corrao, S., Natoli, G., Argano, C. Nonalcoholic cholangiocarcinoma liver disease is associated with intrahepatic cholangiocarcinoma and not with extrahepatic form: definitive evidence from meta-analysis and trial sequential analysis. *European Journal of Gastroenterology & Hepatology*. 2020; **33**(1): 62–68.

58. Hwang, S.T., Cho, Y.K., Park, J.H., Kim, H.J., Park, D.I., Sohn, C.I., Jeon, W.K., Kim, B.I., Won, K.H., Jin, W. Relationship of non-alcoholic fatty liver disease to colorectal adenomatous polyps. *Journal of Gastroenterology and Hepatology*. 2010; **25**(3): 562–567.

59. Lee, Y.I., Lim, Y.-S., Park, H.S. Colorectal neoplasms in relation to non-alcoholic fatty liver disease in Korean women: a retrospective cohort study. *Journal of Gastroenterology and Hepatology*. 2012; **27**(1): 91–95.

60. Wong, V.W.-S., Wong, G.L., Tsang, S.W., Fan, T., Chu, W.C., Woo, J., Chan, A.W., Choi, P.C., Chim, A.M., Lau, J.Y. High prevalence of colorectal neoplasm in patients with non-alcoholic steatohepatitis. *Gut*. 2011; **60**(6): 829–836.

61. Huang, K.W., Leu, H.B., Wang, Y.J., Luo, J.C., Lin, H.C., Lee, F.Y., Chan, W.L., Lin, J.K., Chang, F.Y. Patients with nonalcoholic fatty liver disease have higher risk of colorectal adenoma after negative baseline colonoscopy. *Colorectal Disease*. 2013; **15**(7): 830–835.

62. Sørensen, H.T., Mellemkjær, L., Jepsen, P., Thulstrup, A.M., Baron, J., Olsen, J.H., Vilstrup, H. Risk of cancer in patients hospitalized with fatty liver: a Danish cohort study. *Journal of Clinical Gastroenterology*. 2003; **36**(4): 356–359.

63. Chen, J., Bian, D., Zang, S., Yang, Z., Tian, G., Luo, Y., Yang, J., Xu, B., Shi, J. The association between nonalcoholic fatty liver disease and risk of colorectal adenoma and cancer incident and recurrence: a meta-analysis of observational studies. *Expert Review of Gastroenterology & Hepatology*. 2019; **13**(4): 385–395.

64. Mantovani, A., Dauriz, M., Byrne, C.D., Lonardo, A., Zoppini, G., Bonora, E., Targher, G. Association between nonalcoholic fatty liver disease and colorectal tumours in asymptomatic adults undergoing screening colonoscopy: a systematic review and meta-analysis. *Metabolism*. 2018; **87**: 1–12.

65. Shaukat, A., Kahi, C.J., Burke, C.A., Rabeneck, L., Sauer, B.G., Rex, D.K. ACG clinical guidelines: colorectal cancer screening 2021. *Official Journal of the American College of Gastroenterology | ACG*. 2021; **116**(3): 458–479.

66. Lv, Y., Zhang, H.J. Effect of non-alcoholic fatty liver disease on the risk of synchronous liver metastasis: analysis of 451 consecutive patients of newly diagnosed colorectal cancer. *Frontiers in Oncology*. 2020; **10**: 251.

67. VanSaun, M.N., Lee, I.K., Washington, M.K., Matrisian, L., Gorden, D.L. High fat diet induced hepatic steatosis establishes a permissive microenvironment for colorectal metastases and promotes primary dysplasia in a murine model. *The American Journal of Pathology*. 2009; **175**(1): 355–364.

68. Ohashi, K., Wang, Z., Yang, Y.M., Billet, S., Tu, W., Pimienta, M., Cassel, S.L., Pandol, S.J., Lu, S.C., Sutterwala, F.S. NOD-like receptor C4 inflammasome regulates the growth of colon cancer liver metastasis in NAFLD. *Hepatology*. 2019; **70**(5): 1582–1599.

69. Hayashi, S., Masuda, H., Shigematsu, M. Liver metastasis rare in colorectal cancer patients with fatty liver. *Hepato-gastroenterology*. 1997; **44**(16): 1069–1075.

70. XI, Z., Fan, Z., Qiu, D., Zeng, M. The relationship between fatty liver disease and liver metastases from colorectal cancer. *Chinese Journal of Digestion*. 2009; 157–160.

71. Ahmed, O.T., Allen, A.M. Extrahepatic malignancies in nonalcoholic fatty liver disease. *Current Hepatology Reports*. 2019; **18**(4): 455–472.

72. Kim, G.-A., Lee, H.C., Choe, J., Kim, M.J., Lee, M.J., Chang, H.S., Bae, I.Y., Kim, H.K., An, J., Shim, J.H. Association between non-alcoholic fatty liver disease and cancer incidence rate. *Journal of Hepatology*. 2018; **68**(1): 140–146.

73. Allen, A.M., Hicks, S.B., Mara, K.C., Larson, J.J., Therneau, T.M. The risk of incident extrahepatic cancers is higher in non-alcoholic fatty liver disease than obesity—a longitudinal cohort study. *Journal of Hepatology*. 2019; **71**(6): 1229–1236.

74. Sun, L.-M., Lin, M.C., Lin, C.L., Liang, J.A., Jeng, L.B., Kao, C.H., Lu, C.Y. Nonalcoholic cirrhosis increased risk of digestive tract malignancies: a population-based cohort study. *Medicine*. 2015; **94**(49).

75. Watanabe, D., Horiguchi, A., Tasaki, S., Kuroda, K., Sato, A., Asakuma, J., Ito, K., Asano, T., Shinmoto, H. Clinical implication of ectopic liver lipid accumulation in renal cell carcinoma patients without visceral obesity. *Scientific Reports*. 2017; **7**(1): 1–7.

76. Choi, Y.J., Lee, D.H., Han, K.D., Yoon, H., Shin, C.M., Park, Y.S., Kim, N. Is nonalcoholic fatty liver disease associated with the development of prostate cancer? A nationwide study with 10,516,985 Korean men. *PLoS ONE*. 2018; **13**(9): e0201308.

77. Chu, C.-H., Lin, S.C., Shih, S.C., Kao, C.R., Chou, S.Y. Fatty metamorphosis of the liver in patients with breast cancer: possible associated factors. *World Journal of Gastroenterology: WJG*. 2003; **9**(7): 1618.

78. Wijarnpreecha, K., Aby, E.S., Ahmed, A., Kim, D. Evaluation and management of extrahepatic manifestations of nonalcoholic fatty liver disease. *Clinical and Molecular Hepatology*. 2021; **27**(2): 221.

79. Stadlmayr, A., Aigner, E., Steger, B., Scharinger, L., Lederer, D., Mayr, A., Strasser, M., Brunner, E., Heuberger, A., Hohla, F. Nonalcoholic fatty liver disease: an independent risk factor for colorectal neoplasia. *Journal of Internal Medicine*. 2011; **270**(1): 41–49.

80. Lin, X.-F., Shi, K.Q., You, J., Liu, W.Y., Luo, Y.W., Wu, F.L., Chen, Y.P., Wong, D.K.H., Yuen, M.F., Zheng, M.H. Increased risk of colorectal malignant neoplasm in patients with nonalcoholic fatty liver disease: a large study. *Molecular Biology Reports*. 2014; **41**(5): 2989–2997.

81. Bhatt, B.D., Lukose, T., Siegel, A.B., Brown Jr, R.S., Verna, E.C. Increased risk of colorectal polyps in

patients with non-alcoholic fatty liver disease undergoing liver transplant evaluation. *Journal of Gastrointestinal Oncology*. 2015; **6**(5): 459.

82. Lee, T., Yun, K.E., Chang, Y., Ryu, S., Park, D.I., Choi, K., Jung, Y.S. Risk of colorectal neoplasia according to fatty liver severity and presence of gall bladder polyps. *Digestive Diseases and Sciences*. 2016; **61**(1): 317–324.

83. Yang, Y.J., Bang, C.S., Shin, S.P., Baik, G.H. Clinical impact of non-alcoholic fatty liver disease on the occurrence of colorectal neoplasm: propensity score matching analysis. *PLoS ONE*. 2017; **12**(8): e0182014.

84. Ahn, J., Sinn, D.H., Min, Y.W., Hong, S.N., Kim, H.S., Jung, S.H., Gu, S., Rhee, P.L., Paik, S.W., Son, H.J. Non-alcoholic fatty liver diseases and risk of colorectal neoplasia. *Alimentary Pharmacology & Therapeutics*. 2017; **45**(2): 345–353.

85. Kim, M.C., Park, J.G., Jang, B.I., Lee, H.J., Lee, W.K. Liver fibrosis is associated with risk for colorectal adenoma in patients with nonalcoholic fatty liver disease. *Medicine*. 2019; **98**(6).

86. Cho, Y., Lim, S.K., Joo, S.K., Jeong, D.H., Kim, J.H., Bae, J.M., Park, J.H., Chang, M.S., Lee, D.H., Jung, Y.J. Nonalcoholic steatohepatitis is associated with a higher risk of advanced colorectal neoplasm. *Liver International*. 2019; **39**(9): 1722–1731.

87. Uzel, M., Sahiner, Z., Filik, L. Non-alcoholic fatty liver disease, metabolic syndrome and gastric cancer: Single center experience. *Journal of BU ON.: Official Journal of the Balkan Union of Oncology*. 2015; **20**(2): 662–662.

88. Chang, C.-F., Tseng, Y.C., Huang, H.H., Shih, Y.L., Hsieh, T.Y., Lin, H.H. Exploring the relationship between nonalcoholic fatty liver disease and pancreatic cancer by computed tomographic survey. *Internal and Emergency Medicine*. 2018; **13**(2): 191–197.

89. Kwak, M.-S., Yim, J.Y., Yi, A., Chung, G.E., Yang, J.I., Kim, D., Kim, J.S., Noh, D.Y. Nonalcoholic fatty liver disease is associated with breast cancer in non-obese women. *Digestive and Liver Disease*. 2019; **51**(7): 1030–1035.

SECTION V
NAFLD IN SPECIAL POPULATIONS

21 NAFLD in Children

Unique Aspects and Controversies

Samar H. Ibrahim and Rohit Kohli

CONTENTS

21.1 INTRODUCTION

21.1.1 Definition and Nosology

"A rose by any other name would smell as sweet." We have all heard if not read this often quoted Shakespearean line of prose. When we speak to fatty liver disease in children, however, nosology and the definitions (see Table 21.1) it encompasses are both critically important.

We are particularly torn by the nosology whereby "non-alcoholic" continues to be used as a defining element for a disease afflicting an increasingly large pediatric population worldwide. Each child that is provided this definition must understand, at some point, the associated stigma inherent with the term "alcoholic." Given that most will agree that children should not—and the vast majority do not—partake in the consumption of alcohol, a change in the terminology is the need of the hour. We propose the usage of the prefix "Nutrition associated," thus keeping the acronym "NAFLD/NASH" unchanged. This shift in focus to the crux of the problem, "nutrition," will allow us to pivot away from the pejorative and negative connotations associated with "nonalcoholic" and hopefully help refocus the efforts of the family on improving the child's "nutrition."

21.1.2 Epidemiology and Significance

The prevalence and incidence of NAFLD in children have been an awakening for pediatric care providers. What was once an obscure diagnosis bringing to mind a slew of metabolic and inborn errors of metabolism, excess fat in a child's liver is now, unfortunately, extremely common. The rise of childhood obesity has paralleled the shifts in lifestyles of our children over the past 4 decades. The identification of this disorder in the early 1980s (1) was followed by a focus on understanding its epidemiology through population-based cohorts in the early 2000s (2).

The epidemiological facts accepted broadly today are listed in Table 21.2.

NAFLD in children is truly a significant result of the public health tsunami of childhood obesity. We therefore have to acknowledge the limitations of what can be achieved in the four walls of our health care units. With that said, there is clear import to the collaboration of the primary care provider or the gastrointestinal (GI) specialist in making a difference in the lives of these children.

Our current suggested approach is outlined in detail here and is encapsulated in an educational video produced by the joint efforts of the Fatty Liver Clinic and the marketing department at Children's Hospital Los Angeles (https://youtu.be/4CFYMAx5-7E).

21.2 CURRENT APPROACH

Patients with NAFLD are often asymptomatic and incidentally identified by the elevation of liver enzymes or hepatic steatosis on abdominal imaging studies performed for different indications. Although screening for pediatric

Table 21.1: Definitions

Fatty liver disease (NAFLD)	>5% liver steatosis
Fatty liver (NAFL)	NAFLD – [inflammation ± fibrosis]
Steatohepatitis (NASH)	NAFLD + [inflammation ± fibrosis]

Table 21.2: Key Points in NAFLD Epidemiology

Overall NAFLD rates have been increasing (3).

Boys have a higher prevalence of NAFLD (3).

Genetics plays a significant role in defining the prevalence of the severe form of the disease spectrum, NASH (4).

Children of Hispanic and Asian heritage are at increased risk of NASH.

Children of African heritage have a lower prevalence of NASH (5).

Sugar-sweetened beverage consumption is linked to increased rates of hepatic fibrosis (6)

DOI: 10.1201/9781003386698-26

NAFLD is an area of controversy that lacks consensus among different societies (7–9) an ever increasing number of patients are now identified through screening protocols. We believe that preventive screening in pediatric NAFLD is impactful given the high prevalence, the wide availability of an inexpensive screening tool (alanine aminotransferase [ALT]) and, most importantly, an effective although challenging-to-implement therapy (lifestyle intervention). Furthermore, early intervention in childhood will prevent the onset of end-stage liver disease and improve the patient's outcome. The North American Society of Pediatric Gastroenterology Hepatology and Nutrition (NASPGHAN) practice guideline recommends screening for NAFLD beginning between ages 9 and 11 years for all obese and overweight children with additional risk factors (e.g., insulin resistance, hyperlipidemia, hypertension, polycystic ovarian syndrome, obstructive sleep apnea, family history of NAFLD) (8). An earlier screening age is warranted in patients with panhypopituitarism given the high prevalence of rapidly progressive fibrosing NASH in this subset of patients (10). The recommended screening test is ALT using sex-specific upper limits of normal (females, 22 U/L; males, 26 U/L) that represent the 97th percentiles for a healthy lean population, as determined from the National Health and Nutrition Examination Survey (11).

It's important to acknowledge that ALT has some limitations as a screening tool, with advanced fibrosis detected in patients even with mild ALT elevation (12). Screening for gamma-glutamyltransferase (GGT) elevation in addition to ALT will improve the diagnostic accuracy and help identify patients at increased risk of progression. The use of abdominal ultrasound is not recommended as a screening tool for NAFLD (8).

Clinical assessment is of utmost importance in guiding management and is geared to identify:

1. *Pediatric NAFLD-causing disorders*: Including hypothyroidism (goiter), partial lipodystrophy (abnormal body fat distribution), lysosomal acid lipase (LAL) deficiency (xanthelasmas) (13), panhypopituitarism (neurological deficit, short stature and severe obesity);

2. *Associated metabolic comorbidities*: Hypertension and insulin resistance (assessed by the presence of acanthosis nigricans)

3. *Other signs*: Of portal hypertension (splenomegaly and spider angioma) and advanced liver disease (sarcopenia, clubbing).

Further management is guided by the extent and the duration of the ALT elevation and the response to lifestyle intervention overtime as outlined in Figure 21.1.

Indications for referral to the pediatric gastroenterology and hepatology subspecialist are highlighted in Figure 21.1. A comprehensive evaluation is often undertaken by the specialists and aims to rule out other causes of chronic elevation of liver enzymes, to screen for comorbidities, to confirm the diagnosis, and to stage and grade NASH (see Table 21.3).

Ultrasound-based shear wave elastography such as FibroScan® is gaining broader use as a noninvasive technique to screen and monitor fibrosis. FibroScan® accurately detects significant liver fibrosis. However, the accuracy is reduced with mild liver fibrosis, and the technical failure rate is higher in patients with severe central adiposity (14).

The magnetic resonance imaging proton density fat fraction (MRI-PDFF) provides an accurate, validated marker of hepatic steatosis and, when coupled with magnetic

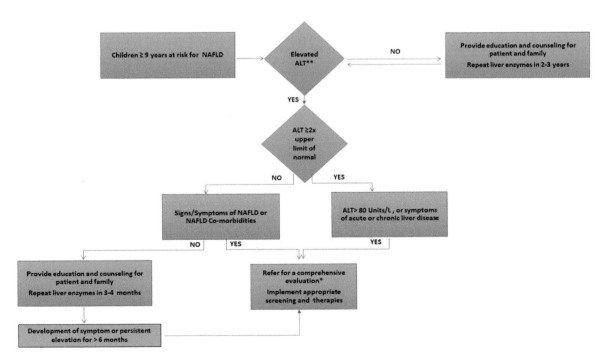

Figure 21.1 Algorithm for the screening and management of pediatric patients with suspected NAFLD

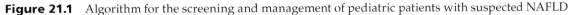

* The comprehensive evaluation is outlined in Table 21.3.
** Normal ALT is defined as ≤22 U/L in females and ≤ 26 U/L in males.

Table 21.3: Compressive Evaluation of Patients with Suspected NAFLD

Screening laboratory studies
- CBC with differential, AST, GGT, alkaline phosphatase, bilirubin total and direct, albumin, total protein, INR, hemoglobin A1C, and fasting glucose and lipid panel

Laboratory evaluation for common cause of chronic elevation of liver enzymes
- *Autoimmune liver disease*: Autoantibody profile (ASMA, ANA, ALKM)
- *Genetic*: Alpha 1 antitrypsin deficiency (alpha 1 antitrypsin phenotype); Wilson disease (ceruloplasmin and 24-hour urine copper quantification); juvenile hemochromatosis (serum iron, total iron binding capacity, ferritin); lysosomal acid lipase (LAL) deficiency (enzymatic assay and genetic study); abetalipoproteinemia (lipoprotein electrophoresis) (19,20)
- *Viral hepatitis*: Hepatitis C antibody, HBsAg and HBsAb
- *Celiac disease*: Tissue transglutaminase antibody (TTG) IgA, total IgA
- *Hypothyroidism*: TSH, FT4

Imaging studies
- *Abdominal ultrasound*: To rule out anatomical abnormalities and to assess for signs of portal hypertension (splenomegaly and nodular liver)
- FibroScan®: Considered when available to assess liver fibrosis
- *MRI-PDFF*: When available, considered to measure liver fat and MR elastography to assess liver fibrosis

Liver biopsy
- To confirm the diagnosis and consider vitamin E
- To assess the severity of steatosis, grade the inflammation and stage the fibrosis
- To rule out alternate liver diseases: Wilson's disease by copper quantification, and autoimmune hepatitis in patients with positive autoantibodies
- To support the bariatric surgery indication in select candidates with advanced liver fibrosis

resonance elastography (MRE), serves as a promising noninvasive tool to identify patients with hepatic steatosis and advanced liver fibrosis and to optimize risk stratification. However, the MRE does not discriminate between absence of fibrosis and mild fibrosis (15). Furthermore, the high cost and limited availability render it inappropriate as an NAFLD screening tool. Nonetheless, the three-dimensional MRE has the potential to assess steatosis (PDFF), inflammation (dampening ratio), and fibrosis (elastography) and is emerging as a noninvasive diagnostic and monitoring tool in patients with NASH (16).

Indications for a liver biopsy in patients with suspected NAFLD have not been uniformly established, and practice varies. There is a low likelihood that a liver biopsy would change the diagnosis in the majority of pediatric patients suspected to have NAFLD. However, there is merit in identifying a diagnosis of NASH, which opens up the potential for use of vitamin E as a temporary pharmacotherapy (17), details of which are discussed later in this chapter. Hence the decision to pursue a liver biopsy should be made on a case-by-case basis, after discussion of the benefits and risks and shared with the patients and their families.

Pediatric patients with NAFLD often have unique histological features that include portal inflammation and fibrosis in the absence of hepatocellular ballooning; this pattern is referred to as "type 2" NAFLD, while the pattern typically seen in adults is referred to as "type 1" NAFLD (18).

The management of pediatric NAFLD is geared to improving the outcome, achieving NASH resolution and fibrosis regression. The treatment is a three-pronged approach with lifestyle intervention, medical therapy and bariatric surgery.

Lifestyle intervention with diet and exercise to achieve 7–10% weight loss remains the cornerstone in the management of NASH. In a relatively recent systemic review and meta-analysis of 19 studies that included 923 patients, aerobic exercise and diet were the most used interventions, and in two studies aerobic exercise was the only intervention. The age of participants ranged from 6 to 18 years. The diet employed was normo-caloric ranging from 1,300 to 1,900 Kcal/day (50–65% from carbohydrates, 10–30% from fat and 12–20% from protein). All studies assessed aerobic exercise, ranging from once a week to daily workouts of 60 minutes on average, mostly 3–7 times per week. The duration of intervention ranged between 4 and 52 weeks. lifestyle changes to treat NAFLD in this study showed significant improvements in BMI, ALT levels and hepatic steatosis (21).

Emerging studies suggest that a low-glycemic, low-added-sugar diet (22) is beneficial in patients with NAFLD when adopted by the whole family. Recently, there has been increased interest in employing the Mediterranean diet in NAFLD patients due to the high-fiber, polyunsaturated-fatty-acids, and antioxidants content (23). Adult, randomized clinical trials using the Mediterranean diet showed significant weight loss, greater improvement in ALT and liver stiffness and higher adherence (24).

In addition, training with aerobic plus resistance exercise led to greater changes in ALT and greater resolution of hepatic steatosis than aerobic training alone (25). Hence physical activity is essential in the management of NASH and may be beneficial in the absence of weight loss supporting the importance of limiting screen time to no more than 2 hours a day.

The frequency of the visit and the accountability system, as well as the management by a multidisciplinary team, are essential in achieving and maintaining weight loss in patients with NAFLD (26). Children and adolescents with NAFLD should be counseled that alcohol consumption may exacerbate NAFLD. Assuring immunity after vaccination for hepatitis B and hepatitis A is important in NAFLD patients to eliminate the risk of vaccine preventable viral hepatitis.

Medications approved for weight loss in adolescents and adults include liraglutide and orlistat, but these have not been studied as NAFLD therapy in children. Although pediatric NAFLD lacks regulatory agency-approved therapy, here we will focus on medical agents in clinical use in pediatrics rather than in the pipeline.

The Treatment of NAFLD in Children (TONIC) trial evaluating vitamin E or metformin in 173 children ages 8 to 17 years with biopsy-proven NAFLD showed that daily vitamin E (800 IU) enhanced NASH resolution when compared to placebo without significant change in ALT (17). The same study did not show efficacy of metformin therapy. Hence, we recommend vitamin E in patients with biopsy-proven NASH.

The potential for *n*-3 PUFA supplementation in reducing hepatic steatosis and blood triglyceride level in children with NAFLD is well-established (27). However, there was no improvement in ALT or components of the metabolic syndrome to recommend supplementation with *n*-3 PUFA as a treatment of NAFLD (28).

Although small studies in pediatrics using probiotic have shown improvement of ALT and hepatic steatosis over the short period of administration (29), the beneficial role of probiotic as NAFLD therapy has not been established, and additional randomized controlled trial are required (30) before probiotics are recommended.

Selection criteria for bariatric surgery include a BMI 35–39 or 120% of the 95th percentile with comorbidities (type 2 diabetes mellitus, obstructive sleep apnea, advanced NASH, pseudotumor cerebri, Blount's disease, slipped capital femoral epiphysis, gastroesophageal reflux, and hypertension) or a BMI ≥40 or 140% of 95th percentile without any additional comorbidities requirement to qualify for bariatric surgery. The bariatric surgery evaluation includes a multidisciplinary team assessment of ability and motivation to adhere to pre- and postoperative treatment recommendations, including micronutrient supplements (31). Operations used in adolescents include restrictive surgeries (when the stomach volume is surgically reduced) and malabsorptive (when the small bowel absorptive area is bypassed). Sleeve gastrectomy (SG) and gastric band (GB) are restrictive surgeries while Roux-en-Y gastric bypass (RYGB) is malabsorptive and restrictive. A comparative study that included adolescents with RYGB (*n* = 177), SG (*n* = 306) and laparoscopic adjustable gastric banding (*n* = 61) showed that since 2005 the use of the SG bariatric surgery approach has gradually increased, while the RYGB and GB approaches have declined.

Furthermore, the mean BMI changes were respectively −31% for RYGB, −28% for SG and −10% for GB at 1 year. Similar trends were seen at 3 years, suggesting that laparoscopic adjustable gastric banding was significantly less effective for BMI reduction than SG and RYGB (32). Bariatric surgery in adolescents is associated with significant improvements in weight loss, diabetes, prediabetes, dyslipidemia, hypertension and kidney disfunction, and weight-related quality of life at 3 years after the procedure. Risks associated with surgery included low ferritin and the need for additional complication-related abdominal procedures (33).

Endoscopic bariatric surgery has been established in adults with some emerging literature supporting safety and efficacy of endoscopically an inserted gastric balloon in adolescents (34) (Figure 21.2). This is a potential therapeutic strategy that puts together the benefits of weight loss surgery sans the surgery!

21.3 UNIQUE ASPECTS AND GAPS IN KNOWLEDGE

The natural history and long-term risk of mortality in children and young adults with biopsy-confirmed NAFLD is poorly defined. Emerging data suggest progression of NAFLD in patients receiving lifestyle intervention (35), as well as higher rates of cancer, liver- and cardiometabolic-specific mortality (36). In a nationwide, matched cohort of all Swedish children and young adults (≤25 years) with biopsy-confirmed NAFLD, the 20-year absolute risk of overall mortality was 7.7 % among NAFLD vs. 1.1% in the general population (36).

While screening tools for NAFLD are evolving, the precision of some including the FibroScan® requires further validation, and MR elastography is more available than before but is still not very widely available. Therefore, the role of noninvasive monitoring is crucial in the pediatric population to abrogate the risks of a liver biopsy performed usually under anesthesia in the pediatric age group.

Furthermore, pediatric NAFLD is a heterogeneous disease influenced by age, sex, genetic variants, metabolic comorbidities and the microbiota composition. The heterogeneous nature of NAFLD results from a different contributions of numerous pathogenic mechanisms manifesting as multiple disease phenotypes with different natural history, prognosis and response to therapy (37).

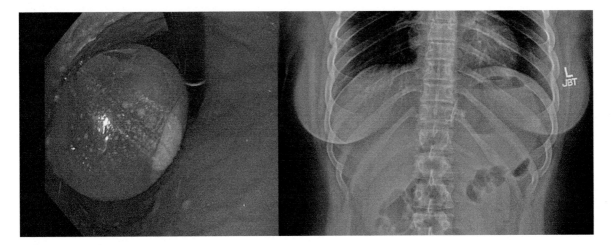

Figure 21.2   Endoscopically inserted gastric balloon, appropriate position confirmed by X-ray (Courtesy of Dr. Imad Absah, Mayo Clinic.)

The role of disease modifier in the severity of NASH is unraveling. A well-described example is alpha-1 antitrypsin deficiency, where the heterozygotes (MZ) genotype may contribute to the severity of NAFLD and the need of liver transplantation (38). In addition, intestinal dysbiosis plays a critical role in the development of pediatric NAFLD but is not clinically used in the diagnosis and management. A subset of patients with rapidly progressive NASH associated with panhypopituitarism may require liver transplantation in adolescence or young adulthood and are at high risk of recurrence in the graft (39,40). All these factors account for the modest response to therapies applied on a diverse patient population without stratification.

Adding to the challenges of managing pediatric NAFLD is that weight loss and maintenance are not achieved without family-based, patient-centered intensive interventions.

Increased awareness and advocacy for the development of public health policies that support healthy school meals and the design of cities that incorporate space for children's outdoor activities are essential in the journey to prevent and treat pediatric NAFLD.

21.4 CONCLUSION AND FUTURE DIRECTIONS

In summation, we are faced with a challenge that is society's own making. The genes that predispose us to the severe form of this disease, NASH, have been in existence for millennia, but the change in our nutritional environment that has been brought to bear on these genes is no more than a few decades in the making. We liken this challenge to our dependence as a society on fossil fuels. There is a way out through green energy for the latter, and there is a way out by reversing our current mal-lifestyle for the former.

While we await the population-based public health endeavors to bear fruit, we will still have to take care of the children with NASH and their progressive fibrosis leading to end-stage liver disease and the need for liver transplant in early adulthood. To those children we need to deliver safe and effective medications and/or weight loss strategies. These may even include, for the very extreme scenarios, weight loss surgical techniques that are currently exclusive to adults, such as endoscopic bariatric surgery or devices. These medications and procedures are, of course, not ready for "prime time" yet; however, we should not be surprised to see them brought up in our pediatric practices and discussed by families as therapeutic options for their children who may unfortunately have NASH. When that does happen, we better be prepared to discuss the *smell of these new roses!*

REFERENCES

1. Ludwig J, Viggiano TR, McGill DB, Oh BJ. Nonalcoholic steatohepatitis: Mayo clinic experiences with a hitherto unnamed disease. *Mayo Clin Proc.* 1980;55(7):434–438. Epub 1980/07/01. PubMed PMID: 7382552.

2. Schwimmer JB, Deutsch R, Kahen T, Lavine JE, Stanley C, Behling C. Prevalence of fatty liver in children and adolescents. *Pediatrics.* 2006;118(4):1388–1393. Epub 2006/10/04. doi:10.1542/peds.2006-1212. PubMed PMID: 17015527.

3. Zhang X, Wu M, Liu Z, Yuan H, Wu X, Shi T, et al. Increasing prevalence of NAFLD/NASH among children, adolescents and young adults from 1990 to 2017: A population-based observational study. *BMJ Open.* 2021;11(5):e042843. Epub 2021/05/06. doi:10.1136/bmjopen-2020-042843. PubMed PMID: 33947727; PubMed Central PMCID: PMCPMC8098935.

4. Trepo E, Valenti L. Update on NAFLD genetics: From new variants to the clinic. *J Hepatol.* 2020;72(6):1196–1209. Epub 2020/03/08. doi:10.1016/j.jhep.2020.02.020. PubMed PMID: 32145256.

5. Yu EL, Schwimmer JB. Epidemiology of pediatric non-alcoholic fatty liver disease. *Clin Liver Dis (Hoboken).* 2021;17(3):196–199. Epub 2021/04/20. doi:10.1002/cld.1027. PubMed PMID: 33868665; PubMed Central PMCID: PMCPMC8043694.

6. Moran-Lev H, Cohen S, Webb M, Yerushalmy-Feler A, Amir A, Gal DL, et al. Higher BMI predicts liver fibrosis among obese children and adolescents with NAFLD—an interventional pilot study. *BMC Pediatr.* 2021;21(1):385. Epub 2021/09/05. doi:10.1186/s12887-021-02839-1. PubMed PMID: 34479517; PubMed Central PMCID: PMCPMC8414665.

7. Chalasani N, Younossi Z, Lavine JE, Charlton M, Cusi K, Rinella M, et al. The diagnosis and management of nonalcoholic fatty liver disease: Practice guidance from the American Association for the Study of Liver Diseases. *Hepatology.* 2018;67(1):328–357. Epub 2017/07/18. doi:10.1002/hep.29367. PubMed PMID: 28714183.

8. Vos MB, Abrams SH, Barlow SE, Caprio S, Daniels SR, Kohli R, et al. NASPGHAN clinical practice guideline for the diagnosis and treatment of nonalcoholic fatty liver disease in children: Recommendations from the expert committee on NAFLD (ECON) and the North American society of pediatric gastroenterology, hepatology and nutrition (NASPGHAN). *J Pediatr Gastroenterol Nutr.* 2017;64(2):319–334. Epub 2017/01/21. doi:10.1097/MPG.0000000000001482. PubMed PMID: 28107283; PubMed Central PMCID: PMCPMC5413933.

9. Koot BGP, Nobili V. Screening for non-alcoholic fatty liver disease in children: Do guidelines provide enough guidance? *Obes Rev.* 2017;18(9):1050–1060. Epub 2017/05/26. doi:10.1111/obr.12556. PubMed PMID: 28544608.

10. Gilliland T, Dufour S, Shulman GI, Petersen KF, Emre SH. Resolution of non-alcoholic steatohepatitis after growth hormone replacement in a pediatric liver transplant patient with panhypopituitarism. *Pediatr Transplant.* 2016;20(8):1157–1163. Epub 2016/10/21. doi:10.1111/petr.12819. PubMed PMID: 27762491.

11. Schwimmer JB, Dunn W, Norman GJ, Pardee PE, Middleton MS, Kerkar N, et al. SAFETY study: Alanine aminotransferase cutoff values are set too high for reliable detection of pediatric chronic liver disease. *Gastroenterology.* 2010;138(4):1357–1364, 64 e1–2. Epub 2010/01/13. doi:10.1053/j.gastro.2009.12.052. PubMed PMID: 20064512; PubMed Central PMCID: PMCPMC2846968.

12. Molleston JP, Schwimmer JB, Yates KP, Murray KF, Cummings OW, Lavine JE, et al. Histological abnormalities in children with nonalcoholic fatty liver disease and normal or mildly elevated alanine aminotransferase levels. *J Pediatr.* 2014;164(4):707–713 e3. Epub 2013/12/24. doi:10.1016/j.jpeds.2013.10.071. PubMed PMID: 24360992; PubMed Central PMCID: PMCPMC3962701.

13. Burton BK, Deegan PB, Enns GM, Guardamagna O, Horslen S, Hovingh GK, et al. Clinical features of

lysosomal acid lipase deficiency. *J Pediatr Gastroenterol Nutr*. 2015;61(6):619–625. Epub 2015/08/08. doi:10.1097/MPG.0000000000000935. PubMed PMID: 26252914; PubMed Central PMCID: PMCPMC4645959.

14. Garcovich M, Veraldi S, Di Stasio E, Zocco MA, Monti L, Toma P, et al. Liver stiffness in pediatric patients with fatty liver disease: Diagnostic accuracy and reproducibility of shear-wave elastography. *Radiology*. 2017;283(3):820–827. Epub 2016/12/17. doi:10.1148/radiol.2016161002. PubMed PMID: 27982761.

15. Schwimmer JB, Behling C, Angeles JE, Paiz M, Durelle J, Africa J, et al. Magnetic resonance elastography measured shear stiffness as a biomarker of fibrosis in pediatric nonalcoholic fatty liver disease. *Hepatology*. 2017;66(5):1474–1485. Epub 2017/05/12. doi:10.1002/hep.29241. PubMed PMID: 28493388; PubMed Central PMCID: PMCPMC5650504.

16. Allen AM, Shah VH, Therneau TM, Venkatesh SK, Mounajjed T, Larson JJ, et al. The role of three-dimensional magnetic resonance elastography in the diagnosis of nonalcoholic steatohepatitis in obese patients undergoing bariatric surgery. *Hepatology*. 2020;71(2):510–521. Epub 2018/12/26. doi:10.1002/hep.30483. PubMed PMID: 30582669; PubMed Central PMCID: PMCPMC6591099.

17. Lavine JE, Schwimmer JB, Van Natta ML, Molleston JP, Murray KF, Rosenthal P, et al. Effect of vitamin e or metformin for treatment of nonalcoholic fatty liver disease in children and adolescents the TONIC randomized controlled trial. *Jama-J Am Med Assoc*. 2011;305(16):1659–1668. doi:10.1001/jama.2011.520. PubMed PMID: WOS:000289890500019.

18. Schwimmer JB, Behling C, Newbury R, Deutsch R, Nievergelt C, Schork NJ, et al. Histopathology of pediatric nonalcoholic fatty liver disease. *Hepatology*. 2005;42(3):641–649. Epub 2005/08/24. doi:10.1002/hep.20842. PubMed PMID: 16116629.

19. Welty FK. Hypobetalipoproteinemia and abetalipoproteinemia. *Curr Opin Lipidol*. 2014;25(3):161–168. Epub 2014/04/23. doi:10.1097/MOL.0000000000000072. PubMed PMID: 24751931; PubMed Central PMCID: PMCPMC4465983.

20. Peretti N, Sassolas A, Roy CC, Deslandres C, Charcosset M, Castagnetti J, et al. Guidelines for the diagnosis and management of chylomicron retention disease based on a review of the literature and the experience of two centers. *Orphanet J Rare Dis*. 2010;5:24. Epub 2010/10/06. doi:10.1186/1750-1172-5-24. PubMed PMID: 20920215; PubMed Central PMCID: PMCPMC2956717.

21. Utz-Melere M, Targa-Ferreira C, Lessa-Horta B, Epifanio M, Mouzaki M, Mattos AA. Non-alcoholic fatty liver disease in children and adolescents: Lifestyle change—a systematic review and meta-analysis. *Ann Hepatol*. 2018;17(3):345–354. Epub 2018/05/08. doi:10.5604/01.3001.0011.7380. PubMed PMID: 29735796.

22. Schwimmer JB, Ugalde-Nicalo P, Welsh JA, Angeles JE, Cordero M, Harlow KE, et al. Effect of a low free sugar diet vs usual diet on nonalcoholic fatty liver disease in adolescent boys: A randomized clinical trial. *JAMA*. 2019;321(3):256–265. Epub 2019/01/23. doi:10.1001/jama.2018.20579. PubMed PMID: 30667502; PubMed Central PMCID: PMCPMC6440226.

23. Anania C, Perla FM, Olivero F, Pacifico L, Chiesa C. Mediterranean diet and nonalcoholic fatty liver disease. *World J Gastroenterol*. 2018;24(19):2083–2094. Epub 2018/05/23. doi:10.3748/wjg.v24.i19.2083. PubMed PMID: 29785077; PubMed Central PMCID: PMCPMC5960814.

24. Katsagoni CN, Papatheodoridis GV, Ioannidou P, Deutsch M, Alexopoulou A, Papadopoulos N, et al. Improvements in clinical characteristics of patients with non-alcoholic fatty liver disease, after an intervention based on the Mediterranean lifestyle: A randomised controlled clinical trial. *Br J Nutr*. 2018;120(2):164–175. Epub 2018/06/28. doi:10.1017/S000711451800137X. PubMed PMID: 29947322.

25. de Piano A, de Mello MT, Sanches Pde L, da Silva PL, Campos RM, Carnier J, et al. Long-term effects of aerobic plus resistance training on the adipokines and neuropeptides in nonalcoholic fatty liver disease obese adolescents. *Eur J Gastroenterol Hepatol*. 2012;24(11):1313–1324. Epub 2012/08/31. doi:10.1097/MEG.0b013e32835793ac. PubMed PMID: 22932160.

26. Mameli C, Krakauer JC, Krakauer NY, Bosetti A, Ferrari CM, Schneider L, et al. Effects of a multidisciplinary weight loss intervention in overweight and obese children and adolescents: 11 years of experience. *PLoS ONE*. 2017;12(7):e0181095. Epub 2017/07/14. doi:10.1371/journal.pone.0181095. PubMed PMID: 28704494; PubMed Central PMCID: PMCPMC5509286.

27. Nobili V, Alisi A, Della Corte C, Rise P, Galli C, Agostoni C, et al. Docosahexaenoic acid for the treatment of fatty liver: Randomised controlled trial in children. *Nutr Metab Cardiovasc Dis*. 2013;23(11):1066–1070. Epub 2012/12/12. doi:10.1016/j.numecd.2012.10.010. PubMed PMID: 23220074.

28. Chen LH, Wang YF, Xu QH, Chen SS. Omega-3 fatty acids as a treatment for non-alcoholic fatty liver disease in children: A systematic review and meta-analysis of randomized controlled trials. *Clin Nutr*. 2018;37(2):516–521. doi:10.1016/j.clnu.2016.12.009. PubMed PMID: WOS:000428483200012.

29. Famouri F, Shariat Z, Hashemipour M, Keikha M, Kelishadi R. Effects of probiotics on nonalcoholic fatty liver disease in obese children and adolescents. *J Pediatr Gastroenterol Nutr*. 2017;64(3):413–417. Epub 2017/02/24. doi:10.1097/MPG.0000000000001422. PubMed PMID: 28230607.

30. Sharpton SR, Maraj B, Harding-Theobald E, Vittinghoff E, Terrault NA. Gut microbiome-targeted therapies in nonalcoholic fatty liver disease: A systematic review, meta-analysis, and meta-regression. *Am J Clin Nutr*. 2019;110(1):139–149. Epub 2019/05/28. doi:10.1093/ajcn/nqz042. PubMed PMID: 31124558; PubMed Central PMCID: PMCPMC6599739.

31. Armstrong SC, Bolling CF, Michalsky MP, Reichard KW, Section on Obesity SOS. Pediatric metabolic and bariatric surgery: Evidence, barriers, and best practices. *Pediatrics*. 2019;144(6). Epub 2019/10/28. doi:10.1542/peds.2019-3223. PubMed PMID: 31656225.

32. Inge TH, Coley RY, Bazzano LA, Xanthakos SA, McTigue K, Arterburn D, et al. Comparative effectiveness of bariatric procedures among adolescents: The PCORnet bariatric study. *Surg Obes Relat Dis*. 2018;14(9):1374–1386. Epub 2018/05/26. doi:10.1016/j.soard.2018.04.002. PubMed PMID: 29793877; PubMed Central PMCID: PMCPMC6165694.

33. Inge TH, Courcoulas AP, Jenkins TM, Michalsky MP, Helmrath MA, Brandt ML, et al. Weight loss and health status 3 years after bariatric surgery in adolescents. *N Engl J Med*. 2016;374(2):113–123. Epub 2015/11/07. doi:10.1056/NEJMoa1506699. PubMed PMID: 26544725; PubMed Central PMCID: PMCPMC4810437.

34. De Peppo F, Caccamo R, Adorisio O, Ceriati E, Marchetti P, Contursi A, et al. The Obalon swallowable intragastric balloon in pediatric and adolescent morbid obesity. *Endosc Int Open*. 2017;5(1):E59–E63. Epub 2017/02/10. doi:10.1055/s-0042-120413. PubMed PMID: 28180149; PubMed Central PMCID: PMCPMC5283171.

35. Xanthakos SA, Lavine JE, Yates KP, Schwimmer JB, Molleston JP, Rosenthal P, et al. Progression of fatty liver disease in children receiving standard of care lifestyle advice. *Gastroenterology*. 2020;159(5):1731–1751 e10. Epub 2020/07/28. doi:10.1053/j.gastro.2020.07.034. PubMed PMID: 32712103; PubMed Central PMCID: PMCPMC7680281.

36. Simon TG, Roelstraete B, Hartjes K, Shah U, Khalili H, Arnell H, et al. Non-alcoholic fatty liver disease in children and young adults is associated with increased long-term mortality. *J Hepatol*. 2021;75(5):1034–1041. Epub 2021/07/06. doi:10.1016/j.jhep.2021.06.034. PubMed PMID: 34224779; PubMed Central PMCID: PMCPMC8530955.

37. Arrese M, Arab JP, Barrera F, Kaufmann B, Valenti L, Feldstein AE. Insights into nonalcoholic fatty-liver disease heterogeneity. *Semin Liver Dis*. 2021;41(4):421–434. Epub 2021/07/08. doi:10.1055/s-0041-1730927. PubMed PMID: 34233370; PubMed Central PMCID: PMCPMC8492194 present study. L.V. has received speaking fees from MSD, Gilead, AlfaSigma, and AbbVie, served as a consultant for Gilead, Pfizer, AstraZeneca, Novo Nordisk, Intercept, Diatech Pharmacogenetics and Ionis Pharmaceuticals, and received research grants from Gilead.

38. Regev A, Guaqueta C, Molina EG, Conrad A, Mishra V, Brantly ML, et al. Does the heterozygous state of alpha-1 antitrypsin deficiency have a role in chronic liver diseases? Interim results of a large case-control study. *J Pediatr Gastroenterol Nutr*. 2006;43(Suppl 1):S30–35. Epub 2006/07/05. doi:10.1097/01.mpg.0000226387.56612.1e. PubMed PMID: 16819398.

39. Adams LA, Feldstein A, Lindor KD, Angulo P. Nonalcoholic fatty liver disease among patients with hypothalamic and pituitary dysfunction. *Hepatology*. 2004;39(4):909–914. doi:10.1002/hep.20140. PubMed PMID: WOS:000220539300006.

40. Bhanji RA, Watt KD. Fatty allograft and cardiovascular outcomes after liver transplantation. *Liver Transpl*. 2017;23(S1):S76–S80. Epub 2017/08/18. doi:10.1002/lt.24843. PubMed PMID: 28815935.

22 NAFLD in HIV Patients

Giada Sebastiani

CONTENTS

Key Points

- Aging-related comorbidities, including liver disease, represent the main drivers of morbidity and mortality in people with HIV (PWH). This trend is driven by the successful implementation of effective antiretroviral therapy (ART), with PWH now reaching a life expectancy similar to that of the general population.

- Nonalcoholic fatty liver disease (NAFLD) is a frequent aging-related comorbidity, affecting 35% of HIV mono-infected patients.

- PWH are at higher risk not only of NAFLD but also of NASH and associated liver fibrosis. Multiple pathogenic mechanisms may be involved, including excess metabolic comorbidities, hepatotoxic effect of lifelong ART and immunoactivation due to chronic HIV infection.

- Noninvasive diagnostic tests, such as serum biomarkers and elastography, may help case finding of PWH with NAFLD-related fibrosis. This will improve risk stratification and enhancement of clinical management decisions, including prompt initiation of interventions such as lifestyle changes and a few pharmacologic interventions, as well as surveillance for hepatocellular carcinoma and esophageal varices.

22.1 INTRODUCTION

HIV continues to be a major global public health issue. In 2018, there were approximately 37.9 million people with HIV (PWH) worldwide (1). The advent of combination antiretroviral therapy (ART) has considerably improved the health of PWH: 50% of PWH in North America are now over 50 years old (2). As a consequence, the focus in the management of PWH is shifting to chronic noninfectious comorbidities as both chronic HIV infection itself and long-term ART may affect the trajectory of aging-related conditions (3). Nowadays, mortality from liver disease is higher than that from cardiovascular diseases and second only to AIDS-related mortality (4). Over the last decade,

the proportion of deaths attributed to liver-related causes has increased between 8- and 10-fold in the post-ART era while AIDS-related mortality has fallen more than 90-fold (5, 6). While coinfection with hepatitis B (HBV) and C (HCV) viruses is believed to have driven this trend in the past, risk factors unique to this population, combined with frequent metabolic comorbidities, may contribute to nonalcoholic fatty liver disease (NAFLD) in HIV mono-infected patients, who represent 86–89% of PWH (7).

22.2 DEFINITION OF NAFLD IN HIV

NAFLD is an umbrella term that encompasses a spectrum of clinical and pathologic features characterized by a fatty overload involving over 5% of the liver weight in the absence of other causes of liver disease. Nonalcoholic fatty liver or simple steatosis can evolve to nonalcoholic steatohepatitis (NASH), significant scarring (fibrosis) and liver cirrhosis, eventually resulting in end-stage complications (8). Metabolic-associated fatty liver disease (MAFLD) is a novel concept proposed in 2020 aiming to replace the term NAFLD (9). Unlike NAFLD, MAFLD is not a diagnosis of exclusion of other liver diseases, such as excessive alcohol consumption or viral hepatitis. MAFLD is a positive diagnosis done in patients when they have both hepatic steatosis and any of the following three metabolic conditions: overweight/obesity, diabetes mellitus or evidence of metabolic dysregulation in lean individuals. This novel concept has also been proposed in HIV, especially considering that lean NAFLD seems more prevalent and severe in the setting of HIV infection (10,11). However further data on its natural history and utility in clinical practice are needed in the setting of HIV infection (12).

22.3 PATHOGENESIS OF NAFLD IN THE CONTEXT OF HIV INFECTION

22.3.1 Classic Pathogenic Factors

The pathogenesis of NAFLD in PWH encompasses multiple complex mechanisms, including frequent metabolic

DOI: 10.1201/9781003386698-27

pathogenic factors and risk factors specific to HIV infection. These mechanisms are only partially understood and include comorbid metabolic conditions, direct viral effects and adverse effects of ART (see Figure 22.1). In HIV-negative NAFLD, insulin resistance represents the major driver of disease pathogenesis. Moreover, any element constituting the metabolic syndrome, such as obesity, type 2 diabetes mellitus (T2DM), hypertension or dyslipidemia, is linked to progression of NAFLD, and 85% of patients with NAFLD have at least one such condition (13). These classic components of the metabolic syndrome are more frequent in PWH. Diabetes is four times more prevalent in PWH compared to HIV-negative men. A longitudinal study with a median follow-up of 4 years found a cumulative incidence of T2DM of 10% in PWH, compared to 3% in uninfected controls (14). A meta-analysis of 44 studies reported a pooled incidence rate of overt diabetes and prediabetes at 13.7 per 1000 person-years (PY) of follow-up (95% confidence interval [CI] 13–20; I = 98.1%) among 396,496 PY and 125 per 1000 PY (95% CI 0–123; I = 99.4%) among 1,532 PY, respectively (15). In PWH, dyslipidemia is a complex condition due to multiple contributing factors including the HIV virus itself, individual genetic characteristics and ART-induced metabolic changes (16). There is evidence of an abnormal HDL cholesterol metabolism in PWH compared with uninfected persons. The prevalence of dyslipidemia in PWH ranges from 35 to 63% (17,18). Among ART regimens, protease inhibitors (PIs) generally increase LDL cholesterol and triglycerides, most notably when paired with ritonavir as a pharmacological booster (16). A study of 13,632 adults reported an incidence rate of dyslipidemia higher in ART-treated compared to ART-naïve and matched non-HIV groups (24.55 per 1,000 PY vs. 14.32 vs. 23.23, respectively). Multivariable analysis suggested a higher risk of dyslipidemia in the ART-treated HIV-infected group (adjusted hazard ratio [aHR],=,1.18; 95% CI 1.07–1.30] and a lower risk in the ART-naïve HIV-infected group (aHR = 0.66; 95% CI 0.53–0.82) compared to the control non-HIV-infected group (19). Hypertension is also very common in PWH. A recent systematic review and meta-analysis including 194 studies (396,776 PWH from 61 countries) reported a global prevalence of hypertension at 23.6% (95% CI 21.6–25.5). The prevalence was higher in high-income countries and in PWH taking ART (20). Finally, the increased prevalence of NAFLD in PWH is paralleled by the concomitant increase in overweight and obesity rate (21). Interestingly, lean NAFLD, defined as NAFLD affecting patients with body mass index (BMI) less than 25 kg/m², seems more frequent in the setting of HIV infection. Indeed, NAFLD affects 1 in 4 lean PWH, representing 35% of all PWH with NAFLD. Lean PWH with NAFLD have also more metabolic derangements, such as higher triglyceride and alanine aminotransferase (ALT) levels, and lower HDL levels than lean patients without NAFLD. Finally, they also have longer duration of HIV infection and higher CD4 lymphocyte counts and are more likely to be virally suppressed (22). Besides insulin resistance, the pathophysiology of NAFLD is influenced by multiple factors (environmental and genetics) in a multiple parallel-hit model, in which oxidative stress may play a primary role. The homeostasis of fat and energy in hepatic cells is regulated by mitochondrial activities, including beta-oxidation of free fatty acids, electron transfer and production of adenosine triphosphate and reactive oxygen species (ROS) (23). Mitochondrial abnormalities alter the balance between pro-oxidant and antioxidant mechanisms, leading to an increase of fatty acids as a result of the blockade of beta-oxidation and the consequent production of ROS (23). A decreased activity of several antioxidant enzymes is also observed. Glutathione peroxidase activity is reduced in NAFLD, and mitochondrial cytochrome P450 2E1, a potential direct source of ROS, has an increased activity in NASH patients. Some cytochrome P450 2E1 polymorphisms have been shown to be associated with the development of NASH in obese, nondiabetic subjects (23). Overall, oxidative stress triggers production of inflammatory cytokines (such as interleukin 6 and cytokeratin 18) and stimulates fibrogenesis and cell death (8) in NAFLD. Of note, PWH have high levels of markers of oxidative stress (24). Genetic predisposition also contributes to NAFLD pathogenesis. A genome-wide association scan of sequence variations (n = 9,229) in a multiethnic population identified an allele variant of the patatin-like phospholipase domain containing 3 (PNPLA3) gene (rs738409; I148M) as strongly linked to more hepatic inflammation and fat content deposition (25). In the Multicenter AIDS Cohort Study, PNPLA3 (rs738409) non-CC genotype was associated with a higher prevalence of fatty liver (odds ratio 3.30, 95% CI 1.66–6.57), although this was not confirmed by a subsequent study (26,27). Gut microbiota has emerged as a potential player in the pathogenesis of NASH. In a study of 81 PWH, Yanavich and colleagues found that those with steatosis or fibrosis had distinct microbial profiles, specifically PWH with steatosis had depletions of Akkermansia muciniphila and Bacteroides dorei and enrichment of Prevotella copri, Finegoldia magna and Ruminococcus bromii, while PWH with fibrosis had depletions of Bacteroides stercoris and Parabacteroides distasonis and enrichment of Sneathia sanguinegens (28). Finally, monocyte/macrophage activation (soluble CD163 and CD14) may affect development of NAFLD and fibrosis, suggesting a Kupffer cell activation in the development of liver fibrosis. Soluble CD163 and CD14 have been associated with immune dysfunction, all-cause mortality and liver fibrosis in PWH (29, 30).

22.3.2 Pathogenic Factors Specific to HIV

Factors unique to PWH may further contribute to the increased frequency and severity of NAFLD. Direct viral effects may contribute to NAFLD. Chronic HIV infection and associated inflammation may lead to immune-activating and pro-apoptotic effects of HIV on hepatocytes, including low-level HIV replication in hepatocytes inducing liver fibrosis (31,32). Indeed, HIV viremia from ART interruptions is an independent risk factors for chronic elevated transaminases (33). Depletion of CD4+ lymphocytes in the gut causes disruption of the gut epithelial barrier, facilitating microbial translocation into the portal and systemic translocation. This promotes liver fibrosis by activation of hepatic Kupffer cells and induction of proinflammatory cytokines (34). HIV-induced mitochondrial dysfunction results in the production of ROS, which causes oxidative stress increasing fat accumulation in hepatocytes (35). Certain ART regimens may also contribute to the pathogenesis of NAFLD. Chronic elevation of ALT is noted in 20–30% of PWH on ART and is associated with histologic abnormalities, including NASH and fibrosis, in up to 60% of cases (31,36). Older nucleoside reverse transcriptase inhibitors (NRTIs), particularly zidovudine, stavudine and didanosine, can induce mitochondrial

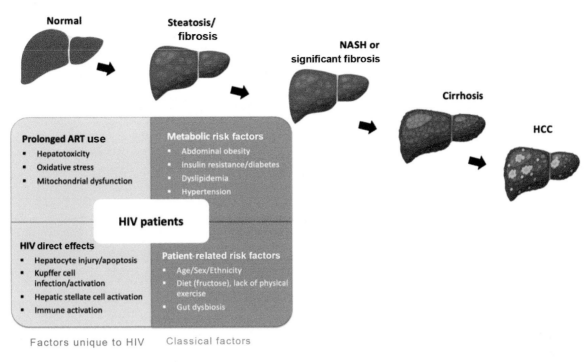

Figure 22.1 Adverse effects of ART

damage leading to impaired fatty acid oxidation and microvesicular steatosis. Although these drugs are no longer recommended, associated insults on the liver persist after discontinuation and may be irreversible (16,37,38). PIs increase central adiposity, decrease hepatic clearance of very-low-density lipoproteins, increase hepatic triglyceride production and potentially contribute to NAFLD (39). Use of ritonavir-boosted PIs (darunavir, indinavir, lopinavir) is commonly associated with elevation in transaminases and direct hepatocyte stress (40). Although less frequent with more modern ART regimens, lipodystrophy is also a potential pathogenetic contributor to NAFLD in PWH. Lipodystrophy is a constellation of body composition and metabolic alterations characterized by a pathological accumulation of adipose tissue in the abdominal region, insulin resistance and dyslipidemia (41). Lipodystrophy may occur in up to 80% of PWH treated with old ART regimens, particularly PIs, and persists after their discontinuation. NAFLD may coexist as integral part of this clinical entity. ART has been associated with weight gain and with metabolic consequences still not known (42). In a US study, nearly half of PWH were obese at the time of starting ART, and in the following 2 years, 20% moved up to a higher BMI category (43). Achhra and colleagues showed that weight gain in the first year after initiation of ART was associated with increased risk of cardiovascular disease and diabetes (44). Despite integrase inhibitors being associated with a safer metabolic profile and less frequent dyslipidemia, recent data suggest increased weight gain, especially in Black African women (45). In a single-center, prospective study of 301 PWH followed for a median of 41.8 months, participants who received integrase inhibitors and tenofovir alafenamide-based ART demonstrated a significantly faster steatosis development or progression by transient elastography (TE) with associated controlled attenuation parameter (CAP) (46). Overall, the pathogenesis of NAFLD in the setting of HIV infection is complex

and only partly understood, due to both HIV itself and the long-lasting exposure to ART, combined with frequent metabolic comorbidities.

22.4 EPIDEMIOLOGY OF NAFLD IN PEOPLE WITH HIV

With longer life expectancy and declining AIDS-associated mortality, non-AIDS-related comorbidities have emerged as major diagnostic and treatment concerns in PWH. Chronic liver disease is now the second most common cause of non-AIDS-related mortality in PWH (4). Results of a US study of 47,062 PWH from 2006 to 2016 showed that 22% had some form of liver disease (47). The increased prevalence of liver disease is multifactorial, but an important component is likely attributable to NAFLD. The prevalence of NAFLD among PWH ranges widely from 13 to 65%, likely due to differences in study population characteristics and diagnostic tools adopted (Table 22.1) (38,48–52). For instance, the proportion of PWH with elevated ALT, distribution of sex and ethnicity, as well as frequency of metabolic comorbidities and HIV characteristics—particularly type and duration of ART exposure and HIV infection—affect this reported prevalence. Older studies included mostly PWH with chronic elevation of liver transaminases, selected to undergo liver biopsy. In those studies, the prevalence of NAFLD was as high as 65% (36,53). Most recently, studies employing noninvasive diagnostic tools in consecutive PWH without viral hepatitis coinfection reported a prevalence ranging between 30 and 40% (54–56). Histologic studies reporting the prevalence of NASH in HIV mono-infection mostly included patients with elevated ALT, thus introducing a selection bias (57). A study from UK including 97 HIV mono-infected patients reported a prevalence of 8.2% (58). In a study of 55 patients with elevated ALT, Crum–Cianflone et al. found a prevalence of NASH at 7.3% (59). The largest histology-based study including 116 PWH

Table 22.1a: Prevalence of NAFLD/NASH and Significant Liver Fibrosis/Cirrhosis in HIV Mono-Infected Patients

	Design/ Country	N	Diagnostic Method	Age (years)	Male (%)	Alcohol Excess (%)	BMI (Kg/m2)	Diabetes (%)	ALT Elevation (%)	Duration HIV Infection (years)	Time on ART (years)	NAFLD/ NASH (%)	≥F2 Fibrosis/ cirrhosis (%)	NAFLD Predictors
Benmassaoud (63)	Prospective/ Canada	202	CAP/TE, CK-18	53.8± 10.5	77.7	0	NA	13.4	75	NA	NA	53.9/11.4	10.9/4.5	NASH: HOMA-IR, ↑ALT
Crum-Cianflone (59)	Prospective/ USA	216 (Biopsy $n = 55$)	US (liver biopsy in a subgroup)	41 (IQR 30–46)	96.2	12.5	26.0±4.1	5.1	100	14 (IQR 6–20)	NA	31/7.3	3.6	NA
Guaraldi (38)	Prospective/ Italy	255	CT scan	48 (range 19–74)	72.4	0	23.7±3.4	12.2	28	12.3±5.0	NA	36.9/NA	NA	AST/ALT ratio, male sex, waist circumference, NRTI exposure
Ingiliz (36)	Prospective/ France	30	Liver biopsy	46 (range 31–67)	97	0	23.0±3.1	NA	100	13 (IQR 9–15)	NA	60/53.3	20	NASH: ↑TG, hyperglycemia, HOMA-IR
Lemoine(61)	Prospective/ France	14	Liver biopsy	43.5 (range 31–58)	86	0	23.0±3.4	NA	100	10.6 (median)	NA	57.1/57.1	28.6	NA
Lombardi(51)	Retrospective/ UK	20 (out of 156)	Liver biopsy	47.5±8.5	91.7	0	NA	11	100	14 (IQR 2–30)	11 (IQR 0–26)	65/NA	NA/5	NA
Lombardi (66)	Retrospective/ UK	125	US/TE	39.6±10.3	91	6.5	24.6±2.9	5.6	16.8	6 (IQR 0–26)	3 (IQR 0–17)	55/NA	17.6/NA	Male sex, age, HOMA-IR, GGT
Lui (50)	Prospective/ China	80	H-MRS/ CK-18/TE	53.9±11.2	92.5	1	23.6±3.9	48.8	NA	8 (IQR 4–13)	NA	28.7/NA	13.8/5	↑TG
Macias (49)	Prospective/ Spain	505	CAP	46 (IQR 41–49)	69	11	23.2 (IQR 20.9–26)	4.4	NA	NA	NA	40/NA	NA	BMI
Mohr (56)	Prospective/ Germany	289	CAP/TE	45 (IQR 20–75)	78	NA	24 (range 16–41)	4	NA	8 (range 0–29)	6 (range 0–23)	40.8/NA	NA	BMI, haemoglobin glycosylated, TG
Morse (53)	Prospective/ USA	62	Liver biopsy	50 (range 17–67)	94	0	27.6 (range 15.3–47.1)	9.7	100	17.5 (range 2.3–27.8)	12.9 (range 1.7–22.8)	72.6/54.8	19.4	NASH: obesity, insulin resistance, PNPLA3
Nishijima (48)	Prospective/ Japan	435	US	10 (range 35–50)	93	0	22.1 (IQR 20.2–24.9)	5.1	NA	NA	1.4 (range 0–5.6)	31/NA	NA	BMI, dyslipidaemia, AST/ALT ratio

Perazzo (68)	Prospective/ Brazil	395	CAP/TE	45 (IQR 35.52)	40	23	25.7 (IQR 23.2–29.4)	10	3	10 (6–16)	7 (range 4–14)	35/NA	9/4.9	Central obesity, diabetes, dyslipidemia, metabolic syndrome
Prat (58)	Retrospective/ UK	97	Liver biopsy	47±10	93	20	27±6	11	100	10.5±9.3	8.3±7.2	28.7/8.2	20	NA
Price (52)	Prospective/ USA	122	H-MRS	51 (IQR 47–57)	53	14	26 (IQR 24–30)	8.2	NA	NA	7.9 (IQR 3.3–12.5)	28/NA	NA/2.5	HIV RNA, HOMA-IR
Sterling (57)	Prospective/ USA	14	Liver biopsy	45±10	71	0	29.9±7.4	0	100	NA	NA	64.3/28.6	14.3	NAFLD: ↑GGT NASH: HOMA-IR
Vodkin (65)	Prospective/ USA	33	Liver biopsy	44.8±9.8	78.8	0	29.8±6.0	18.2	NA	NA	NA	100/63.6	33.3/6	NASH: HIV duration
Vuille-Lessard (54)	Prospective/ Canada	300	CAP/TE	50	43.3	0	NA	11.3	NA	NA	NA	48/NA	15/2.3	BMI, ↑ALT

Legend: Continuous variables are expressed as mean + standard deviation or median (interquartile range or range), and categorical variables are presented as percentages. Significant liver fibrosis is defined as stage >F2 or equivalent.

ALT: Alanine aminotransferase; ART: Antiretroviral therapy; BMI: Body mass index; CAP: Controlled attenuation parameter; CK-18: Cytokeratin 18; CT: Computed tomography; HIV: Human immunodeficiency virus; IQR: Interquartile range; GGT: Gamma glutamyl transferase; H-MRS: Proton magnetic resonance spectroscopy; HOMA-IR: Homeostatic model assessment of insulin resistance; NA: Not available; NAFLD: Nonalcoholic fatty liver disease; NASH: Nonalcoholic steatohepatitis; NRTI: Nucleoside reversal transcriptase inhibitors; PNPLA3: Patatin-like phospholipase domain-containing protein 3; TE: Transient elastography; TG: Triglycerides; US: Ultrasound.

Table 22.1b: Incidence of NAFLD and/or Significant/Advanced Liver Fibrosis in HIV-Infected Patients

Design/Country	N	Age (years)	Duration HIV Infection (years)	Diagnostic Method	Duration Follow-up	NAFLD	Liver Fibrosis	Predictor of Progression	
								Steatosis	Fibrosis
Rivero-Juarez (43)	Prospective/ Spain 2013	210	44.3 ±9.7	8.89 ±5.3	TE>7.2 kPa	18 months (IQR 12–26)	NA	10.9% (end of follow-up)	NA	No association with ART drugs and length of exposure to drugs
Sebastiani (41)	Prospective/ Canada 2015	796	43.5 (IQR 36–49.7)	6.3 (IQR 1.7–13.3)	Hepatic steatosis index >36; FIB-4 >3.25	4.9 years (IQR 2.2–6.4)	6.9 per 100 PY (95% CI, 5.9–7.9)	0.9 per 100 PY (95% CI, 0.6–1.3)	Black ethnicity Lower level of albumin	Hyperglycemia Lower level of albumin
Pembroke (40)	Prospective/ Canada 2017	313 (HIV and HIV/HCV)	50 (43–54)	15 (IQR 8–22)	CAP > 248 dB/m or transition to > 292 TE > 7.1 kPa or transition to >12.5	15.4 months (IQR 8.5–23.0)	37.8 per 100 PY (95% CI, 29.2–49.0)	12.7 per 100 PY (95% CI, 9.5–17.1)	NA	In HIV mono-infected: HIV duration, any grade of NAFL; In HIV/HCV: ↑ALT, HCV RNA
Lallukka-Bruck (42)	Retrospective-prospective/ Finland 2019	42	41.9 ±1.3	23.5 ±0.7	H-MRS, LFAT > 5.56% TE > 8.7kPa/ MRE>3.62	15.7 years (range 12.3–16.4)	Prevalence baseline vs. end of follow-up: 35% vs. 32%	9.5% (end of follow-up)	NA	NA

Legend: Continuous variables are expressed as mean ± standard deviation or median (interquartile range or range), and categorical variables are presented as percentages. ALT: Alanine aminotransferase; ART: Antiretroviral therapy; CAP: Controlled attenuation parameter; CI: Confidence interval; HIV: Human immunodeficiency virus; HCV: Hepatitis C virus; H-MRS: Proton magnetic resonance spectroscopy; IQR: Interquartile range; LFAT: Liver fat; MRE: Magnetic resonance elastography; NA: Not available; NAFLD: Nnonalcoholic fatty liver disease; PY: Person-years; TE: Transient elastography.

with abnormal liver transaminases found a prevalence of NASH at 49% (60). Other studies found even higher prevalences of NASH, ranging from 53 to 64% (36,53,61,62). A case-control study from US found that, compared to age- and sex-matched HIV-negative NAFLD, patients with HIV-associated NAFLD had significantly higher rates of steatohepatitis (37 vs. 63%) and more hepatocyte injury (62). A Canadian study from our team used the biomarker of hepatocyte apoptosis cytokeratin 18 to screen 202 consecutive PWH for NASH (63). The prevalence of NASH was at 11.4%, confirmed in a subgroup by available liver histology. Increased severity of liver disease in PWH, as indicated by higher prevalence of significant liver fibrosis and cirrhosis, has also been reported. The prevalence of significant liver fibrosis due to NAFLD in HIV mono-infected ranges widely from 3.6 to 35.7% (64,65). Across studies employing TE, this prevalence ranges between 9 and 18%(66–68). Similar results were obtained by Guaraldi et al. when the biomarker FIB-4 was used (38). A study employing AST-to-platelet ratio index (APRI) found a prevalence of liver cirrhosis at 2.5% (52). In a meta-analysis of 10 studies in PWH, the prevalence of NAFLD, biopsy-proven NASH, and significant liver fibrosis were 35, 42 and 22%, respectively, all higher than in the general population (37).

22.5 NATURAL HISTORY OF HIV-ASSOCIATED NAFLD

The key histopathological event in the natural history of NAFLD is the development of liver fibrosis, that is, the excessive accumulation of extracellular matrix proteins including collagen that occurs in most types of chronic liver diseases. This eventually leads to progressive distortion of the hepatic architecture and evolution to cirrhosis. The staging of liver fibrosis is essential for risk stratification and prognostication. Presence of stage 2 or higher liver fibrosis is an independent predictor of liver-related complications and all-cause mortality (69). Few studies investigated the natural history of NAFLD in the setting of HIV infection, and all of them are based on noninvasive diagnostic modalities rather than liver histology. The incidence rate of NAFLD reported in the general population varies from ranging from 2.8 to 5.2 per 100 PY (70). In HIV mono-infected patients, a few studies on the incidence of NAFLD have been performed so far. The incidence rate has been reported between 0 and 6.9 per 100 PY (95% CI, 5.9–7.9) (71,72). As for progression of liver fibrosis over time, the incidence of significant liver fibrosis was reported at 0.9 per 100 PY by the serum biomarker FIB-4, while the transition rate to significant liver fibrosis or liver cirrhosis by TE was determined at 12.7 per 100 PY (67,71). These figures are higher than the general, uninfected population. Scarce data exist on clinical outcomes related to NAFLD in HIV mono-infected patients. In the general HIV-uninfected population, the 10-year mortality reported in 3,869 NAFLD subjects was 10.2%, higher than controls (7.6%) (73). A study of 1,092 patients from the LIVEr disease in HIV (LIVEHIV) Cohort reported an incidence rate of liver-related events of 8.6 per 1,000 PY, without difference between HIV mono-infected and HIV/HCV coinfected patients (74). Due to its systemic pathogenesis, NAFLD is a risk factor for all-cause mortality attributable to cardiovascular disease and extrahepatic cancer, as well as for incident T2DM, chronic kidney disease, vasculopathy (69,75–77). HIV itself and ART carry higher risk of these conditions (78). A study of 485 patients from the LIVEHIV

Cohort followed for a median of 40.1 months reported an increased incidence of T2DM and dyslipidemia in HIV mono-infected patients with NAFLD compared to those without NAFLD (79). The interplay between two multisystem diseases, HIV and NAFLD, could be responsible for these findings.

22.6 DIAGNOSTIC TOOLS FOR NAFLD, LIVER FIBROSIS AND ESOPHAGEAL VARICES IN HIV MONO-INFECTED PATIENTS

Several noninvasive tools for the diagnosis of hepatic steatosis and fibrosis have been extensively studies in NAFLD. These methods rely on two different approaches: a biological approach, based on the quantification of biomarkers in the serum, and a physical approach, based on the measurement of liver stiffness by either ultrasonographic or magnetic resonance elastography (80). Few of these methods have been validated against liver histology in the specific setting of HIV infection. In 66 HIV mono-infected patients, Morse et al. found that TE outperformed the simple serum biomarkers APRI, FIB-4 and NAFLD fibrosis score to diagnose significant liver fibrosis. The reported area under the curve (AUC) for TE was 0.93, with associated sensitivity and specificity of 93 and 73%, respectively, for a cutoff value of 7.1 kPa (81). Lemoine and colleagues reported on the diagnostic accuracy of several noninvasive diagnostic tests for hepatic steatosis, NASH and fibrosis in 49 HIV mono-infected patients with available histology (82). For the diagnosis of hepatic steatosis, the AUC for magnetic resonance imaging derived proton density fat fraction (MRI-PDFF) and CAP was 0.98 and 0.87, respectively. Interestingly, an ALT cutoff value of 36 had an AUC of 0.88 to diagnose NASH, with 91 and 77% sensitivity and specificity, respectively. In this study the serum fibrosis biomarkers APRI and FIB-4 had higher performance than TE for the diagnosis of significant liver fibrosis. A poor concordance between serum fibrosis biomarkers and TE in the specific setting of HIV infection has also been reported (83). CAP was also validated against MRI-PDFF in a study by Ajmera et al. including 70 HIV mono-infected patients, reporting an AUC of 0.82 and identifying an optimal cutoff value of 285 dB/m for CAP to detect at least 5% hepatic steatosis (84). The Baveno VII guidelines were proposed to reduce the number of unnecessary endoscopies: patients with compensated advanced chronic liver disease can forego esophagogastroduodenoscopy if the TE value is <20 kPa and the platelet count >150,000/μL (85). In a multicenter study, we validated these criteria in 507 PWH with TE >10 kPa, including 42 HIV mono-infected patients with suspected NAFLD. The Baveno VII criteria could save at least 33.3% screening endoscopy (86). These findings can be used for resource optimization in HIV clinics.

22.7 MODELS OF CARE FOR HIV-ASSOCIATED NAFLD

NAFLD is often asymptomatic until patients develop hepatic decompensation, with significant morbidity and mortality and related socioeconomic burden (8). There is a need for personalized medicine and implementation of strategies to identify those who have advanced liver fibrosis and who are at risk of adverse outcomes. The guidelines from the European AIDS Clinical Society (EACS) recommend the case finding of advanced liver fibrosis in PWH with metabolic conditions or persistent elevated transaminases (87). These recommendations are in line with other at-risk populations for NAFLD-related liver fibrosis, such as patients with T2DM (88). In PWH, diagnosing liver fibrosis is challenging due to the large population at risk for NAFLD, as well as the additional resources of delivering TE with CAP, which is often not readily accessible in clinics practicing HIV care. Clinical pathways have been proposed in HIV-negative NAFLD to screen for liver fibrosis in at-risk populations and reduce the need for specialist tests. In these models, readily available and inexpensive fibrosis biomarkers, such as FIB-4, with high negative predictive value are used as first-tier tests, while more specialized tests, such as TE with CAP, are second-tier tests reserved to cases in which fibrosis cannot be excluded by the simple biomarker (87). A recent international study in PWH applied several models based on serum fibrosis biomarkers as first-tier tests, followed by TE with CAP. This care pathway would result in up to 86.3% reduction in need for TE examination, with increased accessibility and reduced costs (89).

22.8 TREATMENT OF HIV-ASSOCIATED NAFLD

Lifestyle modifications are the cornerstone of treatment for NAFLD, while limited pharmacologic options are available for patients with significant liver fibrosis.

22.8.1 Lifestyle Changes

The first line treatment for NASH is weight loss, through a combination of lifestyle changes including calorie reductions, exercise and healthy eating. In the general NAFLD population, suggested interventions for weight loss include 500–1,000 kcal energy defect to induce a weight loss of 500–1,000 g/week (88). Weight loss of >7% can lead to resolution of NASH, while a weight loss >10% can regress liver fibrosis (88). Few ad hoc studies investigated the effect of lifestyle interventions on HIV-associated NAFLD. However, considering that BMI is a frequently reported predictor of NAFLD in PWH, these interventions may also be effective in PWH (87). A randomized controlled trial of PWH with NAFLD investigated telemedicine as a tool for dietary intervention during the COVID-19 pandemic. Fifty-five PWH with NAFLD were allocated to dietary intervention vs. standard of care. During lockdown, 93.3% of patients in the standard of care group referred that the "diet got worse" vs. 6.7% in the intervention group, and 35.3% vs. 15.7% reported increase in appetite, respectively. PWH in the standard of care group gained more weight than in the intervention group (90). Another study evaluated the relationship between food intake of lipids with NAFLD in PWH. Participants with higher intake of total fat were associated with higher odds for NAFLD compared to those with lower consumption (adjusted odds ratio = 1.91, 95% CI 1.06–3.44) (91). Other important components of dietary interventions in the context of NAFLD include reducing alcohol intake, avoiding fructose-containing beverages and food, and limiting the consumption of processed red meat (88).

22.8.2 ART-Related Interventions

The EACS guidelines recommend considering the use of metabolically neutral ART regimens in PWH at risk for or with NAFLD. In a randomized controlled trial, Macias and colleagues investigated the effect of switching efavirenz to raltegravir on hepatic steatosis diagnosed by TE with CAP among 39 HIV/HCV coinfected patients. At week 48, resolution of hepatic steatosis was observed in 47% patients who were switched to raltegravir compared to only 15% of

patients who were maintained on efavirenz (92). Similar results were obtained by an Italian observational study of 61 PWH, of whom those switched from ritonavir-boosted PIs to raltegravir had a significant decrease in hepatic steatosis (93). However, recent data suggest that regimens containing integrase inhibitors, in particular dolutegravir, may be associated with weight gain (45). Further studies with larger sample sizes and longer follow-up are warranted. In a retrospective cohort study, maraviroc, a chemokine receptor 5 antagonist, showed a potential protective role in reducing the incidence of NAFLD in PWH (94).

22.8.3 Pharmacologic Therapy

Few pharmacologic approaches have been tested in the specific context of HIV infection as PWH are currently excluded from global NASH clinical trials (39). In the context of HIV-associated lipodystrophy, pioglitazone reduced liver fat and lobular inflammation in 13 PWH but did not achieve the primary endpoint of improvement or resolution of NASH (95). The ARRIVE trial, a double-blind, randomized, placebo-controlled trial, tested the efficacy of 12 weeks of treatment with Aramchol vs. placebo in 25 PWH with NAFLD. Over a 12-week period, there was no significant change of hepatic fat or body fat assessed by MRI-PDFF (96). In a phase 4 open-label clinical trial, vitamin E 800 IU daily for 24 weeks reduced ALT (–27 units/L), steatosis estimated by CAP (–22 dB/m), and cytokeratin 18 (–123 units/L) (24). A randomized multicenter trial including 61 PWH with NAFLD assessed the therapeutic potential of tesamorelin, a synthetic form of growth hormone-releasing hormone approved for the treatment of excess abdominal fat in HIV-associated lipodystrophy (97). After 12 months of treatment, steatosis had decreased by 32% from baseline in patients on the treatment arm, while it had increased by 5% in placebo patients. Moreover, 35% of patients in the tesamorelin group resolved steatosis in comparison to only 4% of patients on placebo.

22.8.4 Bariatric Surgery

Bariatric surgery is an option for durable weight loss in obese NAFLD patients, with significant improvement in both associated metabolic syndrome comorbidities and liver fibrosis. Weight loss surgery is being increasingly considered in morbidly obese PWH (98). However, consideration should be provided to variable ART absorption after weight loss surgery (99).

22.9 CONCLUSION/SUMMARY POINTS

NAFLD is frequent and more severe in the setting of HIV infection. A complex multifactorial pathogenesis underlines this epidemiologic evidence. Progression to NASH should be highly suspected in case of elevated ALT, overweight and confirmation by serum fibrosis biomarkers or TE. A case finding of NAFLD-related liver fibrosis should be implemented at in PWH with metabolic comorbidities or persistently elevated ALT. A therapeutic approach in PWH should be based on lifestyle modification and a few pharmacologic options in the presence of NASH or significant liver fibrosis. Future research directions should target longitudinal studies characterizing the natural history of NASH and fibrosis progression, the identification of biomarkers to diagnose NASH in the specific setting of HIV, along with targeted interventions to improve liver-related clinical outcomes in PWH.

22.10 CONFLICT OF INTEREST

GS has acted as speaker for Merck, Gilead, Abbvie, Novonordisk, Novartis, served as an advisory board member for Merck, Novonordisk, Novartis, Gilead, Allergan and Intercept and has received unrestricted research funding from Theratec.

22.11 ACKNOWLEDGMENT

GS is supported by a Senior Salary Award from FRQS (#296306).

REFERENCES

1. Organization WH. www.who.int/gho/hiv/en/ Last access 9th May 2020, 2020.
2. CDC. Monitoring selected national HIV prevention and care objectives by using HIV surveillance data—United States and 6 dependent areas—2015. *HIV Surveillance Suppl. Rep.* 2017;22(2).
3. Lewden C, May T, Rosenthal E, Burty C, Bonnet F, Costagliola D, et al. Changes in causes of death among adults infected by HIV between 2000 and 2005: The "Mortalite 2000 and 2005" surveys (ANRS EN19 and Mortavic). *J Acquir Immune Defic Syndr.* 2008;48(5):590–598.
4. Smith CJ, Ryom L, Weber R, Morlat P, Pradier C, Reiss P, et al. Trends in underlying causes of death in people with HIV from 1999 to 2011 (D:A:D): A multicohort collaboration. *Lancet.* 2014;384(9939):241–248.
5. Rosenthal E, Salmon-Ceron D, Lewden C, Bouteloup V, Pialoux G, Bonnet F, et al. Liver-related deaths in HIV-infected patients between 1995 and 2005 in the French GERMIVIC joint study group network (Mortavic 2005 study in collaboration with the mortalite 2005 survey, ANRS EN19). *HIV Med.* 2009;10(5):282–289.
6. Croxford S, Kitching A, Desai S, Kall M, Edelstein M, Skingsley A, et al. Mortality and causes of death in people diagnosed with HIV in the era of highly active antiretroviral therapy compared with the general population: An analysis of a national observational cohort. *Lancet Pub Health.* 2017;2(1):e35–e46.
7. Kaspar MB, Sterling RK. Mechanisms of liver disease in patients infected with HIV. *BMJ Open Gastroenterol.* 2017;4(1):e000166.
8. Chalasani N, Younossi Z, Lavine JE, Charlton M, Cusi K, Rinella M, et al. The diagnosis and management of nonalcoholic fatty liver disease: Practice guidance from the American Association for the study of liver diseases. *Hepatology.* 2018;67(1):328–357.
9. Eslam M, Sanyal AJ, George J, International Consensus P. MAFLD: A consensus-driven proposed nomenclature for metabolic associated fatty liver disease. *Gastroenterology.* 2020;158(7):1999–2014 e1.
10. Cervo A, Milic J, Mazzola G, Schepis F, Petta S, Krahn T, et al. Prevalence, predictors and severity of lean non-alcoholic fatty liver disease in HIV-infected patients. *Clin Infect Dis.* 2020.
11. Lake JE, Overton T, Naggie S, Sulkowski M, Loomba R, Kleiner DE, et al. Expert panel review on nonalcoholic fatty liver disease in persons with human immunodeficiency virus. *Clin Gastroenterol Hepatol.* 2020.
12. Liu D, Shen Y, Zhang R, Xun J, Wang J, Liu L, et al. Prevalence and risk factors of metabolic associated fatty liver disease among people living with HIV in China. *J Gastroenterol Hepatol.* 2021;36(6):1670–1678.
13. Gariani K, Philippe J, Jornayvaz FR. Non-alcoholic fatty liver disease and insulin resistance: From bench to bedside. *Diabetes Metab.* 2013;39(1):16–26.
14. Brown TT, Cole SR, Li X, Kingsley LA, Palella FJ, Riddler SA, et al. Antiretroviral therapy and the prevalence and incidence of diabetes mellitus in the multicenter AIDS cohort study. *Arch Intern Med.* 2005;165(10):1179–1184.
15. Nansseu JR, Bigna JJ, Kaze AD, Noubiap JJ. Incidence and risk factors for prediabetes and diabetes mellitus among HIV-infected adults on antiretroviral therapy: A systematic review and meta-analysis. *Epidemiology.* 2018;29(3):431–441.
16. Guaraldi G, Lonardo A, Maia L, Palella FJ, Jr. Metabolic concerns in aging HIV-infected persons: From serum lipid phenotype to fatty liver. *AIDS.* 2017;31(Suppl 2):S147–S56.
17. Myerson M, Poltavskiy E, Armstrong EJ, Kim S, Sharp V, Bang H. Prevalence, treatment, and control of dyslipidemia and hypertension in 4278 HIV outpatients. *J Acquir Immune Defic Syndr.* 2014;66(4):370–377.
18. Manuthu EM, Joshi MD, Lule GN, Karari E. Prevalence of dyslipidemia and dysglycaemia in HIV infected patients. *East Afr Med J.* 2008;85(1):10–17.
19. Tripathi A, Jerrell JM, Liese AD, Zhang J, Rizvi AA, Albrecht H, et al. Association of clinical and therapeutic factors with incident dyslipidemia in a cohort of human immunodeficiency virus-infected and non-infected adults: 1994–2011. *Metab Syndr Relat Disord.* 2013;11(6):417–426.
20. Bigna JJ, Ndoadoumgue AL, Nansseu JR, Tochie JN, Nyaga UF, Nkeck JR, et al. Global burden of hypertension among people living with HIV in the era of increased life expectancy: A systematic review and meta-analysis. *J Hypertens.* 2020;38(9):1659–1668.
21. Crum-Cianflone N, Roediger MP, Eberly L, Headd M, Marconi V, Ganesan A, et al. Increasing rates of obesity among HIV-infected persons during the HIV epidemic. *PLoS ONE.* 2010;5(4):e10106.
22. Cervo A, Milic J, Mazzola G, Schepis F, Petta S, Krahn T, et al. Prevalence, predictors, and severity of lean nonalcoholic fatty liver disease in patients living with human immunodeficiency virus. *Clin Infect Dis.* 2020;71(10):e694–e701.
23. Masarone M, Rosato V, Dallio M, Gravina AG, Aglitti A, Loguercio C, et al. Corrigendum to 'Role of oxidative stress in pathophysiology of nonalcoholic fatty liver disease'. *Oxid Med Cell Longev.* 2021;2021:9757921.
24. Sebastiani G, Saeed S, Lebouche B, de Pokomandy A, Szabo J, Haraoui LP, et al. Vitamin E is an effective treatment for nonalcoholic steatohepatitis in HIV mono-infected patients. *AIDS.* 2020;34(2):237–244.
25. Romeo S, Kozlitina J, Xing C, Pertsemlidis A, Cox D, Pennacchio LA, et al. Genetic variation in PNPLA3 confers susceptibility to nonalcoholic fatty liver disease. *Nature Genetics.* 2008;40(12):1461–1465.
26. Dold L, Luda C, Schwarze-Zander C, Boesecke C, Hansel C, Nischalke HD, et al. Genetic polymorphisms associated with fatty liver disease and fibrosis in HIV positive patients receiving combined antiretroviral therapy (cART). *PLoS ONE.* 2017;12(6):e0178685.
27. Price JC, Seaberg EC, Latanich R, Budoff MJ, Kingsley LA, Palella FJ, Jr., et al. Risk factors for fatty liver in the multicenter AIDS cohort study. *Am J Gastroenterol.* 2014;109(5):695–704.

28. Yanavich C, Perazzo H, Li F, Tobin N, Lee D, Zabih S, et al. A pilot study of microbial signatures of liver disease in those with HIV mono-infection in Rio de Janeiro, Brazil. *AIDS.* 2022;36(1):49–58.

29. Lemoine M, Lacombe K, Bastard JP, Sebire M, Fonquernie L, Valin N, et al. Metabolic syndrome and obesity are the cornerstones of liver fibrosis in HIV-monoinfected patients: Results of the METAFIB study. *AIDS.* 2017.

30. Kirkegaard-Klitbo DM, Mejer N, Knudsen TB, Moller HJ, Moestrup SK, Poulsen SD, et al. Soluble CD163 predicts incident chronic lung, kidney and liver disease in HIV infection. *AIDS.* 2017;31(7):981–988.

31. Kovari H, Weber R. Influence of antiretroviral therapy on liver disease. *Curr Opin HIV AIDS.* 2011;6(4):272–277.

32. Kong L, Cardona Maya W, Moreno-Fernandez ME, Ma G, Shata MT, Sherman KE, et al. Low-level HIV infection of hepatocytes. *Virol J.* 2012;9:157.

33. El-Sadr WM, Lundgren JD, Neaton JD, Gordin F, Abrams D, Arduino RC, et al. CD4+ count-guided interruption of antiretroviral treatment. *N Engl J Med.* 2006;355(22):2283–2296.

34. Brenchley JM, Price DA, Schacker TW, Asher TE, Silvestri G, Rao S, et al. Microbial translocation is a cause of systemic immune activation in chronic HIV infection. *Nat Med.* 2006;12(12):1365–1371.

35. Perez-Matute P, Perez-Martinez L, Blanco JR, Oteo JA. Role of mitochondria in HIV infection and associated metabolic disorders: Focus on nonalcoholic fatty liver disease and lipodystrophy syndrome. *Oxid Med Cell Longev.* 2013;2013:493413.

36. Ingiliz P, Valantin MA, Duvivier C, Medja F, Dominguez S, Charlotte F, et al. Liver damage underlying unexplained transaminase elevation in human immunodeficiency virus-1 mono-infected patients on antiretroviral therapy. *Hepatology.* 2009;49(2):436–442.

37. Maurice JB, Patel A, Scott AJ, Patel K, Thursz M, Lemoine M. Prevalence and risk factors of nonalcoholic fatty liver disease in HIV-monoinfection. *AIDS.* 2017;31(11):1621–1632.

38. Guaraldi G, Squillace N, Stentarelli C, Orlando G, D'Amico R, Ligabue G, et al. Nonalcoholic fatty liver disease in HIV-infected patients referred to a metabolic clinic: Prevalence, characteristics, and predictors. *Clin Infect Dis: An Official Publication of the Infectious Diseases Society of America.* 2008;47(2):250–257.

39. Guaraldi G, Maurice JB, Marzolini C, Monteith K, Milic J, Tsochatzis E, et al. New drugs for NASH and HIV infection: Great expectations for a great need. *Hepatology.* 2020;71(5):1831–1844.

40. Sulkowski MS, Mehta SH, Chaisson RE, Thomas DL, Moore RD. Hepatotoxicity associated with protease inhibitor-based antiretroviral regimens with or without concurrent ritonavir. *AIDS.* 2004;18(17):2277–2284.

41. Falutz J. Management of fat accumulation in patients with HIV infection. *Curr HIV/AIDS Rep.* 2011;8(3):200–208.

42. Sax PE, Erlandson KM, Lake JE, McComsey GA, Orkin C, Esser S, et al. Weight gain following initiation of antiretroviral therapy: Risk factors in randomized comparative clinical trials. *Clin Infect Dis.* 2020;71(6):1379–1389.

43. Tate T, Willig AL, Willig JH, Raper JL, Moneyham L, Kempf MC, et al. HIV infection and obesity: Where did all the wasting go? *Antivir Ther.* 2012;17(7):1281–1289.

44. Achhra AC, Mocroft A, Reiss P, Sabin C, Ryom L, de Wit S, et al. Short-term weight gain after antiretroviral therapy initiation and subsequent risk of cardiovascular disease and diabetes: The D:A:D study. *HIV Med.* 2016;17(4):255–268.

45. Bourgi K, Rebeiro PF, Turner M, Castilho JL, Hulgan T, Raffanti SP, et al. Greater weight gain in treatment naive persons starting dolutegravir-based antiretroviral therapy. *Clin Infect Dis.* 2019.

46. Bischoff J, Gu W, Schwarze-Zander C, Boesecke C, Wasmuth JC, van Bremen K, et al. Stratifying the risk of NAFLD in patients with HIV under combination antiretroviral therapy (cART). *EClinicalMedicine.* 2021;40:101116.

47. Paik JM, Henry L, Golabi P, Alqahtani SA, Trimble G, Younossi ZM. Presumed nonalcoholic fatty liver disease among Medicare beneficiaries with HIV, 2006–2016. *Open Forum Infect Dis.* 2020;7(1):ofz509.

48. Nishijima T, Gatanaga H, Shimbo T, Komatsu H, Nozaki Y, Nagata N, et al. Traditional but not HIV-related factors are associated with nonalcoholic fatty liver disease in Asian patients with HIV-1 infection. *PLoS ONE.* 2014;9(1):e87596.

49. Macias J, Gonzalez J, Tural C, Ortega-Gonzalez E, Pulido F, Rubio R, et al. Prevalence and factors associated with liver steatosis as measured by transient elastography with controlled attenuation parameter in HIV-infected patients. *AIDS.* 2014;28(9):1279–1287.

50. Lui G, Wong VW, Wong GL, Chu WC, Wong CK, Yung IM, et al. Liver fibrosis and fatty liver in Asian HIV-infected patients. *Aliment Pharmacol Ther.* 2016;44(4):411–421.

51. Lombardi R, Lever R, Smith C, Marshall N, Rodger A, Bhagani S, et al. Liver test abnormalities in patients with HIV mono-infection: Assessment with simple noninvasive fibrosis markers. *Ann Gastroenterol.* 2017;30(3):349–356.

52. Price JC, Ma Y, Scherzer R, Korn N, Tillinghast K, Peters MG, et al. Human immunodeficiency virus-infected and uninfected adults with non-genotype 3 hepatitis C virus have less hepatic steatosis than adults with neither infection. *Hepatology.* 2017;65(3):853–863.

53. Morse CG, McLaughlin M, Matthews L, Proschan M, Thomas F, Gharib AM, et al. Nonalcoholic steatohepatitis and hepatic fibrosis in HIV-1-Monoinfected adults with elevated aminotransferase levels on antiretroviral therapy. *Clin Infect Dis.* 2015;60(10):1569–1578.

54. Vuille-Lessard E, Lebouche B, Lennox L, Routy JP, Costiniuk CT, Pexos C, et al. Nonalcoholic fatty liver disease diagnosed by transient elastography with controlled attenuation parameter in unselected HIV monoinfected patients. *AIDS.* 2016;30(17):2635–2643.

55. Jongraksak T, Sobhonslidsuk A, Jatchavala J, Warodomwichit D, Kaewduang P, Sungkanuparph S. Prevalence and predicting factors of metabolic-associated fatty liver disease diagnosed by transient elastography with controlled attenuation parameters in HIV-positive people. *Int J STD AIDS.* 2021;32(3):266–275.

56. Mohr R, Boesecke C, Dold L, Schierwagen R, Schwarze-Zander C, Wasmuth JC, et al. Return-to-health effect of modern combined antiretroviral therapy potentially predisposes HIV patients to hepatic steatosis. *Medicine.* 2018;97(17):e0462.

57. Sterling RK, Smith PG, Brunt EM. Hepatic steatosis in human immunodeficiency virus: A prospective study

in patients without viral hepatitis, diabetes, or alcohol abuse. *J Clin Gastroenterol.* 2013;47(2):182–187.

58. Prat LI, Roccarina D, Lever R, Lombardi R, Rodger A, Hall A, et al. Aetiology and severity of liver disease in HIV positive patients with suspected NAFLD: Lessons from a cohort with available liver biopsies. *J Acquir Immune Defic Syndr.* 2018.

59. Crum-Cianflone N, Collins G, Medina S, Asher D, Campin R, Bavaro M, et al. Prevalence and factors associated with liver test abnormalities among human immunodeficiency virus-infected persons. *Clin Gastroenterol Hepatol.* 2010;8(2):183–191.

60. Maurice JB, Goldin R, Hall A, Price JC, Sebastiani G, Morse CG, et al. Increased body mass index and type 2 diabetes are the main predictors of nonalcoholic fatty liver disease and advanced fibrosis in liver biopsies of patients with human immunodeficiency virus monoinfection. *Clin Infect Dis.* 2021;73(7):e2184–2193.

61. Lemoine M, Barbu V, Girard PM, Kim M, Bastard JP, Wendum D, et al. Altered hepatic expression of SREBP-1 and PPARgamma is associated with liver injury in insulin-resistant lipodystrophic HIV-infected patients. *AIDS.* 2006;20(3):387–395.

62. Vodkin I, Valasek MA, Bettencourt R, Cachay E, Loomba R. Clinical, biochemical and histological differences between HIV-associated NAFLD and primary NAFLD: A case-control study. *Aliment Pharmacol Ther.* 2015;41(4):368–378.

63. Benmassaoud A, Ghali P, Cox J, Wong P, Szabo J, Deschenes M, et al. Screening for nonalcoholic steatohepatitis by using cytokeratin 18 and transient elastography in HIV mono-infection. *PLoS ONE.* 2018;13(1):e0191985.

64. Cai J, Sebastiani G. HIV, elevated transaminases, fatty liver: The perfect storm? *J Acquir Immune Defic Syndr.* 2019;81(1):e23–25.

65. Cai J, Osikowicz M, Sebastiani G. Clinical significance of elevated liver transaminases in HIV-infected patients. *AIDS.* 2019;33(8):1267–1282.

66. Lombardi R, Sambatakou H, Mariolis I, Cokkinos D, Papatheodoridis GV, Tsochatzis EA. Prevalence and predictors of liver steatosis and fibrosis in unselected patients with HIV mono-infection. *Dig Liver Dis.* 2016;48(12):1471–1477.

67. Pembroke T, Deschenes M, Lebouche B, Benmassaoud A, Sewitch M, Ghali P, et al. Hepatic steatosis progresses faster in HIV mono-infected than HIV/HCV co-infected patients and is associated with liver fibrosis. *J Hepatol.* 2017;67(4):801–808.

68. Perazzo H, Cardoso SW, Yanavich C, Nunes EP, Morata M, Gorni N, et al. Predictive factors associated with liver fibrosis and steatosis by transient elastography in patients with HIV mono-infection under long-term combined antiretroviral therapy. *J Int AIDS Soc.* 2018;21(11):e25201.

69. Dulai PS, Singh S, Patel J, Soni M, Prokop LJ, Younossi Z, et al. Increased risk of mortality by fibrosis stage in nonalcoholic fatty liver disease: Systematic review and meta-analysis. *Hepatology.* 2017;65(5):1557–1565.

70. Younossi ZM. The epidemiology of nonalcoholic steatohepatitis. *Clin Liver Dis (Hoboken).* 2018;11(4):92–94.

71. Sebastiani G, Rollet-Kurhajec KC, Pexos C, Gilmore N, Klein MB. Incidence and predictors of hepatic steatosis and fibrosis by serum biomarkers in a large cohort of human immunodeficiency virus mono-infected patients. *Open Forum Infect Dis.* 2015;2(1):ofv015.

72. Lallukka-Bruck S, Isokuortti E, Luukkonen PK, Hakkarainen A, Lundbom N, Sutinen J, et al. Natural course of nonalcoholic fatty liver disease and type 2 diabetes in patients with human immunodeficiency virus with and without combination antiretroviral therapy-associated lipodystrophy: A 16-year follow-up study. *Clin Infect Dis.* 2020;70(8):1708–1716.

73. Allen AM, Therneau TM, Larson JJ, Coward A, Somers VK, Kamath PS. Nonalcoholic fatty liver disease incidence and impact on metabolic burden and death: A 20 year-community study. *Hepatology.* 2018;67(5):1726–1736.

74. Benmassaoud A, Nitulescu R, Pembroke T, Halme AS, Ghali P, Deschenes M, et al. Liver-related events in human immunodeficiency virus-infected persons with occult cirrhosis. *Clin Infect Dis.* 2019;69(8):1422–1430.

75. Sinn DH, Kang D, Jang HR, Gu S, Cho SJ, Paik SW, et al. Development of chronic kidney disease in patients with non-alcoholic fatty liver disease: A cohort study. *J Hepatol.* 2017;67(6):1274–1280.

76. Petta S, Valenti L, Marchesini G, Di Marco V, Licata A, Camma C, et al. PNPLA3 GG genotype and carotid atherosclerosis in patients with non-alcoholic fatty liver disease. *PLoS ONE.* 2013;8(9):e74089.

77. Mantovani A, Byrne CD, Bonora E, Targher G. Nonalcoholic fatty liver disease and risk of incident type 2 diabetes: A meta-analysis. *Diabetes Care.* 2018;41(2):372–382.

78. Boyd MA, Mocroft A, Ryom L, Monforte AD, Sabin C, El-Sadr WM, et al. Cardiovascular disease (CVD) and chronic kidney disease (CKD) event rates in HIV-positive persons at high predicted CVD and CKD risk: A prospective analysis of the D:A:D observational study. *PLoS Med.* 2017;14(11):e1002424.

79. Krahn T, Martel M, Sapir-Pichhadze R, Kronfli N, J F, G G, et al. Non-alcoholic fatty liver disease predicts development of metabolic comorbidities in HIV-infected patients. *J Infect Dis.* 2020.

80. Patel K, Sebastiani G. Limitations of non-invasive tests for assessment of liver fibrosis. *JHEP Rep.* 2020;2(2):100067.

81. Morse CG, McLaughlin M, Proschan M, Koh C, Kleiner DE, Heller T, et al. Transient elastography for the detection of hepatic fibrosis in HIV-monoinfected adults with elevated aminotransferases on antiretroviral therapy. *AIDS.* 2015;29(17):2297–2302.

82. Lemoine M, Assoumou L, De Wit S, Girard PM, Valantin MA, Katlama C, et al. Diagnostic accuracy of noninvasive markers of steatosis, NASH, and liver fibrosis in HIV-Monoinfected individuals at risk of nonalcoholic fatty liver disease (NAFLD): Results from the ECHAM study. *J Acquir Immune Defic Syndr.* 2019;80(4):e86-e94.

83. Kirkegaard-Klitbo DM, Bendtsen F, Lundgren J, Nielsen SD, Benfield T, group Cs. Poor concordance between liver stiffness and noninvasive fibrosis scores in HIV infection without viral hepatitis. *Clin Gastroenterol Hepatol.* 2019.

84. Ajmera VH, Cachay ER, Ramers CB, Bassirian S, Singh S, Bettencourt R, et al. Optimal threshold of controlled attenuation parameter for detection of HIV-Associated NAFLD with magnetic resonance imaging as the reference standard. *Clin Infect Dis.* 2021;72(12):2124–2131.

85. Franchis Rd, Bosch J, Garcia-Tsao G, Reiberger T, Ripoll C, Faculty obotV. Baveno VII—Renewing consensus in portal hypertension. *J Hepatol*. 2021.

86. Merchante N, Saroli Palumbo C, Mazzola G, Pineda JA, Tellez F, Rivero-Juarez A, et al. Prediction of esophageal varices by liver stiffness and platelets in persons with HIV infection and compensated advanced chronic liver disease. *Clin Infect Dis*. 2019.

87. Ryom L, Cotter A, De Miguel R, Beguelin C, Podlekareva D, Arribas JR, et al. 2019 update of the European AIDS clinical society guidelines for treatment of people living with HIV version 10.0. *HIV Med*. 2020;21(10):617–624.

88. European Association for the Study of the L, European Association for the Study of D, European Association for the study of O. EASL-EASD-EASO clinical practice guidelines for the management of non-alcoholic fatty liver disease. *J Hepatol*. 2016;64(6):1388–1402.

89. Sebastiani G, Milic J, Cervo A, Saeed S, Krahn T, Kablawi D, et al. Two-tier care pathways for liver fibrosis associated to non-alcoholic fatty liver disease in HIV mono-infected patients. *J Pers Med*. 2022;12(2).

90. Policarpo S, Machado MV, Cortez-Pinto H. Telemedicine as a tool for dietary intervention in NAFLD-HIV patients during the COVID-19 lockdown: A randomized controlled trial. *Clin Nutr ESPEN*. 2021;43:329–334.

91. de Almeida CF, da Silva PS, Cardoso CSA, Moreira NG, Antunes JC, de Andrade MM, et al. Relationship between dietary fatty acid intake with nonalcoholic fatty liver disease and liver fibrosis in people with HIV. *Nutrients*. 2021;13(10).

92. Macias J, Mancebo M, Merino D, Tellez F, Montes-Ramirez ML, Pulido F, et al. Changes in liver steatosis after switching from efavirenz to raltegravir among human immunodeficiency virus-infected patients with nonalcoholic fatty liver disease. *Clin Infect Dis*. 2017;65(6):1012–1019.

93. Calza L, Colangeli V, Borderi M, Coladonato S, Tazza B, Fornaro G, et al. Improvement in liver steatosis after the switch from a ritonavir-boosted protease inhibitor to raltegravir in HIV-infected patients with non-alcoholic fatty liver disease. *Infect Dis (Lond)*. 2019;51(8):593–601.

94. Piconi S, Foschi A, Malagoli A, Carli F, Zona S, Milic J, et al. Impact of prolonged maraviroc treatment on non-AIDS-related comorbidities in HIV-positive patients: A retrospective cohort study. *J Antimicrob Chemother*. 2019;74(9):2723–2731.

95. Matthews L, Kleiner DE, Chairez C, McManus M, Nettles MJ, Zemanick K, et al. Pioglitazone for hepatic steatosis in HIV/Hepatitis C virus coinfection. *AIDS Res Hum Retrov*. 2015;31(10):961–966.

96. Ajmera VH, Cachay E, Ramers C, Vodkin I, Bassirian S, Singh S, et al. MRI assessment of treatment response in HIV-associated NAFLD: A randomized trial of a Stearoyl-Coenzyme-A-Desaturase-1 inhibitor (Arrive trial). *Hepatology*. 2019;70(5):1531–1545.

97. Stanley TL, Fourman LT, Feldpausch MN, Purdy J, Zheng I, Pan CS, et al. Effects of tesamorelin on non-alcoholic fatty liver disease in HIV: A randomised, double-blind, multicentre trial. *Lancet HIV*. 2019;6(12):e821–830.

98. Sharma P, McCarty TR, Ngu JN, O'Donnell M, Njei B. Impact of bariatric surgery in patients with HIV infection: A nationwide inpatient sample analysis, 2004–2014. *AIDS*. 2018;32(14):1959–1965.

99. Amouyal C, Buyse M, Lucas-Martini L, Hirt D, Genser L, Torcivia A, et al. Sleeve gastrectomy in morbidly obese HIV Patients: Focus on anti-retroviral treatment absorption after surgery. *Obes Surg*. 2018;28(9):2886–2893.

23 NAFLD in Liver Transplant Recipients

Liyun Yuan and Norah Terrault

CONTENTS

Key Points

1. In the United States, the proportion of liver transplants (LT) performed for nonalcoholic steatohepatitis (NASH) more than quadrupled in the past 2 decades.

2. The post-LT survival of patients with a pre-LT diagnosis of NASH is similar or better than other indications such as alcohol and hepatitis C. Recurrent steatosis is common, but recurrent NASH cirrhosis is infrequent with follow-up durations of up to 10 years.

3. Post-transplant metabolic syndrome is very common, reflecting comorbidities present in NASH patients pre-LT and the heightened risk of metabolic complications post-LT due to effects of immunosuppression and weight gain.

4. Monitoring for recurrent NAFLD and NASH is best accomplished using elastography with liver biopsy used to distinguish recurrent NAFLD/NASH from other post-LT liver complications, such as rejection and biliary disease.

5. As in nontransplant patients, the cornerstone of prevention of recurrent and de novo NAFLD is optimization of weight via lifestyle measures and treatment of metabolic comorbidities. Bariatric surgery in highly selected LT patients has yielded positive outcomes, but more data are needed.

6. Cardio- and cerebrovascular diseases and nonhepatic malignancies are the most frequent causes of death post-LT, so attention to surveillance and risk mitigation strategies is important.

23.1 INTRODUCTION

Nonalcoholic fatty liver disease (NAFLD) is one of the most common chronic liver diseases globally (1), and NAFLD-associated cirrhosis is becoming a leading indication for liver transplantation (LT). In the United States, the proportion of liver transplant performed for nonalcoholic steatohepatitis (NASH) more than quadrupled between 2002 and 2019 from 5 to 28%. The rise in LT for NASH-associated hepatocellular carcinoma is noteworthy also, now the second most frequent cause of HCC among LT recipients in the US and the leading etiology of HCC among women undergoing LT (2). As the number of transplant recipients with NASH rises, attention has turned to understanding the unique risks of this population, who are older (3,4) at the time of LT and have higher rates of metabolic comorbidities such as obesity, diabetes and hypertension. These comorbidities add complexity to transplant management and heighten the risk of post-LT complications such as cardiovascular disease, renal disease and malignancy (5). Additionally, post-transplant NAFLD is well-recognized, both recurrent (6) and de novo (7), with endogenous and exogenous factors contributing to its development and progression. Identification of potentially modifiable risks and therapeutic strategies are important to improving post-transplant outcomes.

23.2 GRAFT AND PATIENT SURVIVAL

The post-LT survival of patients with a pre-LT diagnosis of NASH is similar or better than other indications such as alcohol and hepatitis C. (8). In a recent analysis of the Scientific Registry of Transplant Recipients of 6,515 LT

DOI: 10.1201/9781003386698-28

for NASH cirrhosis between 2002 and 2019, the overall 5-year survival was 79% (9). In multivariable analysis, the independent predictors of lower survival were pre-LT diabetes, ventilator dependence, hemodialysis within a week of transplant, poor functional status and age older than 70; patients with all 5 of these factors had a 5-year survival less than 65%. Another study (10) using registry data found higher mortality among NASH vs. alcohol and hepatitis C etiologies within the first year post-LT, with NASH patients having higher rates of death from cardiovascular and cerebrovascular diseases and age being a strong predictor of mortality: HR 1.31 (95% CI 1.04, 1.66) for patients 50–59 years, 1.66 (95% CI 1.31, 2.11) for patients 60–64 years, 2.08 (95% CI 1.63, 2.64) for patients 65–69 years, and 2.66 ((5% CI 1.98, 3.57) for patients and ≥70 years. Similarly, the US NailNASH consortium emphasized the importance of nonhepatic causes of death among patients transplanted for NASH. Among 938 patients followed for a median of 3.8 years post-LT and with 95 deaths, 19% were ascribed to infection, 18% to cardiovascular disease and 17% to cancer, with only 11% liver-related (11). Only 2.6% of deaths were attributable to recurrent NASH cirrhosis. In multivariable analysis, older age, end-stage renal disease and Black race were associated with inferior outcomes, and statin use with reduced risk of death (11). These studies highlight the importance of nonhepatic complications in patients transplanted for NASH and the need to consider means to modulate risk via patient selection and management to metabolic comorbidities.

23.3 PREVALENCE OF METABOLIC RISKS AFTER LIVER TRANSPLANTATION

Metabolic syndrome is common post-LT, with prevalence increasing with time from LT (12). A recent meta-analysis, including 3,539 patients, reported a post-LT prevalence of metabolic syndrome of 39%, with pretransplant diabetes and obesity the only risk factors associated with its presence post-LT (13). However, it should be noted that this meta-analysis was focused on studies published prior to 2016 when NASH contributed only 10% or less to the study populations and were not representative of current LT cohorts, where NASH typically accounts for 25–30% of the LT recipients (2). Patients with NASH undergoing LT will have a higher likelihood of having obesity, diabetes, hypertension and dyslipidemia than patients with other etiologies (4). Thus it is not surprising that metabolic syndrome is exceedingly common among NASH transplant recipients— with a prevalence at 5 years post-LT of 90% (14).

23.3.1 Diabetes

The vast majority of NASH patients with pre-LT DM will have persistent post-LT. A large retrospective study from Canada found NASH patients without diabetes pre-LT had a 2-fold higher likelihood of developing post-LT DM than non-NASH etiologies (15). In a national US cohort study of LT recipients without pre-LT DM, more with NASH vs. non-NASH (40 vs. 27%) had any documentation of de novo DM post-LT, with two-thirds within the first 6 months ($p < 0.0001$) (16). Overall, NASH patients had a 30% higher risk of de novo DM than non-NASH, non-HCV controls, after accounting for other recognized risks including older age, use of calcineurin inhibitors, and body weight (aHR: 1.29, 95% CI: 1.18–1.42) (16).

23.3.2 Obesity

Patients on the waiting list suffer from poor appetite, micronutrient deficiencies and protein-calorie malnutrition, reflecting the hypercatabolic state of advanced cirrhosis. However, post-LT patients rapidly regain their appetite and rediscover the joys of eating after months to years of early satiety due to ascites, dietary sodium restrictions and other factors, resulting in the risk of excess weight gain (17). In the first 1–3 years after LT, average weight gain is 5–10 kg (18–20). Interestingly, the surgery itself may be a factor, with transection of the autonomic nerves of the liver, both the anterior plexus around the hepatic artery and the posterior plexus around the portal vein and bile duct (21). Potential effects on appetite and homeostasis are suggested by studies comparing LT and kidney transplant recipients, with LT patients having higher fat but lower carbohydrate intake, hyperphagia and loss of increased thermogenesis despite increasing body mass, all of which contribute to excessive weight gain (22).

Additionally, the majority of patients do not resume or achieve normal levels of physical activity, thus compounding the risk for excessive weight gain post-LT. In a cross-sectional study of 156 patients more than a year from LT, 63% had metabolic syndrome, and there was an inverse correlation between presence of metabolic syndrome and level of physical activity (aOR = 0.69, 95% 0.54–0.89) (23). A small study comparing fuel utilization in NASH vs. non-NASH LT recipients showed that NASH patients have impaired fatty acid utilization that was correlated with fat free muscle volume and visceral adiposity (24). The authors proposed that this was a marker of reduced metabolic flexibility that may predispose to development of recurrent NAFLD. Whether patients with NASH are at greater risk for weight gain post-LT than patients with other etiologies has not been rigorously evaluated. Two single-center studies from Europe found no difference in overweight/obesity at 5 years post-LT in NASH compared to alcohol-associated liver disease (19, 25).

23.3.3 Hyperlipidemia

The prevalence of hyperlipidemia is estimated to vary from 27 to 71% among LT recipients (26). Atherogenic dyslipidemia, defined as elevated small dense LDL-C and the increased size and concentration of VLDL particles, is very common among LT recipients with NAFLD or metabolic syndrome with reported prevalence of up to 80% (6,26,27). A prospective study of 130 enrolled LT recipients (28) showed serum small dense LDL-C >25 mg/dl was a strong predictor for post-LT cardiovascular events (hazard ratio 6.4, 95% CI 2.7, 15.3; $P < 0.001$), while LDL-C cutoff of 100 mg/dl was unable to identify of CVD risk among this group. The development of post-LT atherogenic dyslipidemia is influenced by post-LT weight gain, insulin resistance, de novo NAFLD, abnormal renal function and genetic predisposition in a couple of the impact of immunosuppression (29,30), specifically cyclosporin, which affects lipid metabolisms by increasing triglyceride secretion, reducing bile acid synthesis and reducing lipolysis (28,31).

23.4 IMMUNOSUPPRESSION IN NAFLD AND POST-TRANSPLANT METABOLIC SYNDROME

The need for chronic immunosuppression for prevention of allograft rejection and insuring long-term graft survival places patients at risk for metabolic complications. Most of the drug classes commonly used for immunosuppression have some metabolic consequences (Table 23.1), and for patients with preexisting metabolic comorbidities, immunosuppressive drugs can exacerbate risk of metabolic complications post-LT.

Table 23.1: Metabolic Side Effects of Immunosuppressive Drugs

Immunosuppressions	Actions	Metabolic Consequences
Corticosteroids	Hyperphagia ↑Appetite ↑De novo lipogenesis ↑Glucogenesis ↑Insulin resistance ↑Vascular resistance	Weight gain DMII and HTN
Calcineurin inhibitors (CNIs)	↓β cell function ↓Peripheral glucose utilization ↓Mitochondrial β oxidation ↓Triglyceride secretion ↓Bile acid synthesis ↑Renal arterial vasocontriction ↓GFR and ↑sodium retention	Weight gain Insulin resistance/type 1 diabetes Renal dysfunction Hyperlipidemia
Mammalian target of rapamycin (mTOR) inhibitor	↓β cell mass ↓Hepatic insulin clearance ↑Hepatic gluconeogenesis ↑Hepatic synthesis of triglyceride ↑Secretion of VLDL ↑FFA release from adipose	Hyperlipidemia Insulin resistance

23.4.1 Corticosteroids

Corticosteroids are commonly used in the early post-LT period to treat episodes of acute rejection. Excess exogenous or endogenous glucocorticoid has been implicated across all the stages of NAFLD pathogenesis. Glucocorticoid binds to glucocorticoid receptors, acting upon both liver and adipose tissues by regulating lipid metabolism (32). In adipose tissue, it promotes lipolysis, increases the delivery of free fatty acids for de novo lipogenesis and drives peripheral insulin resistance. Within the liver, glucocorticoid promotes gluconeogenesis and glycogenolysis, increasing the availability of glucose as a substrate for de novo lipogenesis. Steroid avoidance or minimization is viewed as a favorable strategy to prevent excessive weight gain, though data supporting such a benefit are mixed (33–35).

23.4.2 Calcineurin Inhibitors (CNIs)

CNIs are the backbone of immunosuppression for LT recipients but can exacerbate multiple facets of post-transplant metabolic syndrome. In the US, tacrolimus is the most widely prescribed CNI, with cyclosporine use very infrequently. Diabetes is more frequent with tacrolimus than cyclosporine (36), whereas hypertension and renal dysfunction are more common with cyclosporine than tacrolimus (37). CNIs promote insulin resistance by impairing beta cell function, decreasing insulin secretion and enhancing insulin sensitivities. They affect lipid metabolism by impairing mitochondrial beta-oxidation and decreasing TG secretion (38). CNIs cause hypertension through arteriolar vasoconstriction, and calcium blockades are the most effective antihypertensive agent for CNIs-induced hypertension. Direct comparison of CNIs side effects in NASH vs. non-NASH post-LT recipients is lacking, but since NASH patients have a higher prevalence of metabolic syndrome pre-LT, an increased risk for CNI-related toxicities post-LT should be anticipated. Minimization of CNI dosage to reduce the long-term metabolic consequences is the goal in any LT patient but is particularly important for the NASH LT recipient.

23.4.3 Mammalian Target of Rapamycin (mTOR) Inhibitor

The mTOR inhibitors, including sirolimus and everolimus, were initially introduced as renal-sparing immunosuppression. The early use of everolimus (started at 1 month post-transplant), in combination with reduced dose tacrolimus, has been shown to have a beneficial effect on renal function, particularly in those with reduced eGFR. Their antineoplastic effects are viewed as potentially beneficial to patients who have undergone LT for liver cancer (39, 40), with a recent metanalysis showing a survival benefit (41). As the proportion of patients with NASH undergoing LT with HCC as their primary indication increases, there may be reason to consider an immunosuppressive regimen that includes an MTOR inhibitor. Yet adverse effects are recognized, with dyslipidemia observed in over 50% patients (42). Thus, for NAFLD patients, the benefits of preserving renal function and potentially reducing HCC recurrence needs to be balanced with the worsening dyslipidemia.

23.5 RECURRENT OR DE NOVO NAFLD: Incidence and Natural History

Both recurrent NAFLD and de novo NAFLD are recognized post-LT, with the distinction dependent upon whether or not there was a pre-LT diagnosis of NASH. A pretransplant diagnosis is typically based on the presence of risk factors and exclusion of other causes, with liver biopsy often not done. The loss of classic histologic features of NASH with advanced cirrhosis is recognized. In a detailed study of explants form 2014 to 2016, 3 of 20 patients (15%) with a pre-LT diagnosis of NASH lacked histologic features to confirm the diagnosis, and, on the flip side, of 37 patients labeled as cryptogenic cirrhosis, 7 (19%) had histologic features of NASH (43). Accurate pre-LT diagnosis may be relevant in predicting the risk of post-LT NASH. In a single-center study of 258 patients with a pretransplant diagnosis of cryptogenic cirrhosis or NASH who underwent protocol biopsies post-LT, recurrent steatosis was more frequent in the NASH (45%) than cryptogenic (23%) group at 5 years (44). This suggests that the evaluation of explants for evidence of NASH may help to predict the likelihood of recurrent disease.

The histopathology features of allograft NASH are the same as the native liver, with immunosuppression per se not believed to alter the histologic presentation. However, concurrent allograft complications, such as chronic rejection or chronic biliary strictures, may influence the risk for fibrosis progression. For patients with pretransplant NASH, allograft steatosis typically appears within the first year (45) (Figure 23.1). This rapid development of steatosis within the first year post-LT is not surprising, given that LT reverses the chronic catabolic state of advanced cirrhosis and there is increased appetite and associated weight gain starting soon after LT and that the doses of immunosuppressive drugs are higher in the early vs. late post-LT period. These factors set the stage for metabolic derangements that favor steatosis. In a meta-analysis of 17 retrospective studies and including 2,378 patients, the estimated incidence of recurrent NAFLD at 1, 3 and 5 years was 59, 57 and 82% and for recurrent NASH was 53, 57.4 and 38%, respectively, but with low confidence in these estimates due to study heterogeneity (46). In contrast, de novo recurrent NASH was infrequent with an estimated incidence of only 17% at 5 years. A higher frequency of advanced fibrosis (F3/F4) at 5 years has been reported in those with recurrent vs. de novo NASH (72% vs. 13%, $p < 0.01$) (45).

Whether disease progression is accelerated post-LT in those who develop recurrent NASH is unclear. Though recurrent NASH is very common, development of allograft dysfunction or cirrhosis is very low (Figure 23.1). In a retrospective cohort of 226 patients, with 75% undergoing at least 1 biopsy during post-LT follow-up, 49% developed recurrence of NASH at an average 3 years, with 23% developing advanced fibrosis and 1.8% progressing to cirrhosis at a mean of 9 years follow-up (47). Reflecting this low rate of cirrhosis at 10 years post-LT, studies of post-LT survival show no difference for those with NAFLD vs. other indications (48). While the risk of recurrent cirrhosis and its complications may be a threat to patient and graft survival with longer duration of follow-up (beyond 10 years), competing risks of mortality among patients with NAFLD are likely to continue to be the primary drivers of post-LT mortality—specifically cardio- and cerebrovascular diseases (11, 49). Moreover, as the proportion of NASH LT recipients with HCC as a primary indication for LT increases, outcomes will be strongly influenced by rates of recurrent HCC (50, 51).

23.6 RISK FACTORS FOR DEVELOPMENT OF ALLOGRAFT NAFLD/NASH (FIGURE 23.1)

23.6.1 Donor Factors

The prevalence of NAFLD among donors is increasing, and up to 70% of utilized donors have some degree of steatosis. Whether the presence of donor steatosis is a risk factor for de novo or recurrent NAFLD is unclear. In a biopsy-based study from France, with 31% of 599 patients having steatosis (53% grade 1; 16% grade 3), the presence of donor steatosis was an independent risk factor for post-NAFLD (52). Similarly, in a study of 155 Korean LT recipients with a liver biopsy beyond 1 year, donor steatosis was associated with a 3-fold higher odds of recipient NAFLD (OR 3.15, $p = 0.02$) (53). However, a US study conducted with paired donor–recipient liver biopsies (only 14% with pre-LT NASH) found no association between donor steatosis and subsequent NAFLD with follow-up an average 704 days post-LT (54).

Donor genetic polymorphisms increase the likelihood of liver allograft fat content after LT (55). In a single-center study from the Czech Republic (56,57) consisting of 268 adult LT donors/recipients with genotyping and at least 1 liver biopsy taken 6–30 months after LT, the carrier state for the donor *TM6SF2* A and the *PNPLA3* G alleles, recipient age, pretransplant BMI, and presence of DM were strong predictors of increased liver graft steatosis after LT. The frequency of allograft steatosis was 36.7, 53.2, 58.3, and 77.8% in those without risk alleles, with donor *PNPLA3* G, with donor *TM6SF2* A, and both risk alleles, respectively (56,57). In another study where the prevalence of donor

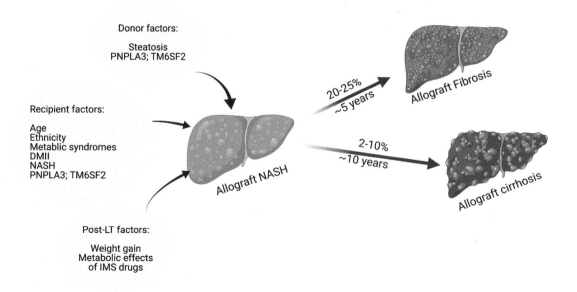

Figure 23.1 Donor, recipient and post-transplant factors related to immunosuppressive drugs influence the natural history of NAFLD after liver transplant. Approximately 20-25% will develop recurrent NASH within 5 years, with rates of cirrhosis infrequent in first 10 years post-transplant.

PNPLA3 G allele was low, recipients homozygous for G alleles had a 13.7-fold higher risk of graft steatosis than recipients with normal PNPLA3 CC genotype (P = 0.022), independent of recipient age, weight gain after liver transplantation, or the underlying disease (58). Thus the future risk predictor for the LT recipient may need to consider donor and recipient genetic polymorphisms.

23.6.2 Recipient Factors

As in the nontransplant setting, the metabolic syndrome is associated with recurrent and de novo steatosis. The majority of NASH LT recipients have preexisting obesity, diabetes, dyslipidemia and history of hypertension. These persist and are often exacerbated post-LT. Rapid weight gain after liver transplantation is an important contributing factor to de novo NAFLD or recurrent NAFLD. Richards et al. (59) shows the greatest weight gain occurred within 6 months after transplant. Post-transplant weight gain is associated with increased risk of hypertension, hypercholesterolemia, hypertriglyceridemia and insulin resistance. In a meta-regression of factors associated with post-LT NASH, post-LT body mass index, dyslipidemia, and history of alcohol use were identified (26). Whether specific metabolic risk increases the likelihood of NASH (vs. steatosis only) is unclear, as the overall proportion of patients developing NASH is modest, and there are limited longitudinal biopsy studies upon which to evaluate the relative contributions of weight gain, diabetes, dyslipidemia and hypertension over time—especially as patients may experience periods of exacerbation and control.

Among nontransplant patients, disparities in natural history are evident by sex and race-ethnicity. Latinx have the highest prevalence of NAFLD, followed by Caucasians and Asian (60). Although African Americans have a high prevalence of metabolic syndrome, NAFLD prevalence is low. Women have lower rates of NASH progression until menopause, after which the gender gap closes (61). Whether these disparities influence rates of recurrent or de novo NASH post-LT requires further investigation. As most NASH LT recipients are over the age 50, sex differences are unlikely, but race-ethnicity disparities warrant additional study.

23.7 MONITORING FOR RECURRENT OR DE NOVO NAFLD

Liver biopsy remains the gold standard for diagnosis of NAFLD and quantifying stage of fibrosis in the post-LT setting. For patients with elevated liver tests, the need to exclude other potential allograft complications, including acute rejection or viral infections, requires the use of liver biopsy. However, beyond the early transplant period, risk for other allograft complications declines and monitoring for recurrent NASH is typically done using noninvasive methods. Noninvasive serum biomarkers, such as APRI and FIB4 are not accurate in the post-LT setting (62), primarily because platelet counts may be affected by immunosuppression and residual portal hypertension, and AST/ALT levels may be increased by other non-NAFLD post-transplant allograft complications, such as biliary strictures. The use of elastography offers more promise, though the presence of concurrent liver conditions may lead to erroneous measures. Liver stiffness may be affected by cholestasis (from chronic rejection), vascular compromise, biliary obstruction or anatomic variability. However, in patients without those allograft complications (the majority), elastography measures of steatosis and fibrosis may be useful.

Published series suggest the liver stiffness cutoffs for significant or advanced fibrosis are different for liver allograft compared to the native liver. In a single-center study (63) of 150 LT recipients evaluated using transient elastography (TE) with controlled attenuation parameter (CAP) a mean of 10 years post-LT and using CAP cutoff of 222 dB/m to define steatosis, 70% of patients were affected, with 28% of patients meeting the criteria for severe steatosis (CAP of ≥290 dB), and most patients had normal liver enzymes. Advanced fibrosis was identified in 12.7%, and of the 5 patients who underwent liver biopsy, none showed cirrhosis but all had evidence of chronic rejection. A systemic review suggests higher cutoffs of liver stiffness for advanced fibrosis in LT recipients, varying from 10.5 to 26.5 kPa (64), but much of the published studies focus on patients with hepatitis C. In a recent large prospective study of 259 LT recipients who had TE at the time of liver biopsy, the optimal cutoff values were suggested to be 15.1 kPa for F3 and 16.7 kPa for F4 for LT recipients for all etiologies (65). More studies are needed, but available data suggest that TE has value in identifying steatosis, and an elevated liver stiffness measure should prompt consideration of liver biopsy to evaluate for cause.

The magnetic resonance elastography (MRE) and proton density fat fraction (PDFF) methods have high accuracy in detection of liver fibrosis and steatosis in the nontransplant setting (66,67). In a systemic review by Singh et al. including 6 cohorts and 141 LT recipients with MRE and liver biopsy, a mean AUROC value of MRE for advanced fibrosis and cirrhosis were 0.83 (95% CI: 0.61–0.88) and 0.96 (0.93–0.98), respectively, whereas the accuracy of mild to moderate fibrosis was lower, AUROC was 0.73 (0.66–0.81) and 0.69 (0.62–0.74) (68). However, almost all included patients had HCV or alcohol-associated liver diseases. A cross-sectional study of 126 LT patients (50% for HBV, only 9% for NAFLD) who underwent TE and MRE at a mean of 75 months post-LT, showed that MRI-PDFF and TE CAP were moderately correlated (r = 0.44) but higher for identifying significant fibrosis (r = 0.79) (69).

Thus MRE/PDFF or TE/CAP can be considered for monitoring steatosis and fibrosis post-LT. Given that most patients have normal liver enzymes, reliance on liver test abnormalities to trigger evaluation will miss patients with significant disease. We proposed an algorithm of surveillance (Figure 23.2). We favor the use of TE/CAP due to its ease and lower cost than MRE/PDFF and suggest that programs consider a protocolized approach with imaging done at 1 year and then every 2–3 years depending on initial findings. Patients with severe steatosis warrant closer follow-up, as do those with evidence of increased liver stiffness. Liver biopsy still has a role to play, particularly in distinguishing recurrent or de novo NASH from other post-LT complications.

23.8 MANAGEMENT APPROACH FOR NAFLD POST-LT

Prevention of recurrent or de novo NAFLD depends first and foremost on prevention and optimization of metabolic complications (Figure 23.2). Immunosuppression warrants careful attention, as most of the drugs used to prevent rejection have adverse metabolic side effects. Lifestyle measures that focus on attaining a more ideal body weight through healthy diet and exercise are important with approaches similar to that used in nontransplant settings, though one must acknowledge that studies on the efficacy of dietary and exercise measures in LT recipients are lacking. Bariatric surgery may be considered in the setting of LT. Repurposed drugs, such as semaglutide, may have a role. Finally, given the heightened

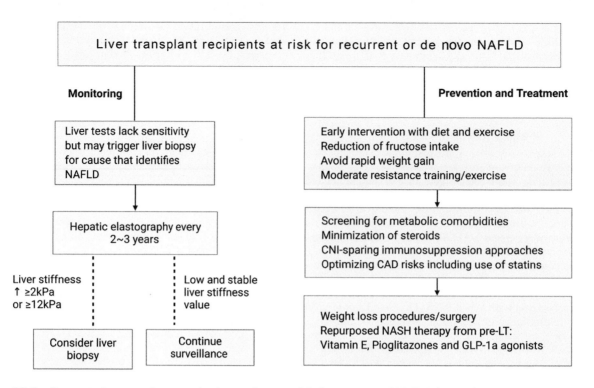

Figure 23.2 Suggested approach to monitoring patients at risk for recurrent NAFLD focused on use of hepatic elastography. Prevention requires attention to lifestyle measures starting early after liver transplantation to avoid rapid weight gain, screening and treating metabolic comorbidities that are more frequent post-LT, and use of NAFLD-specific treatments when recurrent NAFLD occurs.

cardiovascular risk of LT recipients, particularly those with metabolic comorbidities, transplant physician plays an important role in advocating for use of medications to reduce risk, such as statins, and to assist in managing drug–drug interactions.

23.8.1 Immunosuppression

While corticosteroids are often used at high doses in the early post-LT period and for treatment of acute rejection, long-term corticosteroids are to be avoided. As CNIs carry the greatest risk of metabolic complications and risk for renal dysfunction, strategies to minimize CNIs are desirable in this population. Reduction of CNIs has been shown to improve post-LT metabolic syndrome (70, 71). Reduced dose CNIs in combination with mTOR inhibitors or with mycophenolate are potential approaches. A randomized study of LT patients **(72)** was divided into 3 treatment groups: everolimus plus reduced tacrolimus ($n = 245$); tacrolimus control ($n = 243$); and tacrolimus elimination with everolimus alone ($n = 231$). The groups with tacrolimus reduction/elimination achieved less weight gain, better renal function and improved metabolic profiles. Reduction of CNI by replacement with mycophenolate mofetil has been shown to improve posttransplant dyslipidemia, renal function and hypertension (70).

23.8.2 Lifestyle Modifications and Exercise

Lifestyle modification remains the mainstay and first-line therapy for prevention and treatment of post-LT NAFLD. Establishing healthy eating patterns early post-LT is important, particularly for individuals with pre-LT NASH. Nutritional consultation in the early post-LT period may be beneficial. A well-balanced Mediterranean diet with whole grain, vegetable, fruits, fish, beans and nuts diet and elimination of fructose are among the key recommendations. Coffee is beneficial for many liver-related outcomes and drinking 3 or more cups per day may be beneficial (73)—though data specific to LT patients are lacking.

Exercise is pivotal for improving overall post-transplant health, as well as reduction in risk of metabolic syndrome. LT recipients often experience an initial downward trajectory in frailty in the immediate post-LT periods, typically the low point being at month 3, followed by a gradual modest improvement by 12 months post-LT (74). In a study of 204 LT recipients, exercise intensity was inversely associated with development of post-LT metabolic syndrome (OR = 0.69, 95% CI = 0.54–0.89). Three randomized trials of post-transplant exercises demonstrated that any forms of resistance exercise, such as home-based exercise or structured exercise programs or aerobic fitness, when adhered to for a long period of time, provides benefit in improving global muscle strength, pulmonary function and body composites (75–77). An exercise program needs to be individualized, as each LT recipient has a distinct course of recovery, influenced by age, fragility, comorbidities and post-transplant complications. US population guidelines recommend 150 minutes/week of moderate-to-vigorous activity, along with resistance exercise training for 15–20 minutes twice a week (78), and this is a reasonable target for post-transplant recipients. A personized training program tailored to the need of the transplant recipients is ideal, but an emphasis on physical activities from care givers, providers and social groups is indispensable to success.

23.8.3 Role of Bariatric Surgery in Obese LT Recipients

Data are limited to single-center experiences but highlight the potential metabolic benefits as well as weight improvements. The University of California–San Francisco has the largest experience with pre-LT laparoscopic sleeve gastrectomy in highly select patients with stable cirrhosis and well-controlled complications (79,80). In long-term follow-up (mean 5 years) of patients with pre-LT sleeve gastrectomy who subsequently underwent LT, those who had bariatric surgery had a significantly lower risk post-LT of diabetes (OR 0.04, 95% CI 0.00–0.41, $p = 0.01$), hypertension (OR 0.15, 95% CI 0.04–0.67, $p = 0.01$), and recurrent and de novo NAFLD (HR 0.19, 95% CI 0.04–0.91, $p = 0.04$) that matched patients who were managed medically. The Mayo Clinic has the largest experience with simultaneous sleeve gastrectomy and LT (81). In a highly selective group of morbidly obese candidates, weight loss of 20 to 50% of initial body weight was achieved after 3 years of follow-up, and none of the patients had major complications. Finally, the largest single-center experience post-LT bariatric surgery comes from the University of Cincinnati and included 15 patients with median time from LT to laparoscopic sleeve gastrectomy of 2.2 years (82). They showed BMI decreased from 42.7 to 35.9 kg/m^2 with a reduction of insulin doses among insulin-dependent diabetics with follow-up period of 2.6 years. While these early experiences are encouraging, it must be emphasized that this represents the results of highly experienced centers and in highly select patients only.

In a meta-analysis (83) including a total of 96 patients from 8 studies who underwent bariatric surgery, 28 were prior to the transplant, 29 simultaneous with LT, and 39 after LT. The bariatric surgery-related morbidity and mortality rates were 37 and 0.6%, respectively. Importantly, improvement of hypertension and diabetes were seen in 61 and 45% of patients, respectively. Sleeve gastrectomy was the preferred technique in most studies and is favored because it preserves the anatomical continuity with the duodenum allowing for ease of biliary tree access and lowers the risk of malnutrition and malabsorption, and absorption of immunosuppressive medications is largely unaffected. Unresolved issues include the best timing of the procedure (pre-LT, concurrent with LT or post-LT), defining the criteria for optimal candidates and full characterization of short- and long-term risks.

23.8.4 Repurposed Drugs for Treatment of Post-LT NASH

There are no published clinical trials of therapies for prevention or treatment of allograft NASH. However, data gleaned from the non-LT populations may be considered. The PIVENS clinical trial showed that both vitamin E 800 IU daily and pioglitazone are associated with improvement in histologic features of NASH, supporting a potential role in post-LT care (84). Neither drug interacts with calcineurin inhibitors. Cautions with vitamin E include avoidance in those with diabetes (less well-studied) and in those without risk for prostate cancer or stroke. Pioglitazone (85) is limited by the side effects of edema and weight gain, which many patients find difficult to accept, given emphasis on weight optimization. Glucagon-like peptide-1 receptor agonists (GLP-1RAs), liraglutide and semaglutide are FDA-approved medical therapy for obesity or type II DM. In a 72-week, double-blinded phase 2 trial involving biopsy-confirmed NASH and fibrosis (86), 59% patients with 0.4 mg once-daily subcutaneous semaglutide achieved NASH resolution, compared to 17% in the placebo group. A dose-dependent weight reduction is seen with treatment with semaglutide. Seventy-two-week treatment with 0.4 mg daily dose achieves 13% body weight loss along with improvement of metabolic syndromes.

Weekly subcutaneous dose, 2.4 mg of semaglutide was also approved for obesity treatment, and approximately average 16% body weight reduction was observed with a 68-week course (87). Gastrointestinal adverse effects are very common, including nausea, abdominal pain and diarrhea. Although the clinical trials have not been extended to post-transplant recipients, owing to the therapeutic efficacy in weight loss, improvement of lipid panel, insulin resistance and type 2 DM, semaglutide may be a consideration in LT recipients with NASH.

23.9 MANAGEMENT OF NONHEPATIC RISKS AMONG LT RECIPIENTS

Among NASH LT recipients, morbidity and mortality related to nonhepatic complications are noteworthy. In a multicenter US study of NASH recipients followed for a median of 3.8 years (IQR 1.6–7.1), the rank order of causes of death were infection, cardiovascular disease and cancer, with liver-related mortality ranking 4th and accounting for only 11% of deaths (11). In multivariable analysis, older age, end-stage renal disease and Black race were associated with inferior outcomes, and statin use reduced risk of death. Such studies highlight the importance of transplant physicians supporting a strategy of risk mitigation for cardiovascular, infectious and cancer complications in NASH recipients.

23.9.1 Infections

The risks for heightened morbidity and mortality from infectious complications are likely multifactorial, including older age, greater frailty after LT (88), concurrent diabetes and higher rates of renal dysfunction. Prevention of frailty through dietary and physical activity interventions may be of particular importance to NASH patients.

23.9.2 Cardio- and Cerebrovascular Diseases

In the NailNASH multicenter study, the most common cardiovascular complications seen post-LT were atrial fibrillation (11%), cardiac dysrhythmia (18%), ischemic heart disease (3%) and congestive heart failure (10%) (11). The authors highlight that, despite careful pretransplant cardiac evaluation and exclusion of those with significant atherosclerotic disease, events rates related to ischemic heart disease doubled (from 1.4 to 2.7%) over the study period of ~4 years follow-up. Moreover, statins were shown to have a positive influence on post-LT outcomes.

Statin therapy is the cornerstone for prevention of atherosclerotic cardiovascular disease. The development of dyslipidemia accelerates after LT with the prevalence increasing from 23% pretransplant to 55.5% at 5 years (89). Up to 70% patients on mTOR inhibitors will develop elevated triglycerides and low-density lipoprotein cholesterol. This highlights the importance of statin therapy after LT to optimize lipid panel and decrease risk of cardiovascular events. A potential additional benefit of statin therapy among LT recipients includes risk reduction of venous thromboembolic events and hepatic artery complication **(90)**. However, less than half of statin-eligible LT recipients receive statin therapy, and doses of statins are often underprescribed (91). Statins are well-tolerated among LT recipients, but attention to potential drug–drug interactions is necessary. CNIs, particularly cyclosporin, have a dominant inhibitory effect on a liver-specific statin transporter and increases the level of most statins as they share the common cytochrome P450 metabolism pathway. Pravastatin and rosuvastatin are less affected through the P450 systems and thus are favorable choice post-organ transplantation.

Beyond this, there may be potential hepatic benefit of statin therapy across all the stages of NAFLD spectrum. Population-based studies in nontransplant patients show that statin treatment decreases the risk of NAFLD development and progression (92) and is associated with reduced risk of HCC among patients with NAFLD (93). Even among patients with cirrhosis, statins appear to be beneficial in improving portal hypertension, reducing risk of HCC and improving overall mortality (94,95). Collectively, these data serve to support the use of statins in post-LT patients, with indications similar to non-LT recipients.

23.9.3 Nonliver Malignancies Post-LT

NASH LT recipients have a heightened risk of de novo malignancy, which has been underappreciated. Data from the SRTR found that patients transplanted for NASH had the highest rates of de novo malignancies post-LT at 16.3% (95% CI, 13.9–18.7) at 10 years and driven principally by the higher risk of skin and solid organ malignancies (96). Recipients who underwent transplant for NASH had the highest risk of breast cancer, colon cancer (among non-PSC etiologies) and pancreatic cancer. The NailNASH US cohort of 938 NASH patients transplanted 1997–2007, de novo malignancies accounted for 17% of deaths. As NASH LT recipients are older, on average, than non-NASH recipients, the increased rate of nonliver malignancies, in part, reflects age-related risk. However, as nonliver malignancies occur at higher rates among non-LT NASH patients than among non-NASH, there is likely a true increase in risk of nonliver malignancies among NASH LT recipients, and vigilance for de novo malignancies is warranted (96).

23.10 SUMMARY

NASH-associated cirrhosis and HCC are increasingly prevalent among LT candidates. As a patient population, these patients are older and more frequently have metabolic comorbidities that can contribute to post-LT morbidity and mortality. Recurrent NAFLD is common, though progression to NASH and NASH-associated cirrhosis is slow, with few developing liver disease complications within the first decade post-LT. Cardio- and cerebrovascular complications and nonliver malignancies are more frequent causes of death post-LT, highlighting the need for post-LT surveillance and prevention strategies to maximize long-term survival. Interventions are modeled after the practices in non-LT patients with NASH, with focus on weight optimization through diet and exercise and on aggressive management of hypertension, dyslipidemia and diabetes. Attention to immunosuppression is key. Bariatric surgery can be a consideration in select patients. NASH-specific therapies are understudied in LT recipients, and consideration of this special population for future clinical trials is important—with the goal of preventing NASH progression and insuring long-term graft survival.

REFERENCES

1. Z. Younossi et al., Global burden of NAFLD and NASH: Trends, predictions, risk factors and prevention. *Nat Rev Gastroenterol Hepatol* **15**, 11–20 (2018).
2. Z. M. Younossi et al., Nonalcoholic steatohepatitis is the most rapidly increasing indication for liver transplantation in the United States. *Clin Gastroenterol Hepatol* **19**, 580–589.e585 (2021).
3. J. B. Henson et al., Transplant outcomes in older patients with nonalcoholic steatohepatitis compared to alcohol-related liver disease and hepatitis C. *Transplantation* **104**, e164-e173 (2020).
4. S. S. Patel et al., Coronary artery disease in decompensated patients undergoing liver transplantation evaluation. *Liver Transpl* **24**, 333–342 (2018).
5. L. B. Vanwagner et al., Patients transplanted for nonalcoholic steatohepatitis are at increased risk for postoperative cardiovascular events. *Hepatology* **56**, 1741–1750 (2012).
6. C. Bhati et al., Long-term outcomes in patients undergoing liver transplantation for nonalcoholic steatohepatitis-related cirrhosis. *Transplantation* **101**, 1867–1874 (2017).
7. G. Losurdo et al., Systematic review with meta-analysis: De novo non-alcoholic fatty liver disease in liver-transplanted patients. *Aliment Pharmacol Ther* **47**, 704–714 (2018).
8. G. Cholankeril et al., Liver transplantation for nonalcoholic steatohepatitis in the US: Temporal trends and outcomes. *Dig Dis Sci* **62**, 2915–2922 (2017).
9. R. S. Karnam et al., Predicting long-term survival after liver transplantation in patients with NASH cirrhosis. *Clin Gastroenterol Hepatol* **20**, 704–705 (2022).
10. S. Nagai et al., Increased risk of death in first year after liver transplantation among patients with nonalcoholic steatohepatitis vs liver disease of other etiologies. *Clin Gastroenterol Hepatol* **17**, 2759–2768.e2755 (2019).
11. M. E. Rinella et al., Factors impacting survival in those transplanted for NASH cirrhosis: Data from the NailNASH consortium. *Clin Gastroenterol Hepatol*, (2022).
12. L. R. Anastácio et al., Prospective evaluation of metabolic syndrome and its components among long-term liver recipients. *Liver Int* **34**, 1094–1101 (2014).
13. L. B. Thoefner, A. A. Rostved, H. C. Pommergaard, A. Rasmussen, Risk factors for metabolic syndrome after liver transplantation: A systematic review and meta-analysis. *Transplant Rev (Orlando)* **32**, 69–77 (2018).
14. M. Laryea et al., Metabolic syndrome in liver transplant recipients: Prevalence and association with major vascular events. *Liver Transpl* **13**, 1109–1114 (2007).
15. A. D. Aravinthan et al., The impact of preexisting and post-transplant diabetes mellitus on outcomes following liver transplantation. *Transplantation* **103**, 2523–2530 (2019).
16. M. Stepanova et al., Risk of de novo post-transplant type 2 diabetes in patients undergoing liver transplant for non-alcoholic steatohepatitis. *BMC Gastroenterol* **15**, 175 (2015).
17. M. Giusto et al., Changes in nutritional status after liver transplantation. *World J Gastroenterol* **20**, 10682–10690 (2014).
18. J. E. Everhart et al., Weight change and obesity after liver transplantation: Incidence and risk factors. *Liver Transpl Surg* **4**, 285–296 (1998).
19. V. J. Canzanello et al., Evolution of cardiovascular risk after liver transplantation: A comparison of cyclosporine A and tacrolimus (FK506). *Liver Transpl Surg* **3**, 1–9 (1997).
20. S. Beckmann et al., New-onset obesity after liver transplantation-outcomes and risk factors: The swiss transplant cohort study. *Transpl Int* **31**, 1254–1267 (2018).
21. I. Colle, H. Van Vlierberghe, R. Troisi, B. De Hemptinne, Transplanted liver: Consequences of denervation for liver functions. *Anat Rec A Discov Mol Cell Evol Biol* **280**, 924–931 (2004).
22. R. A. Richardson, O. J. Garden, H. I. Davidson, Reduction in energy expenditure after liver transplantation. *Nutrition* **17**, 585–589 (2001).

23. E. R. Kallwitz *et al.*, Physical activity and metabolic syndrome in liver transplant recipients. *Liver Transpl* **19**, 1125–1131 (2013).

24. M. S. Siddiqui *et al.*, Differential fuel utilization in liver transplant recipients and its relationship with development of NAFLD. *Liver Int*, (2022).

25. J. van Son *et al.*, Post-transplant obesity impacts long-term survival after liver transplantation. *Metabolism* **106**, 154204 (2020).

26. I. Laish *et al.*, Metabolic syndrome in liver transplant recipients: Prevalence, risk factors, and association with cardiovascular events. *Liver Transpl* **17**, 15–22 (2011).

27. S. Patel *et al.*, Association between lipoprotein particles and atherosclerotic events in nonalcoholic fatty liver disease. *Clin Gastroenterol Hepatol* **19**, 2202–2204 (2021).

28. M. B. Siddiqui *et al.*, Small dense low-density lipoprotein cholesterol predicts cardiovascular events in liver transplant recipients. *Hepatology* **70**, 98–107 (2019).

29. F. Bril *et al.*, Hepatic steatosis and insulin resistance, but not steatohepatitis, promote atherogenic dyslipidemia in NAFLD. *J Clin Endocrinol Metab* **101**, 644–652 (2016).

30. T. Syed, M. S. Siddiqui, Atherogenic dyslipidemia after liver transplantation: Mechanisms and clinical implications. *Liver Transpl* **27**, 1326–1333 (2021).

31. O. Heisel, R. Heisel, R. Balshaw, P. Keown, New onset diabetes mellitus in patients receiving calcineurin inhibitors: A systematic review and meta-analysis. *Am J Transplant* **4**, 583–595 (2004).

32. A. J. Peckett, D. C. Wright, M. C. Riddell, The effects of glucocorticoids on adipose tissue lipid metabolism. *Metabolism* **60**, 1500–1510 (2011).

33. C. B. Ramirez, C. Doria, A. M. Frank, S. T. Armenti, I. R. Marino, Completely steroid-free immunosuppression in liver transplantation: A randomized study. *Clin Transplant* **27**, 463–471 (2013).

34. S. J. Pelletier *et al.*, A prospective, randomized trial of complete avoidance of steroids in liver transplantation with follow-up of over 7 years. *HPB (Oxford)* **15**, 286–293 (2013).

35. M. Charlton *et al.*, Everolimus is associated with less weight gain than tacrolimus 2 years after liver transplantation: Results of a randomized multicenter study. *Transplantation* **101**, 2873–2882 (2017).

36. S. Kotha *et al.*, Impact of immunosuppression on incidence of post-transplant diabetes mellitus in solid organ transplant recipients: Systematic review and meta-analysis. *World J Transplant* **11**, 432–442 (2021).

37. J. Noble, F. Terrec, P. Malvezzi, L. Rostaing, Adverse effects of immunosuppression after liver transplantation. *Best Pract Res Clin Gastroenterol* **54–55**, 101762 (2021).

38. N. D. Vaziri, K. Liang, H. Azad, Effect of cyclosporine on HMG-CoA reductase, cholesterol 7alpha-hydroxylase, LDL receptor, HDL receptor, VLDL receptor, and lipoprotein lipase expressions. *J Pharmacol Exp Ther* **294**, 778–783 (2000).

39. A. A. Schnitzbauer *et al.*, mTOR inhibition is most beneficial after liver transplantation for hepatocellular carcinoma in patients with active tumors. *Ann Surg* **272**, 855–862 (2020).

40. E. Cholongitas, C. Mamou, K. I. Rodríguez-Castro, P. Burra, Mammalian target of rapamycin inhibitors are associated with lower rates of hepatocellular carcinoma recurrence after liver transplantation: A systematic review. *Transpl Int* **27**, 1039–1049 (2014).

41. X. Yan *et al.*, Sirolimus or everolimus improves survival after liver transplantation for hepatocellular carcinoma: A systematic review and meta-analysis. *Liver Transpl*, (2021).

42. Y. Gueguen *et al.*, Compared effect of immunosuppressive drugs cyclosporine A and rapamycin on cholesterol homeostasis key enzymes CYP27A1 and HMG-CoA reductase. *Basic Clin Pharmacol Toxicol* **100**, 392–397 (2007).

43. M. Jain *et al.*, Explant liver evaluation decodes the mystery of cryptogenic cirrhosis! *JGH Open* **4**, 39–43 (2020).

44. K. Yalamanchili, S. Saadeh, G. B. Klintmalm, L. W. Jennings, G. L. Davis, Nonalcoholic fatty liver disease after liver transplantation for cryptogenic cirrhosis or nonalcoholic fatty liver disease. *Liver Transpl* **16**, 431–439 (2010).

45. M. Vallin *et al.*, Recurrent or de novo nonalcoholic fatty liver disease after liver transplantation: Natural history based on liver biopsy analysis. *Liver Transpl* **20**, 1064–1071 (2014).

46. N. Saeed *et al.*, Incidence and risks for nonalcoholic fatty liver disease and steatohepatitis post-liver transplant: Systematic review and meta-analysis. *Transplantation* **103**, e345–e354 (2019).

47. S. Kakar *et al.*, Incidence of recurrent NASH-related allograft cirrhosis. *Dig Dis Sci* **64**, 1356–1363 (2019).

48. J. W. Yu *et al.*, Obesity does not significantly impact outcomes following simultaneous liver kidney transplantation: Review of the UNOS database—a retrospective study. *Transpl Int* **32**, 206–217 (2019).

49. V. Bhagat *et al.*, Outcomes of liver transplantation in patients with cirrhosis due to nonalcoholic steatohepatitis versus patients with cirrhosis due to alcoholic liver disease. *Liver Transpl* **15**, 1814–1820 (2009).

50. B. Castelló *et al.*, Post-transplantation outcome in nonalcoholic steatohepatitis cirrhosis: Comparison with alcoholic cirrhosis. *Ann Hepatol* **18**, 855–861 (2019).

51. L. Yuan *et al.*, Portrait of regional trends in liver transplantation for nonalcoholic steatohepatitis in the United States. *Am J Gastroenterol* **117**, 433–444 (2022).

52. J. Ong, Z. M. Younossi, Non-alcoholic fatty liver disease after liver transplantation: A case of nurture and nature. *Am J Gastroenterol* **105**, 621–623 (2010).

53. H. Kim *et al.*, Histologically proven non-alcoholic fatty liver disease and clinically related factors in recipients after liver transplantation. *Clin Transplant* **28**, 521–529 (2014).

54. O. Shaked *et al.*, Impact of donor and recipient clinical characteristics and hepatic histology on steatosis/fibrosis following liver transplantation. *Transplantation* **106**, 106–116 (2022).

55. U. Iqbal, B. Perumpail, D. Akhtar, D. Kim, A. Ahmed, The epidemiology, risk profiling and diagnostic challenges of nonalcoholic fatty liver disease.

56. P. Trunečka *et al.*, Donor PNPLA3 rs738409 genotype is a risk factor for graft steatosis. A post-transplant biopsy-based study. *Dig Liver Dis* **50**, 490–495 (2018).

57. I. Míková *et al.*, Donor PNPLA3 and TM6SF2 variant alleles confer additive risks for graft steatosis after liver transplantation. *Transplantation* **104**, 526–534 (2020).

58. A. Finkenstedt *et al.*, Patatin-like phospholipase domain-containing protein 3 rs738409-G in recipients of liver transplants is a risk factor for graft steatosis. *Clin Gastroenterol Hepatol* **11**, 1667–1672 (2013).

59. J. Richards, B. Gunson, J. Johnson, J. Neuberger, Weight gain and obesity after liver transplantation. *Transpl Int* **18**, 461–466 (2005).

60. S. R. Weston *et al.*, Racial and ethnic distribution of nonalcoholic fatty liver in persons with newly diagnosed chronic liver disease. *Hepatology* **41**, 372–379 (2005).

61. J. D. Yang *et al.*, Gender and menopause impact severity of fibrosis among patients with nonalcoholic steatohepatitis. *Hepatology* **59**, 1406–1414 (2014).
62. I. Mikolasevic *et al.*, Noninvasive markers of liver steatosis and fibrosis after liver transplantation—Where do we stand? *World J Transplant* **11**, 37–53 (2021).
63. M. Chayanupatkul, D. B. Dasani, K. Sogaard, T. D. Schiano, The utility of assessing liver allograft fibrosis and steatosis post-liver transplantation using transient elastography with controlled attenuation parameter. *Transplant Proc* **53**, 159–165 (2021).
64. K. Kohda, N. Sawada, Y. Kawazoe, Formation of O6,7-dimethylguanine residues in calf thymus deoxyribonucleic acid treated with carcinogenic N-methyl-N-nitrosourea in vitro. *Chem Pharm Bull (Tokyo)* **39**, 801–802 (1991).
65. B. Della-Guardia *et al.*, Diagnostic accuracy of transient elastography for detecting liver fibrosis after liver trannsplantation: A specific cut-off value is really needed? *Dig Dis Sci* **62**, 264–272 (2017).
66. C. C. Park *et al.*, Magnetic resonance elastography vs transient elastography in detection of fibrosis and noninvasive measurement of steatosis in patients with biopsy-proven nonalcoholic fatty liver disease. *Gastroenterology* **152**, 598–607.e592 (2017).
67. B. Taouli, L. Serfaty, Magnetic resonance imaging/elastography is superior to transient elastography for detection of liver fibrosis and fat in nonalcoholic fatty liver disease. *Gastroenterology* **150**, 553–556 (2016).
68. S. Singh *et al.*, Diagnostic accuracy of magnetic resonance elastography in liver transplant recipients: A pooled analysis. *Ann Hepatol* **15**, 363–376 (2016).
69. Z. Melekoglu Ellik *et al.*, Evaluation of magnetic resonance elastography and transient elastography for liver fibrosis and steatosis assessments in the liver transplant setting. *Turk J Gastroenterol* **33**, 153–160 (2022).
70. D. D'Avola *et al.*, Cardiovascular morbidity and mortality after liver transplantation: The protective role of mycophenolate mofetil. *Liver Transpl* **23**, 498–509 (2017).
71. K. D. Watt, Metabolic syndrome: Is immunosuppression to blame? *Liver Transpl* **17(Suppl 3)**, S38–S42 (2011).
72. P. De Simone *et al.*, Everolimus with reduced tacrolimus improves renal function in de novo liver transplant recipients: A randomized controlled trial. *Am J Transplant* **12**, 3008–3020 (2012).
73. J. W. Molloy *et al.*, Association of coffee and caffeine consumption with fatty liver disease, nonalcoholic steatohepatitis, and degree of hepatic fibrosis. *Hepatology* **55**, 429–436 (2012).
74. J. C. Lai *et al.*, Physical frailty after liver transplantation. *Am J Transplant* **18**, 1986–1994 (2018).
75. A. M. Garcia, C. E. Veneroso, D. D. Soares, A. S. Lima, M. I. Correia, Effect of a physical exercise program on the functional capacity of liver transplant patients. *Transplant Proc* **46**, 1807–1808 (2014).
76. D. Moya-Nájera *et al.*, Combined resistance and endurance training at a moderate-to-high intensity improves physical condition and quality of life in liver transplant patients. *Liver Transpl* **23**, 1273–1281 (2017).
77. J. C. Jones, J. S. Coombes, G. A. Macdonald, Exercise capacity and muscle strength in patients with cirrhosis. *Liver Transpl* **18**, 146–151 (2012).
78. C. J. Lavie *et al.*, Exercise and the cardiovascular system: Clinical science and cardiovascular outcomes. *Circ Res* **117**, 207–219 (2015).
79. S. R. Sharpton, N. A. Terrault, M. M. Tavakol, A. M. Posselt, Sleeve gastrectomy prior to liver transplantation is superior to medical weight loss in reducing posttransplant metabolic complications. *Am J Transplant* **21**, 3324–3332 (2021).
80. S. R. Sharpton, N. A. Terrault, A. M. Posselt, Outcomes of sleeve gastrectomy in obese liver transplant candidates. *Liver Transpl* **25**, 538–544 (2019).
81. D. Zamora-Valdes *et al.*, Long-term outcomes of patients undergoing simultaneous liver transplantation and sleeve gastrectomy. *Hepatology* **68**, 485–495 (2018).
82. M. C. Morris *et al.*, Delayed sleeve gastrectomy following liver transplantation: A 5-year experience. *Liver Transpl* **25**, 1673–1681 (2019).
83. V. Lopez-Lopez *et al.*, Are we ready for bariatric surgery in a liver transplant program? A meta-analysis. *Obes Surg* **31**, 1214–1222 (2021).
84. A. J. Sanyal *et al.*, Pioglitazone, vitamin E, or placebo for nonalcoholic steatohepatitis. *N Engl J Med* **362**, 1675–1685 (2010).
85. K. Cusi *et al.*, Long-term pioglitazone treatment for patients with nonalcoholic steatohepatitis and prediabetes or type 2 diabetes mellitus: A randomized trial. *Ann Intern Med* **165**, 305–315 (2016).
86. P. N. Newsome *et al.*, A placebo-controlled trial of subcutaneous semaglutide in nonalcoholic steatohepatitis. *N Engl J Med* **384**, 1113–1124 (2021).
87. D. M. Rubino *et al.*, Effect of weekly subcutaneous semaglutide vs daily liraglutide on body weight in adults with overweight or obesity without diabetes: The STEP 8 randomized clinical trial. *JAMA* **327**, 138–150 (2022).
88. R. A. Bhanji *et al.*, Differing impact of sarcopenia and frailty in nonalcoholic steatohepatitis and alcoholic liver disease. *Liver Transpl* **25**, 14–24 (2019).
89. S. S. Patel *et al.*, The impact of coronary artery disease and statins on survival after liver transplantation. *Liver Transpl* **25**, 1514–1523 (2019).
90. P. E. Frasco *et al.*, Statin therapy and the incidence of thromboembolism and vascular events following liver transplantation. *Liver Transpl* **27**, 1432–1442 (2021).
91. P. T. Campbell, L. B. VanWagner, Mind the gap: Statin underutilization and impact on mortality in liver transplant recipients. *Liver Transpl* **25**, 1477–1479 (2019).
92. J. I. Lee, H. W. Lee, K. S. Lee, H. S. Lee, J. Y. Park, Effects of statin use on the development and progression of nonalcoholic fatty liver disease: A nationwide nested case-control study. *Am J Gastroenterol* **116**, 116–124 (2021).
93. B. Zou, M. C. Odden, M. H. Nguyen, Statin use and reduced hepatocellular carcinoma risk in patients with non-alcoholic fatty liver disease. *Clin Gastroenterol Hepatol*, (2022).
94. F. M. Chang *et al.*, Statins decrease the risk of decompensation in hepatitis B virus- and hepatitis C virus-related cirrhosis: A population-based study. *Hepatology* **66**, 896–907 (2017).
95. A. Mohanty, J. P. Tate, G. Garcia-Tsao, Statins are associated with a decreased risk of decompensation and death in veterans with hepatitis C-related compensated cirrhosis. *Gastroenterology* **150**, 430–440.e431 (2016).
96. M. Bhat, K. Mara, R. Dierkhising, K. D. Watt, Gender, Race and disease etiology predict de novo malignancy risk after liver transplantation: Insights for future individualized cancer screening guidance. *Transplantation* **103**, 91–100 (2019).

24 NAFLD in Lean Individuals

Donghee Kim and Vincent Wai-Sun Wong

CONTENTS

Key Points

- NAFLD is strongly associated with obesity and the related metabolic disorders. Nonetheless, NAFLD may be present in 5–27% of patients with a relatively normal body mass index (BMI).

- Long thought to be an Asian phenomenon, NAFLD has now been reported in lean individuals of different ethnic backgrounds.

- Despite normal BMI, lean individuals with NAFLD tend to have visceral obesity and other metabolic risk factors. Genetic predisposition (e.g., *PNPLA3* and *TM6SF2* gene polymorphism) and gut microbiota dysbiosis also contribute to NAFLD development. More research is needed to define which pathogenic mechanisms are specific to the development of NAFLD in lean individuals.

- In general, lean individuals have less severe NAFLD. Data on disease progression are conflicting, with a few studies suggesting that a subset of lean patients may be at a higher risk of liver-related morbidity and mortality in the long run than obese patients.

- Noninvasive tests of fibrosis such as simple fibrosis scores, specific biomarkers and imaging techniques perform similarly in lean and obese patients and can be used for initial assessment.

- Lean patients with NAFLD also benefit from lifestyle intervention but can achieve improvements in liver fat at a smaller degree of weight reduction than obese patients. Few if any studies examined the effect of pharmacological treatment in lean patients with NASH. The latter should be addressed in future studies.

24.1 INTRODUCTION

Nonalcoholic fatty liver disease (NAFLD) is strongly associated with obesity and metabolic syndrome.[1] In particular, insulin resistance is almost universal in NAFLD patients even before the development of diabetes.[2] Nonetheless, it is clear from numerous observational and epidemiological studies that a proportion of patients with NAFLD may have relatively normal body mass index (BMI). This is often referred to as "lean" or "nonobese" NAFLD. In the early 2000s, it was generally believed that this was an Asian phenomenon as most publications on this topic came from Asia, and Asians tended to have central obesity at a lower BMI.[3] However, subsequent studies showed that the same could be seen in Western countries.

In this chapter, we will first discuss the definitions of obesity and leanness and then review the epidemiology, pathogenesis, clinical features and outcomes of NAFLD in lean patients. Based on the knowledge, we discuss the implications on the assessment and treatment of this condition.

24.2 WHAT IS LEAN?

According to the World Health Organization (WHO), BMI is a crude measure of overweight and obesity.[4] BMI is calculated as body weight (kg) divided by body height (m) squared. Using BMI, people's nutritional status can be classified into underweight (BMI <18.5 kg/m^2), normal weight (18.5–24.9 kg/m^2), overweight (25.0–29.9 kg/m^2), obesity class I (30.0–34.9 kg/m^2), obesity class II (35.0–39.9 kg/m^2) and obesity class III (>40 kg/m^2). People with BMI <25.0 kg/m^2 are considered lean.

However, it has been apparent since the use of BMI that there are major differences in BMI across ethnic groups. In particular, Asians have lower BMI in general but tend to have central obesity and cardiometabolic complications at a lower BMI.[3] After the original BMI classification in adult Europids published in 1998, the WHO proposed BMI classification in adult Asians as follows: underweight (BMI <18.5 kg/m^2), normal weight (18.5–22.9 kg/m^2), overweight (23.0–24.9 kg/m^2), obesity class I (25.0–29.9 kg/m^2) and obesity class II (≥30 kg/m^2).[5] However, there is considerable heterogeneity across ethnic groups. For instance, Pacific

DOI: 10.1201/9781003386698-29

Islanders have a higher BMI than East Asians. Studies from different countries have also adopted different BMI cutoffs.

BMI is easy to measure and can be readily adopted in clinical practice and epidemiological studies. Nonetheless, its limitations should also be recognized. BMI does not distinguish between fat and muscle mass. Besides, BMI tends to be high and out of proportion to the degree of adiposity in people with extreme body heights.

Among other methods to measure adiposity, the waist circumference and waist-to-hip ratio are more widely used. They reflect the degree of visceral adiposity and have been shown to predict cardiovascular events and mortality.[6] The International Diabetes Federation defined central obesity as waist circumference ≥94 cm in male and ≥80 cm in female Europids and ≥90 cm in male and ≥80 cm in female South Asians, Chinese and Japanese.[7] The downside is the standardization and interobserver variability in waist circumference measurement. Examples of other anthropometric adiposity measures include waist-to-height ratio, waist-thigh ratio, body fat percentage and skinfold thickness. Despite its crudeness, waist circumference was superior to several common adiposity measures

in predicting cardiovascular risk in a meta-analysis of 20 studies in Caucasians.[8]

As will be discussed, BMI is only one of the many ways to measure adiposity, and most patients with NAFLD are insulin resistant and have central obesity despite normal BMI. Thus, the term "lean NAFLD" disregards the metabolic dysfunction in such patients and is potentially misleading. A better way to describe the disease is "NAFLD in lean individuals."

24.3 PREVALENCE OF NAFLD IN LEAN OR NONOBESE INDIVIDUALS

Despite its more conventionally recognized clinical phenotype, NAFLD is also reported in nonobese populations. Estimates in the prevalence of NAFLD among lean individuals are confounded by differences in sample selection methods, ethnic disparities in metabolic syndrome, variable diagnostic modalities, in addition to the unique impact of lifestyle and dietary habits across global populations. Epidemiologic data on NAFLD in lean individuals between Asians and other races is not directly compared due to the different BMI cutoffs employed between

Table 24.1: Prevalence of Nonalcoholic Fatty Liver Disease (NAFLD) in Lean or Nonobese Individuals

Author, Year	Population	N	Detection	BMI Cutoff (kg/m²)	Prevalence Lean or Nonobese NAFLD	NAFLD
Western						
Lean NAFLD						
Bellentani, 2000[12]	Italy, community-based (nonobese)	257	US	<25	16.4%	
Kim, 2012[10]	USA, Population-based (NHANES III)	11,277	US	<25	21.2%	34.0%
Nonobese NAFLD						
Browning, 2004[9]	USA, Population-based (The Dallas Heart Study)	2,287	MRS	<30	16.7%	34%
Foster, 2013[11]	USA, population-based (MESA)	3,056	CT	<30	11.3%	17.0%
Eastern						
Lean NAFLD						
Das, 2010[13]	India, community-based study	1,911	US, liver biopsy	<23 <25	5.05% 6.92%	8.7% (0.2% cirrhosis)
Sinn, 2012[15]	Korea, community-based study (nonobese, nondiabetic)	5,878	US	≥18.5, <25 ≥18.5, <23	27.4% 16.0%	
Nonobese NAFLD						
Kwon, 2012[14]	Korea, community-based study	29,994	US	<25	12.6%	20.1%
Wei, 2015[16]	Hong Kong, community-based study	911	MRS	<25	19.3%	28.8%
Meta-analysis						
Young, 2020[17]	Meta-analysis of 53 studies	314,573		<23 (Eastern) <25 (Western)	11.2%	20.6%
Ye, 2020[18]	Meta-analysis of 93 studies	10,530,308		<23 (Eastern) <25 (Western)	10.6%	
Lu, 2020[19]	Meta-analysis of 33 studies	205,307		<23 (Eastern) <25 (Western)	9.7%	

BMI: Body mass index; NAFLD: Nonalcoholic fatty liver disease; US: Ultrasonography; MRS: Magnetic resonance spectroscopy; CT: Computed tomography.

studies. The various prevalences of NAFLD in lean individuals are summarized in Table 24.1.

Among studies in Western populations, the differential prevalences of NAFLD are likely driven by a lack of standardization in the diagnostic technologies used for establishing the burden of steatosis. The Dallas Heart Study estimated hepatic triglyceride content with proton nuclear magnetic resonance spectroscopy (^{1}H-MRS), finding the prevalence of hepatic steatosis in nonobese individuals to be 16.7%, compared with 34% in the total population.[9] Based on the third National Health and Nutrition Examination Survey (NHANES) from 1988 to 1994, the prevalence of ultrasonography-detected NAFLD in lean individuals was 21%.[10] A study based on the Multi-Ethnic Study of Atherosclerosis (MESA) reported that the prevalence of nonobese, as assessed by computed tomography, was 11%, including 9% among Caucasians, 6% among African Americans, and 18% among Hispanics.[11] The Dionysus Study from Italy demonstrated similar findings, estimating the prevalence of ultrasonography-detected NAFLD in lean individuals to be 16%.[12]

Stark differences in the prevalence of NAFLD in lean individuals from Asian populations is appreciated in a community-based study from rural India, whereby the prevalence in lean and nonobese patients was estimated at 5.5 and 7.4%, respectively.[13] A community-based Korean study of 29,994 individuals recruited for general medical screening programs reported a slightly higher prevalence for nonobese individuals, more in keeping with Western estimates at 12.6%.[14] In a similar study analyzing 5,878 nonobese, nondiabetic individuals, the prevalence of NAFLD in lean individuals remained high at 16%.[15] A population-based study from Hong Kong using ^{1}H-MRS showed that the prevalence of NAFLD was 19.3% in the nonobese population and 60.5% in the obese population.[16] In this study, 2.6 % nonobese NAFLD and 5.1% obese NAFLD had a similarly high probability of advanced fibrosis by transient elastography, although liver stiffness was slightly higher in obese NAFLD.[16]

In 2020, three systematic reviews with meta-analyses estimating the prevalence of NAFLD in lean individuals were published simultaneously. The first meta-analysis estimated the prevalence of lean NAFLD from a general population (n = 314,573) to be 11.2% (95% confidence interval [CI]: 9.6–13.0%).[17] This estimate was obtained using pooled data from 30 studies, and 9.2% (95% CI: 7.4–11.3%) from 15 studies that contributed sample sizes of greater than 1,000 participants.[17] Among individuals with established NAFLD, the prevalence of NAFLD in lean individuals was 25.3%.[17] A second meta-analysis including 30 studies (n = 218,106) reported similar findings, whereby the prevalence of nonobese NAFLD in the general population was estimated at 12.1% (95% CI: 9.3–15.6%) with the prevalence of overweight NAFLD of 8.6% (95% CI: 6.7–11.0%) and NAFLD in lean individuals 4.9% (95% CI: 3.1–7.7%), respectively.[18] Among the NAFLD population (35 studies, n = 36,529), 19.2% (95% CI: 15.9–23.0%) were considered to have NAFLD in lean individuals.[18] Among the general population (23 studies, n = 113,394), the prevalence of NAFLD in lean individuals was 5.1% (95% CI: 3.7–7.0%), whereas among the lean population (19 studies, n = 49,503), the prevalence of NAFLD in lean individuals was 10.6% (95% CI: 7.8–14.1%).[18] The incidence of nonobese NAFLD was 24.6 (95% CI: 13.4–39.2%) per 1,000 person-years (n = 8,827) and was similar to the incidence of NAFLD in lean individuals (23.2% [95% CI: 7.3–48.0%], n = 3,925, p= 0.92),

while the incidence of obese NAFLD was 77.5% (95% CI: 28.3–150.6%, n = 1,969).[18] The third meta-analysis, including 33 studies, showed that the global prevalence of NAFLD in lean individuals was 4.1% (95% CI: 3.4–4.8%).[19] In the lean population, the prevalence of NAFLD was 9.7% (95% CI: 7.7–11.8%). The highest prevalence of NAFLD in lean individuals (4.8%, 95% CI: 4.0–5.6%) in Asia, while the lower prevalence of NAFLD in lean individuals was 3.1% (95% CI: 2.3–3.8%) in US studies and 2.2% (95% CI: 2.3–3.8%) in European studies.[19] The prevalence of NAFLD in lean individuals showed an upward trend between 1988 and 2017, especially in Asia.[19]

Acknowledging major differences in BMI cutoffs employed for characterizing population weight categories, epidemiological data indicate that the prevalence of NAFLD in lean individuals was 4–11% in the general population. When measuring within exclusive NAFLD populations, the lean individuals accounted for 25%. Variations in prevalence should be interpreted with caution and are presumed to be influenced by ethnic variation and lack of standardization in the accepted definition for BMI as well as diagnostic measurement modalities.

24.3.1 Prevalence of Nonalcoholic Steatohepatitis (NASH) and Fibrosis in Lean Individuals

Estimating the prevalence of nonalcoholic steatohepatitis (NASH) and fibrosis utilizing pathologic specimens can be limited due to the invasive testing required to confirm the histologic presence of fibrosis with associated cellular damage. According to a recent meta-analysis, 39.0% (95% CI: 24.1–56.3%) had NASH, 29.2% (95% CI: 21.9–37.9%) had significant fibrosis and 3.2% (95% CI: 1.5–5.7%) had cirrhosis among NAFLD in lean or nonobese individuals.[18] Morphological features of NAFLD in lean individuals and obese NAFLD are presumed to be indistinguishable from each other, displaying features of NASH with or without fibrosis. An Italian study that included 669 individuals with biopsy-proven NAFLD determined that NAFLD in lean individuals had a lower prevalence of NASH (17 vs. 40%) and significant fibrosis (17 vs. 42%) compared to obese or overweight NAFLD.[20] A prospective cohort study with biopsy-proven NAFLD (n = 307) from Hong Kong showed similar findings such that nonobese NAFLD had a lower NAFLD activity score and fibrosis stage than obese patients.[21] However, there was no difference in the histologic severity of NASH or fibrosis between lean NAFLD and overweight NAFLD in the nonobese population.[21] In contrast, a Korean prospective cohort study with biopsy-proven NAFLD (n = 664) showed no significant difference in histology between nonobese NAFLD and obese NAFLD except for higher severity of hepatic fibrosis in nonobese NASH.[22] Consistently, an Austrian study (n = 466) showed that biopsy-proven NAFLD in lean individuals had a comparable degree of inflammation, ballooning and fibrosis and a similar proportion of NASH to obese NAFLD.[23] A recent multicenter study based on the GOASIA (Gut and Obesity in Asia) database (n = 1,812) determined that nonobese NAFLD had lower proportions of NASH (50.5 vs. 56.5%) and advanced fibrosis (14.0 vs. 18.7%) compared to obese NAFLD.[24] Finally, a multicenter study of Caucasians with biopsy-confirmed NAFLD (n = 1,339) showed similar results that NAFLD in lean individuals had less severe histological disease (NASH: 54.1 vs. 71.2%; advanced fibrosis: 10.1 vs. 25.2%) compared to counterparts.[25] Overall, a substantial proportion of NAFLD in nonobese or lean individuals still exhibited features of NASH and/or advanced fibrosis, while NAFLD in nonobese or lean individuals had relatively less severe histologic findings.

24.4 PATHOGENESIS

A distinct subgroup of lean individuals have been known to exhibit excess visceral adiposity, insulin resistance and metabolic abnormalities, typically observed in those with obesity—metabolically obese, normal-weight (MONW).[22,26] Therefore, it is essential to determine the presence of metabolic abnormalities, including NAFLD, that are present in a significant proportion of lean individuals. NAFLD in lean individuals may represent a subset phenotype of NAFLD in MONW subjects. Different mechanisms underlie the various NAFLD phenotypes (obese NAFLD vs. NAFLD in lean individuals), including genetic, clinical and behavioral factors, some of which may be modifiable.

24.4.1 Visceral Adiposity and Sarcopenia

The distribution of adiposity is thought to be more critical to the development of NAFLD than the total adipose mass. In fact, visceral adiposity accounts for a greater risk for developing NAFLD than BMI among lean individuals.[27] Although visceral adiposity accounts for only 7–15% of the total body fat, it carries significant prognostic value, consequential to the pathogenesis of NAFLD and insulin resistance.[26,27] A prospective cohort study demonstrated that visceral adiposity was dose-dependently associated with incident nonobese NAFLD, with significant associations with subcutaneous adiposity for regressed nonobese NAFLD independent of visceral adiposity.[27] Visceral adiposity has also confirmed a predictor for NASH and significant fibrosis in nonobese NAFLD.[22] The association between visceral adiposity and NAFLD was differentially stronger in nonobese NASH than in obese NASH (63 vs. 38% increased risk of NASH per 1-standard deviation [SD] increase of visceral fat).[22] Likewise, nonobese NAFLD with a 1-SD increase of visceral fat had 57% greater odds of significant fibrosis; however, visceral adiposity was not associated with significant fibrosis in the obese population.[22]

The structural integrity of the skeletal muscle compartment could affect metabolic homeostasis. Several studies showed an increased risk of NAFLD, NASH and fibrosis among individuals with sarcopenia, independent of obesity, insulin resistance and inflammatory marker.[28,29] Because sarcopenia and visceral adiposity could often coexist in NAFLD in lean individuals, sarcopenia and visceral adiposity might have a synergistic effect on the development and progression of NAFLD in lean individuals.

24.4.2 Other Metabolic Risk Factors

In lean individuals, various metabolic risk factors in NAFLD are consistent with obese NAFLD. However, the association with components of metabolic syndrome was stronger for NAFLD in lean individuals than for obese NAFLD.[14] Nonobese NAFLD had higher prevalence ratios for specific components of metabolic syndrome (high triglycerides for both genders, high blood pressure, low high-density-lipoprotein cholesterol and impaired fasting glucose for women) than those with obese NAFLD. Nonobese NAFLD was associated with insulin resistance, regardless of other components of metabolic syndrome in the nondiabetic population.[15] In addition, several cohort studies reported the association between weight gain within the normal weight range and incident NAFLD in lean individuals.[30] A prospective cohort study from Hong Kong showed increased waist circumference and serum triglycerides during the follow-up were associated with incident NAFLD in lean individuals.[31] Therefore, susceptible lean individuals may be triggered into developing NAFLD with relatively minor changes in their metabolic profile because the current definitions for metabolic syndrome are not sufficiently sensitive to characterize their metabolic risk.

24.4.3 Diet

As several studies suggest that a high cholesterol diet is associated with NAFLD in lean individuals, cholesterol metabolism is thought to contribute to the pathogenesis of NAFLD in lean individuals than in obese individuals.[26] A high-cholesterol diet may stimulate de novo lipogenesis by increasing the level of oxysterol, a metabolite in the sterol-regulatory element-binding protein-1c (SREBP-1c) pathway,[32] even when the total caloric intake may not be excessive in lean individuals. Fructose-sweetened soft drinks consumption is associated with nonobese NAFLD.[33] To the degree that NAFLD in lean individuals occurs at a younger age than obese NAFLD and that young adults tend to consume more soft drinks than older adults, fructose ingestion such as soft drink consumption may play a more prominent role in NAFLD in lean individuals than in obese individuals.[10] Therefore, the dietary composition may represent a readily modifiable environmental factor, particularly in young NAFLD in lean individuals, although interventional data are not available at present.

24.4.4 Genetic Risk Factors

Although visceral obesity, dietary composition and metabolic abnormalities are the most prevalent risk factors for NAFLD in lean individuals, genetic factors may be necessary in determining the risk of NAFLD in lean individuals.

24.4.4.1 PNPLA3

Variation in the patatin-like phospholipase domain-containing 3 (PNPLA3) gene is strongly linked to differences in hepatic triglycerides content and susceptibility to NAFLD in lean individuals. PNPLA3 is not mediated through insulin resistance and related metabolic comorbidities such as obesity. Thus individuals with variant PNPLA3 are associated with NAFLD without insulin resistance or adipose tissue inflammation.[34,35] These data suggest that the PNPLA3 variant may play an essential role in the pathogenesis of NAFLD in lean individuals. A population-based study determined that a higher proportion of nonobese NAFLD carried the variant PNPLA3 allele than obese NAFLD (78.4 vs. 59.8%) and that the PNPLA3 polymorphism remained an independent predictor for nonobese NAFLD.[16] A recent meta-analysis reported that the variant PNPLA3 rs738409 gene polymorphism is more prevalent in NAFLD in lean or nonobese individuals than in obese individuals (CG + GG vs. CC; OR 1.72, 95% CI 1.21–2.44).[36]

24.4.4.2 TM6SF2

Single nucleotide polymorphism in TM6SF2, transmembrane 6 superfamily member 2 was associated with hepatic triglyceride content in The Dallas Heart Study.[37] Subsequently, this TM6SF2 minor allele was associated with hepatic fibrosis independent of age, diabetes, obesity and the PNPLA3 genotype.[38] A study including a cohort of Caucasian patients with biopsy-proven NAFLD (n = 538) determined that NAFLD in lean individuals had a significantly higher prevalence of carriage of the *TM6SF2* T allele than obese counterparts.[39] *TM6SF2* T allele still associated with NAFLD in lean individuals after adjusting for age, sex, alanine aminotransferase, diabetes, total cholesterol level, fibrosis, steatosis and *PNPLA3* genotype (odds ratio, 2.57; 95% CI (confidence intervals): 1.43–4.62).[39] Another study also showed a higher expression of the variant in NAFLD in lean individuals compared to overweight/obese NAFLD (4 vs. 0.3%).[20]

24.4.5 Gut Microbiome

The mechanisms by which the gut microbiome contributes to NAFLD in lean individuals consist of altered gut permeability, endogenous ethanol production, endotoxemia, increased energy harvest from food and alterations in bile acid and choline metabolism.[40] A Chinese study showed that nonobese NAFLD had a lower abundance of *Firmicutes*, including *Lachnospiraceae*, *Ruminococcaceae* and *Lactobacillacea* and an increase in lipopolysaccharide-producing gram-negative bacteria.[41] A Brazilian study revealed a trend toward NASH differences in lean individuals compared to the obese NAFLD, with a 3-fold lower abundance of *Fecalibacterium* and *Ruminococcus* species and a relative deficiency in *Lactobacillus*.[42] Regarding fibrosis, *Ruminococcaceae* and *Veillonellaceae* are the central microbiota associated with fibrosis severity in nonobese, nonobese, individuals.[43] However, data regarding the impact of the gut microbiome on NAFLD in lean individuals is still in development.

24.5 CLINICAL FEATURES

Lean individuals with NAFLD are by no means metabolically healthy. Compared with lean individuals without NAFLD, those with NAFLD have higher BMI, waist circumference, visceral fat, insulin resistance and a higher prevalence of diabetes, hypertension and dyslipidemia.[26] Even among those with persistently normal BMI, people who develop incident NAFLD often have a history of weight gain.[31] The fact that BMI remains a risk factor of NAFLD in lean and nonobese individuals suggests that the risk is a continuum by BMI. In a retrospective study using the 1999–2016 NHANES databases, nonobese individuals with NAFLD were older and more likely to be male than those without NAFLD.[44] Foreign-born Asians were at increased risk, whereas Blacks had a lower risk, even when ethnic-specific BMI cutoffs were applied.

One interesting question is that lean patients develop NAFLD because their other metabolic risk factors are more severe, thus compensating for the effect of relatively normal BMI. This hypothesis turns out to be wrong. Studies have consistently shown that, among patients with NAFLD, those who were obese had higher insulin resistance and more severe metabolic diseases than those who were nonobese or lean.[16]

Studies using noninvasive tests in general showed that lean patients with NAFLD had less severe liver fibrosis than obese patients.[16] Likewise, lean patients with NAFLD have less severe histological features than obese patients in terms of steatosis, lobular inflammation, hepatocyte ballooning and fibrosis.[45] That being said, severe liver disease can be found in lean and nonobese individuals. Among various histologic cohorts, around 44–54% of lean and nonobese patients had NASH, and 10–26% had advanced liver fibrosis.[25,39,45] Because not every NAFLD patient would undergo a liver biopsy, histologic studies are limited by selection bias and tend to include patients with more severe liver disease, but the bottom line is that severe liver disease can occur in this population.

The association between NAFLD and metabolic disorders, particularly type 2 diabetes, is well-established.[46] This appears to be a bidirectional relationship, with NAFLD preceding other metabolic comorbidities in some cases and metabolic risk factors preceding NAFLD in others. The same is true in lean subjects. In a longitudinal study of 51,463 Koreans undergoing health examinations, lean individuals (BMI <23 kg/m^2) with NAFLD had a hazard ratio of incident diabetes of 1.18 (95% CI: 1.03–1.35), compared with those without NAFLD, at a median follow-up of 4 years.[47] In another community study of 2,985 participants from Sri Lanka, 24, 66, 82 and 79% of lean individuals with NAFLD developed incident diabetes, hypertension, hypertriglyceridemia and decreased high-density lipoprotein-cholesterol, respectively, after 7 years of follow-up.[48]

24.6 CLINICAL OUTCOMES

Whether NAFLD in lean individuals is a distinct entity with an increased risk of adverse clinical outcomes is a matter of hot debate. Intuitively, if lean individuals have a lower metabolic burden and less severe liver disease at baseline, their cardiovascular and liver-related outcomes should be more favorable. However, a multicenter retrospective study of 1,090 patients with biopsy-proven NAFLD (125 had BMI <25 kg/m^2) first suggested that lean patients had higher overall mortality at a mean follow-up of 133 months.[49] Unfortunately, the study remains in abstract form, and it is unclear if confounding factors and misclassifications have been adequately addressed. In another study of 646 patients with biopsy-proven NAFLD from Sweden (19% were lean), lean patients did not have increased mortality but had an increased risk of progressing to severe liver disease (defined as decompensated liver disease, liver failure, hepatocellular carcinoma or cirrhosis; hazard ratio 1.48 [95% CI: 0.75–2.91]; adjusted hazard ratio 2.69 [95% CI: 1.31–5.50] after adjusting for age, sex, type 2 diabetes and fibrosis at baseline).[50] Although the results are intriguing, the high hazard ratio after adjustment clearly indicates that the lean group had more favorable risk profiles, and the apparent increase in risk was the result of statistical modeling that deserves validation in further studies. In contrast, studies from Italy, the United Kingdom, Spain, Australia and Hong Kong did not observe an increase in overall mortality or liver-related events in lean or nonobese individuals with NAFLD.[25,39,45]

Cardiovascular disease and extrahepatic malignancies are the leading causes of death in NAFLD patients. However, current data have not shown a definitive association between NAFLD and these complications in lean individuals. In the 1999–2016 NHANES cohort, compared with people without NAFLD, obese subjects with NAFLD had increased cancer-related mortality, but nonobese subjects with NAFLD had similar cardiovascular disease-related (adjusted hazard ratio 0.83; 95% CI: 0.55–1.25) and cancer-related mortality (adjusted hazard ratio 1.12; 95% CI: 0.71–1.79).[44]

In 2020, a group of hepatologists proposed to rename NAFLD as metabolic-associated or metabolic dysfunction-associated fatty liver disease (MAFLD).[51] The new definition of MAFLD requires the presence of overweight or obesity, type 2 diabetes or 2 other metabolic risk factors. Since then, a number of studies showed that patients who had fatty liver but did not meet the metabolic criteria of

MAFLD (i.e., NAFLD but not MAFLD) were less likely to have advanced liver fibrosis or to develop cardiovascular events.[52,53] Likewise, data from NHANES III showed that MAFLD but not NAFLD increased all-cause mortality at a median follow-up of 23 years.[54] Since overweight and obese individuals with fatty liver would fulfill the definition of MAFLD, these data further support the notion that lean individuals with NAFLD tend to have a better prognosis.

24.7 ASSESSMENT

The three components of assessment of NAFLD are (1) establishing the diagnosis, (2) assessing the severity of liver disease, and (3) evaluating the cardiometabolic profile. The diagnosis of NAFLD relies on the detection of fatty liver and exclusion of other concomitant liver diseases and secondary causes of fatty liver. In clinical practice, fatty liver is mainly detected by abdominal ultrasonography, whereas quantification of hepatic steatosis by imaging biomarkers (e.g., controlled attenuation parameter by vibration-controlled transient elastography [VCTE] and magnetic resonance imaging proton density fat fraction) is used in research settings.[55] Abdominal ultrasonography is more challenging in obese patients, though dedicated studies on the accuracy of ultrasonography for the diagnosis of fatty liver in nonobese patients are lacking.

Because lean individuals with NAFLD tend to have less severe liver histology, noninvasive tests are preferred to liver biopsy as initial assessment of the severity of liver disease. Among the histologic features of NAFLD, fibrosis has the strongest correlation with clinical outcomes. Noninvasive tests of fibrosis are also more widely available and robust, though combined scores such as the MACK-3, NIS4 and FAST scores have recently been developed for the detection of NASH with significant fibrosis.

Noninvasive tests of fibrosis can be divided into simple fibrosis scores, specific blood fibrosis biomarkers (e.g., enhanced liver fibrosis panel, Pro-C3), and imaging biomarkers (ultrasound and magnetic resonance elastography).[55] Some simple fibrosis scores (e.g., Fibrosis-4 index and aspartate aminotransferase-to-platelet ratio index) were initially derived and validated in patients with chronic viral hepatitis, whereas others (e.g., the NAFLD fibrosis score and BARD score) were specifically developed for NAFLD patients. In both real-world cohorts and clinical trials, the performance of these scores was as good in lean patients as in obese patients with NAFLD, even though some scores (e.g., the NAFLD fibrosis score) had BMI as one of the components.[56]

Ultrasound elastography (VCTE, point-shear wave elastography, two-dimensional shear wave elastography) has been validated in patients with different liver diseases.[57] The accuracy and applicability of VCTE are higher in lean patients with NAFLD.[56] Because the failure rate of VCTE is higher in obese patients, the manufacturer developed the XL probe to cater for obese patients. When applied on the same patient, the XL probe yields a lower liver stiffness value than the M probe.[58] However, if the M probe is used in patients with BMI <30 kg/m^2 and XL probe in those with BMI ≥30 kg/m^2, the same liver stiffness cutoffs can be used.[59] Currently, the machine has an automatic probe selection tool to recommend the use of M or XL probes based on the skin-to-liver capsule distance.

Magnetic resonance elastography has a higher success rate and overall accuracy than VCTE, and the success rate is not affected by obesity. Data on its use in lean individuals with NAFLD are lacking.

Clinicians should also be alert to secondary causes of fatty liver, particularly in patients with little metabolic burden but rather severe liver disease (Table 24.2).

24.8 TREATMENT

Lifestyle modification is the cornerstone in the management of NAFLD and NASH. One interesting question is whether nonobese patients with NAFLD should still lose weight. To this end, a secondary analysis of a randomized controlled trial in Hong Kong showed that 67% of the patients with BMI <25 kg/m^2 achieved remission of NAFLD (intrahepatic triglyceride content <5% by proton-magnetic resonance spectroscopy) after 12 months of lifestyle intervention, compared with 18% in the control group.[60] In addition, there was a dose–response relationship between the degree of weight reduction and remission of NAFLD in both nonobese and obese patients, though nonobese patients did not need to lose as much weight to achieve the same beneficial effects (Figure 24.1).

At the moment, there is no registered drug for the treatment of NASH, though various guidelines support the use of vitamin E, pioglitazone or glucagon-like peptide-1 receptor agonists (GLP-1 RA) in selected patients.[1] In particular, GLP-1 RA improves insulin sensitivity, reduces the appetite centrally and slows gastric emptying, and is one of the most effective pharmacological treatments for weight reduction and diabetic control.[61] Importantly, this class of drug improves cardiovascular outcomes in long-term studies. In a phase 2b study, semaglutide at a dose of 0.4 mg daily for 72 weeks led to resolution of NASH in 59% of patients, compared with 17% in the placebo group.[62] It is unclear whether the treatment effects differ in lean patients, though BMI does not appear to affect the glucose-lowering effects of GLP-1 RA in patients with type 2 diabetes. Likewise, future studies should determine the safety and efficacy of new NASH drugs in the lean population.

In patients with severe obesity, bariatric surgery is currently the most effective method for weight reduction. It also reverses histologic NASH and fibrosis and prevents the development of cirrhosis and hepatic decompensation.[63] For obvious reasons, bariatric surgery cannot be recommended for lean individuals.

24.9 CONCLUSION

In the past two decades, accumulated data have shed light on the epidemiology, clinical characteristics, pathogenesis and management of NAFLD in lean individuals. It is now clear that the condition can be found in both Western and

Table 24.2: Secondary Causes of Fatty Liver

Endocrine disorders (e.g., hypothyroidism, hypogonadism, growth hormone deficiency)

Disorders of lipid metabolism

Total parenteral nutrition

Hepatitis C virus infection

Severe weight loss

Medications (e.g., tamoxifen, methotrexate, systemic steroids)

Lipodystrophy

Wilson's disease

Celiac disease

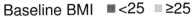

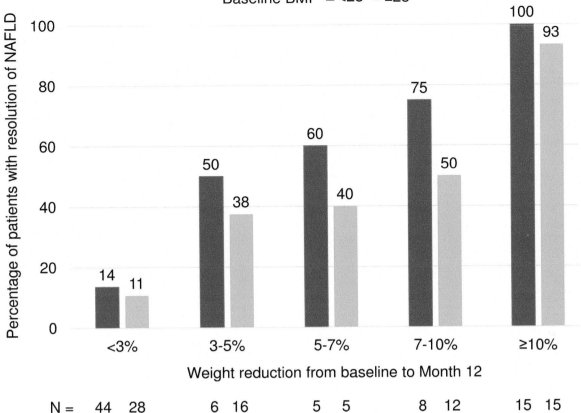

Figure 24.1 Degree of weight reduction and resolution of NAFLD at 12 months in nonobese individuals (Modified with permission from Wong et al.[60])

Asian countries. Although lean individuals usually have mild liver disease, NASH and advanced fibrosis can be seen in selected cases. Noninvasive tests should be used for initial assessment, and their performance is equally good in lean and obese patients. Because lean patients are underrepresented in clinical trials, future studies should define the safety and efficacy of new NASH drugs in this special population.

REFERENCES

1. Powell EE, Wong VW, Rinella M. Non-alcoholic fatty liver disease. *Lancet* 2021;397:2212–2224.
2. Bugianesi E, Moscatiello S, Ciaravella MF, et al. Insulin resistance in nonalcoholic fatty liver disease. *Curr Pharm Des* 2010;16:1941–1951.
3. Fan JG, Kim SU, Wong VW. New trends on obesity and NAFLD in Asia. *J Hepatol* 2017;67:862–873.
4. World Health Organization. *Obesity and overweight.* www.who.int/news-room/fact-sheets/detail/obesity-and-overweight (accessed on 7 January 2022).
5. World Health Organization Western Pacific Region, International Association for the Study of Obesity, International Obesity TaskForce. *The Asia-Pacific perspective: Redefining obesity and its treatment.* February 2000 chrome-extension://efaidnbmnnnibpcajpcglclefindm-kaj/viewer.html?pdfurl=https%3A%2F%2Fapps.who.int%2Firis%2Fbitstream%2Fhandle%2F10665%2F206936%2F0957708211_eng.pdf%3Fsequence%3D1%26tnqh_x0026%3BisAllowed%3Dy&clen=2539548&chunk=true (accessed on 7 January 2022).
6. Pischon T, Boeing H, Hoffmann K, et al. General and abdominal adiposity and risk of death in Europe. *N Engl J Med* 2008;359:2105–2120.
7. Alberti KG, Zimmet P, Shaw J. Metabolic syndrome—a new world-wide definition. A consensus statement from the international diabetes federation. *Diabet Med* 2006;23:469–480.
8. van Dijk SB, Takken T, Prinsen EC, et al. Different anthropometric adiposity measures and their association with cardiovascular disease risk factors: A meta-analysis. *Neth Heart J* 2012;20:208–218.
9. Browning JD, Szczepaniak LS, Dobbins R, et al. Prevalence of hepatic steatosis in an urban population in the United States: Impact of ethnicity. *Hepatology* 2004;40:1387–1395.
10. Kim D, Kim W. Non-overweight fatty liver disease (NOFLD): A distinct entity? *Hepatology* 2012;56:A886–A887.
11. Foster T, Anania FA, Li D, et al. The prevalence and clinical correlates of nonalcoholic fatty liver disease (NAFLD) in African Americans: The multi-ethnic study of atherosclerosis (MESA). *Dig Dis Sci* 2013;58:2392–2398.
12. Bellentani S, Saccoccio G, Masutti F, et al. Prevalence of and risk factors for hepatic steatosis in Northern Italy. *Ann Intern Med* 2000;132:112–117.
13. Das K, Das K, Mukherjee PS, et al. Nonobese population in a developing country has a high prevalence of nonalcoholic fatty liver and significant liver disease. *Hepatology* 2010;51:1593–1602.

14. Kwon YM, Oh SW, Hwang SS, et al. Association of nonalcoholic fatty liver disease with components of metabolic syndrome according to body mass index in Korean adults. *Am J Gastroenterol* 2012;107:1852–1858.

15. Sinn DH, Gwak GY, Park HN, et al. Ultrasonographically detected non-alcoholic fatty liver disease is an independent predictor for identifying patients with insulin resistance in nonobese, non-diabetic middle-aged Asian adults. *Am J Gastroenterol* 2012;107:561–567.

16. Wei JL, Leung JC, Loong TC, et al. Prevalence and severity of nonalcoholic fatty liver disease in non-obese patients: A population study using proton-magnetic resonance spectroscopy. *Am J Gastroenterol* 2015;110:1306–1314; quiz 1315.

17. Young S, Tariq R, Provenza J, et al. Prevalence and profile of nonalcoholic fatty liver disease in lean adults: Systematic review and meta-analysis. *Hepatol Commun* 2020;4:953–972.

18. Ye Q, Zou B, Yeo YH, et al. Global prevalence, incidence, and outcomes of nonobese or lean non-alcoholic fatty liver disease: A systematic review and meta-analysis. *Lancet Gastroenterol Hepatol* 2020;5:739–752.

19. Lu FB, Zheng KI, Rios RS, et al. Global epidemiology of lean non-alcoholic fatty liver disease: A systematic review and meta-analysis. *J Gastroenterol Hepatol* 2020;35:2041–2050.

20. Fracanzani AL, Petta S, Lombardi R, et al. Liver and cardiovascular damage in patients with lean nonalcoholic fatty liver disease, and association with visceral obesity. *Clin Gastroenterol Hepatol* 2017;15:1604–1611 e1.

21. Leung JC, Loong TC, Wei JL, et al. Histological severity and clinical outcomes of nonalcoholic fatty liver disease in nonobese patients. *Hepatology* 2017;65:54–64.

22. Kim D, Kim W, Joo SK, et al. Predictors of nonalcoholic steatohepatitis and significant fibrosis in nonobese nonalcoholic fatty liver disease. *Liver Int* 2019;39:332–341.

23. Denkmayr L, Feldman A, Stechemesser L, et al. Lean patients with non-alcoholic fatty liver disease have a severe histological phenotype similar to obese patients. *J Clin Med* 2018;7.

24. Tan EX, Lee JW, Jumat NH, et al. Nonobese non-alcoholic fatty liver disease (NAFLD) in Asia: An international registry study. *Metabolism* 2022;126:154911.

25. Younes R, Govaere O, Petta S, et al. Caucasian lean subjects with non-alcoholic fatty liver disease share long-term prognosis of non-lean: Time for reappraisal of BMI-driven approach? *Gut* 2022;71:382–390.

26. Kim D, Kim WR. Nonobese fatty liver disease. *Clin Gastroenterol Hepatol* 2017;15:474–485.

27. Kim D, Chung GE, Kwak MS, et al. Body fat distribution and risk of incident and regressed nonalcoholic fatty liver disease. *Clin Gastroenterol Hepatol* 2016;14:132–138 e4.

28. Koo BK, Kim D, Joo SK, et al. Sarcopenia is an independent risk factor for non-alcoholic steatohepatitis and significant fibrosis. *J Hepatol* 2017;66:123–131.

29. Wijarnpreecha K, Kim D, Raymond P, et al. Associations between sarcopenia and nonalcoholic fatty liver disease and advanced fibrosis in the USA. *Eur J Gastroenterol Hepatol* 2019;31:1121–1128.

30. Chang Y, Ryu S, Sung E, et al. Weight gain within the normal weight range predicts ultrasonographically detected fatty liver in healthy Korean men. *Gut* 2009;58:1419–1425.

31. Wong VW, Wong GL, Yeung DK, et al. Incidence of non-alcoholic fatty liver disease in Hong Kong: A population study with paired proton-magnetic resonance spectroscopy. *J Hepatol* 2015;62:182–189.

32. McCarthy EM, Rinella ME. The role of diet and nutrient composition in nonalcoholic fatty liver disease. *J Acad Nutr Diet* 2012;112:401–409.

33. Assy N, Nasser G, Kamayse I, et al. Soft drink consumption linked with fatty liver in the absence of traditional risk factors. *Can J Gastroenterol* 2008;22:811–816.

34. Lallukka S, Sevastianova K, Perttila J, et al. Adipose tissue is inflamed in NAFLD due to obesity but not in NAFLD due to genetic variation in PNPLA3. *Diabetologia* 2013;56:886–892.

35. Shen J, Wong GL, Chan HL, et al. PNPLA3 gene polymorphism accounts for fatty liver in community subjects without metabolic syndrome. *Aliment Pharmacol Ther* 2014;39:532–539.

36. Zou ZY, Wong VW, Fan JG. Epidemiology of non-alcoholic fatty liver disease in nonobese populations: Meta-analytic assessment of its prevalence, genetic, metabolic, and histological profiles. *J Dig Dis* 2020;21:372–384.

37. Kozlitina J, Smagris E, Stender S, et al. Exome-wide association study identifies a TM6SF2 variant that confers susceptibility to nonalcoholic fatty liver disease. *Nat Genet* 2014;46:352–356.

38. Liu YL, Reeves HL, Burt AD, et al. TM6SF2 rs58542926 influences hepatic fibrosis progression in patients with non-alcoholic fatty liver disease. *Nat Commun* 2014;5:4309.

39. Chen F, Esmaili S, Rogers GB, et al. Lean NAFLD: A distinct entity shaped by differential metabolic adaptation. *Hepatology* 2020;71:1213–1227.

40. Kuchay MS, Martinez-Montoro JI, Choudhary NS, et al. Non-alcoholic fatty liver disease in lean and nonobese individuals: Current and future challenges. *Biomedicines* 2021;9.

41. Wang B, Jiang X, Cao M, et al. Altered fecal microbiota correlates with liver biochemistry in nonobese patients with non-alcoholic fatty liver disease. *Sci Rep* 2016;6:32002.

42. Duarte SMB, Stefano JT, Miele L, et al. Gut microbiome composition in lean patients with NASH is associated with liver damage independent of caloric intake: A prospective pilot study. *Nutr Metab Cardiovasc Dis* 2018;28:369–384.

43. Lee G, You HJ, Bajaj JS, et al. Distinct signatures of gut microbiome and metabolites associated with significant fibrosis in nonobese NAFLD. *Nat Commun* 2020;11:4982.

44. Zou B, Yeo YH, Nguyen VH, et al. Prevalence, characteristics and mortality outcomes of obese, nonobese and lean NAFLD in the United States, 1999–2016. *J Intern Med* 2020;288:139–151.

45. Leung JC, Loong TC, Wei JL, et al. Histological severity and clinical outcomes of nonalcoholic fatty liver disease in nonobese patients. *Hepatology* 2017;65:54–64.

46. Lee HW, Wong GL, Kwok R, et al. Serial transient elastography examinations to monitor patients with type 2 diabetes: A prospective cohort study. *Hepatology* 2020;72:1230–1241.

47. Sinn DH, Kang D, Cho SJ, et al. Lean non-alcoholic fatty liver disease and development of diabetes: A cohort study. *Eur J Endocrinol* 2019;181:185–192.

48. Niriella MA, Kasturiratne A, Pathmeswaran A, et al. Lean non-alcoholic fatty liver disease (lean NAFLD): Characteristics, metabolic outcomes and risk factors from a 7-year prospective, community cohort study from Sri Lanka. *Hepatol Int* 2019;13:314–322.

49. Dela Cruz AC, Bugianesi E, George J, et al. Characteristics and long-term prognosis of lean patients with nonalcoholic fatty liver disease. *Gastroenterology* 2014;146:S-909.

50. Hagstrom H, Nasr P, Ekstedt M, et al. Risk for development of severe liver disease in lean patients with nonalcoholic fatty liver disease: A long-term follow-up study. *Hepatol Commun* 2018;2:48–57.

51. Eslam M, Newsome PN, Sarin SK, et al. A new definition for metabolic dysfunction-associated fatty liver disease: An international expert consensus statement. *J Hepatol* 2020;73:202–209.

52. Wong VW, Wong GL, Woo J, et al. Impact of the new definition of metabolic associated fatty liver disease on the epidemiology of the disease. *Clin Gastroenterol Hepatol* 2021;19:2161–2171 e5.

53. Lee H, Lee YH, Kim SU, et al. Metabolic dysfunction-associated fatty liver disease and incident cardiovascular disease risk: A nationwide cohort study. *Clin Gastroenterol Hepatol* 2021;19:2138–2147 e10.

54. Kim D, Konyn P, Sandhu KK, et al. Metabolic dysfunction-associated fatty liver disease is associated with increased all-cause mortality in the United States. *J Hepatol* 2021;75:1284–1291.

55. Wong VW, Adams LA, de Ledinghen V, et al. Noninvasive biomarkers in NAFLD and NASH—current progress and future promise. *Nat Rev Gastroenterol Hepatol* 2018;15:461–478.

56. Fu C, Wai JW, Nik Mustapha NR, et al. Performance of simple fibrosis scores in nonobese patients with nonalcoholic fatty liver disease. *Clin Gastroenterol Hepatol* 2020;18:2843–2845 e2.

57. Zhang X, Wong GL, Wong VW. Application of transient elastography in nonalcoholic fatty liver disease. *Clin Mol Hepatol* 2020;26:128–141.

58. Wong VW, Vergniol J, Wong GL, et al. Liver stiffness measurement using XL probe in patients with nonalcoholic fatty liver disease. *Am J Gastroenterol* 2012;107:1862–1871.

59. Wong VW, Irles M, Wong GL, et al. Unified interpretation of liver stiffness measurement by M and XL probes in non-alcoholic fatty liver disease. *Gut* 2019;68:2057–2064.

60. Wong VW, Wong GL, Chan RS, et al. Beneficial effects of lifestyle intervention in nonobese patients with nonalcoholic fatty liver disease. *J Hepatol* 2018;69:1349–1356.

61. Shi Q, Wang Y, Hao Q, et al. Pharmacotherapy for adults with overweight and obesity: A systematic review and network meta-analysis of randomised controlled trials. *Lancet* 2022;399:259–269.

62. Newsome PN, Buchholtz K, Cusi K, et al. A placebo-controlled trial of subcutaneous semaglutide in nonalcoholic steatohepatitis. *N Engl J Med* 2021;384:1113–1124.

63. Aminian A, Al-Kurd A, Wilson R, et al. Association of bariatric surgery with major adverse liver and cardiovascular outcomes in patients with biopsy-proven nonalcoholic steatohepatitis. *JAMA* 2021;326:2031–2042.

Index

Note: Page locators in **bold** indicate a table and page locators in *italics* indicate a figure.